Nursing Theories & Nursing Practice
Fourth Edition

Nursing Theories & Nursing Practice
Fourth Edition

Marlaine C. Smith, PhD, RN, AHN-BC, FAAN

Marilyn E. Parker, PhD, RN, FAAN

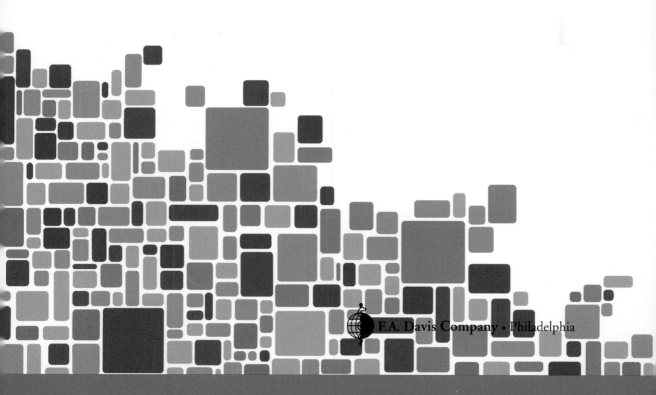

F.A. Davis Company • Philadelphia

F. A. Davis Company
1915 Arch Street
Philadelphia, PA 19103
www.fadavis.com

Copyright © 2015 by F. A. Davis Company

Printed in the United States of America

Last digit indicates print number: 10 9 8 7 6 5 4 3 2 1

Publisher, Nursing: Joanne Patzek DaCunha, RN, MSN; Susan Rhyner
Developmental Editor: Marcia Kelley
Director of Content Development: Darlene D. Pedersen
Content Project Manager: Echo K. Gerhart
Manager of Art and Design: Carolyn O'Brien

As new scientific information becomes available through basic and clinical research, recommended treatments and drug therapies undergo changes. The author(s) and publisher have done everything possible to make this book accurate, up to date, and in accord with accepted standards at the time of publication. The author(s), editors, and publisher are not responsible for errors or omissions or for consequences from application of the book, and make no warranty, expressed or implied, in regard to the contents of the book. Any practice described in this book should be applied by the reader in accordance with professional standards of care used in regard to the unique circumstances that may apply in each situation. The reader is advised always to check product information (package inserts) for changes and new information regarding dose and contraindications before administering any drug. Caution is especially urged when using new or infrequently ordered drugs.

Library of Congress Cataloging-in-Publication Data

Nursing theories and nursing practice.
  Nursing theories & nursing practice / [edited by] Marlaine C. Smith, Marilyn E. Parker. — Fourth edition.
     p. ; cm.
  Preceded by Nursing theories and nursing practice / [edited by] Marilyn E. Parker, Marlaine C. Smith. 3rd ed. c2010.
  Includes bibliographical references and index.
  ISBN 978-0-8036-3312-4 (alk. paper)
  I. Smith, Marlaine C. (Marlaine Cappelli), editor. II. Parker, Marilyn E., editor. III. Title.
  [DNLM: 1. Nursing Theory—Biography. 2. Nurses—Biography. WY 86]
  RT84.5
  610.7301—dc23
                        2014047296

Preface to the Fourth Edition

This book offers the perspective that nursing is a professional discipline with a body of knowledge that guides its practice. Nursing theories are an important part of this body of knowledge, and regardless of complexity or abstraction, they reflect phenomena central to the discipline, and should be used by nurses to frame their thinking, action, and being in the world. As guides, nursing theories are practical in nature and facilitate communication with those we serve as well as with colleagues, students, and others practicing in health-related services. We hope this book illuminates for the readers the interrelationship between nursing theories and nursing practice, and that this understanding will transform practice to improve the health and quality of life of people who are recipients of nursing care.

This very special book is intended to honor the work of nursing theorists and nurses who use these theories in their day-to-day practice. Our foremost nursing theorists have written for this book, or their theories have been described by nurses who have comprehensive knowledge of the theorists' ideas and who have a deep respect for the theorists as people, nurses, and scholars. To the extent possible, contributing authors have been selected by theorists to write about their work. Three middle-range theories have been added to this edition of the book, bringing the total number of middle-range theories to twelve. Obviously, it was not possible to include all existing middle-range theories in this volume; however, the expansion of this section illustrates the recent growth in middle-range theory development in nursing. Two chapters from the third edition, including Levine's conservation

theory and Paterson & Zderad's humanistic nursing have been moved to supplementary online resources at http://davisplus.fadavis.com.

This book is intended to help nursing students in undergraduate, masters, and doctoral nursing programs explore and appreciate nursing theories and their use in nursing practice and scholarship. In addition, and in response to calls from practicing nurses, this book is intended for use by those who desire to enrich their practice by the study of nursing theories and related illustrations of nursing practice. The contributing authors describe theory development processes and perspectives on the theories, giving us a variety of views for the twenty-first century and beyond. Each chapter of the book includes descriptions of a theory, its applications in both research and practice, and an example that reflects how the theory can guide practice. We anticipate that this overview of the theory and its applications will lead to deeper exploration of the theory, leading students to consult published works by the theorists and those working closely with the theory in practice or research.

There are six sections in the book. The first provides an overview of nursing theory and a focus for thinking about evaluating and choosing a nursing theory for use in practice. For this edition, the evolution of nursing theory was added to Chapter 1. Section II introduces the work of early nursing scholars whose ideas provided a foundation for more formal theory development. The nursing conceptual models and grand theories are clustered into three parts in Sections III, IV, and V. Section III contains those theories classified within the interactive-integrative paradigm, and those in the unitary-transformative paradigm are included in Section IV. Grand theories that are focused on the phenomena of care or caring appear in Section V. The final section contains a selection of middle-range theories.

An outline at the beginning of each chapter provides a map for the contents. Major points are highlighted in each chapter. Since this book focuses on the relationship of nursing theory to nursing practice, we invited the authors to share a practice exemplar. You will notice that some practice exemplars were written by someone other than the chapter author. In this edition the authors also provided content about research based on the theory. Because of page limitations you can find additional chapter content online at http://davisplus.fadavis.com. While every attempt was made to follow a standard format for each of the chapters throughout the book, some of the chapters vary from this format; for example, some authors chose not to include practice exemplars.

The book's website features materials that will enrich the teaching and learning of these nursing theories. Materials that will be helpful for teaching and learning about nursing theories are included as online resources. For example, there are case studies, learning activities, and PowerPoint presentations included on both the instructor and student websites. Other online resources include additional content, more extensive bibliographies and longer biographies of the theorists. Dr. Shirley Gordon and a group of doctoral students from Florida Atlantic University developed these ancillary materials for the third edition. For this edition, the ancillary materials for students and faculty were updated by Diane Gullett, a PhD candidate at Florida Atlantic University. She developed all materials for the new chapters as well as updating ancillary materials for chapters that appeared in the third edition. We are so grateful to Diane and Shirley for their creativity and leadership and to the other doctoral students for their thoughtful contributions to this project .

We hope that this book provides a useful overview of the latest theoretical advances of many of nursing's finest scholars. We are grateful for their contributions to this book. As

editors we've found that continuing to learn about and share what we love nurtures our growth as scholars, reignites our passion and commitment, and offers both fun and frustration along the way. We continue to be grateful for the enthusiasm for this book shared by many nursing theorists and contributing authors and by scholars in practice and research who bring theories to life. For us, it has been a joy to renew friendships with colleagues who have contributed to past editions and to find new friends and colleagues whose theories enriched this edition.

Nursing Theories and Nursing Practice, now in the fourth edition, has roots in a series of nursing theory conferences held in South Florida, beginning in 1989 and ending when efforts to cope with the aftermath of Hurricane Andrew interrupted the energy and resources needed for planning and offering the Fifth South Florida Nursing Theory Conference. Many of the theorists in this book addressed audiences of mostly practicing nurses at these conferences. Two books stimulated by those conferences and published by the National League for Nursing are *Nursing Theories in Practice* (1990) and *Patterns of Nursing Theories in Practice* (1993).

For me (Marilyn), even deeper roots of this book are found early in my nursing career, when I seriously considered leaving nursing for the study of pharmacy. In my fatigue and frustration, mixed with youthful hope and desire for more education, I could not answer the question "What is nursing?" and could not distinguish the work of nursing from other tasks I did every day. Why should I continue this work? Why should I seek degrees in a field that I could not define? After reflecting on these questions and using them to examine my nursing, I could find no one who would consider the questions with me. I remember being asked, "Why would you ask that question? You are a nurse; you must surely know what nursing is." Such responses, along with a drive for serious consideration of my questions, led me to the library. I clearly remember reading several descriptions of nursing that, I thought, could just as well have been about social work or physical therapy. I then found nursing defined and explained in a book about education of nurses written by Dorothea Orem. During the weeks that followed, as I did my work of nursing in the hospital, I explored Orem's ideas about why people need nursing, nursing's purposes, and what nurses do. I found a fit between her ideas, as I understood them, with my practice, and I learned that I could go even further to explain and design nursing according to these ways of thinking about nursing. I discovered that nursing shared some knowledge and practices with other services, such as pharmacy and medicine, and I began to distinguish nursing from these related fields of practice. I decided to stay in nursing and made plans to study and work with Dorothea Orem. In addition to learning about nursing theory and its meaning in all we do, I learned from Dorothea that nursing is a unique discipline of knowledge and professional practice. In many ways, my earliest questions about nursing have guided my subsequent study and work. Most of what I have done in nursing has been a continuation of my initial experience of the interrelations of all aspects of nursing scholarship, including the scholarship that is nursing practice. Over the years, I have been privileged to work with many nursing scholars, some of whom are featured in this book. My love for nursing and my respect for our discipline and practice have deepened, and knowing now that these values are so often shared is a singular joy.

Marlaine's interest in nursing theory had similar origins to Marilyn's. As a nurse pursuing an interdisciplinary master's degree in public health, I (Marlaine) recognized that while all the other public health disciplines had some unique perspective to share, public health nursing seemed to lack a clear identity. In search of the identity of nursing I pursued a second master's in nursing. At that time nursing theory was beginning to garner attention, and I learned about it from my teachers and mentors Sr. Rosemary Donley, Rosemarie Parse, and Mary Jane Smith. This discovery was the answer I was seeking, and it both expanded and focused my thinking about nursing. The question of "What is nursing?" was answered for me by these theories and I couldn't get

enough! It led to my decision to pursue my PhD in Nursing at New York University where I studied with Martha Rogers. During this same time I taught at Duquesne University with Rosemarie Parse and learned more about Man-Living-Health, which is now humanbecoming. I conducted several studies based on Rogers' conceptual system and Parse's theory. At theory conferences I was fortunate to dialogue with Virginia Henderson, Hildegard Peplau, Imogene King, and Madeleine Leininger. In 1988 I accepted a faculty position at the University of Colorado when Jean Watson was Dean. The School of Nursing was guided by a caring philosophy and framework and I embraced caring as a central focus of the discipline of nursing. As a unitary scholar, I studied Newman's theory of health as expanding consciousness and was intrigued by it, so for my sabbatical I decided to study it further as well as learn more about the unitary appreciative inquiry process that Richard Cowling was developing.

We both have been fortunate to hold faculty appointments in universities where nursing theory has been valued, and we are fortunate today to hold positions at the Christine E. Lynn College of Nursing at Florida Atlantic University, where faculty and students ground their teaching scholarship and practice on caring theories, including nursing as caring, developed by Dean Anne Boykin and a previous faculty member at the College, Savina Schoenhofer. Many faculty colleagues and students continue to help us study nursing and have contributed to this book in ways we would never have adequate words to acknowledge. We are grateful to our knowledgeable colleagues who reviewed and offered helpful suggestions for chapters of this book, and we sincerely thank those who contributed to the book as chapter authors. It is also our good fortune that many nursing theorists and other nursing scholars live in or visit our lovely state of Florida. Since the first edition of this book was published, we have lost many nursing theorists. Their work continues through those refining, modifying, testing, and expanding the theories. The discipline of nursing is expanding as research and practice advances existing theories and as new theories emerge. This is especially important at a time when nursing theory can provide what is missing and needed most in health care today.

All four editions of this book have been nurtured by Joanne DaCunha, an expert nurse and editor for F. A. Davis Company, who has shepherded this project and others because of her love of nursing. Near the end of this project Joanne retired, and Susan Rhyner, our new editor, led us to the finish line. We are both grateful for their wisdom, kindness, patience and understanding of nursing. We give special thanks to Echo Gerhart, who served as our contact and coordinator for this project. Marilyn thanks her husband, Terry Worden, for his abiding love and for always being willing to help,

and her niece, Cherie Parker, who represents many nurses who love nursing practice and scholarship and thus inspire the work of this book. Marlaine acknowledges her husband Brian and her children, Kirsten, Alicia, and Brady, and their spouses, Jonathan Vankin and Tori Rutherford, for their love and understanding. She honors her parents, Deno and Rose Cappelli, for instilling in her the love of learning, the value of hard work, and the importance of caring for others, and dedicates this book to her granddaughter Iyla and the new little one who is scheduled to arrive as this book is released.

Marilyn E. Parker,
Olathe, Kansas

Marlaine C. Smith,
Boca Raton, Florida

Nursing Theorists

Elizabeth Ann Manhart Barrett, PhD, RN, FAAN
Professor Emerita
Hunter College
City University of New York
New York, New York

Charlotte D. Barry, PhD, RN, NCSN, FAAN
Professor of Nursing
Christine E. Lynn College of Nursing
Florida Atlantic University
Boca Raton, Florida

Anne Boykin, PhD, RN*
Dean and Professor Emerita
Christine E. Lynn College of Nursing
Florida Atlantic University
Boca Raton, Florida

Barbara Montgomery Dossey, PhD, RN, AHN-BC, FAAN,
  HWNC-BC
*Co-Director, International Nurse Coach
  Association*
Core Faculty, Integrative Nurse Coach
  Certificate Program
Miami, Florida

Joanne R. Duffy, PhD, RN, FAAN
*Endowed Professor of Research and
  Evidence-based Practice and Director
  of the PhD Program*
West Virginia University
Morgantown, West Virginia

Helen L. Erickson*
Professor Emerita
University of Texas at Austin
Austin, Texas

Lydia Hall†

Virginia Henderson†

Dorothy Johnson†

Imogene King†

Katharine Kolcaba, PhD, RN
Associate Professor Emeritus Adjunct
The University of Akron
Akron, Ohio

Madeleine M. Leininger†

Patricia Liehr, PhD, RN
Professor
Christine E. Lynn College of Nursing
Florida Atlantic University
Boca Raton, Florida

Rozzano C. Locsin, PhD, RN
Professor Emeritus
Christine E. Lynn College of Nursing
Florida Atlantic University
Boca Raton, Florida

Afaf I. Meleis, PhD, DrPS(hon), FAAN
Professor of Nursing and Sociology
University of Pennsylvania
Philadelphia, Pennsylvania

Betty Neuman, PhD, RN, PLC, FAAN
Beverly, Ohio

Margaret Newman, RN, PhD, FAAN
Professor Emerita
University of Minnesota College of Nursing
Saint Paul, Minnesota

Dorothea E. Orem†

Ida Jean Orlando (Pelletier)†

Marilyn E. Parker, PhD, RN, FAAN
Professor Emerita
Christine E. Lynn College of Nursing
Florida Atlantic University
Boca Raton, Florida

ix

Rosemarie Rizzo Parse, PhD, FAAN
Distinguished Professor Emeritus
Marcella Niehoff School of Nursing
Loyola University Chicago
Chicago, Illinois

Hildegard Peplau†

Marilyn Anne Ray, PhD, RN, CTN
Professor Emerita
Christine E. Lynn College of Nursing
Florida Atlantic University
Boca Raton, Florida

Pamela G. Reed, PhD, RN, FAAN
Professor
University of Arizona
Tucson, Arizona

Martha E. Rogers†

Sister Callista Roy, PhD, RN, FAAN
Professor and Nurse Theorist
William F. Connell School of Nursing
Boston College
Chestnut Hill, Massachusetts

Savina O. Schoenhofer, PhD, RN
Professor of Nursing
University of Mississippi
Oxford, Mississippi

Marlaine C. Smith, PhD, RN, AHN-BC, FAAN
Dean and Helen K. Persson Eminent Scholar
Christine E. Lynn College of Nursing
Florida Atlantic University
Boca Raton, Florida

Mary Jane Smith, PhD, RN
Professor
West Virginia University
Morgantown, West Virginia

Mary Ann Swain, PhD
Professor and Director, Doctoral Program
Decker School of Nursing
Binghamton University
Binghamton, New York

Kristen M. Swanson, PhD, RN, FAAN
Dean
Seattle University
Seattle, Washington

Evelyn Tomlin*

Joyce Travelbee†

Meredith Troutman-Jordan, PhD, RN
Associate Professor
University of North Carolina
Chapel Hill, North Carolina

Jean Watson, PhD, RN, AHN-BC, FAAN
Distinguished Professor Emeritus
University of Colorado at Denver—Anschutz
   Campus
Aurora, Colorado

Ernestine Wiedenbach†

*Retired
†Deceased

Contributors

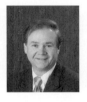

Patricia Deal Aylward, MSN, RN, CNS
Assistant Professor
Santa Fe Community College
Gainesville, Florida

Howard Karl Butcher, PhD, RN, PMHCNS-BC
Associate Professor
University of Iowa
Iowa City, Iowa

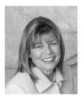

Lynne M. Hektor Dunphy, PhD, APRN-BC
*Associate Dean for Practice and Community
    Engagement*
Christine E. Lynn College of Nursing
Florida Atlantic University
Boca Raton, Florida

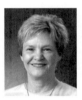

Laureen M. Fleck, PhD, FNP-BC, FAANP
Associate Faculty
Christine E. Lynn College of Nursing
Florida Atlantic University
Boca Raton, Florida

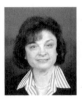

Maureen A. Frey, PhD, RN*

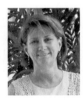

Shirley C. Gordon, PhD, RN
*Professor and Assistant Dean Graduate Practice
    Programs*
Christine E. Lynn College of Nursing
Florida Atlantic University
Boca Raton, Florida

---

*Retired.

Diane Lee Gullett, RN, MSN, MPH
Doctoral Candidate
Christine E. Lynn College of NursingFlorida
   Atlantic University
Boca Raton, Florida

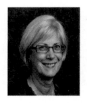

Beth M. King, PhD, RN, PMHCNS-BC
Assistant Professor and RN–BSN Coordinator
Christine E. Lynn College of Nursing
Florida Atlantic University
Boca Raton, Florida

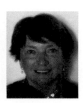

Donna L. Hartweg, PhD, RN
Professor Emerita and Former Director
Illinois Wesleyan University
Bloomington, Illinois

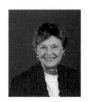

Lois White Lowry, DNSc, RN*
Professor Emerita
East Tennessee State University
Johnson City, Tennessee

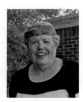

Bonnie Holaday, PhD, RN, FAAN
Professor
Clemson University
Clemson, South Carolina

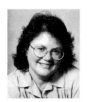

Violet M. Malinski, PhD, MA, RN
Associate Professor
College of New Rochelle
New Rochelle, New York

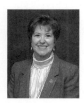

Mary B. Killeen, PhD, RN, NEA-BC
Consultant
Evidence Based Practice Nurse Consultants,
   LLC
Howell, Michigan

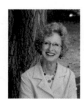

Ann R. Peden, RN, CNS, DSN
Professor and Chair
Capital University
Columbus, Ohio

Margaret Dexheimer Pharris, PhD, RN, CNE, FAAN
Associate Dean for Nursing
St. Catherine University
St. Paul, Minnesota

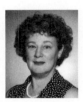

Maude Rittman, PhD, RN
Associate Chief of Nursing Service for Research
Gainesville Veteran's Administration
   Medical Center
Gainesville, Florida

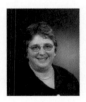

Pamela Senesac, PhD, SM, RN
Assistant Professor
University of Massachusetts
Shrewsbury, Massachusetts

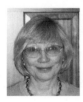

Christina L. Sieloff, PhD, RN
Associate Professor
Montana State University
Billings, Montana

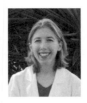

Jacqueline Staal, MSN, ARNP, FNP-BC
PhD Candidate
Christine E. Lynn College of Nursing
Florida Atlantic University
Boca Raton, Florida

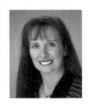

Marian C. Turkel, PhD, RN, NEA-BC, FAAN
Director of Professional Nursing Practice
Holy Cross Medical Center
Fort Lauderdale, Florida

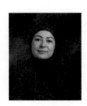

Hiba Wehbe-Alamah, PhD, RN, FNP-BC, CTN-A
Associate Professor
University of Michigan-Flint
Flint, Michigan

Kelly White, RN, PhD, FNP-BC
Assistant Professor
South University
West Palm Beach, Florida

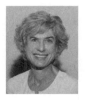

Terri Kaye Woodward, MSN, RN, CNS, AHN-BC, HTCP
Founder
Cocreative Wellness
Denver, Colorado

Reviewers

Ferrona Beason, PhD, ARNP
Assistant Professor in Nursing
Barry University – Division of Nursing
Miami Shores, Florida

Abimbola Farinde, PharmD, MS
Clinical Pharmacist Specialist
Clear Lake Regional Medical Center
Webster, Texas

Lori S. Lauver, PhD, RN, CPN, CNE
Associate Professor
Jefferson School of Nursing
Thomas Jefferson University
Philadelphia, Pennsylvania

Elisheva Lightstone, BScN, MSc
Professor
Department of Nursing
Seneca College
King City, Ontario, Canada

Carol L. Moore, PhD, APRN, CNS
Assistant Professor of Nursing, Coordinator,
    Graduate Nursing Studies
Fort Hays State University
Hays, Kansas

Kathleen Spadaro, PhD, PMHCNS, RN
MSN Program Co-coordinator & Assistant
    Professor of Nursing
Chatham University
Pittsburgh, Pennsylvania

Contents

Section I An Introduction to Nursing Theory, 1

Chapter 1 Nursing Theory and the Discipline of Nursing, 3
Marlaine C. Smith and Marilyn E. Parker

Chapter 2 A Guide for the Study of Nursing Theories for Practice, 19
Marilyn E. Parker and Marlaine C. Smith

*Chapter 3 Choosing, Evaluating, and Implementing Nursing Theories
for Practice, 23*
Marilyn E. Parker and Marlaine C. Smith

Section II Conceptual Influences on the Evolution of Nursing Theory, 35

Chapter 4 Florence Nightingale's Legacy of Caring and Its Applications, 37
Lynne M. Hektor Dunphy

Chapter 5 Early Conceptualizations About Nursing, 55
Shirley C. Gordon

Chapter 6 Nurse-Patient Relationship Theories, 67
Ann R. Peden, Jacqueline Staal, Maude Rittman, and Diane Lee Gullett

Section III Conceptual Models/Grand Theories in the Integrative-Interactive Paradigm, 87

*Chapter 7 Dorothy Johnson's Behavioral System Model and Its
Applications, 89*
Bonnie Holaday

Chapter 8 Dorothea Orem's Self-Care Deficit Nursing Theory, 105
Donna L. Hartweg

Chapter 9 Imogene King's Theory of Goal Attainment, 133
Christina L. Sieloff and Maureen A. Frey

Chapter 10 Sister Callista Roy's Adaptation Model, 153
Pamela Sensac and Sister Callista Roy

Chapter 11 Betty Neuman's Systems Model, 165
Lois White Lowry and Patricia Deal Aylward

Chapter 12 Helen Erickson, Evelyn Tomlin, and Mary Ann Swain's Theory of Modeling and Role Modeling, 185
Helen L. Erickson

Chapter 13 Barbara Dossey's Theory of Integral Nursing, 207
Barbara Montgomery Dossey

Section IV Conceptual Models and Grand Theories in the Unitary–Transformative Paradigm, 235

Chapter 14 Martha E. Rogers Science of Unitary Human Beings, 237
Howard Karl Butcher and Violet M. Malinski

Chapter 15 Rosemarie Rizzo Parse's Humanbecoming Paradigm, 263
Rosemarie Rizzo Parse

Chapter 16 Margaret Newman's Theory of Health as Expanding Consciousness, 279
Margaret Dexheimer Pharris

Section V Grand Theories about Care or Caring, 301

Chapter 17 Madeleine Leininger's Theory of Culture Care Diversity and Universality, 303
Hiba Wehbe-Alamah

Chapter 18 Jean Watson's Theory of Human Caring, 321
Jean Watson

Chapter 19 Theory of Nursing as Caring, 341
Anne Boykin and Savina O. Schoenhofer

Section VI Middle-Range Theories, 357

Chapter 20 Transitions Theory, 361
Afaf I. Meleis

Chapter 21 Katharine Kolcaba's Comfort Theory, 381
Katharine Kolcaba

Chapter 22 Joanne Duffy's Quality-Caring Model©, 393
Joanne R. Duffy

Chapter 23 Pamela Reed's Theory of Self-Transcendence, 411
Pamela G. Reed

Chapter 24 Patricia Liehr and Mary Jane Smith's Story Theory, 421
Patricia Liehr and Mary Jane Smith

Chapter 25 The Community Nursing Practice Model, 435
Marilyn E. Parker, Charlotte D. Barry. and Beth M. King

Chapter 26 Rozzano Locsin's Technological Competency as Caring in Nursing, 449
Rozzano C. Locsin

Chapter 27 Marilyn Anne Ray's Theory of Bureaucratic Caring, 461
Marilyn Anne Ray and Marian C. Turkel

Chapter 28 Troutman-Jordan's Theory of Successful Aging, 483
Meredith Troutman-Jordan

Chapter 29 Barrett's Theory of Power as Knowing Participation in Change, 495
Elizabeth Ann Manhart Barrett

Chapter 30 Marlaine Smith's Theory of Unitary Caring, 509
Marlaine C. Smith

Chapter 31 Kristen Swanson's Theory of Caring, 521
Kristen M. Swanson

Index, 533

An Introduction to Nursing Theory

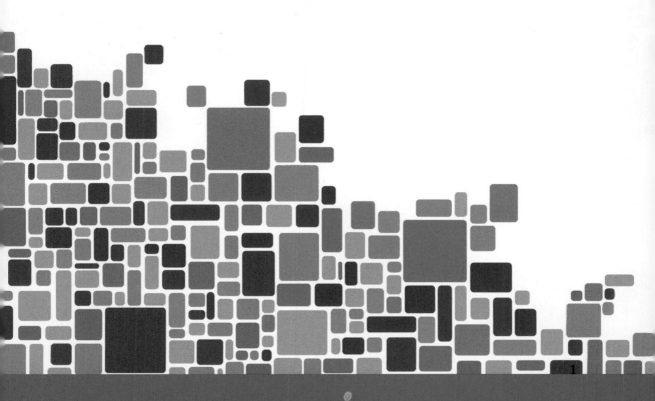

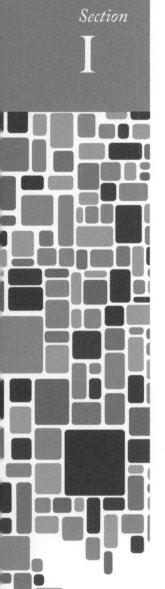

An Introduction to Nursing Theory

In this first section of the book, you will be introduced to the purpose of nursing theory and shown how to study, analyze, and evaluate it for use in nursing practice. If you are new to the idea of theory in nursing, the chapters in this section will orient you to what theory is, how it fits into the evolution and context of nursing as a professional discipline, and how to approach its study and evaluation. If you have studied nursing theory in the past, these chapters will provide you with additional knowledge and insight as you continue your study.

Nursing is a professional discipline focused on the study of human health and healing through caring. Nursing practice is based on the knowledge of nursing, which consists of its philosophies, theories, concepts, principles, research findings, and practice wisdom. Nursing theories are patterns that guide the thinking about nursing. All nurses are guided by some implicit or explicit theory or pattern of thinking as they care for their patients. Too often, this pattern of thinking is implicit and is colored by the lens of diseases, diagnoses, and treatments. This does not reflect practice from the disciplinary perspective of nursing. The major reason for the development and study of nursing theory is to improve nursing practice and, therefore, the health and quality of life of those we serve.

The first chapter in this section focuses on nursing theory within the context of nursing as an evolving professional discipline. We examine the relationship of nursing theory to the characteristics of a discipline. You'll learn new words that describe parts of the knowledge structure of the discipline of nursing, and we'll speculate about the future of nursing theory as nursing, health care, and our global society change. Chapter 2 is a guide to help you study the theories in this book. Use this guide as you read and think about how nursing theory fits in your practice. Nurses embrace theories that fit with their values and ways of thinking. They choose theories to guide their practice and to create a practice that is meaningful to them. Chapter 3 focuses on the selection, evaluation, and implementation of theory for practice. Students often get the assignment of evaluating or critiquing a nursing theory. Evaluation is coming to some judgment about value or worth based on criteria. Various sets of criteria exist for you to use in theory evaluation. We introduce some that you can explore further. Finally, we offer reflections on the process of implementing theory-guided practice models.

Nursing Theory and the Discipline of Nursing

MARLAINE C. SMITH AND
MARILYN E. PARKER

The Discipline of Nursing
Definitions of Nursing Theory
The Purpose of Theory in a Professional
Discipline
The Evolution of Nursing Science
The Structure of Knowledge in the
Discipline of Nursing
Nursing Theory and the Future
Summary
References

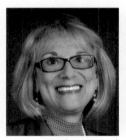

Marlaine C. Smith

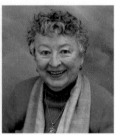

Marilyn E. Parker

What is nursing? At first glance, the question may appear to be one with an obvious answer, but when it is posed to nurses, many define nursing by providing a litany of functions and activities. Some answer with the elements of the nursing process: assessing, planning, implementing, and evaluating. Others might answer that nurses coordinate a patient's care.

Defining nursing in terms of the nursing process or by functions or activities nurses perform is problematic. The phases of the nursing process are the same steps we might use to solve any problem we encounter, from a broken computer to a failing vegetable garden. We assess the situation to determine what is going on and then identify the problem; we plan what to do about it, implement our plan, and then evaluate whether it works. The nursing process does nothing to define nursing.

Defining ourselves by tasks presents other problems. What nurses do—that is, the functions associated with practice—differs based on the setting. For example, a nurse might start IVs, administer medications, and perform treatments in an acute care setting. In a community-based clinic, a nurse might teach a young mother the principles of infant feeding or place phone calls to arrange community resources for a child with special needs. Multiple professionals and nonprofessionals may perform the same tasks as nurses, and persons with the ability and authority to perform certain tasks change based on time and setting. For example, both physicians and nurses may listen to breath sounds and recognize the presence of rales. Both nurses and social workers might do discharge planning. Both nurses and family members might change dressings, monitor vital signs, and administer medications, so defining nursing based solely on functions or activities performed is not useful.

To answer the question "What is nursing?" we must formulate nursing's unique identity as a field of study or discipline. Florence Nightingale is credited as the founder of modern nursing, the one who articulated its distinctive focus. In her book *Notes on Nursing: What It Is and What It Is Not* (Nightingale, 1859/1992), she differentiated nursing from medicine, stating that the two were distinct practices. She defined nursing as putting the person in the best condition for nature to act, insisting that the focus of nursing was on health and the natural healing process, not on disease and reparation. For her, creating an environment that provided the conditions for natural healing to occur was the focus of nursing. Her beginning conceptualizations were the seeds for the theoretical development of nursing as a professional discipline.

In this chapter, we situate the understanding of nursing theory within the context of the discipline of nursing. We define the discipline of nursing, describe the purpose of theory for the discipline of nursing, review the evolution of nursing science, identify the structure of the discipline of nursing, and speculate on the future place of nursing theory in the discipline.

The Discipline of Nursing

Every discipline has a unique focus that directs the inquiry within it and distinguishes it from other fields of study (Smith, 2008, p. 1). Nursing knowledge guides its professional practice; therefore, it is classified as a professional discipline. Donaldson and Crowley (1978) stated that a discipline "offers a unique perspective, a distinct way of viewing . . . phenomena, which ultimately defines the limits and nature of its inquiry" (p. 113). Any discipline includes networks of philosophies, theories, concepts, approaches to inquiry, research findings, and practices that both reflect and illuminate its distinct perspective. **The discipline of nursing is formed by a community of scholars, including**

nurses in all nursing venues, who share a commitment to values, knowledge, and processes to guide the thought and work of the discipline.

The classic work of King and Brownell (1976) is consistent with the thinking of nursing scholars (Donaldson & Crowley, 1978; Meleis, 1977) about the discipline of nursing. These authors have elaborated attributes that characterize all disciplines. As you will see in the discussion that follows, the attributes of King and Brownell provide a framework that contextualizes nursing theory within the discipline of nursing.

Expression of Human Imagination

Members of any discipline imagine and create structures that offer descriptions and explanations of the phenomena that are of concern to that discipline. These structures are the theories of that discipline. Nursing theory is dependent on the imagination of nurses in practice, administration, research, and teaching, as they create and apply theories to improve nursing practice and ultimately the lives of those they serve. To remain dynamic and useful, the discipline requires openness to new ideas and innovative approaches that grow out of members' reflections and insights.

Domain

A professional discipline must be clearly defined by a statement of its domain—the boundaries or focus of that discipline. The domain of nursing includes the phenomena of interest, problems to be addressed, main content and methods used, and roles required of the discipline's members (Kim, 1997; Meleis, 2012). The processes and practices claimed by members of the disciplinary community grow out of these domain statements. Nightingale provided some direction for the domain of the discipline of nursing. Although the disciplinary focus has been debated, there is some degree of consensus. Donaldson and Crowley (1978, p. 113) identified the following as the domain of the discipline of nursing:

1. Concern with principles and laws that govern the life processes, well-being, and

optimal functioning of human beings, sick or well

2. Concern with the patterning of human behavior in interactions with the environment in critical life situations
3. Concern with the processes through which positive changes in health status are affected

Fawcett (1984) described the metaparadigm as a way to distinguish nursing from other disciplines. The metaparadigm is very general and intended to reflect agreement among members of the discipline about the field of nursing. This is the most abstract level of nursing knowledge and closely mirrors beliefs held about nursing. By virtue of being nurses, all nurses have some awareness of nursing's metaparadigm. However, because the term may not be familiar, it offers no direct guidance for research and practice (Kim, 1997; Walker & Avant, 1995). The metaparadigm consists of four concepts: persons, environment, health, and nursing. According to Fawcett, nursing is the study of the interrelationship among these four concepts.

Modifications and alternative concepts for this framework have been explored throughout the discipline (Fawcett, 2000). For example, some nursing scholars have suggested that "caring" replace "nursing" in the metaparadigm (Stevenson & Tripp-Reimer, 1989). Kim (1987, 1997) set forth four domains: client, client–nurse encounters, practice, and environment. In recent years, increasing attention has been directed to the nature of nursing's relationship with the environment (Kleffel, 1996; Schuster & Brown, 1994).

Others have defined nursing as the study of "the health or wholeness of human beings as they interact with their environment" (Donaldson & Crowley, 1978, p. 113), the life process of unitary human beings (Rogers, 1970), care or caring (Leininger, 1978; Watson, 1985), and human–universe–health interrelationships (Parse, 1998). A widely accepted focus statement for the discipline was published by Newman, Sime, and Corcoran-Perry (1991): "Nursing is the study of caring in the human health experience" (p. 3). A consensus statement of philosophical unity in the discipline was published by Roy and Jones (2007). Statements include the following:

• The human being is characterized by wholeness, complexity, and consciousness.
• The essence of nursing involves the nurse's true presence in the process of human-to-human engagement.
• Nursing theory expresses the values and beliefs of the discipline, creating a structure to organize knowledge and illuminate nursing practice.
• The essence of nursing practice is the nurse–patient relationship.

In 2008, Newman, Smith, Dexheimer-Pharris, and Jones revisited the disciplinary focus asserting that relationship was central to the discipline, and the convergence of seven concepts—health, consciousness, caring, mutual process, presence, patterning, and meaning—specified relationship in the professional discipline of nursing. Willis, Grace, and Roy (2008) posited that the central unifying focus for the discipline is facilitating humanization, meaning, choice, quality of life, and healing in living and dying (p. E28). Finally, Litchfield and Jondorsdottir (2008) defined the discipline as the study of humanness in the health circumstance. Smith (1994) defined the domain of the discipline of nursing as "the study of human health and healing through caring" (p. 50). For Smith (2008), "nursing knowledge focuses on the wholeness of human life and experience and the processes that support relationship, integration, and transformation" (p. 3). Nursing conceptual models, grand theories, middle-range theories, and practice theories explicate the phenomena within the domain of nursing. In addition, the focus of the nursing discipline is a clear statement of social mandate and service used to direct the study and practice of nursing (Newman et al., 1991).

Syntactical and Conceptual Structures

Syntactical and conceptual structures are essential to any discipline and are inherent in nursing theories. The conceptual structure delineates the proper concerns of nursing, guides what is to be studied, and clarifies accepted ways of knowing and using content of the discipline. This structure is grounded in the focus of the discipline. The conceptual structure relates concepts within nursing theories. The syntactical structures help nurses and other professionals to understand the talents, skills, and abilities that must be developed within the community. This structure directs descriptions of data needed from research, as well as evidence required to demonstrate the effect on nursing practice. In addition, these structures guide nursing's use of knowledge in research and practice approaches developed by related disciplines. It is only by being thoroughly grounded in the discipline's concepts, substance, and modes of inquiry that the boundaries of the discipline can be understood and possibilities for creativity across disciplinary borders can be created and explored.

Specialized Language and Symbols

As nursing theory has evolved, so has the need for concepts, language, and forms of data that reflect new ways of thinking and knowing specific to nursing. The complex concepts used in nursing scholarship and practice require language that can be specific and understood. The language of nursing theory facilitates communication among members of the discipline. Expert knowledge of the discipline is often required for full understanding of the meaning of these theoretical terms.

Heritage of Literature and Networks of Communication

This attribute calls attention to the array of books, periodicals, artifacts, and aesthetic expressions, as well as audio, visual, and electronic media that have developed over centuries to communicate the nature of nursing knowledge and practice. Conferences and forums on every aspect of nursing held throughout the world are part of this network. Nursing organizations and societies also provide critical communication links. Nursing theories are part of this heritage of literature, and those working with these theories present their work

at conferences, societies, and other communication networks of the nursing discipline.

Tradition

The tradition and history of the discipline is evident in the study of nursing over time. There is recognition that theories most useful today often have threads of connection with ideas originating in the past. For example, many theorists have acknowledged the influence of Florence Nightingale and have acclaimed her leadership in influencing nursing theories of today. In addition, nursing has a rich heritage of practice. Nursing's practical experience and knowledge have been shared and transformed as the content of the discipline and are evident in many nursing theories (Gray & Pratt, 1991).

Values and Beliefs

Nursing has distinctive views of persons and strong commitments to compassionate and knowledgeable care of persons through nursing. Fundamental nursing values and beliefs include a holistic view of person, the dignity and uniqueness of persons, and the call to care. There are both shared and differing values and beliefs within the discipline. The metaparadigm reflects the shared beliefs, and the paradigms reflect the differences.

Systems of Education

A distinguishing mark of any discipline is the education of future and current members of the community. Nursing is recognized as a professional discipline within institutions of higher education because it has an identifiable body of knowledge that is studied, advanced, and used to underpin its practice. Students of any professional discipline study its theories and learn its methods of inquiry and practice. Nursing theories, by setting directions for the substance and methods of inquiry for the discipline, should provide the basis for nursing education and the framework for organizing nursing curricula.

Definitions of Nursing Theory

A *theory* is a notion or an idea that explains experience, interprets observation, describes relationships, and projects outcomes. Parsons (1949), often quoted by nursing theorists, wrote that theories help us know what we know and decide what we need to know. Theories are mental patterns or frameworks created to help understand and create meaning from our experience, organize and articulate our knowing, and ask questions leading to new insights. **As such, theories are not discovered in nature but are human inventions.**

Theories are organizing structures of our reflections, observations, projections, and inferences. Many describe theories as lenses because they color and shape what is seen. The same phenomena will be seen differently depending on the theoretical perspective assumed. For these reasons, "theory" and related terms have been defined and described in a number of ways according to individual experience and what is useful at the time. Theories, as reflections of understanding, guide our actions, help us set forth desired outcomes, and give evidence of what has been achieved. A theory, by traditional definition, is an organized, coherent set of concepts and their relationships to each other that offers descriptions, explanations, and predictions about phenomena.

Early writers on nursing theory brought definitions of theory from other disciplines to direct future work within nursing. Dickoff and James (1968, p. 198) defined theory as a "conceptual system or framework invented for some purpose." Ellis (1968, p. 217) defined theory as "a coherent set of hypothetical, conceptual, and pragmatic principles forming a general frame of reference for a field of inquiry." McKay (1969, p. 394) asserted that theories are the capstone of scientific work and that the term refers to "logically interconnected sets of confirmed hypotheses." Barnum (1998, p. 1) later offered a more open definition of theory as a "construct that accounts for or organizes some phenomenon" and simply stated that a nursing theory describes or explains nursing.

Definitions of theory emphasize its various aspects. Those developed in recent years are more open and conform to a broader conception of science. The following definitions of theory are consistent with general ideas of theory

in nursing practice, education, administration, or research:

• Theory is a set of concepts, definitions, and propositions that project a systematic view of phenomena by designating specific interrelationships among concepts for purposes of describing, explaining, predicting, and/or controlling phenomena (Chinn & Jacobs, 1987, p. 71).
• Theory is a creative and rigorous structuring of ideas that projects a tentative, purposeful, and systematic view of phenomena (Chinn & Kramer, 2004, p. 268).
• Nursing theory is a conceptualization of some aspect of reality (invented or discovered) that pertains to nursing. The conceptualization is articulated for the purpose of describing, explaining, predicting, or prescribing nursing care (Meleis, 1997, p. 12).
• Nursing theory is an inductively and/or deductively derived collage of coherent, creative, and focused nursing phenomena that frame, give meaning to, and help explain specific and selective aspects of nursing research and practice (Silva, 1997, p. 55).
• A theory is an imaginative grouping of knowledge, ideas, and experience that are represented symbolically and seek to illuminate a given phenomenon." (Watson, 1985, p. 1).

The Purpose of Theory in a Professional Discipline

All professional disciplines have a body of knowledge consisting of theories, research, and methods of inquiry and practice. They organize knowledge, guide inquiry to advance science, guide practice and enhance the care of patients. Nursing theories address the phenomena of interest to nursing, human beings, health, and caring in the context of the nurse–person relationship[1]. **On the basis of strongly held values and beliefs about nursing, and within contexts of various worldviews, theories are patterns that guide the thinking about, being, and doing of nursing.**

---

[1]Person refers to individual, family, group, or community.

Theories provide structures for making sense of the complexities of reality for both practice and research. Research based in nursing theory is needed to explain and predict nursing outcomes essential to the delivery of nursing care that is both humane and cost-effective (Gioiella, 1996). Some conceptual structure either implicitly or explicitly directs all avenues of nursing, including nursing education and administration. Nursing theories provide concepts and designs that define the place of nursing in health care. Through theories, nurses are offered perspectives for relating with professionals from other disciplines, who join with nurses to provide human services. Nursing has great expectations of its theories. At the same time, theories must provide structure and substance to ground the practice and scholarship of nursing and must also be flexible and dynamic to keep pace with the growth and changes in the discipline and practice of nursing.

The major reason for structuring and advancing nursing knowledge is for the sake of nursing practice. The primary purpose of nursing theories is to further the development and understanding of nursing practice. Because nursing theory exists to improve practice, the test of nursing theory is a test of its usefulness in professional practice (Colley, 2003; Fitzpatrick, 1997). The work of nursing theory is moving from academia into the realm of nursing practice. Chapters in the remaining sections of this book highlight the use of nursing theories in nursing practice.

Nursing practice is both the source and the goal of nursing theory. From the viewpoint of practice, Gray and Forsstrom (1991) suggested that theory provides nurses with different ways of looking at and assessing phenomena, rationales for their practice, and criteria for evaluating outcomes. Many of the theories in this book have been used to guide nursing practice, stimulate creative thinking, facilitate communication, and clarify purposes and processes in practice. The practicing nurse has an ethical responsibility to use the discipline's theoretical knowledge base, just as it is the nurse scholar's ethical responsibility to develop the knowledge base specific to nursing practice (Cody, 1997,

2003). Engagement in practice generates the ideas that lead to the development of nursing theories.

At the empirical level of theory, abstract concepts are operationalized, or made concrete, for practice and research (Fawcett, 2000; Smith & Liehr, 2013). Empirical indicators provide specific examples of how the theory is experienced in reality; they are important for bringing theoretical knowledge to the practice level. These indicators include procedures, tools, and instruments to determine the effects of nursing practice and are essential to research and management of outcomes of practice (Jennings & Staggers, 1998). The resulting data form the basis for improving the quality of nursing care and influencing health-care policy. Empirical indicators, grounded carefully in nursing concepts, provide clear demonstration of the utility of nursing theory in practice, research, administration, and other nursing endeavors (Allison & McLaughlin-Renpenning, 1999; Hart & Foster, 1998).

Meeting the challenges of systems of care delivery and interprofessional work demands practice from a theoretical perspective. Nursing's disciplinary focus is important within the interprofessional health-care environment (Allison & McLaughlin-Renpenning, 1999); otherwise, its unique contribution to the interprofessional team is unclear. Nursing actions reflect nursing concepts from a nursing perspective. Careful, reflective, and critical thinking are the hallmarks of expert nursing, and nursing theories should undergird these processes. Appreciation and use of nursing theory offer opportunities for successful collaboration with colleagues from other disciplines and provide definition for nursing's overall contribution to health care. Nurses must know what they are doing, why they are doing it, and what the range of outcomes of nursing may be, as well as indicators for documenting nursing's effects. These theoretical frameworks serve as powerful guides for articulating, reporting, and recording nursing thought and action.

One of the assertions referred to most often in the nursing-theory literature is that theory is born of nursing practice and, after examination and refinement through research, must be returned to practice (Dickoff, James, & Wiedenbach, 1968). Nursing theory is stimulated by questions and curiosities arising from nursing practice. Development of nursing knowledge is a result of theory-based nursing inquiry. The circle continues as data, conclusions, and recommendations of nursing research are evaluated and developed for use in practice. Nursing theory must be seen as practical and useful to practice, and the insights of practice must in turn continue to enrich nursing theory.

The Evolution of Nursing Science

Disciplines can be classified as belonging to the sciences or humanities. In any science, there is a search for an understanding about specified phenomena through creating some organizing frameworks (theories) about the nature of those phenomena. These organizing frameworks (theories) are evaluated for their empirical accuracy through research. So science is composed of theories developed and tested through research (Smith, 1994).

The evolution of nursing as a science has occurred within the past 70 years; however, before nursing became a discipline or field of study, it was a healing art. Throughout the world, nursing emerged as a healing ministry to those who were ill or in need of support. Knowledge about caring for the sick, injured, and those birthing, dying, or experiencing normal developmental transitions was handed down, frequently in oral traditions, and comprised folk remedies and practices that were found to be effective through a process of trial and error. In most societies, the responsibility for nursing fell to women, members of religious orders, or those with spiritual authority in the community. With the ascendency of science, those who were engaged in the vocations of healing lost their authority over healing to medicine. Traditional approaches to healing were marginalized, as the germ theory and the development of pharmaceuticals and surgical procedures were legitimized because of their grounding in science.

Although there were healers from other countries who can be acknowledged for their importance to the history of nursing, Florence Nightingale holds the title of the "mother of modern nursing" and the person responsible for setting Western nursing on a path toward scientific advancement. She not only defined nursing as "putting the person in the best condition for nature to act," she also established a phenomenological focus of nursing as caring for and about the human–environment relationship to health. While nursing soldiers during the Crimean War, Nightingale began to study the distribution of disease by gathering data, so she was arguably the first nurse-scientist in that she established a rudimentary theory and tested that theory through her practice and research.

Nightingale schools were established in the West at the turn of the 20th century, but Nightingale's influence on the nursing profession waned as student nurses in hospital-based training schools were taught nursing primarily by physicians. Nursing became strongly influenced by the "medical model" and for some time lost its identity as a distinct profession.

Slowly, nursing education moved into institutions of higher learning where students were taught by nurses with higher degrees. By 1936, 66 colleges and universities had baccalaureate programs (Peplau, 1987). Graduate programs began in the 1940s and grew significantly from the 50s through the 1970s.

The publication of the journal *Nursing Research* in 1952 was a milestone, signifying the birth of nursing as a fledgling science (Peplau, 1987). But well into the 1940s, "many textbooks for nurses, often written by physicians, clergy or psychologists, reminded nurses that theory was too much for them, that nurses did not need to think but rather merely to follow rules, be obedient, be compassionate, do their 'duty' and carry out medical orders" (Peplau, 1987, p. 18). We've come a long way in a mere 70 years.

The development of nursing curricula stimulated discussion about the nature of nursing as distinct from medicine. In the 1950s, early nursing scholars such as Hildegard Peplau, Virginia Henderson, Dorothy Johnson, and

Lydia Hall established the distinct characteristics of nursing as a profession and field of study. Faye Abdellah, Ida Jean Orlando, Joyce Travelbee, Ernestine Wiedenbach, Myra Levine, and Imogene King followed during the 1960s, elaborating their conceptualizations of nursing. During the early 1960s, the federally-funded Nurse Scientist Program was initiated to educate nurses in pursuit of doctoral degrees in the basic sciences. Through this program nurses received doctorates in education, sociology, physiology, and psychology. These graduates brought the scientific traditions of these disciplines into nursing as they assumed faculty positions in schools of nursing.

By the 1970s, nursing theory development became a priority for the profession and the discipline of nursing was becoming established. Martha Rogers, Callista Roy, Dorothea Orem, Betty Newman, and Josephine Paterson and Loraine Zderad published their theories and graduate students began studying and advancing these theories through research. During this time, the National League for Nursing required a theory-based curriculum as a standard for accreditation, so schools of nursing were expected to select, develop, and implement a conceptual framework for their curricula. This propelled the advancement of theoretical thinking in nursing. (Meleis, 1992). A national conference on nursing theory and the Nursing Theory Think Tanks were formed to engage nursing leaders in dialogue about the place of theory in the evolution of nursing science. The linkages between theory, research, and philosophy were debated in the literature, and *Advances in Nursing Science,* the premiere journal for publishing theoretical articles, was launched.

In the 1980s additional grand theories such as Parse's man-living-health (later changed to human becoming); Newman's health as expanding consciousness; Leininger's transcultural nursing; Erickson, Tomlinson, and Swain's modeling and role modeling; and Watson's transpersonal caring were disseminated. Nursing theory conferences were convened, frequently attracting large numbers of participants. Those scholars working with the published theories in research and practice formalized networks into organizations and held conferences. For example the Society for Rogerian Scholars held the first Rogerian Conference; the Transcultural Nursing Society was formed, and the International Association for Human Caring was formed. Some of these organizations developed journals publishing the work of scholars advancing these conceptual models and grand theories. Metatheorists such as Jacqueline Fawcett, Peggy Chinn, and Joyce Fitzpatrick and Ann Whall published books on nursing theory, making nursing theories more accessible to students. Theory courses were established in graduate programs in nursing. The Fuld Foundation supported a series of videotaped interviews of many theorists, and the National League for Nursing disseminated videos promoting theory within nursing. *Nursing Science Quarterly,* a journal focused exclusively on advancing extant nursing theories, published its first issue in 1988.

During the 1990s, the expansion of conceptual models and grand theories in nursing continued to deepen, and forces within nursing both promoted and inhibited this expansion. The theorists and their students began conducting research and developing practice models that made the theories more visible. Regulatory bodies in Canada required that every hospital be guided by some nursing theory. This accelerated the development of nursing theory–guided practice within Canada and the United States. The accrediting bodies of nursing programs pulled back on their requirement of a specified conceptual framework guiding nursing curricula. Because of this, there were fewer programs guided by specific conceptualizations of nursing, and possibly fewer students had a strong grounding in the theoretical foundations of nursing. Fewer grand theories emerged; only Boykin and Schoenhofer's nursing as caring grand theory was published during this time. Middle-range theories emerged to provide more descriptive, explanatory, and predictive models around circumscribed phenomena of interest to nursing. For example, Meleis's transition theory, Mishel's uncertainty theory, Barrett's power theory, and Pender's health promotion model were generating interest.

From 2000 to the present, there has been accelerated development of middle-range theories with less interest in conceptual models and grand theories. There seems to be a devaluing of nursing theory; many graduate programs have eliminated their required nursing theory courses, and baccalaureate programs may not include the development of conceptualizations of nursing into their curricula. This has the potential for creating generations of nurses who have no comprehension of the importance of theory for understanding the focus of the discipline and the diverse, rich legacy of nursing knowledge from these theoretical perspectives.

On the other hand, health-care organizations have been more active in promoting attention to theoretical applications in nursing practice. For example, those hospitals on the magnet journey are required to select a guiding nursing framework for practice. Watson's theory of caring is guiding nursing practice in a group of acute care hospitals. These hospitals have formed a consortium so that best practices can be shared across settings.

Although nursing research is advancing and making a difference in people's lives, the research may not be linked explicitly to theory, and probably not linked to nursing theory. This compromises the advancement of nursing science. All other disciplines teach their foundational theories to their students, and their scientists test or develop their theories through research.

There is a trend toward valuing theories from other disciplines over nursing theories. For example, motivational interviewing is a practice theory out of psychology that nurse researchers and practitioners are gravitating to in large numbers. Arguably, there are several similar nursing theoretical approaches to engaging others in health promotion behaviors that preceded motivational interviewing, yet these have not been explored. Interprofessional practice and interdisciplinary research are essential for the future of health care, but we do not do justice to this concept by abandoning the rich,

distinguishing features of nursing science over others.

If nursing is to advance as a science in its own right, future generations of nurses must respect and advance the theoretical legacy of our discipline. Scientific growth happens through cumulative knowledge development with current research building on previous findings. To survive and thrive, nursing theories must be used in nursing practice and research.

The Structure of Knowledge in the Discipline of Nursing

Theories are part of the knowledge structure of any discipline. The domain of inquiry (also called the metaparadigm or focus of the discipline) is the foundation of the structure. The knowledge of the discipline is related to its general domain or focus. For example, knowledge of biology relates to the study of living things; psychology is the study of the mind; sociology is the study of social structures and behaviors. Nursing's domain was discussed earlier and relates to the disciplinary focus statement or metaparadigm. Other levels of the knowledge structure include paradigms, conceptual models or grand theories, middle-range theories, practice theories, and research and practice traditions. These levels of nursing knowledge are interrelated; each level of development is influenced by work at other levels. Theoretical work in nursing must be dynamic; that is, it must be continually in process and useful for the purposes and work of the discipline. It must be open to adapting and extending to guide nursing endeavors and to reflect development within nursing. Although there is diversity of opinion among nurses about the terms used to describe the levels of theory, the following discussion of theoretical development in nursing is offered as a context for further understanding nursing theory.

Paradigm

Paradigm is the next level of the disciplinary structure of nursing. The notion of paradigm can be useful as a basis for understanding nursing knowledge. A *paradigm* is a global, general framework made up of assumptions about aspects of the discipline held by members to be essential in development of the discipline. Paradigms are particular perspectives on the metaparadigm or disciplinary domain. The concept of paradigm comes from the work of Kuhn (1970, 1977), who used the term to describe models that guide scientific activity and knowledge development in disciplines. Because paradigms are broad, shared perspectives held by members of the discipline, they are often called "worldviews." Kuhn set forth the view that science does not always evolve as a smooth, regular, continuing path of knowledge development over time, but that periodically there are times of revolution when traditional thought is challenged by new ideas, and "paradigm shifts" occur.

Kuhn's ideas provide a way for us to think about the development of science. Before any discipline engages in the development of theory and research to advance its knowledge, it is in a preparadigmatic period of development. Typically, this is followed by a period of time when a single paradigm emerges to guide knowledge development. Research activities initiated around this paradigm advance its theories. This is a time during which knowledge advances at a regular pace. At times, a new paradigm can emerge to challenge the worldview of the existing paradigm. It can be revolutionary, overthrowing the previous paradigm, or multiple paradigms can coexist in a discipline, providing different worldviews that guide the scientific development of the discipline.

Kuhn's work has meaning for nursing and other scientific disciplines because of his recognition that science is the work of a community of scholars in the context of society. Paradigms and worldviews of nursing are subtle and powerful, reflecting different values and beliefs about the nature of human beings, human–environment relationships, health, and caring. Kuhn's (1970, 1977) description of scientific development is particularly relevant to nursing today as new perspectives are being articulated, some traditional views are being strengthened, and some views are taking their places as part of our history. **As we continue to move away from the historical conception of nursing as a part of biomedical science, developments in the nursing discipline are directed by at least two paradigms, or worldviews, outside the medical model.** These are now described.

Several nursing scholars have named the existing paradigms in the discipline of nursing (Fawcett, 1995; Newman et al., 1991; Parse, 1987). Parse (1987) described two paradigms: the totality and the simultaneity. The totality paradigm reflects a worldview that humans are integrated beings with biological, psychological, sociocultural, and spiritual dimensions. Humans adapt to their environments, and health and illness are states on a continuum. In the simultaneity paradigm, humans are unitary, irreducible, and in continuous mutual process with the environment (Rogers, 1970, 1992). Health is subjectively defined and reflects a process of becoming or evolving. In contrast to Parse, Newman and her colleagues (1991) identified three paradigms in nursing: particulate–deterministic, integrative–interactive, and unitary–transformative. From the perspective of the particulate–deterministic paradigm, humans are known through parts; health is the absence of disease; and predictability and control are essential for health management. In the integrative–interactive paradigm, humans are viewed as systems with interrelated dimensions interacting with the environment, and change is probabilistic. The worldview of the unitary–transformative paradigm describes humans as patterned, self-organizing fields within larger patterned, self-organizing fields. Change is characterized by fluctuating rhythms of organization–disorganization toward more complex organization. Health is a reflection of this continuous change. Fawcett (1995, 2000) provided yet another model of nursing paradigms: reaction, reciprocal interaction, and simultaneous action. In the reaction paradigm, humans are the sum of their parts, reaction is causal, and stability is valued. In the reciprocal interaction worldview, the parts are seen within the context of a larger whole, there is a reciprocal nature to the relationship with the environment, and change is based on multiple factors. Finally, the simultaneous-action worldview includes a belief that humans are known by pattern and are in an open ever-changing process with the environment. Change is unpredictable and evolving toward greater complexity (Smith, 2008, pp. 4–5).

It may help you to think of theories being clustered within these nursing paradigms. Many theories share the worldview established by a particular paradigm. At present, multiple paradigms coexist within nursing.

Grand Theories and Conceptual Models

Grand theories and conceptual models are at the next level in the structure of the discipline. They are less abstract than the focus of the discipline and paradigms but more abstract than middle-range theories. Conceptual models and grand theories focus on the phenomena of concern to the discipline such as persons as adaptive systems, self-care deficits, unitary human beings, human becoming, or health as expanding consciousness. The grand theories, or conceptual models, are composed of concepts and relational statements. Relational statements on which the theories are built are called assumptions and often reflect the foundational philosophies of the conceptual model or grand theory. These philosophies are statements of enduring values and beliefs; they may be practical guides for the conduct of nurses applying the theory and can be used to determine the compatibility of the model or theory with personal, professional, organizational, and societal beliefs and values. Fawcett (2000) differentiated conceptual models and grand theories. For her, conceptual models, also called conceptual frameworks or conceptual systems, are sets of general concepts and propositions that provide perspectives on the major concepts of the metaparadigm: person, environment, health, and nursing. Fawcett (1993, 2000) pointed out that direction for research must be described as part of the conceptual model to guide development and testing of nursing theories. We do not differentiate between conceptual models and grand theories and use the terms interchangeably.

Middle-Range Theories

Middle-range theories comprise the next level in the structure of the discipline. Robert Merton

(1968) described this level of theory in the field of sociology, stating that they are theories broad enough to be useful in complex situations and appropriate for empirical testing. Nursing scholars proposed using this level of theory because of the difficulty in testing grand theory (Jacox, 1974). Middle-range theories are narrower in scope than grand theories and offer an effective bridge between grand theories and the description and explanation of specific nursing phenomena. They present concepts and propositions at a lower level of abstraction and hold great promise for increasing theory-based research and nursing practice strategies (Smith & Liehr, 2008). Several middle-range theories are included in this book. Middle-range theories may have their foundations in a particular paradigmatic perspective or may be derived from a grand theory or conceptual model. The literature presents a growing number of middle-range theories. This level of theory is expanding most rapidly in the discipline and represents some of the most exciting work published in nursing today. Some of these new theories are synthesized from knowledge from related disciplines and transformed through a nursing lens (Eakes, Burke, & Hainsworth, 1998; Lenz, Suppe, Gift, Pugh, & Milligan, 1995; Polk, 1997). The literature also offers middle-range nursing theories that are directly related to grand theories of nursing (Ducharme, Ricard, Duquette, Levesque, & Lachance, 1998; Dunn, 2004; Olson & Hanchett, 1997). Reports of nursing theory developed at this level include implications for instrument development, theory testing through research, and nursing practice strategies.

Practice-Level Theories

Practice-level theories have the most limited scope and level of abstraction and are developed for use within a specific range of nursing situations. Theories developed at this level have a more direct effect on nursing practice than do more abstract theories. Nursing practice theories provide frameworks for nursing interventions/activities and suggest outcomes and/or the effect of nursing practice. Nursing actions may be described or developed as nursing practice theories. Ideally, nursing practice theories are interrelated with concepts from middle-range theories or developed under the framework of grand theories. A theory developed at this level has been called a prescriptive theory (Crowley, 1968; Dickoff, James, & Wiedenbach, 1968), a situation-specific theory (Meleis, 1997), and a micro-theory (Chinn & Kramer, 2011). **The day-to-day experience of nurses is a major source of nursing practice theory.**

The depth and complexity of nursing practice may be fully appreciated as nursing phenomena and relations among aspects of particular nursing situations are described and explained. Dialogue with expert nurses in practice can be fruitful for discovery and development of practice theory. Research findings on various nursing problems offer data to develop nursing practice theories. Nursing practice theory has been articulated using multiple ways of knowing through reflective practice (Johns & Freshwater, 1998). The process includes quiet reflection on practice, remembering and noting features of nursing situations, attending to one's own feelings, reevaluating the experience, and integrating new knowing with other experience (Gray & Forsstrom, 1991). The LIGHT model (Andersen & Smereck, 1989) and the attendant nurse caring model (Watson & Foster, 2003) are examples of the development of practice level theories.

Associated Research and Practice Traditions

Research traditions are the associated methods, procedures, and empirical indicators that guide inquiry related to the theory. For example, the theories of health as expanding consciousness, human becoming, and cultural care diversity and universality have specific associated research methods. Other theories have specific tools that have been developed to measure constructs related to the theories. The practice tradition of the theory consists of the activities, protocols, processes, tools, and practice wisdom emerging from the theory. Several conceptual models and grand theories have specific associated practice methods.

Nursing Theory and the Future

Nursing theory is essential to the continuing evolution of the discipline of nursing. Several trends are evident in the development and use of nursing theory. First, there seems to be more agreement on the focus of the discipline of nursing that provides a meaningful direction for our study and inquiry. This disciplinary dialogue has extended beyond the confines of Fawcett's metaparadigm and explicates the importance of caring and relationship as central to the discipline of nursing (Newman et al., 2008; Roy & Jones, 2007; Willis et al., 2008). The development of new grand theories and conceptual models has decreased. Dossey's (2008) theory of integral nursing, included in this book, is the only new theory at this level that has been developed in nearly 20 years. Instead, the growth in theory development is at the middle-range and practice levels. There has been a significant increase in middle-range theories, and many practice scholars are working on developing and implementing practice models based on grand theories or conceptual models.

Several changes in the teaching and learning of nursing theory are troubling. Many baccalaureate programs include little nursing theory in their curricula. Similarly, some graduate programs are eliminating or decreasing their emphasis on nursing theory. This alarming trend deserves our attention. If nursing is to continue to thrive and to make a difference in the lives of people, our practitioners and researchers need to practice and expand knowledge within the structure of the discipline. As health care becomes more interprofessional, the focus of nursing becomes even more important. If nurses do not learn and practice based on the knowledge of their discipline, they may be co-opted into the practice of another discipline. Even worse, another discipline could emerge that will assume practices associated with the discipline of nursing. For example, health coaching is emerging as an area of practice focused on providing people with help as they make health-related changes in their lives. However, this is the practice of nursing, as articulated by many nursing theories.

On a positive note, nursing theories are being embraced by health-care organizations to structure nursing practice. For example, organizations embarking on the journey toward magnet status (www.nursecredentialing .org/magnet) are required to identify a theoretical perspective that guides nursing practice, and many are choosing existing nursing models. This work has great potential to refine and extend nursing theories.

The use of nursing theory in research is inconsistent at best. Often, outcomes research is not contextualized within any theoretical perspective; however, reviewers of proposals for most funding agencies request theoretical frameworks, and scoring criteria give points for having one. This encourages theoretical thinking and organizing findings within a broader perspective. Nurses often use theories from other disciplines instead of their own and this expands the knowledge of another discipline.

We are hopeful about the growth, continuing development, and expanded use of nursing theory. We hope that there will be continued growth in the development of all levels of nursing theory. The students of all professional disciplines study the theories of their disciplines in their courses of study. We must continue to include the study of nursing theories within our baccalaureate, master's, and doctoral programs. Baccalaureate students need to understand the foundations for the discipline, our historical development, and the place of nursing theory in its history and future. They should learn about conceptual models and grand theories. Didactic and practice courses should reflect theoretical values and concepts so that students learn to practice nursing from a theoretical perspective. Middle-range theories should be included in the study of particular phenomena such as self-transcendence, sorrow, and uncertainty. As they prepare to become practice leaders of the discipline, doctor of nursing practice students should learn to develop and test nursing theory-guided models. PhD students will learn to develop and extend nursing theories in their research. New and expanded nursing specialties, such as nursing informatics, call for development and use of nursing theory (Effken, 2003). New, more

open and inclusive ways to theorize about nursing will be developed. These new ways will acknowledge the history and traditions of nursing but will move nursing forward into new realms of thinking and being. Reed (1995) noted the "ground shifting" with the reforming of philosophies of nursing science and called for a more open philosophy, grounded in nursing's values, which connects science, philosophy, and practice. Gray and Pratt (1991, p. 454) projected that nursing scholars will continue to develop theories at all levels of abstraction and that theories will be increasingly interdependent with other disciplines such as politics, economics, and ethics. These authors expect a continuing emphasis on unifying theory and practice that will contribute to the validation of the nursing discipline. Theorists will work in groups to develop knowledge in an area of concern to nursing, and these phenomena of interest, rather than the name of the author, will define the theory (Meleis, 1992). Newman (2003) called for a future in which we transcend competition and boundaries that have been constructed between nursing theories and instead appreciate the links among theories, thus moving toward a fuller, more inclusive, and richer understanding of nursing knowledge.

Nursing's philosophies and theories must increasingly reflect nursing's values for understanding, respect, and commitment to health beliefs and practices of cultures throughout the world. **It is important to question to what extent theories developed and used in one major culture are appropriate for use in other cultures.** To what extent must nursing theory be relevant in multicultural contexts? Despite efforts of many international scholarly societies, how relevant are American nursing theories for the global community? Can nursing theories inform us about how to stand with and learn from peoples of the world? Can we learn from nursing theory how to come to know those we nurse, how to be with them, to truly listen and hear? Can these questions be recognized as appropriate for scholarly work and practice for graduate students in nursing? Will these issues offer direction for studies of doctoral students? If so, nursing theory will prepare nurses for humane leadership in national and global health policy. Perspectives of various times and worlds in relation to present nursing concerns were described by Schoenhofer (1994). Abdellah (McAuliffe, 1998) proposed an international electronic "think tank" for nurses around the globe to dialogue about nursing theory. Such opportunities could lead nurses to truly listen, learn, and adapt theoretical perspectives to accommodate cultural variations.

■ Summary

This chapter focused on the place of nursing theory within the discipline of nursing. The relationship and importance of nursing theory to the characteristics of a professional discipline were reviewed. A variety of definitions of theory were offered, and the evolution and structure of knowledge in the discipline was outlined. Finally, we reviewed trends and speculated about the future of nursing theory development and application. One challenge of nursing theory is that theory is always in the process of developing and that, at the same time, it is useful for the purposes and work of the discipline. This paradox may be seen as ambiguous or as full of possibilities. Continuing students of the discipline are required to study and know the basis for their contributions to nursing and to those we serve; at the same time, they must be open to new ways of thinking, knowing, and being in nursing. Exploring structures of nursing knowledge and understanding the nature of nursing as a professional discipline provide a frame of reference to clarify nursing theory.

References

Allison, S. E., & McLaughlin-Renpenning, K. E. (1999). *Nursing administration in the 21st century: A self-care theory approach*. Thousand Oaks, CA: Sage.

Andersen, M. D., & Smereck, G. A. D. (1989). Personalized nursing LIGHT model. *Nursing Science Quarterly, 2*, 120–130.

Barnum, B. S. (1998). *Nursing theory: Analysis, application, evaluation* (5th ed.). Philadelphia: Lippincott, Williams & Wilkins.

Chinn, P., & Jacobs, M. (1987). *Theory and nursing: A systematic approach*. St. Louis, MO: Mosby.

Chinn, P., & Kramer, M. (2004). *Integrated knowledge development in nursing*. St. Louis, MO: Mosby.

Chinn, P., & Kramer, M. (2011). *Integrated theory and knowledge development in nursing* (8th ed.). St. Louis, MO: Mosby.

Cody, W. K. (1997). Of tombstones, milestones, and gemstones: A retrospective and prospective on nursing theory. *Nursing Science Quarterly, 10*(1), 3–5.

Cody, W. K. (2003). Nursing theory as a guide to practice. *Nursing Science Quarterly, 16*(3), 225–231.

Colley, S. (2003). Nursing theory: Its importance to practice. *Nursing Standard, 17*(56), 33–37.

Crowley, D. (1968). Perspectives of pure science. *Nursing Research, 17*(6), 497–501.

Dickoff, J., & James, P. (1968). A theory of theories: A position paper. *Nursing Research, 17*(3), 197–203.

Dickoff, J., James, P., & Wiedenbach, E. (1968). Theory in a practice discipline. *Nursing Research, 17*(5), 415–435.

Donaldson, S. K., & Crowley, D. M. (1978). The discipline of nursing. *Nursing Outlook, 26*(2), 113–120.

Dossey, B. (2008). Theory of integral nursing. *Advances in Nursing Science, 31*(1), E52–E73.

Ducharme, F., Ricard, N., Duquette, A., Levesque, L., & Lachance, L. (1998). Empirical testing of a longitudinal model derived from the Roy adaptation model. *Nursing Science Quarterly, 11*(4), 149–159.

Dunn, K. S. (2004). Toward a middle-range theory of adaptation to chronic pain. *Nursing Science Quarterly, 17*(1), 78–84.

Eakes, G., Burke, M., & Hainsworth, M. (1998). Middle-range theory of chronic sorrow. *Image: Journal of Nursing Scholarship, 30*(2), 179–184.

Effken, J. A. (2003). An organizing framework for nursing informatics research. *Computers Informatics Nursing, 21*(6), 316–325.

Ellis, R. (1968). Characteristics of significant theories. *Nursing Research, 17*(3), 217–222.

Fawcett, J. (1984). The metaparadigm of nursing: Current status and future refinements. *Image: Journal of Nursing Scholarship, 16*, 84–87.

Fawcett, J. (1993). *Analysis and evaluation of nursing theory*. Philadelphia: F. A. Davis.

Fawcett, J. (1995). *Analysis and evaluation of conceptual models of nursing* (3rd ed.). Philadelphia: F. A. Davis.

Fawcett, J. (2000). *Analysis and evaluation of contemporary nursing knowledge: Nursing models and nursing theories*. Philadelphia: F. A. Davis.

Fitzpatrick, J. (1997). Nursing theory and metatheory. In I. King & J. Fawcett (Eds.), *The language of nursing theory and metatheory*. Indianapolis, IN: Center Nursing Press.

Gioiella, E. C. (1996). The importance of theory-guided research and practice in the changing health care scene. *Nursing Science Quarterly, 9*(2), 47.

Gray, J., & Forsstrom, S. (1991). Generating theory for practice: The reflective technique. In J. Gray & R. Pratt (Eds.), *Towards a discipline of nursing*. Melbourne: Churchill Livingstone.

Gray, J., & Pratt, R. (Eds.). (1991). *Towards a discipline of nursing*. Melbourne: Churchill Livingstone.

Hart, M., & Foster, S. (1998). Self-care agency in two groups of pregnant women. *Nursing Science Quarterly, 11*(4), 167–171.

Jacox, A. (1974). Theory construction in nursing: An overview. *Nursing Research, 23*(1), 4–13.

Jennings, B. M., & Staggers, N. (1998). The language of outcomes. *Advances in Nursing Science, 20*(4), 72–80.

Johns, C., & Freshwater, D. (1998). *Transforming nursing through reflective practice*. London: Oxford University Press.

Kim, H. (1987). Structuring the nursing knowledge system: A typology of four domains. *Scholarly Inquiry for Nursing Practice: An International Journal, 1*(1), 99–110.

Kim, H. (1997). Terminology in structuring and developing nursing knowledge. In I. King & J. Fawcett (Eds.), *The language of nursing theory and metatheory*. Indianapolis, IN: Center Nursing Press.

King, A. R., & Brownell, J. A. (1976). *The curriculum and the disciplines of knowledge*. Huntington, NY: Robert E. Krieger.

Kleffel, D. (1996). Environmental paradigms: Moving toward an ecocentric perspective. *Advances in Nursing Science, 18*(4), 1–10.

Kuhn, T. (1970). *The structure of scientific revolutions* (2nd ed.). Chicago: University of Chicago Press.

Kuhn, T. (1977). *The essential tension: Selected studies in scientific tradition and change*. Chicago: University of Chicago Press.

Leininger, M. (1987). *Transcultural nursing*. New York: Wiley.

Lenz, E. R, Suppe, F., Gift, A. G., Pugh, L. C., & Milligan, R. A. (1995). Collaborative development of middle-range theories: Toward a theory of unpleasant symptoms. *Advances in Nursing Science, 17*(3), 1–13.

Litchfield, M., & Jondorsdottir, H. (2008). The practice discipline that's here and now. *Advances in Nursing Science, 31*(1), E79–91.

McAuliffe, M. (1998). Interview with Faye G. Abdellah on nursing research and health policy. *Image: Journal of Nursing Scholarship, 30*(3), 215–219.

McKay, R. (1969). Theories, models and systems for nursing. *Nursing Research, 18*(5), 393–399.

Meleis, A. (1992). Directions for nursing theory development in the 21st century. *Nursing Science Quarterly, 5*, 112–117.

Meleis, A. (1997). *Theoretical nursing: Development and progress*. Philadelphia: Lippincott.

Meleis, A. (2012). *Theoretical nursing: Development and progress* (5th ed.). Philadelphia: Lippincott, Williams and Wilkins.

Merton, R. (1968). *Social theory and social structure*. New York: The Free Press.

Newman, M. (2003). A world of no boundaries. *Advances in Nursing Science, 26*(4), 240–245.

Newman, M., Sime, A., & Corcoran-Perry, S. (1991). The focus of the discipline of nursing. *Advances in Nursing Science, 14*(1), 1–6.

Newman, M., Smith, M. C., Dexheimer-Pharris, M., & Jones, D. (2008). The focus of the discipline of nursing revisited. *Advances in Nursing Science, 31*(1), E16–E27.

Nightingale, F. (1859/1992). *Notes on nursing: What it is and what it is not*. Philadelphia: Lippincott.

Olson, J., & Hanchett, E. (1997). Nurse-expressed empathy, patient outcomes, and development of a middle-range theory. *Image: Journal of Nursing Scholarship, 29*(1), 71–76.

Parse, R. (1987). *Nursing science: Major paradigms, theories and critiques*. Philadelphia: W. B. Saunders.

Parse, R. (1997). Nursing and medicine: Two different disciplines. *Nursing Science Quarterly, 6*(3), 109.

Parse, R. (1998). *The human becoming school of thought: A perspective for nurses and other health professionals*. Thousand Oaks, CA: Sage.

Parsons, T. (1949). *Structure of social action*. Glencoe, IL: The Free Press.

Peplau, H. E. (1987). Nursing science: A historical perspective. In R. R. Parse (Ed.), *Nursing science: Major paradigms, theories and critiques* (pp. 13–29). Philadelphia: Saunders.

Polk, L. (1997). Toward a middle-range theory of resilience. *Advances in Nursing Science, 19*(3), 1–13.

Reed, P. (1995). A treatise on nursing knowledge development for the 21st century: Beyond postmodernism. *Advances in Nursing Science, 17*(3), 70–84.

Rogers, M. E. (1970). *An introduction to the theoretical basis of nursing*. Philadelphia: F. A. Davis.

Rogers, M. E. (1992). Nursing science and the space age. *Nursing Science Quarterly, 5*, 27–34.

Roy, C., & Jones, D. (Eds). (2007). *Nursing knowledge development and clinical practice*. New York: Springer.

Schoenhofer, S. (1994). Transforming visions for nursing in the timeworld of *Einstein's Dreams. Advances in Nursing Science, 16*(4), 1–8.

Schuster, E., & Brown, C. (1994). *Exploring our environmental connections*. New York: National League for Nursing.

Silva, M. (1997). Philosophy, theory, and research in nursing: A linguistic journey to nursing practice. In I. King & J. Fawcett (Eds.), *The language of nursing theory and metatheory.* Indianapolis, IN: Center Nursing Press.

Smith, M. C. (1994). Arriving at a philosophy of nursing: In J. F. Kikuchi & H. Simmons (Eds.), *Developing a philosophy of nursing* (pp. 43–60). Thousand Oaks, CA: Sage.

Smith, M. C. (2008). Disciplinary perspectives linked to middle range theory. In M. J. Smith & P. R. Liehr (Eds.), *Middle range theory for nursing* (2nd ed., pp. 1–12). New York: Springer.

Smith, M. J., & Liehr, P. R. (2013). *Middle range theory for nursing* (3rd ed.). New York: Springer.

Stevenson, J. S., & Tripp-Reimer, T. (Eds.). (1990). Knowledge about care and caring. In *Proceedings of a Wingspread Conference* (February 1–3, 1989). Kansas City, MO: American Academy of Nursing, 1990.

Walker, L., & Avant, K. (1995). *Strategies for theory construction in nursing.* Norwalk, CT: Appleton-Century-Crofts.

Watson, J. (1985). *Nursing: Human science and human care.* Norwalk, CT: Appleton-Century-Crofts.

Watson, J., & Foster, R. (2003). The attending nurse caring model: Integrating theory, evidence and advanced caring-healing therapeutics for transforming professional practice. *Journal of Clinical Nursing, 12,* 360–365.

Willis, D., Grace, P., & Roy, C. (2008). A central unifying focus for the discipline: Facilitating humanization, meaning, quality of life and healing in living and dying. *Advances in Nursing Science, 31*(1), E28–E40.

A Guide for the Study of Nursing Theories for Practice

Chapter *2*

MARILYN E. PARKER AND
MARLAINE C. SMITH

Study of Theory for Nursing Practice
A Guide for Study of Nursing Theory for
Use in Practice
Summary
References

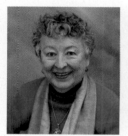

Marilyn E. Parker

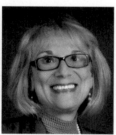

Marlaine C. Smith

Nursing is a professional discipline, a field of study focused on human health and healing through caring (Smith, 1994). The knowledge of the discipline includes nursing science, art, philosophy, and ethics. Nursing science includes the conceptual models, theories, and research specific to the discipline. As in other sciences such as biology, psychology, or sociology, the study of nursing science requires a disciplined approach. This chapter offers a guide to this disciplined approach in the form of a set of questions that facilitate reflection, exploration, and a deeper study of the selected nursing theories.

As you read the chapters in this book, use the questions in the guide to facilitate your study. These chapters offer you an introduction to a variety of nursing theories, which we hope will ignite interest in deeper exploration of some of the theories through reading the books written by the theorists and other published articles related to the use of the theories in practice and research. This book's online resources can provide additional materials as you continue your exploration.[1] The questions in this guide can lead you toward this deeper study of the selected nursing theories.

Rapid and dramatic changes are affecting nurses everywhere. Health-care delivery systems are in crisis and in need of real change. Hospitals continue to be the largest employers of nurses, and some hospitals are recognizing the need to develop nursing theory–guided practice models. A criterion for hospitals seeking magnet hospital designation

---

[1]For additional information please go to bonus chapter content available at FA Davis http://davisplus.fadavis.com

by the American Nurses Credentialing Center (www.nursecredentialing.org/magnet) includes the selection of a theoretical model for practice. The list of questions in this chapter can be useful to nurses as they select theories to guide practice.

Increasingly, nurses are practicing in diverse settings and often develop organized nursing practices through which accessible health care to communities can be provided. Community members may be active participants in selecting, designing, and evaluating the nursing they receive. In these situations, it is important for nurses and the communities they serve to identify the approach to nursing that is most consistent with the community's values. The questions in this chapter can be helpful in the mutual exploration of theoretical approaches to practice.

In the current health-care environment, interprofessional practice is the desired standard. This does not mean that practicing from a nursing-theoretical base is any less important. Interprofessional practice means that each discipline brings its own lens or perspective to the patient care situation. Nursing's lens is essential for a complete picture of the person's health and for the goals of caring and healing. The nursing theory selected will provide this lens, and the questions in this chapter can assist nurses in selecting the theory or theories that will guide their unique contribution to the interprofessional team.

Theories and practices from a variety of disciplines inform the practice of nursing. **The scope of nursing practice is continually being expanded to include additional knowledge and skills from related disciplines, such as medicine and psychology.** Again, this does not diminish the need for practice based on a nursing theory, and these guiding questions help to differentiate the knowledge and practice of nursing from those of other disciplines. For example, nurse practitioners may draw on their knowledge of pathophysiology, pharmacology, and psychology as they provide primary care. Nursing theories will guide the way of viewing the person,[2] inform the way of relating with the person, and direct the goals of practice with the person.

Groups of nurses working together as colleagues to provide care often realize that they share the same values and beliefs about nursing. The study of nursing theories can clarify the purposes of nursing and facilitate building a cohesive practice to meet them. Regardless of the setting of nursing practice, nurses may choose to study nursing theories together to design and articulate theory-guided practice.

The study of nursing theory precedes the activities of analysis and evaluation. The evaluation of a theory involves preparation, judgment, and justification (Smith, 2013). In the preparation phase, the student of the theory spends time coming to know it by reading and reflecting on it. The best approach involves intellectual empathy, curiosity, honesty, and responsibility (Smith, 2013). Through reading and dwelling with the theory, the student tries to understand it from the point of view of the theorist. Curiosity leads to raising questions in the quest for greater understanding. It involves imagining ways the theory might work in practice, as well as the challenges it might present. Honesty involves knowing oneself and being true to one's own values and beliefs in the process of understanding. Some theories may resonate with deeply held values; others may conflict with them. It is important to listen to these inner messages of comfort or discomfort, for they will be important in the selection of theories for practice.

Each member of a professional discipline has a responsibility to take the time and put in the effort to understand the theories of that discipline. In nursing, there is an even greater responsibility to understand and be true to those that are selected to guide nursing practice.

Responses to questions offered and points summarized in the guides may be found in nursing literature, as well as in audiovisual and electronic resources. Primary source material, including the work of nurses who are recognized authorities in specific nursing theories and the use of nursing theory, should be used.

---

[2]"Person" refers to individual, family, groups and communities throughout the chapter.

Study of Theory for Nursing Practice

Four main questions (described in the next section) have been developed and refined to facilitate the study of nursing theories for use in nursing practice (Parker, 1993). They focus on concepts within the theories, as well as on points of interest and general information about each theory. This guide was developed for use by practicing nurses and students in undergraduate and graduate nursing education programs. Many nurses and students have used these questions and contributed to their continuing development. As you study each theory, answer the questions and address the points in the following guide. You will find the information you need in the chapters of this book; other literature, such as books and journal articles authored by the theorists and other scholars working with the theories; and audiovisual and electronic resources.

A Guide for Study of Nursing Theory for Use in Practice

1. **How is nursing conceptualized in the theory?**

Is the focus of nursing stated?
- What does the nurse attend to when practicing nursing?
- What guides nursing observations, reflections, decisions, and actions?
- What illustrations or examples show how the theory is used to guide practice?

What is the purpose of nursing?
- What do nurses do when they are practicing nursing based on the theory?
- What are exemplars of nursing assessments, designs, plans, and evaluations?
- What indicators give evidence of the quality of nursing practice?
- Is the richness and complexity of nursing practice evident?

What are the boundaries or limits for nursing?
- How is nursing distinguished from other health-related professions?
- How is nursing related to other disciplines and services?
- What is the place of nursing in interprofessional practice?
- What is the range of nursing situations in which the theory is useful?

How can nursing situations be described?
- What are the attributes of the recipient of nursing care?
- What are characteristics of the nurse?
- How can interactions between the nurse and the recipient of nursing be described?
- Are there environmental requirements for the practice of nursing? If so, what are they?

2. **What is the context of the theory development?**

Who is the nursing theorist as person and as nurse?
- Why did the theorist develop the theory?
- What is the background of the theorist as a nursing scholar?
- What central values and beliefs does the theorist set forth?

What are major theoretical influences on this theory?
- What previous knowledge influenced the development of this theory?
- What are the relationships between this theory and other theories?
- What nursing-related theories and philosophies influenced this theory?

What were major external influences on development of the theory?
- What were the social, economic, and political influences that informed the theory?
- What images of nurses and nursing influenced the development of the theory?
- What was the status of nursing as a discipline and profession at the time of the theory's development?

3. **Who are authoritative sources for information about development, evaluation, and use of this theory?**

Which nursing authorities speak about, write about, and use the theory?
- What are the professional attributes of these persons?
- What are the attributes of authorities, and how does one become one?
- Which others can be considered authorities?

What major resources are authoritative sources on the theory?
- What books, articles, and audiovisual and electronic media exist to elucidate the theory?
- What nursing organizations share and support work related to the theory?
- What service and academic programs are authoritative sources for practicing and teaching the theory?

4. **How can the overall significance of the nursing theory be described?**

What is the importance of the nursing theory over time?
- What are exemplars of the theory's use that structure and guide individual practice?
- How has the theory been used to guide programs of nursing education?
- How has the theory been used to guide nursing administration and organizations?
- How does published nursing scholarship reflect the significance of the theory?

What is the experience of nurses who report consistent use of the theory?
- What is the range of reports from practice?
- Has nursing research led to further theoretical formulations?
- Has the theory been used to develop new nursing practices?
- Has the theory influenced the design of methods of nursing inquiry?
- What has been the influence of the theory on nursing and health policy?

What are projected influences of the theory on nursing's future?
- How has the theory influenced the community of scholars?
- In what ways has nursing as a professional practice been strengthened by the theory?
- What future possibilities for nursing have been opened because of this theory?
- What will be the continuing social value of the theory?

■ Summary

This chapter contains a guide designed for the study of nursing theory for use in practice. As members of the professional discipline of nursing, nurses must engage in the serious study of the theories of nursing. The implementation of theory-guided practice models is important for nursing practice in all settings. The guide presented in this chapter can lead students on a journey from a beginning to a deeper understanding of nursing theory. The study of nursing theory precedes its analysis and evaluation. Students should approach the study of nursing theory with intellectual empathy, curiosity, honesty, and responsibility. This guide is composed of four main questions to foster reflection and facilitate the study of nursing theory for practice.

References

Parker, M. (1993). *Patterns of nursing theories in practice*. New York: National League for Nursing.

Smith, M. C. (1994). Arriving at a philosophy of nursing: Discovering? Constructing? Evolving? In J. Kikuchi & H. Simmons (Eds.), *Developing a philosophy of nursing* (pp. 43–60). Thousand Oaks, CA: Sage.

Smith, M. C. (2013). Evaluation of middle range theories for the discipline of nursing. In M. J. Smith & P. Liehr (Eds.), *Middle range theory for nursing* (3rd ed., pp. 3–14). New York: Springer.

Choosing, Evaluating, and Implementing Nursing Theories for Practice

Chapter 3

MARILYN E. PARKER AND
MARLAINE C. SMITH

Significance of Nursing Theory
for Practice
Responses to Questions from Practicing
Nurses About Using Nursing Theory
Choosing a Nursing Theory to Study
A Reflective Exercise for Choosing
a Nursing Theory for Practice
Evaluation of Nursing Theory
Implementing Theory-Guided Practice
Summary
References

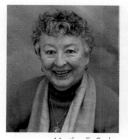
Marilyn E. Parker

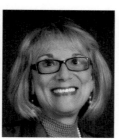
Marlaine C. Smith

The primary purpose of nursing theory is to improve nursing practice and, therefore, the health and quality of life of the persons, families, and communities served. Nursing theories provide coherent ways of viewing and approaching the care of persons in their environment. When a theoretical model is used to organize care in any setting, it strengthens the nursing focus of care and provides consistency to the communication and activities related to nursing care. The development of nursing theories and theory-guided practice models advances the discipline and professional practice of nursing.

One of the most important issues facing the discipline of nursing is the artificial separation of nursing theory and practice. Nursing can no longer afford to see these dimensions as disconnected territories, belonging to either scholars or practitioners. The examination and use of nursing theories are essential for closing the gap between nursing theory and nursing practice. Nurses in practice have a responsibility to study and value nursing theories, just as nursing theory scholars must understand and appreciate the day-to-day practice of nurses. Nursing theory informs and guides the practice of nursing, and nursing practice informs and guides the process of developing theory.

The theories of any professional discipline are useless if they have no effect on practice. Just as psychotherapists, educators, and economists base their approaches and decisions on particular theories, so should nurses be guided by selected nursing theories.

When practicing nurses and nurse scholars work together, both the discipline and practice of nursing benefit, and nursing service to our clients is enhanced. There are many examples throughout this book of how nursing theories have been, or can be, used to guide nursing practice. Many of the nursing theorists in this book developed or refined their theories based on dialogue with nurses who shared descriptions of their practice. This kind of work must continue for nursing theories to be relevant and meaningful to the discipline.

The need to bridge the gap between nursing theory and practice is highlighted by considering the following brief encounter during a question-and-answer period at a conference. A nurse in practice, reflecting her experience, asked a nurse theorist, "What is the meaning of this theory to my practice? I'm in the real world! I want to connect—but how can connections be made between your ideas and my reality?" The nurse theorist responded by describing the essential values and assumptions of her theory. The nurse said, "Yes, I know what you are talking about. I just didn't know I knew it, and I need help to use it in my practice" (Parker, 1993, p. 4). To remain current in the discipline, all nurses must join in community to advance nursing knowledge in practice and must accept their obligations to engage in the continuing study of nursing theories. Today, many health-care organizations that employ nurses adopt a nursing theory as a guiding framework for nursing practice. This decision provides an excellent opportunity for nurses in practice and in administration to study, implement, and evaluate nursing theories for use in practice. Communicating the outcomes of this process with the community of scholars advancing the theories is a useful way to initiate dialogue among nurses and to form new bridges between the theory and practice of nursing.

The purpose of this chapter is to describe the processes leading to implementation of nursing theory-guided practice models. These processes include choosing possible theories for use in practice, analyzing and evaluating these theories, and implementing theory-guided practice models. The chapter begins with responses to the questions: Why study nursing theory? What do practicing nurses gain from nursing theory? Then, methods of analysis and evaluation of nursing theory set forth in the literature are presented. Finally, steps in implementing nursing theory in practice are described.

Significance of Nursing Theory for Practice

Nursing practice is essential for developing, testing, and refining nursing theory. The development of many nursing theories has been enhanced by reflection and dialogue about actual nursing situations. The everyday practice of nursing enriches nursing theories. When nurses think about nursing, they consider the content and structure of the discipline of nursing. Even if nurses do not conceptualize these elements theoretically, their values and perspectives are often consistent with particular nursing theories. Making these values and perspectives explicit through the use of a nursing theory results in a more scholarly, professional practice.

Creative nursing practice is the direct result of ongoing theory-based thinking, decision-making, and action. Nursing practice must continue to contribute to thinking and theorizing in nursing, just as nursing theory must be used to advance practice.

Nursing practice and nursing theory often reflect the same abiding values and beliefs. Nurses in practice are guided by their values and beliefs, as well as by knowledge. These values, beliefs, and knowledge often are reflected in the literature about nursing's metaparadigm, philosophies, and theories. In addition, nursing theorists and nurses in practice think about and work with the same phenomena, including the person, the actions and relationships in the nurse–person (family/community) relationship, and the context of nursing. It is no wonder that nurses often sense a connection and familiarity with many of the concepts in nursing theories. They often say, "I knew this, but I didn't have the words for it." This is another value of nursing theory. It provides a vehicle for us to share and communicate the important concepts within nursing practice.

It is not possible to practice without some theoretical frame of reference. The question is what frame of reference is being used in practice. As stated in Chapter 1, theories are ways to organize our thinking about the complexities of any situation. Theories are lenses we select that will color the way that we view reality. In the case of nursing, the theories we choose to use will frame the way we think about a particular person and his or her health situation. It will inform the ways that we approach the person, how we relate, and what we do. Many nurses practice according to ideas and directions from other disciplines, such as medicine, psychology, and public health. If your approach to a person is framed by his or her medical diagnosis, you are influenced by the medical model that focuses your attention on diagnosis, treatment, and cure. If you are thinking about disease prevention as you work with a community group, you are influenced by public health theory and approaches. Although we use this knowledge in practice, nursing theory focuses us on the distinctive perspective of the discipline, which is more than, and different from, these approaches.

Historically, nursing practice has been deeply rooted in the medical model, and this model continues today. The depth and scope of the practice of nurses who follow notions about nursing held by other disciplines are limited to practices understood and accepted by those disciplines. Nurses who learn to practice from nursing perspectives are awakened to the challenges and opportunities of practicing nursing more fully and with a greater sense of autonomy, respect, and satisfaction for themselves. Hopefully, they also provide different and more expansive opportunities for health and healing for those they serve. Nurses who practice from a nursing perspective approach clients and families in ways unique to nursing. They ask questions, receive and process information about needs for nursing differently, and create nursing responses that are more holistic and client-focused. These nurses learn to reframe their thinking about nursing knowledge and practice and are then able to bring knowledge from other disciplines within the context of their practice—not to direct, their practice.

Nurses who practice from a nursing theoretical base see beyond immediate facts and

delivery systems; they can integrate other health sciences and technologies as the background or context and not the essence of their practice. Nurses who study nursing theory realize that although no group actually owns ideas, professional disciplines do claim a unique perspective that defines their practice. In the same way, no group actually owns the technologies of practice, although disciplines do claim them for their practice. For example, before World War II, nurses rarely took blood pressure readings and did not give intramuscular injections. This was not because nurses lacked the skill, but because they did not claim the use of these techniques within nursing practice. Such a realization can also lead to understanding that the things nurses do that are often called nursing are not nursing at all. The skills and technologies used by nurses, such as taking blood pressure readings, giving injections, and auscultating heart sounds, are actually activities that are part of the context, but not the essence, of nursing practice. Nursing theories provide an organizing framework that directs nurses to the essence of their purpose and places the use of knowledge from other disciplines in their proper perspective.

If nursing theory is to be useful—or practical—it must be brought into practice. At the same time, nurses can be guided by nursing theory in a full range of nursing situations. Nursing theory can change nursing practice: It provides direction for new ways of being present with clients, helps nurses realize ways of expressing caring, and provides approaches to understanding needs for nursing and designing care to address these needs. The chapters of this book affirm the use of nursing theory in practice and the study and assessment of theory to ultimately use in practice.

Responses to Questions from Practicing Nurses about Using Nursing Theory

Study of nursing theory may either precede or follow selection of a nursing theory for use in nursing practice. Analysis and evaluation of nursing theory follow the study of a nursing theory. These activities are demanding and deserve the full commitment of nurses who undertake the work. Because it is understood that the study of nursing theory is not a simple, short-term endeavor, nurses often question doing such work. The following questions about studying and using nursing theory have been collected from many conversations with nurses about nursing theory. These queries also identify specific issues that are important to nurses who consider the study of nursing theory.

My Nursing Practice

• Does this theory reflect nursing practice as I know it? Can it be understood in relation to my nursing practice? Will it support what I believe to be excellent nursing practice?

Conceptual models and grand theories can guide practice in any setting and situation. Middle-range theories address circumscribed phenomena in nursing that are directly related to practice. These levels of theory can enrich perspectives on practice and should foster an excellent professional level of practice.

• Is the theory specific to my area of nursing? Can the language of the theory help me explain, plan, and evaluate my nursing? Will I be able to use the terms to communicate with others?
• Can this theory be considered in relation to a wide range of nursing situations? How does it relate to more general views of nursing people in other settings?
• Will my study and use of this theory support nursing in my interprofessional setting?
• Will those from other disciplines be able to understand, facilitating cooperation?
• Will my work meet the expectations of those I serve? Will other nurses find my work helpful and challenging?

Conceptual models and grand theories are not specific to any nursing specialty. Theories in any discipline introduce new terminology that is not part of general language. For example, the id, ego, and superego are familiar terms in a particular psychological theory but were unknown at the time of the theory's introduction. The language of the theory facilitates thinking differently through naming new concepts or ideas. Members of disciplines do share specific language that may be less familiar to members outside the discipline. In interprofessional communication, new terms should be defined and explained to facilitate communication as needed. Nursing's unique perspective needs to be represented clearly within the interprofessional team. The diversity of each discipline's perspective is important to provide the best care possible for patients. People deserve and expect high-quality care. Nursing theory has the potential to bring to bear the importance of relationship and caring in the process of health and healing; the interrelationship of the environment and health; an understanding of the wholeness of persons in their life situations; and an appreciation of the person's experiences, values, and choices in care. These are essential contributions to a multidisciplinary perspective.

My Personal Interests, Abilities, and Experiences

• Is the study of nursing theories consistent with my talents, interests, and goals? Is this something I want to do?
• Will I be stimulated by thinking about and trying to use this theory? Will my study of nursing be enhanced by use of this theory?
• What will it be like to think about nursing theory in nursing practice?
• Will my work with nursing theory be worth the effort?

The study of nursing theory does take an investment in time and attention. It is a responsibility of a professional nurse who engages in a scholarly level of practice. Learning about nursing theory is a conceptual activity that can be challenging and intellectually stimulating. We need nurses who will invest in these activities so that knowledgeable theory-guided practice is the standard in all health-care settings.

Resources and Support

• Will this be useful to me outside the classroom?
• What resources will I need to understand fully the terms of the theory?

- Will I be able to find the support I need to study and use the theory in my practice?

The purpose of nursing theory goes beyond its study within courses. Nursing theory becomes alive when the ideas are brought to practice. The usefulness of theory in practice is one way that we judge its value and worth. It is helpful to read about the theory from primary sources or the most notable scholars and practitioners who have studied the theory. Nurses interested in particular theories can join online discussion groups where issues related to the theory are discussed. Many of the theory groups have formed professional societies and hold conferences that support lifelong learning and growing with those applying the theory in practice, administration, research, and education.

The Theorist, Evidence, and Opinion

- Who is the author of this theory? What background of nursing education and experience does the theorist bring to this work? Is the author an authoritative nursing scholar?
- How is the theorist's background of nursing education and experience brought to this work?
- What is the evidence that use of the theory may lead to improved nursing care? Has the theory been useful to guide nursing organizations and administrations? What about influencing nursing and health-care policy?
- What is the evidence that this nursing theory has led to nursing research, including questions and methods of inquiry? Did the theory grow out of research findings or out of practice issues and concerns?
- Does the theory reflect the latest thinking in nursing? Has the theory kept pace with the times in nursing? Is this a nursing theory for the future?

Approaching the study of nursing theory with openness, curiosity, imagination, and skepticism is important. Evaluation of any theory should include evidence that practicing based on the theory makes a difference in the lives of people. Theories must have pragmatic value; that is, they need to generate research questions and provide models that can be applied in practice. In the nursing literature, you will find examples of how a theory has been used in research and in practice. In some cases, especially with newly formed theories, this evidence may be unavailable. In these situations, you will need to imagine how the theory might work in practice. Theories have heuristic, or problem-solving, value in that they can lead to new ways of thinking about situations. Consider the heuristic value of the theory as you read it. The theory should ignite your passion about nursing.

Choosing a Nursing Theory to Study

It is important to give adequate attention to the selection of theories. Results of this decision will have lasting influences on your nursing practice. It is not unusual for nurses who begin to work with nursing theory to realize that their practice is changing and that their future efforts in the discipline and practice of nursing are markedly altered.

There is always some measure of hope mixed with anxiety as nurses seriously explore nursing theory for the first time. Individual nurses who practice with a group of colleagues often wonder how to select and study nursing theories. Nurses in practice and nursing students in theory courses have similar questions. Nurses in new practice settings designed and developed by nurses have the same concerns about getting started as do nurses in hospital organizations who want more from their practice.

The following exercise is grounded in the belief that the study and use of nursing theory in nursing practice must have roots in the practice of the nurses involved. Moreover, the nursing theory used by particular nurses must reflect elements of practice that are essential to those nurses, while at the same time bringing focus and freshness to that practice. This exercise calls on the nurse to think about the major components of nursing and bring forth the values and beliefs most important to nurses. In these ways, the exercise begins to parallel knowledge development reflected in the nursing metaparadigm (focus of the discipline) and nursing philosophies described in Chapter 1. Throughout the rest of this book, the reader is guided to connect nursing theory and nursing practice in the context of nursing situations.

A Reflective Exercise for Choosing a Nursing Theory for Practice

Select a comfortable, private, and quiet place to reflect and write. Relax by taking some deep, slow breaths. Think about the reasons you went into nursing in the first place. Bring your nursing practice into focus. Consider your practice today. Continue to reflect and, while avoiding distractions, make notes to record your thoughts and feelings. When you have been thinking for a time and have taken the opportunity to reflect on your practice, proceed with the following questions. Continue to reflect and to make notes as you consider each one.

Enduring Values

• What are the enduring values and beliefs that brought me to nursing?
• What beliefs and values keep me in nursing today?
• What are the personal values that I hold most dear?
• How do my personal and nursing values connect with what is important to society?

Reflect on an instance of nursing in which you interacted with a person, family, or community for nursing purposes. This can be a situation from your current practice or may be from your nursing in years past. Consider the purpose or hoped-for outcome.

Nursing Situations

• Who was this person, family, or community? How did I come to know him, her, or them as unique?
• What were the person's, family's, or community's hopes and dreams for their own health and healing?
• Who was I as a person in the nursing situation?
• Who was I as a nurse in the situation?

• What was the relationship between the person, family, or community and myself?
• What nursing actions emerged in the context of the relationship?
• What other nursing actions might have been possible?
• What was the environment of the nursing situation?
• What about the environment was important to the person, family or community's hopes and dreams for health and healing and my nursing actions?

Nursing can change when we consciously connect values and beliefs to nursing situations. Consider that values and beliefs are the basis for our nursing. Briefly describe the connections of your values and beliefs with your chosen nursing situation.

Connecting Values and the Nursing Situation

• How are my values and beliefs reflected in any nursing situation?
• Are my values and beliefs in conflict or frustrated in this situation?
• Do my values come to life in the nursing situation?

Cultivating Awareness and Appreciation

In reflecting and writing about values and nursing situations that are important to us, we often come to a fuller awareness and appreciation of our practice. Make notes about your insights. You might consider these initial notes the beginning of a journal in which you record your study of nursing theories and their use in nursing practice. This is a valuable way to follow your progress and is a source of nursing questions for future study. You may want to share this process and experience with your colleagues. Sharing is a way to explore and clarify views about nursing and to seek and offer support for nursing values and situations that are critical to your practice. If you are doing this exercise in a group, share your essential values and beliefs with your colleagues.

Multiple Ways of Knowing and Reflecting on Nursing Theory

Multiple ways of knowing are used in theory-guided nursing practice. Carper (1978) studied the nursing literature and described four essential patterns of knowing in nursing. Using the Phenix (1964) model of realms of meaning, Carper described personal, empirical, ethical, and aesthetic ways of knowing in nursing. Chinn and Kramer (2011) use Carper's patterns of knowing and a fifth pattern, called emancipatory knowing, to develop an integrated framework for nursing knowledge development. Additional patterns of knowing in nursing have been explored and described, and the initial four patterns have been the focus of much consideration in nursing (Boykin, Parker, & Schoenhofer, 1994; Leight, 2002; Munhall, 1993; Parker, 2002; Pierson, 1999; Ruth-Sahd, 2003; Thompson, 1999; White, 1995). Each of the patterns of knowing and its relationship to theory-guided practice are articulated in the following paragraphs.

Empirical knowing is the most familiar of the ways of knowing in nursing. Empirical knowing is how we come to know the science of nursing and other disciplines that are used in nursing practice. This includes knowing the actual theories, concepts, principles, and research findings from nursing, pathophysiology, pharmacology, psychology, sociology, epidemiology, and other fields. Nursing theory is within the pattern of empirical knowing. The theoretical framework for practice integrates the concepts, principles, laws, and facts essential for practice.

Personal knowing is about striving to know the self and to actualize authentic relationships between the nurse and person. Using this pattern of knowing in nursing, the client is not seen as an object but as a person moving toward fulfillment of potential (Carper, 1978). The nurse is recognized as continuously learning and growing as a person and practitioner. Reflecting on a person as a client and a person as a nurse in the nursing situation can enhance understanding of nursing practice and the centrality of relationships in nursing. These insights are useful for choosing and studying nursing theory. Knowing the self is essential in selecting a nursing theory to guide practice. Ultimately, the choice of theoretical perspective reflects personal values and beliefs.

Ethical knowing is increasingly important to the study and practice of nursing today. According to Carper (1978), ethics in nursing is the moral component guiding choices within the complexity of health care. Ethical knowing informs us of what is right, what is obligatory, and what is desirable in any nursing situation. Ethical knowing is essential in every action of the nurse in day-to-day practice.

Aesthetic knowing is described by Carper (1978) as the art of nursing; it is the creative and imaginative use of nursing knowledge in practice (Rogers, 1988). Although nursing is often referred to as art, this aspect of nursing may not be as highly valued as the science and ethics of nursing. Each nurse is an artist, expressing and interpreting the guiding theory uniquely in his or her practice. Reflecting on the *experience* of nursing is primary in understanding aesthetic knowing. Through such reflection, the nurse understands that nursing practice has in fact been *created*, that each instance of nursing is unique, and that outcomes of nursing cannot be precisely predicted. Besides the art of nursing, knowing through artistic forms is part of aesthetic knowing. Often human experiences and relationships can best be appreciated and understood through art forms such as stories, paintings, music, or poetry. Some assert that aesthetic knowing allows for understanding the wholeness of experience. Examples of this most complete knowing are frequent in nursing situations in which even momentary connection and genuine presence between the nurse and the person, family, or community is realized.

Emancipatory knowing as described by Chinn and Kramer (2011) is realized in praxis, the integration of knowing, doing and being. Paulo Freire's (1970) definition of praxis is simultaneous reflection and action intended to transform the world. In this pattern knowing is inseparable from action and is integral to the being of the nurse. The transformative action alters the power dynamics that maintain disadvantage for some and privilege for others, and is directed toward goals for social justice (Kagan, Smith, & Chinn, 2014). The nurse using this pattern cultivates awareness of how social, political and economic forces shape assumptions and opinions about knowledge and truth. Unveiling the dynamics that sustain inequity creates freedom to see and act in a way that improves the health of all. Emancipatory knowing reminds us of the contextual nature of knowing, and that through praxis (reflection and action) all patterns of knowing are integrated.

Using Insights to Choose Theory

The notes describing your experience will help in selecting a nursing theory to study and consider for guiding practice. You will want to answer these questions:

- What nursing theory seems consistent with the values and beliefs that guide my practice?
- What theories are consistent with my personal values and beliefs?
- What do I hope to achieve from the use of nursing theory?
- Given my reflection on a nursing situation, how can I use theory to support this description of my practice?
- How can I use nursing theory to improve my practice for myself and for my patients?

Evaluation of Nursing Theory

Evaluation of nursing theory follows its study and analysis and is the process of making a determination about its value, worth, and significance (Smith, 2013). There are many sets of criteria for evaluating conceptual models and grand theories (Chinn & Kramer, 2007; Fawcett, 2004; Fitzpatrick & Whall, 2004; Parse, 1987; Stevens, 1998). Smith (2013) has published criteria for evaluating middle-range theories. After reading and studying the primary sources of the theory, the research and practice applications of the theory, and other critiques and evaluations of the theory, it is important for the evaluator to come to his or her own judgments supported by logical analysis and examples from the theory.

The whole theory must be studied. Parts of the theory without the whole will not be fully meaningful and may lead to misunderstanding.

Before selecting a guide for theory evaluation, consider the level and scope of the theory. Is the theory a conceptual model or grand nursing theory? A middle-range nursing theory? A practice theory? Not all aspects of theory described in an evaluation guide will be evident in all levels of theory. Whall (2004) recognized this in offering particular guides for analysis and evaluation that vary according to three types of nursing theory: models, middle-range theories, and practice theories. Fawcett's (2004; Fawcett & DeSanto-Madeya, 2012) criteria for analysis and evaluation pertain to conceptual models and grand theories. Smith's (2013) criteria specifically address the evaluation of middle-range theories.

Theory analysis and evaluation may be thought of as one process or as a two-step sequence. It may be helpful to think of analysis of theory as necessary for in-depth study of a nursing theory and evaluation of theory as the assessment of a theory's significance, structure, and utility. Guides for theory evaluation are intended as tools to inform us about theories and to encourage further development, refinement, and use of theory. No guide for theory analysis and evaluation is adequate and appropriate for every nursing theory.

Johnson (1974) wrote about three basic criteria to guide evaluation of nursing theory. These have continued in use over time and offer direction today. These criteria state that the theory should:

- Define the congruence of nursing practice with societal expectations of nursing decisions and actions
- Clarify the social significance of nursing, or the effect of nursing on persons receiving nursing
- Describe social utility, or usefulness, of the theory in practice, research, and education

Following are summaries of the most frequently used guides for theory evaluation. These guides are components of the entire work about nursing theory of the individual nursing scholar and offer various interesting approaches to theory evaluation. Each guide should be studied in more detail than is offered in this introduction and should be examined in context of the whole work of the individual nurse scholar.

The approach to theory evaluation set forth by Chinn and Kramer (2011) is to use guidelines for describing nursing theory that are based on their definition of theory as "a creative and rigorous structuring of ideas that projects a tentative, purposeful, and systematic view of phenomena" (p. 58). The guidelines set forth questions that clarify the facts about aspects of theory: purpose, concepts, definitions, relationships and structure, and assumptions. These authors suggest that the next step in the evaluation process is critical reflection about whether and how the nursing theory works. Questions are posed to guide this reflection:

• How clear is this theory?
• How simple is this theory?
• How general is this theory?
• How accessible is this theory?
• How important is this theory?

Fawcett (2004; Fawcett & DeSanto-Madeya, 2012) developed two frameworks for the analysis and evaluation of conceptual models and theories. The questions for *analysis* of conceptual models address:

• Origins of the nursing model
• Unique focus of the nursing model
• Content of the nursing model

The questions for *evaluation* of conceptual models address:

• Explication of origins
• Comprehensiveness of content
• Logical congruence
• Generation of theory
• Credibility of nursing model

The framework for *analysis* of grand and middle-range theories includes:

• Theory scope
• Theory context
• Theory content

The questions for *evaluation* of grand and middle-range theories address:

• Significance
• Internal consistency
• Parsimony
• Testability
• Empirical adequacy
• Pragmatic adequacy

Meleis (2011) stated that the structural and functional components of a theory should be studied before evaluation. The structural components are assumptions, concepts, and propositions of the theory. Functional components include descriptions of the following: focus, client, nursing, health, nurse–client interactions, environment, nursing problems, and interventions. After studying these dimensions of the theory, critical examination of these elements may take place, summarized as follows:

• Relations between structure and function of the theory, including clarity, consistency, and simplicity
• Diagram of theory to elucidate the theory by creating a visual representation
• Contagiousness, or adoption of the theory by a wide variety of students, researchers, and practitioners, as reflected in the literature
• Usefulness in practice, education, research, and administration
• External components of personal, professional, social values, and significance

Smith (2013) developed a framework for the evaluation of middle-range theories that includes the following criteria:

Substantive foundation relates to meaning or how the theory corresponds to existing knowledge in the discipline. The questions for evaluation ask about its fit with the disciplinary focus of nursing; its specification of assumptions; its substantive meaning of a phenomenon; and its origins in practice and/or research.
Structural integrity relates to the structure or internal organization of the theory. Questions for evaluation ask about the clarity of definitions of concepts, the consistency of

level of abstraction, the simplicity of the theory, and the logical representation of relationships among concepts.

Functional adequacy refers to the ability of the theory to be used in practice and research. Questions are related to its applicability to practice and client groups, the identification of empirical indicators, the presence of published examples of practice and research using the theory and the evolution of the theory through inquiry (p. 41 x).

Implementing Theory-Guided Practice

Every nurse should develop a practice that is guided by nursing theory. Most conceptual models or grand theories have actual practice methods or processes that can be adopted. The scope and generality of middle-range theories makes them less appropriate to guide nursing practice within a unit or hospital. Instead, they can be used to understand and respond to phenomena that are encountered in nursing situations. For example, Boykin and Schoenhofer's Nursing as Caring theory has been adopted as a practice model by several hospitals (Boykin, Schoenhofer & Valentine, 2013). Reed's middle-range theory of self-transcendence can be used to guide a nurse who is leading a support group for women with breast cancer. Hospital units or entire nursing departments may adopt a model that guides nursing practice within their unit or organization. The following are suggestions that can facilitate this process of adoption and implementation of theory-guided practice within units or organizations:

Gaining administrative support. Organizational leaders need to support the initiative to begin the process of implementing nursing theory-guided practice. Although the impetus to begin this initiative might not originate in formal leadership, the organizational leaders and managers need to be on board. If it is to succeed, the implementation of a model for practice requires the support of administration at the highest levels.

Selecting the theory or model to be used in practice. The entire nursing staff should be fully involved and invested in the process of deciding on the theoretical model that will guide practice. This can be done is several ways. An organization's governance structure can be used to develop the most appropriate selection process. As stated previously, the selection of a nursing theory or model is based on values. Some nursing organizations have used their mission, values, and vision statements as a blueprint that helps them select nursing theories that are most consistent with these values. Another approach is to survey all nurses about the practice models they would like to see implemented. The nursing staff can then study the top three or four in greater detail so that an informed decision can be made. Staff development can be involved in planning educational offerings related to the models. A process of voting or gaining consensus can be used for the final selection.

Launching the initiative. Once the model has been selected, the leaders (formal and informal) begin to plan for its implementation. This involves creating a timeline, planning the phases and stages of implementation including activities, and using all methods of communication to be sure that all are informed of these plans. Unit champions, informal leaders who are enthusiastic and positive about the initiative, can be key to the building excitement for the initiative. A structure to lead and manage the implementation is essential. Consultants who are experts in the theory itself or who have experience in implementing the theory-guided practice model can be very helpful. For example, Watson's International Caritas Consortium[1] consists of hospitals that have experience implementing the theory in practice. New hospitals can join the consortium for consultation and support as they launch initiatives. A kickoff event, such as an inspirational presentation, can build excitement and visibility for the initiative.

Creating a plan for evaluation. It is important to build in a systematic plan for evaluation of the new model from the beginning. An evaluation study should be designed to track

---

For additional information, visit http://watsoncaring-science.org.

process and outcome indicators. Consultation from an evaluation researcher is essential. For example, outcomes of nurse satisfaction, patient satisfaction, nurse retention, and core measures might be considered as outcomes to be measured before and after the implementation of the model. Focus groups might be held at intervals to identify nurses' experiences and attitudes related to implementation of the model.

Consistent and constant support and education. As the model is implemented, a process to support continuing learning and growth with the theory needs to be in place. The nurses implementing the model will have questions and suggestions, so resident experts should be available for this education and support. Those working with the model will grow in their expertise, and their experiences need to be recorded and shared with the community of scholars advancing the theory in practice. Ways to foster staying on track must be developed. Some hospitals have created unit bulletin boards, newsletters, or signage to prevent reverting to old behaviors and to cement new ones. Staff members need opportunities

to dialogue about their experiences: what is working and what is not. They need the freedom to develop new ways of implementing the model so that their scholarship and creativity flourish.

Periodic feedback on outcomes and opportunities for reenergizing is essential. Planned change involves anticipating the ebb and flow of enthusiasm. In the stressful health-care environment, it is important to find opportunities to provide feedback on how the project is going, to reward and celebrate the successes, and to fan any dying embers of enthusiasm for the project. This can be accomplished by inviting study champions to attend regional or national conferences, bringing in speakers, or holding recognition events.

Revisioning of the theory-guided practice model based on feedback. Any theory-guided practice model will become richer through its testing in practice. The nurses working with the model will help to modify and revise the model based on evaluation data. This revisioning should be done in partnership with theorists and other practice scholars working with the model.

■ Summary

This chapter focused on the important connection between nursing theory and nursing practice and the processes of choosing, evaluating, and implementing theory for practice. The selection of a nursing theory for practice is based on values and beliefs, and a reflective process can help to identify the most important qualities of practice that

need to be present in a chosen theory. Evaluation of nursing theory is a judgment of its value or worth. Several models of theory evaluation are available for use. Implementing a theory-based practice model in a health-care setting can be challenging and rewarding. Suggestions for successful implementation were offered.

References

Boykin, A., Parker, M., & Schoenhofer, S. (1994). Aesthetic knowing grounded in an explicit conception of nursing. *Nursing Science Quarterly, 7*(4), 158–161.

Boykin, A., Schoenhofer, S. & Valentine, K. (2013. *Transformation for Nursing and Healthcare Leaders: Implementing a Culture of Caring.* New York, NY: Springer.

Carper, B. A. (1978). Fundamental patterns of knowing in nursing. *Advances in Nursing Science, 1*(1), 13–23.

Chinn, P., & Jacobs, M. (2007). *Integrated theory and knowledge development in nursing.* (7th edition). St. Louis, MO: Mosby.

Chinn, P., & Kramer, M. (2007). *Integrated knowledge development in nursing* (7th ed.). St. Louis, MO: Mosby.

Chinn, P., & Kramer, M. (2011). *Integrated theory and knowledge development in nursing* (8th ed.). St. Louis, MO: Mosby.

Fawcett, J. (2004). *Analysis and evaluation of contemporary nursing knowledge.* Philadelphia: F.A. Davis.

Fawcett, J. & DeSanto-Madeya . (2012). *Analysis and evaluation of contemporary nursing knowledge* (3rd ed.). Philadelphia, PA: F.A. Davis.

Fitzpatrick, J., & Whall, A. (2004). *Conceptual models of nursing.* Stamford, CT: Appleton & Lange.

Friere, Paulo. (1970). *Pedagogy of the oppressed.* New York, NY: Herder and Herder.

Johnson, D. (1974). Development of theory: A requisite for nursing as a primary health profession. *Nursing Research, 23*(5), 372–377.

Kagan, P., Smith, M., & Chinn, P. (Eds). (2014). *Philosophies and practices of emancipatory nursing: Social justice as praxis.* New York, NY: Routledge.

Leight, S. B. (2002). Starry night: Using story to inform aesthetic knowing in women's health nursing. *Journal of Advanced Nursing, 37*(1), 108–114.

Meleis, A. (2011). *Theoretical nursing: Development and progress* (5th ed.). Philadelphia: Lippincott.

Meleis, A. (2004). *Theoretical nursing: Development and progress* (3rd ed.). Philadelphia: Lippincott.

Munhall, P. (1993). Unknowing: Toward another pattern of knowing in nursing. *Nursing Outlook, 41*, 125–128.

Parker, M. (1993). *Patterns of nursing theories in practice.* New York: National League for Nursing.

Parker, M. E. (2002). Aesthetic ways in day-to-day nursing. In D. Freshwater (Ed.), *Therapeutic nursing: Improving patient care through self-awareness and reflection* (pp. 100–120). Thousand Oaks, CA: Sage.

Parse, R. R. (1987). *Nursing science: Major paradigms, theories and critiques.* Philadelphia: W. B. Saunders.

Phenix, P. H. (1964). *Realms of meaning.* New York: McGraw-Hill.

Pierson, W. (1999). Considering the nature of intersubjectivity within professional nursing. *Journal of Advanced Nursing, 30*(2), 294–302.

Rogers, M. E. (1988). Nursing science and art: A prospective. *Nursing Science Quarterly, 1*(3), 99–102.

Ruth-Sahd, L. A. (2003). Intuition: A critical way of knowing in a multicultural nursing curriculum. *Nursing Education Perspectives, 24*(3), 129–134.

Smith, M. C. (2013). Evaluation of middle range theories for the discipline of nursing. In M. J. Smith & P. R. Liehr (Eds.), *Middle range theory for nursing* (pp. 35–50). New York, NY: Springer.

Stevens, B. (1998). *Nursing theory: Analysis, application, evaluation.* Boston: Little, Brown.

Thompson, C. (1999). A conceptual treadmill: The need for "middle ground" in clinical decision making theory in nursing. *Journal of Advanced Nursing, 30*(5), 1222–1229.

Whall, A. (2004). The structure of nursing knowledge: Analysis and evaluation of practice, middle-range, and grand theory. In J. Fitzpatrick & A. Whall (Eds.), *Conceptual models of nursing: Analysis and application* (4th ed., pp. 5–20). Stamford, CT: Appleton & Lange.

White, J. (1995). Patterns of knowing: Review, critique and update. *Advances in Nursing Science, 17*(4), 73–86.

II

Conceptual Influences on the Evolution of Nursing Theory

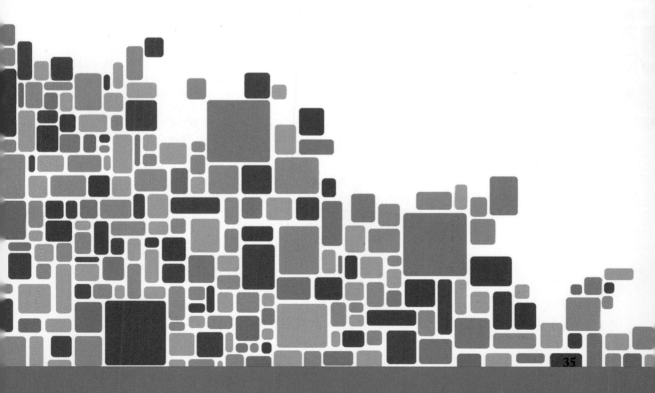

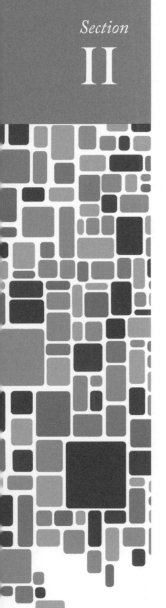

Conceptual Influences on the Evolution of Nursing Theory

The second section of the book has three chapters that describe conceptual influences on the development of nursing theory. Thomas Kuhn calls the stage of scientific development before formal theories are structured the "preparadigm stage." These scholars were working in this stage of our development, planting the seeds that grew into nursing theories. Nursing theorists today have stood on the shoulders of these "giants," building on their brilliant conceptualizations of the nature of nursing and the nurse–patient relationship. In Chapter 4, Dr. Lynne Dunphy, a noted historian and Nightingale scholar, illuminates the core ideas from Nightingale's work that have been essential foundations for the development of nursing theories. Although Nightingale did not develop a theory of nursing, she did provide a direction for the development of the profession and discipline. She believed in the natural or inherent healing ability of human beings and that the goal of nursing was to facilitate the emergence of health and healing by attending to the person–environment relationship. She said that the goal of nursing was to put the patient in the best condition for nature to act, and she identified five environmental components essential to health. Nightingale saw nursing and medicine as separate fields and emphasized the importance of systematic inquiry. Her spiritual nature and vision of nursing as an art continue to influence practice today. The emphasis on optimal healing environments in today's health-care systems can be related to Nightingale's ideas. The quality of the human–environment relationship is related to health and healing.

In Chapter 5, Dr. Shirley Gordon summarized the work of Ernestine Wiedenbach, Virginia Henderson, and Lydia Hall. Wiedenbach emphasized the importance of reverence for life, respect for dignity, autonomy, worth, and uniqueness of each person, and a commitment to act on these values as the essence of a personal philosophy of nursing. Henderson described nursing as "getting into the skin" of the patient so that nurses would be able to provide the strength, will, or knowledge the patient needed to heal or maintain health. Lydia Hall is an inspiration to all who envision nursing as an autonomous discipline and practice. She created a model of nursing consisting of "the core, the cure, and the care" and implemented that model in the Loeb Center for Nursing and Rehabilitation. Physicians referred their patients to the Center, and nurses admitted the patients for nursing care. Nurses worked independently with patients to foster learning, growth, and healing.

Chapter 6, written by a group of authors, focused on three nursing leaders who described the nurse–patient relationship: Hildegard Peplau, Ida Jean Orlando, and Joyce Travelbee. A psychiatric nurse, Peplau viewed the purpose of nursing as helping the patient gain the intellectual and interpersonal competencies necessary to heal. She articulated stages of the nurse–patient relationship, a framework for anxiety and nursing interventions to decrease anxiety. Travelbee emphasized the human-to-human relationship between nurse and person and spoke of the purpose of nursing as assisting the person(s) to prevent or cope with the experience of illness and suffering. Orlando described attributes of the nurse–patient relationship. She valued relationship as central to the practice of nursing and was the first to describe nursing process as identifying and responding to needs.

Chapter 4

Florence Nightingale's Legacy of Caring and Its Applications

LYNNE M. HEKTOR DUNPHY

Introducing the Theorist
Early Life and Education
Spirituality
War
Introducing the Theory
The Medical Milieu
The Feminist Context of Nightingale's Caring
Ideas About Nursing
Nightingale's Legacy for 21st Century Nursing Practice
Summary
References

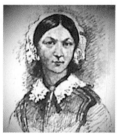

Florence Nightingale

Introducing the Theorist

Florence Nightingale, the acknowledged founder of modern nursing, remains a compelling and transformative figure. Not a year goes by in which new scholarship on Nightingale does not emerge. *Florence Nightingale and the Health of the Raj* was published in 2003 documenting Nightingale's 40-year-long interest and involvement in Indian affairs, a previously not well explored area of scholarship (Gourley, 2003). In 2004, a new biography of Nightingale, *Nightingales: The Extraordinary Upbringing and Curious Life of Miss Florence Nightingale* by Gillian Gill, was published. In 2008, another new biography, *Florence Nightingale: The Making of an Icon* by Mark Bostridge, was published. 2013 saw yet another biography, very finely written and presented, *Florence Nightingale, Feminist* by Judith Lissauer Cromwell. Squarely in the camp of viewing Nightingale as a "feminist"—a term that was non-existent during the years that Nightingale was alive—it is a fine work, told from a post-feminist perspective. Lynn McDonald's prodigious, ambitious, and long overdue *Collected Works of Florence Nightingale* consists of 16 volumes. In 2005, the American Nurses Association published *Florence Nightingale Today: Healing, Leadership, Global Action*, an ambitious casting of Nightingale as 21st century nursing's inspiration and savior. At the time you are perusing this chapter, it will be more than a century since the death of Florence Nightingale in 1910 and almost 200 hundred years since her birth on May 12 in 1820.

Nightingale transformed a "calling from God" and an intense spirituality into a new social role for women: that of nurse. Her caring

37

was a public one. "Work your true work," she wrote, "and you will find God within you" (Woodham-Smith, 1983, p. 74). A reflection on this statement appears in a well-known quote from *Notes on Nursing* (Nightingale, 1859/1992): "Nature [i.e., the manifestation of God] alone cures . . . what nursing has to do . . . is put the patient in the best condition for nature to act upon him" (Macrae, 1995, p. 10). Although Nightingale never defined human care or caring in *Notes on Nursing,* there is no doubt that her life in nursing exemplified and personified an ethos of caring. Jean Watson (1992, p. 83), in the 1992 commemorative edition of *Notes on Nursing,* observed, "Although Nightingale's feminine-based caring-healing model has transcended time and is prophetic for this century's health reform, the model is yet to truly come of age in nursing or the health care system." In a reflective essay, Boykin and Dunphy (2002) extended this thinking and related Nightingale's life, rooted in compassion and caring, as an exemplar of justice making (p. 14). *Justice making* is understood as a manifestation of compassion and caring, "for it is our actions that bring about justice" (p. 16).

This chapter reiterates Nightingale's life from the years 1820 to 1860, delineating the formative influences on her thinking and providing historical context for her ideas about nursing as we recall them today. Part of what follows is a well-known tale, yet it remains one that is irresistible, casting an age-old spell on the reader, like the flickering shadow of Nightingale and her famous lamp in the dark and dreary halls of the Barrack Hospital, Scutari, on the outskirts of Constantinople, circa 1854 to 1856. It is a tale that carries even *more* relevance for nursing practice today.

Early Life and Education

A profession, a trade, a necessary occupation, something to fill and employ all my faculties, I have always felt essential to me, I have always longed for, consciously or not. . . . The first thought I can remember, and the last, was nursing work.
—FLORENCE NIGHTINGALE, CITED IN COOK (1913, p. 106)

Nightingale was born in 1820 in Florence, Italy—the city she was named for. The Nightingales were on an extended European tour, begun in 1818 shortly after their marriage. This was a common journey for those of their class and wealth. Their first daughter, Parthenope, had been born in the city of that name in the previous year.

A legacy of humanism, liberal thinking, and love of speculative thought was bequeathed to Nightingale by her father. His views on the education of women were far ahead of his time. W. E. N., as her father, William, was called, undertook the education of both his daughters. Florence and her sister studied music; grammar; composition; modern languages; classical Greek and Latin; constitutional history and Roman, Italian, German, and Turkish history; and mathematics (Barritt, 1973).

From an early age, Florence exhibited independence of thought and action. The sketch (Fig. 4-1) of W. E. N. and his daughters was

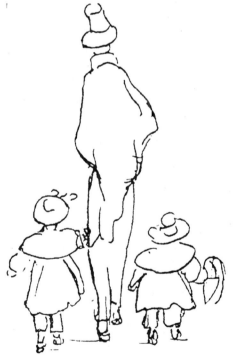

Fig 4 • 1 A sketch of W. E. N. and his daughters by one of his wife Fanny's sisters, Julia Smith.
Source: Woodham-Smith (1983), p. 9, with permission of Sir Henry Verney, Bart.

done by Nightingale's beloved aunt, Julia Smith. It is Parthenope, the older sister, who clutches her father's hand and Florence who, as described by her aunt, "independently stumps along by herself" (Woodham-Smith, 1983, p. 7).

Travel also played a part in Nightingale's education. Eighteen years after Florence's birth, the Nightingales and both daughters made an extended tour of France, Italy, and Switzerland between the years of 1837 and 1838 and later Egypt and Greece (Sattin, 1987). From there, Nightingale visited Germany, making her first acquaintance with Kaiserswerth, a Protestant religious community that contained the Institution for the Training of Deaconesses, with a hospital school, penitentiary, and orphanage. A Protestant pastor, Theodore Fleidner, and his young wife had established this community in 1836, in part to provide training for women deaconesses (Protestant "nuns") who wished to nurse. Nightingale was to return there in 1851 against much family opposition to stay from July through October, participating in a period of "nurse's training" (Cook, Vol. I, 1913; Woodham-Smith, 1983).

Life at Kaiserswerth was spartan. The trainees were up at 5 A.M., ate bread and gruel, and then worked on the hospital wards until noon. Then they had a 10-minute break for broth with vegetables. Three P.M. saw another 10-minute break for tea and bread. They worked until 7 P.M., had some broth, and then Bible lessons until bed. What the Kaiserswerth training lacked in expertise it made up for in a spirit of reverence and dedication. Florence wrote, "The world here fills my life with interest and strengthens me in body and mind" (Huxley, 1975, p. 24).

In 1852, Nightingale visited Ireland, touring hospitals and keeping notes on various institutions along the way. Nightingale took two trips to Paris in 1853; hospital training again was the goal, this time with the sisters of St. Vincent de Paul, an order of nursing nuns. In August 1853, she accepted her first "official" nursing post as superintendent of an "Establishment for Gentlewomen in Distressed Circumstances during Illness," located at 1 Harley Street, London. After 6 months at Harley Street, Nightingale wrote in a letter to her father: "I am in the hey-day of my power" (Nightingale, cited in Woodham-Smith, 1983, p. 77).

By October 1854, larger horizons beckoned.

Spirituality

Today I am 30—the age Christ began his Mission. Now no more childish things, no more vain things, no more love, no more marriage. Now, Lord let me think only of Thy will, what Thou willest me to do. O, Lord, Thy will, Thy will.
—FLORENCE NIGHTINGALE, PRIVATE NOTE, 1850, CITED IN WOODHAM-SMITH (1983, p. 130)

By all accounts, Nightingale was an intense and serious child, always concerned with the poor and the ill, mature far beyond her years. A few months before her 17th birthday, Nightingale recorded in a personal note dated February 7, 1837, that she had been called to God's service. What that service was to be was unknown at that point in time. This was to be the first of four such experiences that Nightingale documented.

The fundamental nature of her religious convictions made her service to God, through service to humankind, a driving force in her life. She wrote: "The kingdom of Heaven is within; but we must make it without" (Nightingale, private note, cited in Woodham-Smith, 1983).

It would take 16 long and torturous years, from 1837 to 1853, for Nightingale to actualize her calling to the role of nurse. This was a revolutionary choice for a woman of her social standing and position, and her desire to nurse met with vigorous family opposition for many years. Along the way, she turned down proposals of marriage, potentially, in her mother's view, "brilliant matches," such as that of Richard Monckton Milnes. However, her need to serve God and to demonstrate her caring through meaningful activity proved stronger. She did not think that she could be married and also do God's will.

Calabria and Macrae (1994) noted that for Nightingale, there was no conflict between science and spirituality; actually, in her view, science is necessary for the development of a mature concept of God. The development of science allows for the concept of one perfect God Who regulates the universe through universal laws as opposed to random happenings. Nightingale referred to these laws, or the organizing principles of the universe, as "Thoughts of God" (Macrae, 1995, p. 9). As part of God's plan of evolution, it was the responsibility of human beings to discover the laws inherent in the universe and apply them to achieve well-being. In *Notes on Nursing* (1860/1969, p. 25), she wrote:

God lays down certain physical laws. Upon his carrying out such laws depends our responsibility (that much abused word). . . . Yet we seem to be continually expecting that He will work a miracle—i.e. break his own laws expressly to relieve us of responsibility.

Influenced by the Unitarian ideas of her father and her extended family, as well as by the more traditional Anglican Church she attended, Nightingale remained for her entire life a searcher of religious truth, studying a variety of religions and reading widely. She was a devout believer in God. Nightingale wrote: "I believe that there is a Perfect Being, of whose thought the universe in eternity is the incarnation" (Calabria & Macrae, 1994, p. 20). Dossey (1998) recast Nightingale in the mode of "religious mystic." However, to Nightingale, mystical union with God was not an end in itself but was the source of strength and guidance for doing one's work in life. For Nightingale, service to God was service to humanity (Calabria & Macrae, 1994, p. xviii).

In Nightingale's view, nursing should be a search for the truth; it should be a discovery of God's laws of healing and their proper application. This is what she was referring to in *Notes on Nursing* when she wrote about the Laws of Health, as yet unidentified. It was the Crimean War that provided the stage for her to actualize these foundational beliefs, rooting forever in her mind certain "truths." In the Crimea, she was drawn closer to those suffering injustice. It was in the Barracks Hospital of Scutari that Nightingale acted justly and responded to a call for nursing from the prolonged cries of the British soldiers (Boykin & Dunphy, 2002, p. 17).

War

I stand at the altar of those murdered men and while I live I fight their cause.
—NIGHTINGALE, CITED IN WOODHAM-SMITH (1951, P. 182)

Nightingale had powerful friends and had gained prominence through her study of hospitals and health matters during her travels. When Great Britain became involved in the Crimean War in 1854, Nightingale was ensconced in her first official nursing post at 1 Harley Street. Britain had joined France and Turkey to ward off an aggressive Russian advance in the Crimea (Fig. 4-2). A successful advance of Russia through Turkey could threaten the peace and stability of the European continent.

The first actual battle of the war, the Battle of Alma, was fought in September 1854. It was written of that battle that it was a "glorious and bloody victory." The best communication technology of the times, the telegraph, was to have an effect on what was to follow. In previous wars, news from the battlefields trickled home slowly. However, the telegraph enabled war correspondents to transmit reports home with rapid speed. The horror of the battlefields was relayed to a concerned citizenry. Descriptions of wounded men, disease, and illness abounded. Who was to care for these men? The French had the Sisters of Charity to care for their sick and wounded. What were the British to do (Goldie, 1987; Woodham-Smith, 1951)?

The minister of war was Sidney Herbert, Lord Herbert of Lea, who was the husband of Liz Herbert; both were close friends of Nightingale. Herbert had an innovative solution: appoint Miss Nightingale and charge her to head a contingent of nurses to the Crimea

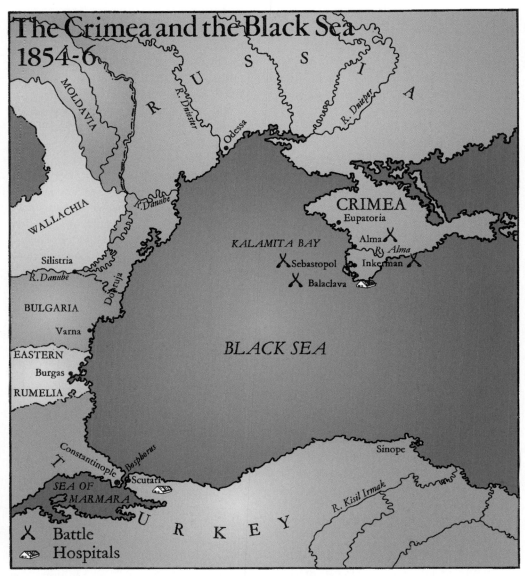

Fig 4 • 2 The Crimea and the Black Sea, 1854 to 1856. *Source: Huxley, E. (1975). Designed by Manuel Lopez Parras.*

to provide help and organization to the deteriorating battlefield situation. It was a brave move on the part of Herbert. Medicine and war were exclusively male domains. To send a woman into these hitherto uncharted waters was risky at best. But, as is well known, Nightingale was no ordinary woman, and she more than rose to the occasion. In a passionate letter to Nightingale, requesting her to accept this post, Herbert wrote:

> Your own personal qualities, your knowledge and your power of administration, and among greater things, your rank and position in society, give you advantages in such a work that no other person possesses. (Dolan, 1971, p. 2)

At the same time, such that their letters actually crossed, Nightingale wrote to Herbert, offering her services. Accompanied by 38 handpicked "nurses" who had no formal training, she arrived on November 4, 1854 to "take charge" and did not return to England until August 1856.

Biographer Woodham-Smith and Nightingale's own correspondence, as cited in a number of sources (Cook, 1913; Goldie, 1987; Huxley, 1975; Summers, 1988; Vicinus & Nergaard, 1990), paint the most vivid picture of the experiences that Nightingale sustained there, experiences that cemented her views on disease and contagion, as well as her commitment to an environmental approach to health and illness:

> The filth became indescribable. The men in the corridors lay on unwashed floors crawling with vermin. As the Rev. Sidney Osborne knelt to take down dying messages, his paper became thickly covered with lice. There were no pillows, no blankets; the men lay, with their heads on their boots, wrapped in the blanket or greatcoat stiff with blood and filth which had been their sole covering for more than a week . . . [S]he [Miss Nightingale] estimated . . . . there were more than 1000 men suffering from acute diarrhea and only 20 chamber pots. . . . [T]here was liquid filth which floated over the floor an inch deep. Huge wooden tubs stood in the halls and corridors for the men to use. In this filth lay the men's food—Miss Nightingale saw the skinned carcass of a sheep lie in a ward all night . . . the stench from the hospital could be smelled outside the walls. (Woodham-Smith, 1983)

On her arrival in the Crimea, the immediate priority of Nightingale and her small band of nurses was not in the sphere of medical or surgical nursing as currently known; rather, their order of business was *domestic management*. This is evidenced in the following exchange between Nightingale and one of her party as they approached Constantinople: "Oh, Miss Nightingale, when we land don't let there be any red-tape delays, let us get straight to nursing the poor fellows!" Nightingale's reply: "The strongest will be wanted at the wash tub" (Cook, 1913; Dolan, 1971).

Although the bulk of this work continued to be done by orderlies after Nightingale's arrival

(with the laundry farmed out to the soldiers' wives), it was accomplished under Nightingale's eagle eye: "She insisted on the huge wooden tubs in the wards being emptied, standing [obstinately] by the side of each one, sometimes for an hour at a time, never scolding, never raising her voice, until the orderlies gave way and the tub was emptied" (Woodham-Smith, 1951, p. 116).

Nightingale set up her own extra "diet kitchen." Small portions, helpings of such things as arrowroot, port wine, lemonade, rice pudding, jelly, and beef tea, whose purpose was to tempt and revive the appetite, were provided to the men. It was therefore a logical sequence from cooking to feeding, from administering food to administering medicines. Because no antidote to infection existed at this time, the provision—by Nightingale and her nurses—of cleanliness, order, encouragement to eat, feeding, clean bed linen, clean bodies, and clean wards was essential to recovery (Summers, 1988).

Mortality rates at the Barrack Hospital in Scutari fell. In February, at Nightingale's insistence, the prime minister had sent to the Crimea a sanitary commission to investigate the high mortality rates. Beginning their work in March, they described the conditions at the Barrack Hospital as "murderous." Setting to work immediately, they opened the channel through which the water supplying the hospital flowed, where a dead horse was found. The commission cleared "556 handcarts and large baskets full of rubbish . . . 24 dead animals and 2 dead horses buried." In addition, they flushed and cleansed sewers, lime-washed walls, tore out shelves that harbored rats, and got rid of vermin. The commission, Nightingale said, "saved the British Army." Miss Nightingale's anti-contagionism was sealed as the mortality rates began showing dramatic declines (Rosenberg, 1979).

Figure 4-3 illustrates Nightingale's own hand-drawn "coxcombs" (as they were referred to), as Nightingale, always aware of the necessity of documenting outcomes of care, kept copious records of all sorts (Cook, 1913; Rosenberg, 1979; Woodham-Smith, 1951).

Diagram Representing the Mortality in the Hospitals
at Scutari and Kulali from Oct. 1st 1854 to Sept. 30th 1855

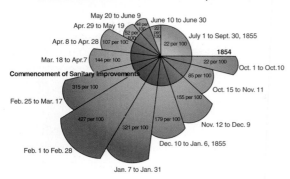

Fig 4 • 3 Diagram by Florence Nightingale showing declining mortality rates. *Source: Cohen (1981).*

Florence Nightingale possessed *moral authority,* so firm because it was grounded in caring and was in a larger mission that came from her spirituality. For Miss Nightingale, spirituality was a much broader, more unifying concept than that of religion. Her spirituality involved the sense of a presence higher than humanity, the divine intelligence that creates, sustains, and organizes the universe, and an awareness of our inner connection to this higher reality. Through this inner connection flows creative endeavors and insight, a sense of purpose and direction. For Miss Nightingale, spirituality was intrinsic to human nature and was the deepest, most potent resource for healing. In *Suggestions for Thought* (Calabria & Macrae, 1994, p. 58), Nightingale wrote that "human consciousness is tending to become what God's consciousness is—to become One with the consciousness of God." This progression of consciousness to unity with the divine was an evolutionary view and not typical of either the Anglican or Unitarian views of the time (Calabria & Macrae, 1994; Macrae, 1995; Rosenberg, 1979; Slater, 1994; Welch, 1986; Widerquist, 1992).

There were 4 miles of beds in the Barrack Hospital at Scutari, a suburb of Constantinople. A letter to the *London Times* dated February 24, 1855, reported the following: "When all the medical officers have retired for the night and silence and darkness have settled upon those miles of prostrate sick, she may be observed, alone with a little lamp in her hand, making her solitary rounds" (Kalisch & Kalisch, 1987, p. 46).

In April 1855, after having been in Scutari for 6 months, Florence wrote to her mother, "[A]m in sympathy with God, fulfilling the purpose I came into the world for" (Woodham-Smith, 1983, p. 97). Henry Wadsworth Longfellow authored "Santa Filomena" to commemorate Miss Nightingale.

Lo! In That House of Misery
A lady with a lamp I see
Pass through the glimmering gloom
And flit from room to room
And slow as if in a dream of bliss
The speechless sufferer turns to kiss
Her shadow as it falls
Upon the darkening walls
As if a door in heaven should be
Opened and then closed suddenly
The vision came and went
The light shone and was spent.
A lady with a lamp shall stand
In the great history of the land
A noble type of good
Heroic womanhood (Longfellow, cited in Dolan, 1971, p. 5)

Miss Nightingale slipped home quietly, arriving at Lea Hurst in Derbyshire on August 7, 1856, after 22 months in the Crimea and after sustained illness from which she was never to recover, after ceaseless work and after witnessing suffering, death, and despair that would haunt her for the remainder of her life. Her hair was shorn; she was pale and drawn (Fig. 4-4). She took her family by surprise. The next morning, a peal of the village church bells and a prayer of Thanksgiving were, her sister wrote, "'all the innocent greeting' except for those provided by the spoils of war that had proceeded her—a one-legged sailor boy, a small Russian orphan, and a large puppy found in some rocks near Balaclava. All England was ringing with her name, but she had left her heart on the battlefields of the Crimea and in the graveyards of Scutari" (Huxley, 1975, p. 147).

Introducing the Theory

In watching disease, both in private homes and public hospitals, the thing which strikes the experienced observer most forcefully is this, that the symptoms or the sufferings generally considered to be inevitable and incident to the disease are very often not symptoms of the disease at all, but of something quite different—of the want of fresh air, or light, or of warmth, or of quiet, or of cleanliness, or of punctuality and care in the administration of diet, of each or of all of these.
—FLORENCE NIGHTINGALE, *NOTES ON NURSING* (1860/1969, p. 8)

The Medical Milieu

To gain a better understanding of Nightingale's ideas on nursing, one must enter the particular world of 19th-century medicine and its views on health and disease. Considerable new medical knowledge had been gained by 1800. Gross anatomy was well known; chemistry promised to shed light on various body processes. Vaccination against smallpox existed. There were some established drugs in the pharmacopoeia: cinchona bark, digitalis, and mercury. Certain major diseases, such as leprosy and the bubonic plague, had almost disappeared. The crude death rate in western Europe was falling, largely related to decreasing infant mortality as a result of improvement in hygiene and standard of living (Ackernecht, 1982; Shyrock, 1959).

Yet, in 1800, physicians still had only the vaguest notion of diagnosis. Speculative philosophies continued to dominate medical thought, although inroads continued to be made that eventually gave way to a new outlook on the nature of disease: from belief in general states common to all illnesses to an understanding of disease-specificity symptoms. It was this shift in thought—a paradigm shift of the first order—that gave us the triumph of 20th-century medicine, with all its attendant glories and concurrent sterility.

The 18th century was host to two major traditions or paradigms in the healing arts: one based on "empirics" or "experience," trial and error, with an emphasis on curative remedies; the other based on Hippocratic notions and learning. Evidence of both these trends persisted into the 19th century and can be found in Nightingale's philosophy.

Consistent with the philosophical nature of her superior education (Barritt, 1973), Nightingale, like many of the physicians of her time, continued to emphatically disavow the

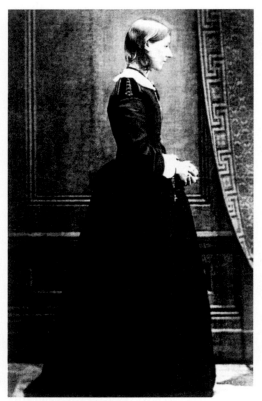

Fig 4 • 4 A rare photograph of Florence taken on her return from the Crimea. Although greatly weakened by her illness, she refused to accept her friends' advice to rest, and pressed on relentlessly with her plans to reform the army medical services. *Source: Huxley (1975), p. 139.*

reality of specific states of disease. She insisted on a view of sickness as an "adjective," not a substantive noun. Sickness was not an "entity" somehow separable from the body. Consistent with her more holistic view, sickness was an aspect or quality of the body as a whole. Some physicians, as she phrased it, taught that diseases were like cats and dogs, distinct species necessarily descended from other cats and dogs. She found such views misleading (Nightingale, 1860/1969).

At this point in time, in the mid-19th century, there were two competing theories regarding the nature and origin of disease. One view was known as "contagionism," postulating that some diseases were communicable, spread via commerce and population migration. A strategic consequence of this explanatory model was *quarantine*, and its attendant bureaucracy aimed at shutting down commerce and trade to keep disease away from noninfected areas. To the new and rapidly emerging merchant classes, quarantine represented government interference and control (Ackernecht, 1982; Arnstein, 1988).

The second school of thought on the nature and origin of disease, of which Nightingale was an ardent champion, was known as "anti-contagionism." It postulated that disease resulted from local environmental sources and arose out of "miasmas"—clouds of rotting filth and matter, activated by a variety of things such as meteorological conditions (note the similarity to elements of water, fire, air, and earth on humors); the filth must be eliminated from *local* areas to prevent the spread of disease. Commerce and "infected" individuals were left alone (Rosenberg, 1979).

William Farr, another Nightingale associate and avid anti-contagionist, was Britain's statistical superintendent of the General Register Office. Farr categorized epidemic and infectious diseases as *zygomatic*, meaning pertaining to or caused by the process of fermentation. The debate as to whether fermentation was a chemical process or a "vitalistic" one had been raging for some time (Swazey & Reed, 1978). The familiarity of the process of fermentation helps to explain its appeal. Anyone who had seen bread rise could immediately grasp

how a minute amount of some contaminating substance could in turn "pollute" the entire atmosphere, the very air that was breathed. What was at issue was the *specificity* of the contaminating substance. Nightingale, and the anti-contagionists, endorsed the position that a "sufficiently intense level of atmospheric contamination could induce both endemic and epidemic ills in the crowded hospital wards [with particular configurations of environmental circumstances determining which]" (Rosenberg, 1979).

Anti-contagionism reached its peak before the political revolutions of 1848; the resulting wave of conservatism and reaction brought contagionism back into dominance, where it remained until its reformulation into the germ theory in the 1870s. Leaders of the contagionists were primarily high-ranking military physicians, politically united. These divergent worldviews accounted in some part for Nightingale's clashes with the military physicians she encountered during the Crimean War.

Given the intellectual and social milieu in which Nightingale was raised and educated, her stance on contagionism seems preordained and logically consistent (Rosenberg, 1979). Likewise, the eclectic religious philosophy she evolved contained attributes of the philosophy of Unitarianism with the fervor of Evangelicalism, all based on an organic view of humans as part of nature. The treatment of disease and dysfunction was inseparable from the nature of man as a whole, and likewise, the environment. And all were linked to God.

The emphasis on "atmosphere" (or "environment") in the Nightingale model is consistent with the views of the "anti-contagionists" of her time. This worldview was reinforced by Nightingale's Crimean experiences, as well as her liberal and progressive political thought. In addition, she viewed all ideas as being distilled through a distinctly *moral* lens (Rosenberg, 1979). As such, Nightingale was typical of a number of her generation's intellectuals. These thinkers struggled to come to grips with an increasingly complex and changing world order and frequently combined a language of two disparate realms of authority: the moral realm and the emerging scientific paradigm that has assumed dominance in the 20th century. Traditional religious and moral assumptions were garbed in a mantle of "scientific objectivity," often spurious at best, but more in keeping with the increasingly rationalized and bureaucratic society accompanying the growth of science.

The Feminist Context of Nightingale's Caring

I have an intellectual nature which requires satisfaction and that would find it in him. I have a passionate nature which requires satisfaction and that would find it in him. I have a moral, an active nature which requires satisfaction and that would not find it in his life.
—FLORENCE NIGHTINGALE, PRIVATE NOTE, 1849, CITED IN WOODHAM-SMITH (1983, p. 51)

Florence Nightingale wrote the following tortured note upon her final refusal of Richard Monckton Milnes's proposal of marriage: "I know I could not bear his life," she wrote, "that to be nailed to a continuation, an exaggeration of my present life without hope of another would be intolerable to me—that voluntarily to put it out of my power ever to be able to seize the chance of forming for myself a true and rich life would seem to be like suicide" (Nightingale, personal note cited in Woodham-Smith, 1983, p. 52). For Miss Nightingale there was no compromise. Marriage and pursuit of her "mission" were not compatible. She chose the mission, a clear repudiation of the mores of her time, which were rooted in the time-honored role of family and "female duty."

The census of 1851 revealed that there were 365,159 "excess women" in England, meaning women who were not married. These women were viewed as redundant, as described in an essay about the census titled "Why Are Women Redundant?" (Widerquist, 1992, p. 52). Many of these women had no acceptable means of support, and Nightingale's development of a suitable occupation for women, that of nursing, was a significant historical development and a major contribution by Nightingale to women's plight in the 19th century. However, in other ways, her views on women and the question of women's rights were quite mixed.

Notes on Nursing: What It Is and What It Is Not (1859/1969) was written not as a manual to teach nurses to nurse but rather to help all women to learn how to nurse.

Nightingale believed all women required this knowledge to take proper care of their families during times of sickness and to promote health—specifically what Nightingale referred to as "the health of houses," that is, the "health" of the environment, which she espoused. Nursing, to her, was clearly situated within the context of female duty.

In *Ordered to Care: The Dilemma of American Nursing*, historian Susan Reverby (1987) traces contemporary conflicts within the nursing profession back to Nightingale herself. She asserts that Nightingale's ideas about female duty and authority, along with her views on disease causality, brought about an independent field—that of nursing—that was separate, and in the view of Nightingale, equal, if not superior, to that of medicine. But this field was dominated by a female hierarchy and insisted on both deference and loyalty to the physician's authority. Reverby (1987) sums it up as follows: "Although Nightingale sought to free women from the bonds of familial demand, in her nursing model she rebound them in a new context." (p. 43)

Does the record support this evidence? Was Nightingale a champion for women's rights or a regressive force? As noted earlier, the answer is far from clear.

The shelter for all moral and spiritual values, threatened by the crass commercialism that was flourishing in the land, as well as the spirit of critical inquiry that accompanied this age of expanding scientific progress, was agreed upon: the home. All considered this to be a "sacred place, a Temple" (Houghton, 1957, p. 343). And who was the head of this home? Woman. Although the Victorian family was patriarchal in nature in that women had virtually no economic and/or legal rights, they nonetheless yielded a major *moral* authority (Arnstein, 1988; Houghton, 1957; Perkins, 1987).

There was hostility on the part of men as well as some women toward women's emancipation. Many intelligent women—for example, Beatrice Webb, George Eliot, and, at times, Nightingale herself—viewed their gender's emancipation with apprehension. In Nightingale's case, the best word might be "ambivalence." There was a fear of weakening women's moral influence, coarsening the feminine nature itself.

This stance is best equated with *cultural feminism,* defined as a belief in inherent gender differences. Women, in contrast to men, are viewed as morally superior, the holders of family values and continuity; they are refined, delicate, and in need of protection. This school of thought, important in the 19th century, used arguments for women's suffrage such as the following: "[W]omen must make themselves felt in the public sphere because their *moral* perspective would improve corrupt masculine politics." In the case of Nightingale, these cultural feminist attitudes "made her impatient with the idea of women seeking rights and activities just because men valued these entities" (Bunting & Campbell, 1990, p. 21).

Nightingale had chafed at the limitations and restrictions placed on women, especially "wealthy" women with nothing to do: "What these [women] suffer—even physically—from the want of such work no one can tell. The accumulation of nervous energy, which has had nothing to do during the day, makes them feel every night, when they go to bed, as if they were going mad." Despite these vivid words, authored by Nightingale (1852/1979) in the fiery polemic "Cassandra," which was used as a rallying cry in many feminist circles, her view of the solution was measured. Her own resolution, painfully arrived at, was to break from her family and actualize her caring mission, that of nurse. One of the many results of this was that a useful occupation for other women to pursue was founded. Although Nightingale approved of this occupation outside of the home for other women, certain other occupations—that of doctor, for example—she

viewed with hostility and as inappropriate for women. Why should these women not be nurses or nurse midwives, a far superior calling in Nightingale's view than that of a medicine "man" (Monteiro, 1984)?

Welch (1990) termed Nightingale a "Christian feminist" on the eve of her departure to the Crimea. She returned even more skeptical of women. Writing to her close friend Mary Clarke Mohl, she described women whom she worked with in the Crimea as being incompetent and incapable of independent thought (Welch, 1990; Woodham-Smith, 1983). According to Palmer (1977), by this time in her life, the concerns of the British people and the demands of service to God took precedence over any concern she had ever had about women's rights.

In other words, Nightingale, despite the clear freedom in which she lived her own life, nonetheless genderized the nursing role, leaving it rooted in 19th-century morality. Nightingale is seen constantly trying to improve the existing order and to work within that order; she was above all a reformer, seeking to improve the existing order, not to change the terrain radically.

In Nightingale's mind, the specific "scientific" activity of nursing—hygiene—was the central element in health care, without which medicine and surgery would be ineffective:

The Life and Death, recovery or invaliding of patients generally depends not on any great and isolated act, but on the unremitting and thorough performance of every minute's practical duty. (Nightingale, 1860/1969)

This "practical duty" was the work of women, and the conception of the proper division of labor resting on work demands internal to each respective "science," nursing and medicine, obscured the professional inequality. The later successes of medical science heightened this inequity. The scientific grounding espoused by Nightingale for nursing was ephemeral at best, as later 19th-century discoveries proved much of her analysis wrong, although nonetheless powerful. Much of her strength was in her rhetoric; if not always logically consistent, it certainly was morally resonant (Rosenberg, 1979).

Despite exceptional anomalies, such as women physicians, what Nightingale effectively accomplished was a genderization of the division of labor in health care: male physicians and female nurses. This appears to be a division that Nightingale supported. Because this "natural" division of labor was rooted in the family, women's work outside the home ought to resemble domestic tasks and complement the "male principle" with the "female." Thus, nursing was left on the shifting sands of a soon-outmoded "science"; the main focus of its authority grounded in an equally shaky moral sphere, also subject to change and devaluation in an increasingly secularized, rationalized, and technological 20th century.

Nightingale failed to provide institutionalized nursing with an autonomous future, on an equal parity with medicine. She did, however, succeed in providing women's work in the public sphere, establishing for numerous women an identity and source of employment. Although that public identity grew out of women's domestic and nurturing roles in the family, the conditions of a modern society required public as well as private forms of care. It is questionable whether more could have been achieved at that point in time (King, 1988).

A woman, Queen Victoria, presided over the age: "Ironically, Queen Victoria, that panoply of family happiness and stubborn adversary of female independence, could not help but shed her aura upon single women." The queen's early and lengthy widowhood, her "relentlessly spreading figure and commensurately increasing empire, her obstinate longevity which engorged generations of men and the collective shocks of history, lent an epic quality to the lives of solitary women" (Auerbach, 1982, pp. 120–121). Both Nightingale and the queen saw themselves as working through men, yet their lives added new, unexpected, and powerful dimensions to the myth of Victorian womanhood, particularly that of a woman alone and in command (Auerbach, 1982, pp. 120–121).

Nightingale's clearly chosen spinsterhood repudiated the Victorian family. Her unmarried life provides a vision of a powerful life lived on her own terms. This is not the spinsterhood of convention—one to be pitied, one of broken hearts—but a *radically* new image. She is freed from the trivia of family complaints and scorns the feminist collectivity; yet in this seemingly solitary life, she finds union not with one man but with all men, personified by the British soldier.

Lytton Strachey's well-known evocation of Nightingale, iconoclastic and bold, is perhaps closest to the decidedly masculine imagery she selected to describe herself, as evidenced in this imaginary speech to her mother written in 1852:

> Well, my dear, you don't imagine with my "talents," and my "European reputation" and my "beautiful letters" and all that, I'm going to stay dangling around my mother's drawing room all my life! . . . [Y]ou must look upon me as your vagabond son . . . I shan't cost you nearly as much as a son would have done, or had I married. You must consider me married or a son. (Woodham-Smith, 1983, p. 66)

Ideas About Nursing

Every day sanitary knowledge, or the knowledge of nursing, or in other words, of how to put the constitution in such a state as that it will have no disease, or that it can recover from disease, takes a higher place.
—FLORENCE NIGHTINGALE, NOTES ON NURSING (1860/1969), PREFACE

Evelyn R. Barritt, professor of nursing and Nightingale scholar, suggested that nursing became a science when Nightingale identified the laws of nursing, also referred to as the laws of health, or nature (Barritt, 1973; Nightingale, 1860/1969). The remainder of all nursing theory may be viewed as mere branches and "acorns," all fruit of the roots of Nightingale's ideas. Early writings of Nightingale, compiled in *Notes on Nursing: What It Is and What It Is Not* (1860/1969), provided the earliest systematic perspective for defining nursing. According to Nightingale, analysis and application of universal "laws" would promote well-being and relieve the suffering of humanity. This was the goal of nursing.

As noted by the caring theorist Madeline Leininger, Nightingale never defined human care or caring in Nightingale's *Notes on Nursing* (1859/1992, p. 31), and she goes on to wonder if Nightingale considered "components of care such as comfort, support, nurturance, and many other care constructs and characteristics and how they would influence the reparative process." Although Nightingale's conceptualizations of nursing, hygiene, the laws of health, and the environment never explicitly identify the construct of caring, an underlying ethos of care and commitment to others echoes in her words and, most importantly, resides in her actions and the drama of her life.

Nightingale did not theorize in the way to which we are accustomed today. Patricia Winstead-Fry (1993), in a review of the 1992 commemorative edition of Nightingale's *Notes on Nursing* (1859/1992, p. 161), states: "Given that theory is the interrelationship of concepts which form a system of propositions that can be tested and used for predicting practice, Nightingale was not a theorist. None of her major biographers present her as a theorist. She was a consummate politician and health care reformer." And our emerging 21st century has never been more in need of nurses who *are* consummate politicians and health-care reformers. Her words and ideas, contextualized in the earlier portion of this chapter, ring differently than those of the other nursing theorists you will study in this book. However, her underlying ideas continue to be relevant and, some would argue, prescient.

Lynn McDonald, Canadian professor of sociology and editor of the *Collected Works of Florence Nightingale,* a 16-volume collection, places Nightingale among the most prominent "Women Methodologists" identified in *The Women Founders of the Social Sciences*

(McDonald, 1994). McDonald notes that Nightingale was firmly committed to "a determined, probabilistic social science" and goes on to state that "Indeed, she [Nightingale] described the laws of social science as God's laws for the right operation of the world" (p. 186). Nightingale was convinced of the necessity for evaluative statistics to underpin rational approaches to public administrations. Consistently she used the presentation of statistical data to prove her case that the costs of disease, crime, and excess mortality was greater than the cost of sanitary improvements. In later life, Nightingale endeavored to establish a chair or readership at Oxford University to teach Quetelet's statistical approaches and probability theory. In today's world, this would translate to a commitment to evidence-based practice as justification for nursing's value.

Karen Dennis and Patricia Prescott (1985) noted that including Nightingale among the nurse theorists has been a recent development. They make the case that nurses today continue to incorporate in their practice the insight, foresight, and, most important, the clinical acumen of Nightingale's more than century and a half vision of nursing. As part of a larger study, they collected a large base of descriptions from both nurses and physicians describing "good" nursing practice. More than 300 individual interviews were subjected to content analysis; categories were named inductively and validated separately by four members of the project staff.

Noting no marked differences in the descriptions obtained from either the nurses or physicians, the authors report that despite their independent derivation, the categories that emerged during the study bore a striking resemblance to nursing practice as described by Nightingale: prevention of illness and promotion of health, observation of the sick, and attention to the physical environment. Also referred to by Nightingale as the "health of houses," this physical environment included ventilation of both the patient's rooms and the larger environment of the "house": light, cleanliness, and the taking of food; attention to the interpersonal milieu, which included variety; and not indulging in superficialities with the sick or giving them false encouragement.

The authors noted that "the words change but the concepts do not" (Dennis & Prescott, 1985, p. 80). In keeping with the tradition established by Nightingale, they noted that nurses continue to foster an interpersonal milieu that focuses on the person while manipulating and mediating the environment to "put the patient in the best condition for nature to act upon him" (Nightingale, 1860/1969, p. 133).

Afaf I. Meleis (1997), nurse scholar, does not compare Nightingale to contemporary nurse theorists; nonetheless, she refers to her frequently. Meleis stated that it was Nightingale's conceptualization of environment as the focus of nursing activity and her de-emphasis of pathology, emphasizing instead the "laws of health" (which she said were yet to be identified), that were the earliest differentiation of nursing and medicine. Meleis (1997, pp. 114–116) described Nightingale's concept of nursing as including "the proper use of fresh air, light, warmth, cleanliness, quiet, and the proper selection and administration of diet, all with the least expense of vital power to the patient." These ideas clearly had evolved from Nightingale's observations and experiences. The art of observation was identified as an important nursing function in the Nightingale model. And this observation was what should form the basis for nursing ideas. Meleis speculates on how differently the theoretical base of nursing might have evolved if we had continued to consider extant nursing practice as a source of ideas.

Pamela Reed and Tamara Zurakowski (1983/1989, p. 33) called the Nightingale model "visionary." They stated: "At the core of all theory development activities in nursing today is the tradition of Florence Nightingale." They also suggest four major factors that influenced her model of nursing: religion, science, war, and feminism, all of which are discussed in this chapter.

The following assumptions were identified by Victoria Fondriest and Joan Osborne (1994).

Nightingale's Assumptions

1. Nursing is separate from medicine.
2. Nurses should be trained.
3. The environment is important to the health of the patient.
4. The disease process is not important to nursing.
5. Nursing should support the environment to assist the patient in healing.
6. Research should be used through observation and empirics to define the nursing discipline.
7. Nursing is both an empirical science and an art.
8. Nursing's concern is with the person in the environment.
9. The person is interacting with the environment.
10. Sickness and wellness are governed by the same laws of health.
11. The nurse should be observant and confidential.

The goal of *nursing* as described by Nightingale is assisting the patient in his or her retention of "vital powers" by meeting his or her needs, and thus, putting the patient in the best condition for nature to act upon (Nightingale, 1860/1969). This must not be interpreted as a "passive state" but rather one that reflects the patient's capacity for self-healing facilitated by nurses' ability to create an environment conducive to health. The focus of this nursing activity was the proper use of fresh air, light, warmth, cleanliness, quiet, proper selection and administration of diet, monitoring the patient's expenditure of energy, and observing. This activity was directed toward the environment and the patient (see Nightingale's Assumptions).

Health was viewed as an additive process—the result of environmental, physical, and psychological factors, not just the absence of disease. Disease was the reparative process of the body to correct a problem and could provide an opportunity for spiritual growth. The laws of health, as defined by Nightingale, were those to do with keeping the person, and the population, healthy. They were dependent on proper environmental control, for example, sanitation. The environment was what the nurse manipulated; it included the physical elements external to the patient.

Nightingale isolated five environmental components essential to an individual's health: clean air, pure water, efficient drainage, cleanliness, and light.

The patient is at the center of the Nightingale model, which incorporates a holistic view of the person as someone with psychological, intellectual, and spiritual components. This is evidenced in her acknowledgment of the importance of "variety." For example, she wrote of "the degree . . . to which the nerves of the sick suffer from seeing the same walls, the same ceiling, the same surroundings" (Nightingale, 1860/1969). Likewise, her chapter on "chattering hopes and advice" illustrates an astute grasp of human nature and of interpersonal relationships. She remarked on the spiritual component of disease and illness, and she felt they could present an opportunity for spiritual growth. In this, all persons were viewed as equal.

A *nurse* was defined as any woman who had "charge of the personal health of somebody," whether well, as in caring for babies and children, or sick, as an "invalid" (Nightingale, 1860/1969). It was assumed that all women, at one time or another in their lives, would nurse. Thus, all women needed to know the laws of health. Nursing proper, or "sick" nursing, was both an art and a science and required organized, formal education to care for those suffering from disease. Above all, nursing was "service to God in relief of man"; it was a "calling" and "God's work" (Barritt, 1973). Nursing activities served as an "art form" through which spiritual development might occur (Reed & Zurakowski, 1983/1989). All nursing actions were guided by the nurses' *caring*, which was guided by underlying ideas about God.

Consistent with this caring base is Nightingale's views on *nursing as an art and a science*. Again, this was a reflection of the marriage, essential to Nightingale's underlying worldview, of science and spirituality. On the surface, these might appear to be odd bedfellows; however, this marriage flows directly from Nightingale's underlying religious and philosophic views, which were operationalized in her nursing practice. Nightingale was an empiricist, valuing the "science" of observation with the intent of using that knowledge to better the life of humankind. The application of that knowledge required an artist's skill, far greater than that of the painter or sculptor:

Nursing is an art; and if it is to be made an art, it requires as exclusive a devotion, as hard a preparation, as any painter's or sculptor's work; for what is the having to do with dead canvas or cold marble, compared with having to do with the living body—the Temple of God's spirit? It is one of the Fine Arts; I had almost said, the finest of the Fine Arts. (Florence Nightingale, cited in Donahue, 1985, p. 469)

Nightingale's ideas about nursing health, the environment, and the person were grounded in experience; she regarded one's sense observations as the only reliable means of obtaining and verifying knowledge. Theory must be reformulated if inconsistent with empirical evidence. This experiential knowledge was then to be transformed into empirically based generalizations, an inductive process, to arrive at, for example, the laws of health. Regardless of Nightingale's commitment to empiricism and experiential knowledge, her early education and religious experience also shaped this emerging knowledge (Hektor, 1992).

According to Nightingale's model, nursing contributes to the ability of persons to maintain and restore health directly or indirectly through managing the environment. The person has a key role in his or her own health, and this health is a function of the interaction among person, nurse, and environment. However, neither the person nor the environment is discussed as influencing the nurse (Fig. 4-5).

Although it is difficult to describe the interrelationship of the concepts in the Nightingale model, Figure 4-6 is a schema that attempts to delineate this. Note the prominence of

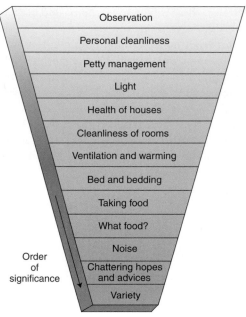

Fig 4 • 5 Perspective on Nightingale's 13 canons. *Illustration developed by V. Fondriest, RN, BSN, and J. Osborne, RN, C BSN in October 1994.*

"observation" on the outer circle (important to all nursing functions) and the interrelationship of the specifics of the interventions, such as "bed and bedding" and "cleanliness of rooms and walls," that go into making up the "health of houses" (Fondriest & Osborne, 1994).

Nightingale's Legacy for 21st Century Nursing Practice

Philip Kalisch and Beatrice Kalisch (1987, p. 26) described the popular and glorified images that arose out of the portrayals of Florence Nightingale during and after the Crimean War—that of nurse as self-sacrificing, refined, virginal, and an "angel of mercy," a far less threatening image than one of educated and skilled professional nurses. They attribute nurses' low pay to the perception of nursing as a "calling," a way of life for devoted women with private means, such as Florence Nightingale (Kalisch & Kalisch, 1987, p. 20). Well over

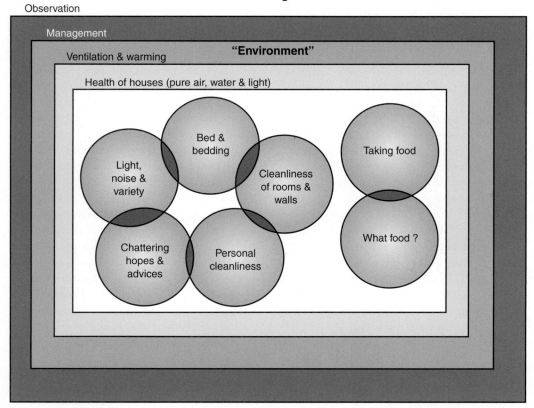

Fig 4 • 6 Nightingale's model of nursing and the environment. *Illustration developed by V. Fondriest, RN, BSN, and J. Osborne, RN, C BSN.*

100 years later, the amount of scholarship on Nightingale provides a more realistic portrait of a complex and brilliant woman. To quote Auerbach (1982) and Strachey (1918), she was "a demon, a rebel."

Florence Nightingale's legacy of caring and the activism it implies is carried on in nursing today. There is a resurgence and inclusion of concepts of spirituality in current nursing practice and a delineation of nursing's caring base that in essence began with the nursing life of Florence Nightingale. Nightingale's caring, as demonstrated in this chapter, extended beyond the individual patient, beyond the individual person. She herself said that the specific business of nursing was the least important of the functions into which she had been forced in the Crimea. Her caring encompassed a broadened sphere—that of the British Army and, indeed, the entire British Commonwealth.

Themes in contemporary nursing practice focusing on evidence-based practice and curricula championing cultures of safety and quality are all found in the life and works of Florence Nightingale. I would venture to say that almost all contemporary nursing practice settings echo some aspect of the ideas—and ideals—of Nightingale. Themes of Nightingale, the environmentalist, are critical to nursing practice for the individual, the community, and global health. An exemplar of practice personifying Nightingale's approach and practice would be a larger-than-life nurse hero or heroine championing current health-care reform by designing health-care systems that are truly responsive to the needs of the populace and that extend cross-culturally and globally.

■ Summary

The unique aspects of Florence Nightingale's personality and social position, combined with historical circumstances, laid the groundwork for the evolution of the modern discipline of nursing. Are the challenges and obstacles that we face today any more daunting than what confronted Nightingale when she arrived in the Crimea in 1854? Nursing for Florence Nightingale was what we might call today her "centering force." It allowed her to express her spiritual values as well as enabled her to fulfill her needs for leadership and authority. As historian Susan Reverby noted, today we are challenged with the dilemma of how to practice our integral values of caring in an unjust health-care system that does not value caring. Let us look again to Florence Nightingale for inspiration, for she remains a role model par excellence on the transformation of values of caring into an *activism* that could potentially transform our current health-care system into a more humanistic and *just* one. Her activism situates her in the context of justice making. *Justice making* is understood as a manifestation of compassion and caring, for it is actions that bring about justice (Boykin & Dunphy, 2002, p. 16). Florence Nightingale's legacy of connecting caring with activism can then truly be said to continue.

References

Ackernecht, E. (1982). *A short history of medicine.* Baltimore: Johns Hopkins University Press.

Arnstein, W. (1988). *Britain: Yesterday and today.* Lexington, MA: Heath.

Auerbach, N. (1982). *Women and the demon: The life of a Victorian myth.* Cambridge, MA: Harvard University Press.

Barritt, E. R. (1973). Florence Nightingale's values and modern nursing education. *Nursing Forum, 12,* 7–47.

Boykin, A., & Dunphy, L. M. (2002). Justice-making: Nursing's call. *Policy, Politics, & Nursing Practice, 3,* 14–19.

Bunting, S., & Campbell, J. (1990). Feminism and nursing: An historical perspective. *Advances in Nursing Science, 12,* 11–24.

Calabria, M., & Macrae, J. (Eds.). (1994). *Suggestions for thought by Florence Nightingale: Selections and commentaries.* Philadelphia: University of Pennsylvania Press.

Cohen, I. B. (1981). Florence Nightingale: The passionate statistician. *Scientific American, 250*(3), 128–137.

Cook, E. T. (1913). *The life of Florence Nightingale* (vols. 1–2). London: Macmillan.

Cromwell, Judith Lissauer (2013). *Florence Nightingale, Feminist.* London: McFarland & Co., Inc., Publishers.

Dennis, K. E., & Prescott, P. A. (1985). Florence Nightingale: Yesterday, today and tomorrow. *Advances in Nursing Science, 7*(2), 66–81.

Dolan, J. (1971). *The grace of the great lady.* Chicago: Medical Heritage Society.

Donahue, P. (1985). *Nursing: The finest art.* St. Louis, MO: Mosby.

Dossey, B. (1998). Florence Nightingale: A 19th century mystic. *Journal of Holistic Nursing, 16*(2), 111–164.

Fondriest, V., & Osborne, J. (1994). A theorist before her time? Presentation, NGR Nursing Graduate Course 5110, Nursing Theory and Advanced Practice Nursing, School of Nursing, Florida International University, North Miami, FL.

Goldie, S. (1987). *I have done my duty: Florence Nightingale in the Crimean War, 1854–1856.* Iowa City: University of Iowa Press.

Gourley, J. (2003). *Florence Nightingale and the health of the Raj.* Cornwall, England: MPG Books.

Hektor, L. M. (1992). *Nursing, science, and gender: Florence Nightingale and Martha E. Rogers.* Unpublished doctoral dissertation, University of Miami.

Houghton, W. (1957). *The Victorian frame of mind.* New Haven, CT: Yale University Press.

Huxley, E. (1975). *Florence Nightingale.* New York: Putnam.

Kalisch, P. A., & Kalisch, B. J. (1987). *The changing image of the nurse.* Menlo Park, CA: Addison-Wesley.

King, M. G. (1988). Gender: A hidden issue in nursing's professionalizing reform movement. Boston: Boston University School of Nursing. In *Strategies for Theory Development V,* March 10–12.

Macrae, J. (1995). Nightingale's spiritual philosophy and its significance for modern nursing. *Image: Journal of Nursing Scholarship, 27,* 8–10.

McDonald, L. (1994). *The women founders of the social sciences.* Quebec, Canada: Carleton University Press.

McDonald, L. (Ed.). (2002–2012). *The collected works of Florence Nightingale Series* (Vols. 1-3, 5-7, 11-16). Ontario, Canada: Wilfrid Laurier University Press.

Meleis, A. I. (1997). *Theoretical nursing: Development and progress* (3rd ed.). Philadelphia: Lippincott.

Monteiro, L. (1984). On separate roads: Florence Nightingale and Elizabeth Blackwell. *Signs: Journal of Women in Culture & Society, 9,* 520–533.

Nightingale, F. (1852/1979). *Cassandra,* with an introduction by Myra Stark. Westbury, NY: Feminist Press.

Nightingale, F. (1859/1992). *Notes on nursing: Commemorative edition with commentaries by contemporary nursing leaders.* Philadelphia: J. B. Lippincott.

Nightingale, F. (1860). *Suggestions for thought to searchers after religious truths* (vols. 2–3). London: George E. Eyre & William Spottiswoode.

Nightingale, F. (1860/1969). *Notes on nursing: What it is and what it is not.* New York: Dover.

Palmer, I. S. (1977). Florence Nightingale: Reformer, reactionary, research. *Nursing Research, 26,* 84–89.

Perkins, J. (1987). *Women and marriage in nineteenth century England.* Chicago: Lyceum Books.

Reed, P. G., & Zurakowski, T. L. (1983/1989). Nightingale: A visionary model for nursing. In J. Fitzpatrick & A. Whall (Eds.), *Conceptual models of nursing: Analysis and application.* Bowie, MD: Robert J. Brady.

Reverby, S. M. (1987). *Ordered to care: The dilemma of American nursing (1865–1945).* New York: Cambridge University Press.

Rosenberg, C. (1979). *Healing and history.* New York: Science History Publications.

Sattin, A. (Ed.). (1987). *Florence Nightingale's letters from Egypt: A journey on the Nile, 1849–1850.* New York: Weidenfeld & Nicolson.

Shyrock, R. (1959). *The history of nursing.* Philadelphia: Saunders.

Slater, V. E. (1994). The educational and philosophical influences on Florence Nightingale, an enlightened conductor. *Nursing History Review, 2,* 137–152.

Strachey, L. (1918). *Eminent Victorians: Cardinal Manning, Florence Nightingale, Dr. Arnold, General Gordon.* London: Chatto & Windus.

Summers, A. (1988). *Angels and citizens: British women as military nurses, 1854–1914.* London: Routledge & Kegan Paul.

Swazey, J., & Reed, K. (1978). Louis Pasteur: Science and the application of science. In J. Swazey & K. Reed (Eds.), *Today's medicine, tomorrow's science* (DHEW Pub. No. NIH 78–244). Washington, DC: U.S. Government Printing Office.

Valle, G. (Ed.). (2003–2007). *The collected works of Florence Nightingale Series* (Vols. 4, 9-10). Ontario, Canada: Wilfrid Laurier University Press.

Vicinus, M., & Nergaard, B. (Eds.). (1990). *Ever yours, Florence Nightingale: Selected letters.* Cambridge, MA: Harvard University Press.

Watson, J. (1992). Commentary. In *Notes on nursing: What it is and what it is not* (pp. 80–85). Commemorative edition. Philadelphia: Lippincott.

Welch, M. (1986). Nineteenth-century philosophic influences on Nightingale's concept of the person. *Journal of Nursing History, 1*(2), 3–11.

Welch, M. (1990). Florence Nightingale: The social construction of a Victorian feminist. *Western Journal of Nursing Research, 12,* 404–407.

Widerquist, J. G. (1992). The spirituality of Florence Nightingale. *Nursing Research, 41,* 49–55.

Winstead-Fry, P. (1993). Book review: *Notes on nursing: What it is and what it is not.* Commemorative edition. *Nursing Science Quarterly, 6*(3), 161–162.

Woodham-Smith, C. (1951). *Florence Nightingale.* New York: McGraw-Hill Book Company

Early Conceptualizations About Nursing

Ernestine Wiedenbach, Virginia Henderson, and Lydia Hall

Shirley C. Gordon

Introducing the Theorists
Overview of Wiedenbach, Henderson, and Hall's Conceptualizations of Nursing
Practice Applications
Practice Exemplars
Summary
References

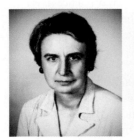

Ernestine Wiederbach

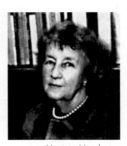

Virginia Henderson

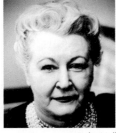

Lydia Hall

Introducing the Theorists

Ernestine Wiedenbach, Virginia Henderson, and Lydia Hall are three of the most important influences on nursing theory development of the 20th century. Indeed, their work continues to ground nursing thought in the new century. The work of each of these nurse scholars was based on nursing practice, and today some of this work might be referred to as *practice theories*. Concepts and terms they first used are heard today around the globe.

This chapter provides a brief introduction to Wiedenbach, Henderson, and Hall; an overview of their nursing conceptualizations; and sections on practice applications and practice exemplars based on their published works. The content of this chapter is partially based on work from scholars who have studied or worked with these theorists and who wrote chapters for the first, second and/or third editions of *Nursing Theories and Nursing Practice* (Gesse, Dombro, Gordon, & Rittman, 2006, 2010; Gordon, 2001; Touhy & Birnbach, 2006, 2010).[1]

Ernestine Wiedenbach

Wiedenbach was born in 1900 in Germany to an American mother and a German father, who immigrated to the United States when Ernestine was a child. She received a bachelor of arts degree from Wellesley College in 1922 and graduated from Johns Hopkins School of Nursing in 1925 (Nickel, Gesse, & MacLaren,

[1]For additional information please see the bonus chapter content available at http://davisplus.fadavis.com.

1992). After completing a master of arts at Columbia University in 1934, she became a professional writer for the *American Journal of Nursing* and played a critical role in the recruitment of nursing students and military nurses during World War II. At age 45, she began her studies in nurse-midwifery. Wiedenbach's roles as practitioner, teacher, author, and theorist were consolidated as a member of the Yale University School of Nursing, where Yale colleagues William Dickoff and Patricia James encouraged her development of prescriptive theory (Dickoff, James, & Wiedenbach, 1968). Even after her retirement in 1966, she and her lifelong friend Caroline Falls offered informal seminars in Miami, always reminding students and faculty of the need for clarity of purpose, based on reality. She even continued to use her gift for writing to transcribe books for the blind, including a Lamaze childbirth manual, which she prepared on her Braille typewriter. Ernestine Wiedenbach died in April 1998 at age 98.

Virginia Henderson

Born in Kansas City, Missouri, in 1897, Virginia Avenel Henderson was the fifth of eight children. With two of her brothers serving in the armed forces during World War I and in anticipation of a critical shortage of nurses, Virginia Henderson entered the Army School of Nursing at Walter Reed Army Hospital. It was there that she began to question the regimentation of patient care and the concept of nursing as ancillary to medicine (Henderson, 1991).

As a member of society during a war, Henderson considered it a privilege to care for sick and wounded soldiers (Henderson, 1960). This wartime experience forever influenced her ethical understanding of nursing and her appreciation of the importance and complexity of the nurse–patient relationship.

After a summer spent with the Henry Street Visiting Nurse Agency in New York City, Henderson began to appreciate the importance of getting to know the patients and their environments. She enjoyed the less formal visiting nurse approach to patient care and became skeptical of the ability of hospital regimes to alter patients' unhealthy ways of living upon returning home (Henderson, 1991). She entered Teachers

College at Columbia University, earning her baccalaureate degree in 1932 and her master's degree in 1934. She continued at Teachers College as an instructor and associate professor of nursing for the next 20 years.

Virginia Henderson presented her definition of the nature of nursing in an era when few nurses had ventured into describing the complex phenomena of modern nursing. Henderson wrote about nursing the way she lived it: focusing on what nurses do, how nurses function, and nursing's unique role in health care. Henderson has been heralded as the greatest advocate for nursing libraries worldwide. Of all her contributions to nursing, Virginia Henderson's work on the identification and control of nursing literature is perhaps her greatest. In the 1950s, there was an increasing interest on the part of the profession to establish a research basis for the nursing practice. After the completion of her revised text in 1955, Henderson moved to Yale University and began what would become a distinguished career in library science research. In 1990, the Sigma Theta Tau International Library was named in her honor.

Lydia Hall

Lydia Hall, born in 1906, was a visionary, risk taker, and consummate professional. She inspired commitment and dedication through her unique conceptual framework.

A 1927 graduate of the York Hospital School of Nursing in Pennsylvania, Hall held various nursing positions during the early years of her career. In the mid-1930s, she enrolled at Teachers College, Columbia University, where she earned a Bachelor of Science degree in 1937, and a Master of Arts degree in 1942. She worked with the Visiting Nurse Service of New York from 1941 to 1947 and was a member of the nursing faculty at Fordham Hospital School of Nursing from 1947 to 1950. Hall was subsequently appointed to a faculty position at Teachers College, where she developed and implemented a program in nursing consultation and joined a community of nurse leaders. At the same time, she was involved in research activities for the U.S. Public Health Service (Birnbach, 1988).

Hall's most significant contribution to nursing practice was the practice model she designed and put into place in the Loeb Center for Nursing and Rehabilitation at Montefiore Medical Center in Bronx, New York. The Loeb Center, which opened in 1963, was the culmination of 5 years of planning and construction under Hall's direction in collaboration with Dr. Martin Cherkasky.

As a visiting nurse, Hall had frequent contact through the Montefiore home care program. Hall and Cherkasky discovered they shared similar philosophies regarding health care and the delivery of quality service (Birnbach, 1988). In 1950, Cherkasky was appointed director of the Montefiore Medical Center. Convalescent treatment was undergoing rapid change owing largely to medical advances, new pharmaceuticals, and technological developments. The emerging trends led to the closing of the Solomon and Betty Loeb Memorial Home in Westchester County, New York, and Cherkasky and Hall convinced the board to join with Montefiore in founding the Loeb Center for Nursing and Rehabilitation. A unique feature of the center was a separate board of trustees that interrelated with the Montefiore board. As a result, Hall had considerable autonomy in developing the center's policies and procedures.

Hall increased the role of nurses in decision making. For example, nurses selected patients for the Loeb Center based on a nursing assessment of an individual patient's potential for rehabilitation. In addition, qualified professional nurses provided direct care to patients and coordinated needed services. Hall frequently described the center as "a halfway house on the road home" (Hall, 1963, p. 2), where the nurse worked with the patients as active participants in achieving desired outcomes that were meaningful to the patients. Over time, the effectiveness of Hall's practice model was validated by the significant decline in the number of readmissions among former Loeb patients compared with those who received other types of posthospital care ("Montefiore cuts," 1966).

Hall died in 1969, and in 1984 she was posthumously inducted into the American Nurses' Association Hall of Fame. Hall is remembered by her colleagues as a force for change; she successfully implemented a professional patient-centered framework at a time when task-oriented team nursing was the preferred practice model in most institutions.

Overview of Wiedenbach, Henderson, and Hall's Conceptualizations of Nursing

Virginia Henderson, sometimes known as the modern-day Florence Nightingale, developed the definition of nursing that is most well known internationally. Ernestine Wiedenbach gave us new ways to think about nursing practice and nursing scholarship, introducing us to the ideas of (1) nursing as a professional practice discipline and (2) nursing practice theory. Lydia Hall challenged us to think conceptually about the key role of professional nursing. Each of these nurse scholars helped us focus on the patient, instead of on the tasks to be done, and to plan care to meet needs of the person. Each emphasized caring based on the perspective of the individual being cared for—through observing, communicating, designing, and reporting. Each was concerned with the unique aspects of nursing practice and scholarship and with the essential question of "What is nursing?"

Wiedenbach's Conceptualizations of Nursing

Initial work on Wiedenbach's prescriptive theory is presented in her article in the *American Journal of Nursing* (1963) and her book *Meeting the Realities in Clinical Teaching* (1969).

Her explanation of prescriptive theory is that **"Account must be taken of the motivating factors that influence the nurse not only in doing what she [*sic*] does, but also in doing it the way she [*sic*] does it with the realities that exist in the situation in which she [*sic*] is functioning"** (Wiedenbach, 1970, p. 2). Three ingredients essential to the prescriptive theory are as follows:

1. The nurse's central purpose in nursing is the nurse's professional commitment. *For Wiedenbach, the central purpose in nursing is to motivate the individual and/or facilitate efforts to overcome the obstacles that may interfere with the ability to respond capably*

to the demands made by the realities within the situation (Wiedenbach, 1970, p. 4). She emphasized that the nurse's goals are grounded in the nurse's philosophy, "those beliefs and values that shape her [sic] attitude toward life, toward fellow human beings and toward herself [sic]." The three concepts that epitomize the essence of such a philosophy are (1) reverence for the gift of life; (2) respect for the dignity, autonomy, worth, and individuality of each human being; and (3) resolution to act dynamically in relation to one's beliefs (Wiedenbach, 1970, p. 4).

She recognized that nurses have different values and various commitments to nursing and that to formulate one's purpose in nursing is a "soul-searching experience." She encouraged each nurse to undergo this experience and be "willing and ready to present your central purpose in nursing for examination and discussion when appropriate" (Wiedenbach, 1970, p. 5).

2. The prescription indicates the broad general action that the nurse deems appropriate to fulfillment of his or her central purpose. *The nurse will have thought through the kind of results to be sought and will take action to obtain these results, accepting accountability for what he/she does and for the outcomes of any action. Nursing action, then, is deliberate action that is mutually understood and agreed on and that is both patient-directed and nurse-directed (Wiedenbach, 1970, p. 5).*

3. The realities are the aspects of the immediate nursing situation that influence the results the nurse achieves through what he or she does (Wiedenbach, 1970, p. 3). *These include the physical, psychological, emotional, and spiritual factors in which nursing action occurs. Within the situation are these components:*

- The agent, who is the nurse supplying the nursing action
- The recipient, or the patient receiving this action or on whose behalf the action is taken
- The framework, comprising situational factors that affect the nurse's ability to achieve nursing results

- The goal, or the end to be attained through nursing activity on behalf of the patient
- The means, the actions and devices through which the nurse is enabled to reach the goal

Henderson's Definition of Nursing and Components of Basic Nursing Care

While working on the 1955 revision of the *Textbook of the Principles and Practice of Nursing*, Henderson focused on the need to be clear about the function of nurses. She opened the first chapter with the following questions: What is nursing and what is the function of the nurse? (Harmer & Henderson, 1955, p. 1). Henderson believed these questions were fundamental to anyone choosing to pursue the study and practice of nursing.

Definition of Nursing

Henderson's often-quoted definition of nursing first appeared in the fifth edition of *Textbook of the Principles and Practice of Nursing* (Harmer & Henderson, 1955, p. 4):

Nursing is primarily assisting the individual (sick or well) in the performance of those activities contributing to health or its recovery (or to a peaceful death), that he [sic] would perform unaided if he [sic] had the necessary strength, will, or knowledge. It is likewise the unique contribution of nursing to help people be independent of such assistance as soon as possible.

In presenting her definition of nursing, Henderson hoped to encourage others to develop their own working concept of nursing and nursing's unique function in society. She believed the definitions of the day were too general and failed to differentiate nurses from other members of the health team, which led to the following questions: "What is nursing that is not also medicine, physical therapy, social work, etc.?" and "What is the unique function of the nurse?" (Harmer & Henderson, 1955, p. 4).

Based on her definition and after coining the term *basic nursing care*, Henderson identified 14 components of basic nursing care that reflect needs pertaining to personal hygiene and healthful living, including helping the patient carry out the physician's therapeutic plan (Henderson, 1960; 1966, pp. 16–17):

1. Breathe normally.
2. Eat and drink adequately.
3. Eliminate bodily wastes.
4. Move and maintain desirable postures.
5. Sleep and rest.
6. Select suitable clothes—dress and undress.
7. Maintain body temperature within normal range by adjusting clothing and modifying the environment.
8. Keep the body clean and well groomed and protect the integument.
9. Avoid dangers in the environment and avoid injuring others.
10. Communicate with others in expressing emotions, needs, fears, or opinions.
11. Worship according to one's faith.
12. Work in such a way that there is a sense of accomplishment.
13. Play or participate in various forms of recreation.
14. Learn, discover, or satisfy the curiosity that leads to normal development and health and use the available health facilities.

Hall's Care, Cure, and Core Model

Hall enumerated three aspects of the person as patient: the person, the body, and the disease (Hall, 1965). She envisioned these aspects as overlapping circles of care, core, and cure that influence each other. It was her belief that

> [e]veryone in the health professions either neglects or takes into consideration any or all of these, but each profession, to be a profession, must have an exclusive area of expertness with which it practices, creates new practices, new theories, and introduces newcomers to its practice. (Hall, 1965, p. 4)

Hall believed that medicine's exclusive area of expertness was disease, which includes pathology and treatment. The area of person, which, according to Hall, had been sadly neglected, belongs to a number of professions, including psychiatry, social work, and the ministry, among others. In contrast, she saw nursing's expertise

as the area of the body. Hall clearly stated that the focus of nursing is the provision of intimate bodily care. She reflected that the public has long recognized this as belonging exclusively to nursing (Hall, 1958, 1964, 1965). In Hall's opinion, to be expert, the nurse must know how to modify the care depending on the pathology and treatment while considering the patient's unique needs and personality.

Based on her view of the person as patient, Hall conceptualized nursing as having three aspects, and she delineated the area that is the specific domain of nursing and those areas that are shared with other professions (Hall, 1955, 1958, 1964, 1965; Fig. 5-1). Hall believed that this model reflected the nature of nursing as a professional interpersonal process. She visualized each of the three overlapping circles as an "aspect of the nursing process related to the patient, to the supporting sciences and to the underlying philosophical dynamics" (Hall, 1958, p. 1). The circles overlap and change in size as the patient progresses through a medical crisis to the rehabilitative phase of the illness. In the acute care phase, the cure circle is the largest. During the evaluation and follow-up phase, the care circle is predominant. Hall's framework for nursing has been described as the Care, Core, and Cure Model.

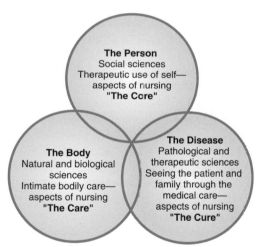

Fig 5 • 1 Care, core, and cure model. *(From Hall, L. [1964, February]. Nursing: What is it? The Canadian Nurse, 60[2], 151. Reproduced with permission from The Canadian Nurse.)*

Care

Hall suggested that the part of nursing that is concerned with intimate bodily care (e.g., bathing, feeding, toileting, positioning, moving, dressing, undressing, and maintaining a healthful environment) belongs exclusively to nursing. From her perspective, nursing is required when people are not able to undertake bodily care activities for themselves. Care provided the opportunity for closeness and required seeing the nursing process as an interpersonal relationship (Hall, 1958). For Hall, the intent of bodily care was to comfort the patient. Through comforting, the patient as a person, as well as his or her body, responds to the physical care. Hall cautioned against viewing intimate bodily care as a task that can be performed by anyone:

To make the distinction between a trade and a profession, let me say that the laying on of hands to wash around a body is an activity, it is a trade; but if you look behind the activity for the rationale and intent, look beyond it for the opportunities that the activity opens up for something more enriching in growth, learning and healing production on the part of the patient—you have got a profession. Our intent when we lay hands on the patient in bodily care is to comfort. While the patient is being comforted, he [*sic*] feels close to the comforting one. At this time, his [*sic*] person talks out and acts out those things that concern him [*sic*]—good, bad, and indifferent. If nothing more is done with these, what the patient gets is ventilation or catharsis, if you will. This may bring relief of anxiety and tension but not necessarily learning. If the individual who is in the comforting role has in her [*sic*] preparation all of the sciences whose principles she [*sic*] can offer a teaching-learning experience around his [*sic*] concerns, the ones that are most effective in teaching and learning, then the comforter proceeds to something beyond—to what I call "nurturer"—someone who fosters learning, someone who fosters growing up emotionally, someone who even fosters healing. (Hall, 1969, p. 86)

Cure

Hall (1958) viewed cure as being shared with medicine and asserted that this aspect of nursing may be viewed as the nurse assisting the doctor by assuming medical tasks/functions or as the nurse helping the patient through his or her medical, surgical, and rehabilitative care in the role of comforter and nurturer. Hall was concerned that the nursing profession was assuming more and more of the medical aspects of care while at the same time relinquishing the nurturing process of nursing to less well-prepared persons. She expressed this concern by stating:

Interestingly enough, physicians do not have practical doctors. They don't need them . . . they have nurses. Interesting, too, is the fact that most nurses show by their delegation of nurturing to others, that they prefer being second class doctors to being first class nurses. This is the prerogative of any nurse. If she [*sic*] feels better in this role, why not? One good reason why not for more and more nurses is that with this increasing trend, patients receive from professional nurses second class doctoring; and from practical nurses, second class nursing. Some nurses would like the public to get first class nursing. Seeing the patient through [his or her] medical care without giving up the nurturing will keep the unique opportunity that personal closeness provides to further [the] patient's growth and rehabilitation. (Hall, 1958, p. 3)

Core

The third area, which Hall believed nursing shared with all of the helping professions, was the core. Hall defined the core as using relationships for therapeutic effect. This area emphasized the social, emotional, spiritual, and intellectual needs of the patient in relation to family, institution, community, and the world (Hall, 1955, 1958, 1965). Knowledge that is foundational to the core is based on the social sciences and on therapeutic use of self. Through the closeness offered by the provision of intimate bodily care, the patient will feel comfortable enough to explore with the nurse "who he [*sic*] is, where he [*sic*] is, where he [*sic*] wants to go, and will take or refuse help in getting there—the patient will make amazingly more rapid progress toward recovery and rehabilitation" (Hall, 1958, p. 3). Hall believed that through this process, the patient would emerge as a whole person.

Knowledge and skills the nurse needs to use self therapeutically include knowing self and learning interpersonal skills. The goals of the interpersonal process are to help patients to understand themselves as they participate in problem focusing and problem-solving. Hall discussed the importance of nursing with the patient as opposed to nursing at, to, or for the patient. Hall reflected on the value of the therapeutic use of self by the professional nurse when she stated:

> The nurse who knows self by the same token can love and trust the patient enough to work *with* him [sic] professionally, rather than for him technically, or at him vocationally.

> Her [sic] goals cease being tied up with "where can I throw my nursing stuff around," or "how can I explain my nursing stuff to get the patient to do what we want him to do," or "how can I understand my patient so that I can handle him better." Instead her goals are linked up with "what is the problem?" and "how can I help the patient understand himself?" as he participates in problem facing and solving. In this way, the nurse recognizes that the power to heal lies in the patient and not in the nurse, unless she is healing herself. She takes satisfaction and pride in her ability to help the patient tap this source of power in his continuous growth and development. She becomes comfortable working cooperatively and consistently with members of other professions, as she meshes her contributions with theirs in a concerted program of care and rehabilitation. (Hall, 1958, p. 5)

Hall believed that the role of professional nursing was enacted through the provision of *care* that facilitates the interpersonal process and invites the patient to learn to reach the *core* of his difficulties while seeing him through the *cure* that is possible. Through the professional nursing process, the patient has the opportunity to see the illness as a learning experience from which he or she may emerge even healthier than before the illness (Hall, 1965).

Practice Applications

The practice of clinical nursing is goal directed, deliberately carried out, and patient centered.
—WIEDENBACH (1964, P. 23)

Wiedenbach

Figure 5-2 represents a spherical model that depicts the "experiencing individual" as the central focus (Wiedenbach, 1964). This model and detailed charts were later edited and published in *Clinical Nursing: A Helping Art* (Wiedenbach, 1964).

In a paper titled "A Concept of Dynamic Nursing," Wiedenbach (1962, p. 7), described the model as follows:

> In its broadest sense, Practice of Dynamic Nursing may be envisioned as a set of concentric circles, with the experiencing individual in the circle at its core. Direct service, with its three components, identification of the individual's experienced need for help, ministration of help needed, and validation that the help provided fulfilled its purpose, fills the circle adjacent to the core. The next circle holds

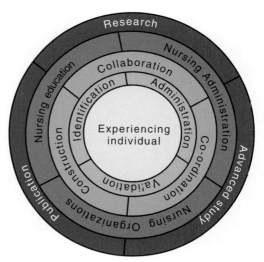

Fig 5 • 2 Professional nursing practice focus and components. *(Reprinted with permission from the Wiedenbach Reading Room [1962], Yale University School of Nursing.)*

the essential concomitants of direct service: coordination, i.e., charting, recording, reporting, and conferring; consultation, i.e., conferencing, and seeking help or advice; and collaboration, i.e., giving assistance or cooperation with members of other professional or nonprofessional groups concerned with the individual's welfare. The content of the fourth circle represents activities which are essential to the ultimate well-being of the experiencing individual, but only indirectly related to him [*sic*]: nursing education, nursing administration, and nursing organizations. The outermost circle comprises research in nursing, publication, and advanced study, the key ways to progress in every area of practice.

Application of Wiedenbach's prescriptive theory was evident in her practice examples and often related to general basic nursing procedures and to maternity nursing practice. The most recent application of Wiedenbach's theory in the literature is a description by VandeVusse (1997) of an educational project designed to guide the nurse midwife in articulating a professional philosophy of nursing.

Henderson

Based on the assumption that nursing has a unique function, Henderson believed that nursing independently initiates and controls activities related to basic nursing care. Relating the conceptualization of basic care components with the unique functions of nursing provided the initial groundwork for introducing the concept of independent nursing practice. In her 1966 publication *The Nature of Nursing*, Henderson stated:

It is my contention that the nurse is, and should be legally, an independent practitioner and able to make independent judgments as long as he, or she, is not diagnosing, prescribing treatment for disease, or making a prognosis, for these are the physician's functions. (Henderson, 1966, p. 22)

Furthermore, Henderson believed that functions pertaining to patient care could be categorized as nursing and nonnursing. She believed that limiting nursing activities to "nursing care" was a useful method of conserving professional nurse power (Harmer & Henderson, 1955). She

defined nonnursing functions as those that are not a service to the person (mind and body) (Harmer & Henderson, 1955). For Henderson, examples of nonnursing functions included ordering supplies, cleaning and sterilizing equipment, and serving food (Harmer & Henderson, 1955).

At the same time, Henderson was not in favor of the practice of assigning patients to lesser trained workers on the basis of complexity level. For Henderson, "all 'nursing care' is essentially complex because it involves constant adaptation of procedures to the needs of the individual" (Harmer & Henderson, 1955, p. 9).

As the authority on basic nursing care, Henderson believed that the nurse has the responsibility to assess the needs of the individual patient, help individuals meet their health needs, and/or provide an environment in which the individual can perform activities unaided. It is the nurse's role, according to Henderson, "to 'get inside the patient's skin' and supplement his [*sic*] strength, will or knowledge according to his needs" (Harmer & Henderson, 1955, p. 5). Conceptualizing the nurse as a substitute for the patient's lack of necessary will, strength, or knowledge to attain good health and to complete or make the patient whole, highlights the complexity and uniqueness of nursing.

Based on the success of *Textbook of the Principles and Practice of Nursing* (fifth edition), Henderson was asked by the International Council of Nurses to prepare a short essay that could be used as a guide for nursing in any part of the world. Despite Henderson's belief that it was difficult to promote a universal definition of nursing, *Basic Principles of Nursing Care* (Henderson, 1960) became an international sensation. To date, it has been published in 29 languages and is referred to as the 20th-century equivalent of Florence Nightingale's *Notes on Nursing*. After visiting countries worldwide, Henderson concluded that nursing varied from country to country and that rigorous attempts to define it have been unsuccessful, leaving the "nature of nursing" largely an unanswered question (Henderson, 1991).

Henderson's definition of nursing has had a lasting influence on the way nursing is practiced around the globe. She was one of the first nurses to articulate that nursing had a unique function yielding a valuable contribution to the health care of individuals. In writing reflections on the nature of nursing, Henderson (1966) stated that her concept of nursing anticipates universally available health care and a partnership among doctors, nurses, and other health-care workers.

The sixth edition of *Principles and Practice of Nursing* (Henderson & Nite, 1978) is considered "the most important single professional document written in the 20th century" (Halloran, 1996, p. 17). In this book, the synthesis of nursing practice, education, theory, and research clearly demonstrated the functions of professional nursing practice.

Henderson was a lifelong supporter of nursing research. In 1964, she published an influential review of nursing research that highlighted the need to increase research studies focusing on the effect of nursing practice on patients (Simmons & Henderson, 1964). This publication resulted in a renewed interest in research studies that focused on the effects of nursing on patient outcomes and the need for research guided by nursing theory (Halloran, 1996). Most recently, Henderson's theory has been applied to the management of the care of patients who donate organs after brain death and their families (Nicely & Delario, 2011).

Hall

In 1963, Lydia Hall was able to actualize her vision of nursing through the creation of the Loeb Center for Nursing and Rehabilitation at Montefiore Medical Center. The center's major orientation was rehabilitation and subsequent discharge to home or to a long-term care institution if further care was needed. Doctors referred patients to the center, and a professional nurse made admission decisions. Criteria for admission were based on the patient's need for rehabilitation nursing. What made the Loeb Center unique was the model of professional nursing that was implemented under Lydia Hall's guidance. The center's guiding philosophy was Hall's belief that during the rehabilitation phase of an illness experience, professional nurses were the best prepared to foster the rehabilitation process, decrease complications and recurrences, and promote health and prevent new illnesses. Hall saw these outcomes being

accomplished by the special and unique way nurses work with patients in a close interpersonal process with the goal of fostering learning, growth, and healing.

PRACTICE EXEMPLARS

Wiedenbach

The focus of practice is the individual for whom the nurse is caring and the way this person perceives his or her condition or situation. Mrs. A was experiencing a red vaginal discharge on her first postpartum day. The doctor recognized it as lochia, a normal concomitant of the phenomenon of involution, and had left an order for her to be up and move about. Instead of trying to get up, Mrs. A remained immobile in her bed. The nurse, who wanted to help her out of bed, expressed surprise at Mrs. A's unwillingness to get up. Mrs. A explained to the nurse that her sister had had a red discharge the day after giving birth 2 years ago and had almost died of hemorrhage. Therefore, to Mrs. A, a red discharge was evidence of the onset of a potentially lethal hemorrhage. The nurse expressed her understanding of the mother's fear and encouraged her to compare her current experience with that of her sister. When the mother did this, she recognized gross differences between her experience and that of her sister and accepted the nurse's explanation that the discharge was normal. The mother voiced her relief and validated it by getting out of bed without further encouragement (Wiedenbach, 1962, pp. 6–7). Wiedenbach considered nursing a "practical phenomenon" that involved action. She believed that this was necessary to understand the theory that underlies the "nurse's way of nursing." This involved "knowing what the nurse wanted to accomplish, how she [*sic*] went about accomplishing it, and in what context she did what she did" (Wiedenbach, 1970, p. 1058).

Henderson

Henderson's definition of nursing and the 14 components of basic nursing care can be useful in guiding the assessment and care of patients preparing for surgical procedures. For example, in assessing Mr. G's preoperative vital signs, the nurse noticed he seemed anxious. The nurse encouraged Mr. G to express his concerns about the surgery. Mr. G told the nurse that he had a fear of not being able to control his body and that he felt general anesthesia represented the extreme limit of loss of bodily control. The nurse recognized this concern as being directly related to Henderson's fourth component of basic nursing care: *Move and maintain desirable postures*. The nurse explained to Mr. G that her role was to "perform those acts he would do for himself if he was not under the influence of anesthesia" (Gillette, 1996, p. 267) and that she would be responsible for maintaining his body in a comfortable and dignified position. She explained how he would need to be positioned during the surgical procedure, what part of his body would be exposed, and how long the procedure was expected to take. Mr. G also told the nurse about an experience he had after an earlier surgical procedure in which he experienced pain in his right shoulder. Mr. G expressed concern that being in one position too long during the surgery would damage his shoulder and result in waking up with shoulder pain again. Together they discussed positions that would be most comfortable for his shoulder during the upcoming procedure, and she assured Mr. G that she would be assessing his position throughout the procedure.

Hall

Hall envisioned that outcomes were accomplished by the special and unique way nurses work with patients in a close interpersonal process with the goal of fostering learning, growth, and healing. Her work at the Loeb Center serves as an administrative exemplar of the application of her theory. At the Loeb Center, nursing was the chief therapy, with medicine and the other disciplines ancillary to nursing. In this new model of organization of nursing services, nursing was in charge of the total health program for the patient and was responsible for integrating all aspects of care. Only registered professional nurses were hired. The 80-bed unit was staffed with 44 professional nurses employed around the clock. Professional nurses gave direct patient care and teaching, and

each nurse was responsible for eight patients and their families. Senior staff nurses were available on each ward as resources and mentors for staff nurses. For every two professional nurses, there was one nonprofessional worker called a "messenger-attendant." The messenger-attendants did not provide hands-on care to the patients. Instead, they performed such tasks as getting linen and supplies, thus freeing the nurse to nurse the patient (Hall, 1964). In addition, there were four ward secretaries. Morning and evening shifts were staffed at the same ratio. Night-shift staffing was less; however, Hall (1965) noted that there were "enough nurses at night to make rounds every hour and to nurse those patients who are awake around the concerns that may be keeping them awake" (p. 2). In most institutions of that time, the number of nurses was decreased during the evening and night shifts because it was felt that larger numbers of nurses were needed during the day to get the work done. Hall took exception to the idea that nursing service was organized around work to be done rather than the needs of the patients.

The patient was the center of care at Loeb and actively participated in all care decisions. Families were free to visit at any hour of the day or night. Rather than strict adherence to institutional routines and schedules, patients at the Loeb Center were encouraged to maintain their own usual patterns of daily activities, thus promoting independence and an easier transition to home. There was no chart section labeled "Doctor's Orders." Hall believed that to order a patient to do something violated the right of the patient to participate in his or her treatment plan. Instead, nurses shared the treatment plan with the patient and helped him or her to discuss his or her concerns and become an active learner in the rehabilitation process. In addition, there were no doctor's progress notes or nursing notes. Instead, all charting was done on a form titled "Patient's Progress Notes." These notes included patients' reaction to care, their concerns and feelings, their understanding of the problems, the goals they have identified, and how they see their progress toward those goals. Patients were also encouraged to keep their own notes to share with their caregivers.

Staff conferences were held at least twice weekly as forums to discuss concerns, problems, or questions. A collaborative practice model between physicians and nurses evolved, and the shared knowledge of the two professions led to more effective team planning (Isler, 1964). The nursing stories published by nurses who worked at Loeb describe nursing situations that demonstrate the effect of professional nursing on patient outcomes. In addition, they reflect the satisfaction derived from practicing in a truly professional role (Alfano, 1971; Bowar, 1971; Bowar-Ferres, 1975; Englert, 1971).

■ Summary

Among other theorists featured in Section II of this book, Wiedenbach, Henderson, and Hall introduced nursing theory to us in the mid-20th century. Each of the nurse theorists presented in this chapter began by reflecting on her personal practice experience to explore the definition of nursing and the importance of nurse–patient interactions. These nurse scholars challenged us to think about nursing in new ways. Their contributions significantly influenced the way nursing was practiced and researched, both in the United States and in other countries around the world. Perhaps most important, each of these scholars stated and responded to the question, "What is nursing?" Their responses helped all who followed to understand that the individual being nursed is a person, not an object, and that the relationship of nurse and patient is valuable to all.

References

Alfano, G. (1971). Healing or caretaking—which will it be? *Nursing Clinics of North America, 6,* 273–280.

Birnbach, N. (1988). Lydia Eloise Hall, 1906–1969. In: V. L. Bullough, O. M. Church, & A. P. Stein (Eds.), *American nursing: A biographical dictionary* (pp. 161–163). New York: Garland.

Bowar, S. (1971). Enabling professional practice through leadership skills. *Nursing Clinics of North America, 6,* 293–301.

Bowar-Ferres, S. (1975). Loeb Center and its philosophy of nursing. *American Journal of Nursing, 75,* 810–815.

Chinn, P. L., & Jacobs, M. K. (1987). *Theory and nursing.* St. Louis, MO: C. V. Mosby.

Dickoff, J., James, P., & Wiedenbach, E. (1968). Theory in a practice discipline. *Nursing Research, 14*(5), 415–437.

Englert, B. (1971). How a staff nurse perceives her role at Loeb Center. *Nursing Clinics of North America, 6*(2), 281–292.

Gesse, T., Dombro, M., Gordon, S. C. & Rittman, M. R. (2006). Twentieth-Century nursing: Wiedenbach, Henderson, and Orlando's theories and their applications. In: M. Parker (Ed.), *Nursing theories and nursing practice* (2nd ed., pp. 70–78). Philadelphia: F. A. Davis.

Gillette, V. A. (1996). Applying nursing theory to perioperative nursing practice. *AORN, 64*(2), 261–270.

Gordon, S. C. (2001). Virginia Avenel Henderson definition of nursing. In: M. Parker (Ed.), *Nursing theories and nursing practice* (pp. 143–149). Philadelphia: F. A. Davis.

Hall, L. E. (1955). *Quality of nursing care.* Manuscript of an address before a meeting of the Department of Baccalaureate and Higher Degree Programs of the New Jersey League for Nursing, February 7, 1955, at Seton Hall University, Newark, New Jersey. Montefiore Medical Center Archives, Bronx, New York.

Hall, L. E. (1958). *Nursing: What is it?* Manuscript. Montefiore Medical Center Archives, Bronx, New York.

Hall, L. E. (1963, March). *Summary of project report: Loeb Center for Nursing and Rehabilitation.* Unpublished report. Montefiore Medical Center Archives, Bronx, New York.

Hall, L. E. (1964). Nursing—what is it? *Canadian Nurse, 60,* 150–154.

Hall, L. E. (1965). *Another view of nursing care and quality.* Address delivered at Catholic University, Washington, DC. Unpublished report. Montefiore Medical Center Archives, Bronx, New York.

Halloran, E. J. (1996). Virgina Hendeson and her timeless writings. *Journal of Advanced Nursing, 23,* 17–23.

Harmer, B., & Henderson, V. A. (1955). *Textbook of the principles and practice of nursing.* New York: Macmillan.

Henderson, V. A. (1960). *Basic principles of nursing care.* Geneva: International Council of Nurses.

Henderson, V. A. (1966). *The nature of nursing.* New York: The National League for Nursing Press.

Henderson, V. A. (1991). *The nature of nursing: Reflections after 25 years.* New York: The National League for Nursing Press.

Henderson, V. A., & Nite, G. (1978). *Principles and practice of nursing* (6th ed.). New York, NY: Macmillan.

Isler, C. (June, 1964). New concept in nursing therapy: Care as the patient improves. *RN,* 58–70.

Montefiore cuts readmissions 80%. (1966, February 23). *The New York Times.*

Nicely, B. & Delario, G. (2011). Virginia Henderson's principles and practice of nursing applied to organ donation after brain death. *Progress in Transplantation,* 21, 72–77

Nickel, S., Gesse, T., & MacLaren, A. (1992). Her professional legacy. *Journal of Nurse Midwifery, 3,* 161.

Simmons, L., & Henderson, V. (1964). *Nursing research: A survey and assessment.* New York: Appleton-Century-Crofts.

Touhy, T., & Birnbach, N. (2006). Lydia Hall: The care, core, and cure model and its applications. In: M. Parker (Ed.), *Nursing theories and nursing practice* (2nd ed., pp. 113–124). Philadelphia: F. A. Davis.

VandeVusse, L. (1997). Education exchange. Sculpting a nurse-midwifery philosophy: Ernestine Wiedenback's Influence. *Journal of Nurse-Midwifery,* 42(1), 43–48.

Wiedenbach, E. (1962). *A concept of dynamic nursing: Philosophy, purpose, practice and process.* Paper presented at the Conference on Maternal and Child Nursing, Pittsburgh, PA. Archives, Yale University School of Nursing, New Haven, CT.

Wiedenbach, E. (1963). The helping art of nursing. *American Journal of Nursing, 63*(11), 54–57.

Wiedenbach, E. (1964). *Clinical nursing: A helping art.* New York: Springer.

Wiedenbach, E. (1969). *Meeting the realities in clinical teaching.* New York: Springer.

Wiedenbach, E. (1970). *A systematic inquiry: Application of theory to nursing practice.* Paper presented at Duke University, Durham, NC (author's personal files).

Chapter 6

Nurse–Patient Relationship Theories

Hildegard Peplau, Joyce Travelbee, and Ida Jean Orlando

ANN R. PEDEN, JACQUELINE STAAL,
MAUDE RITTMAN, AND DIANE
LEE GULLETT

Part One Hildegard Peplau's Nurse–Patient Relationship and Its Applications

Introducing the Theorist
Overview of Peplau's Nurse–Patient
Relationship Theory
Practice Applications
Practice Exemplar
References

Part Two Joyce Travelbee's Human-to-Human Relationship Model and Its Applications

Introducing the Theorist
Overview of Travelbee's Human-to-
Human Relationship Model Theory
Practice Applications
Practice Exemplar
References

Part Three Ida Jean Orlando's Dynamic Nurse–Patient Relationship

Introducing the Theorist
Overview of Orlando's Theory of the
Dynamic Nurse–Patient Relationship
Practice Applications
Practice Exemplar
References

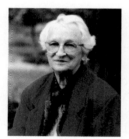

Hildegard Peplau

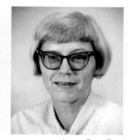

Joyce Travelbee

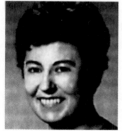

Ida Jean Orlando

The nurse–patient relationship was a significant focus of early conceptualizations of nursing. Hildegard Peplau, Joyce Travelbee, and Ida Jean Orlando were three early nursing scholars who explicated the nature of this relationship. Their work shifted the focus of nursing from performance of tasks to engagement in a therapeutic relationship designed to facilitate health and healing. Each of these conceptualizations will be described in Parts One, Two, and Three of the chapter.

Part One   Peplau's Nurse–Patient Relationship
ANN R. PEDEN[1]

Introducing the Theorist

Hildegard Peplau (1909–1999) was an outstanding leader and pioneer in psychiatric nursing whose career spanned 7 decades. A review of the events in her life also serves as an introduction to the history of modern psychiatric nursing. With the publication of *Interpersonal Relations in Nursing* in 1952, Peplau provided a framework for the practice of psychiatric nursing that would result in a paradigm shift in this specialty. Before this, patients were viewed as objects to be observed. Peplau taught that psychiatric nurses must participate with the patients, engaging in the nurse–patient relationship. Although *Interpersonal Relations in Nursing* was not well received when first published, the book's influence later became widespread. It was reprinted in 1988 and has been translated into at least six languages.

During World War II, Peplau serving in the Army Nurse Corps, was assigned to the School of Military Neuropsychiatry in England. This experience introduced her to the psychiatric problems of soldiers at war. After the war, Peplau attended Columbia University on the GI Bill, earning her master's degree in psychiatric–mental health nursing.

After graduating, Peplau remained at Columbia to teach in their master's program. At that time, there was no direction for what to include in graduate nursing programs. Taking educational experiences from psychiatry and psychology, she adapted them to her conceptualization of nursing. Peplau described this as a time of "innovation or nothing."

Peplau arranged clinical experiences at Brooklyn State Hospital so that her students met twice weekly with the same patient for a session lasting 1 hour. Using carbon paper, the students took verbatim notes during the session. Students then met individually with Peplau to review the interaction in detail. Through this process, both Peplau and her students began to learn what was helpful and what was harmful in the interaction.

In 1955, Peplau left Columbia for Rutgers, where she began the clinical nurse specialist program in psychiatric–mental health nursing. Students were prepared as nurse psychotherapists, developing expertise in individual, group, and family therapies. Peplau required her students to examine their own verbal and nonverbal communication and its effects on the nurse–patient relationship.

In addition to being an educator, researcher, and clinician, Peplau is the only person to serve as both executive director and president of the American Nurses Association. Holding 11 honorary degrees, in 1994, she was inducted into the American Academy of Nursing's (ANA) Living Legends Hall of Fame. She was named one of the 50 great Americans by *Marquis Who's Who* in 1995. In 1997, Peplau received the Christiane Reiman Prize. In 1998, she was inducted into the ANA Hall of Fame. Hildegard Peplau died in March 1999 at her home in Sherman Oaks, California.

Overview of Peplau's Nurse–Patient Relationship Theory

Peplau (1952) defined nursing as a "significant, therapeutic, interpersonal process" that is an "educative instrument, a maturing

---

[1]The author would like to acknowledge the contributions of Kennetha Curtis who assisted in updating the literature.

force, that aims to promote forward movement of personality in the direction of creative, constructive, productive, personal, and community living" (p. 16). Peplau was the first nursing theorist to identify the nurse–patient relationship as being central to all nursing care. In fact, nursing cannot occur if there is no relationship, or connection, between the patient and the nurse. Her work, although written for all nursing specialties, provides specific guidelines for the psychiatric nurse.

The nurse brings to the relationship professional expertise, which includes clinical knowledge. Peplau valued knowledge, believing that the psychiatric nurse must possess extensive knowledge about the potential problems that emerge during a nurse–patient interaction. The nurse must understand psychiatric illnesses and their treatments (Peplau, 1987). The nurse interacts with the patients as both a resource person and a teacher (Peplau, 1952). Through education and supervision, the nurse develops the knowledge base required to select the most appropriate nursing intervention. To engage fully in the nurse–patient relationship, the nurse must possess intellectual, interpersonal, and social skills. These are the same skills often diminished or lacking in psychiatric patients. For nurses to promote growth in patients, they must themselves use these skills competently (Peplau, 1987).

There are four components of the nurse–patient relationship: two individuals (nurse and patient), professional expertise, and patient need (Peplau, 1992). The goal of the nurse–patient relationship is to further the personal development of the patient (Peplau, 1960). Nurse and patient meet as "strangers" who interact differently than friends would. The role of stranger implies respect and positive interest in the patient as an individual. The nurse "accepts the patients as they are and interacts with them as emotionally able strangers and relating on this basis until evidence shows otherwise" (Peplau, 1992, p. 44). Peplau valued therapeutic communication as a key component of nurse–patient

interactions. She advised strongly against the use of "social chit-chat." In fact, she would view this as wasting valuable time with your patient. Every interaction must focus on being therapeutic. Even something as simple as sharing a meal with psychiatric patients can be a therapeutic encounter.

The nurse–patient relationship, viewed as growth-promoting with forward movement, is enhanced when nurses are aware of how their own behavior affects the patient. The "behavior of the nurse-as-a-person interacting with the patient-as-a person has significant effect on the patient's well-being and the quality and outcome of nursing care" (Peplau, 1992, p. 14). An essential component of this relationship is the continuing process of the nurse becoming more self-aware. This occurs via supervision.

Peplau (1989) recommended that nurses participate in weekly supervision meetings with an expert nurse clinician. The focus of the supervisory meetings is on the nurses' interactions with patients. The primary purpose is to review observations and interpersonal patterns that the nurse has made or used. The goal is always to develop the nurse's skills as an expert in interpersonal relations. Peplau (1989) emphasized "the slow but sure growth of nurses" (p. 166) as they developed their competencies in working with patients. Not only are patient problems reviewed but treatment options and the nurses' own pattern of responding to the patient are explored. If an interaction between a nurse and a patient has not gone well, the nurse's response is to examine his or her own behaviors first. Asking questions such as, "Did my own anxiety interfere with this interaction?" or "Is there something in my experiences that influenced how I interacted with this patient?" leads to continual growth and development as a skilled clinician. This process also ensures the delivery of quality care in psychiatric settings. Supervision continues to be an important aspect in advanced practice psychiatric nursing and is a requirement for certification as a psychiatric clinical specialist or nurse practitioner. Supervision is essential as the nurse assumes the role of counselor. In this role, the nurse assists the patient in integrating the thoughts and feelings associated with the illness into the patient's own life experiences (Lakeman, 1999).

The nurse–patient relationship is objective, and its focus is on the needs of the patient. To focus on the patient's needs, the nurse must be a skilled listener and able to respond in ways that foster the patient's growth and return to health. Active listening facilitates the nurse–patient relationship. As Peplau wrote in 1960, nursing is an "opportunity to further the patient's learning about himself [*sic*], the focus in the nurse–patient relationship will be upon the patient —his [*sic*] needs, difficulties, lack in interpersonal competence, interest in living" (p. 966). Within the nurse–patient relationship, the nurse works "to create a mood that encourages clients to reflect, to restructure perceptions and views of situations as needed, to get in touch with their feelings, and to connect interpersonally with other people" (Peplau, 1988, p. 10). Although the nurse–patient relationship is "time-limited in both duration and frequency, the aim is to create an interpersonally intimate encounter, however brief, as if two whole persons are involved in a purposive, enduring relationship; this requires discipline and skill on the part of the nurse" (p. 11). Peplau continued to emphasize that nurses must possess "well-developed intellectual competencies, and disciplined attention to the work at hand" (p. 13).

Communication, both verbal and nonverbal, is an essential component of the nurse–patient relationship. However, in Peplau's view, verbal communication is required for the nurse–patient relationship to develop. She wrote, "[A]nything clients act out with nurses will most probably not be talked about, and that which is not discussed cannot be understood" (Peplau, 1989, p. 197). One objective of the nurse–patient relationship is to talk about the problem or need that has resulted in the patient interacting with the nurse. Peplau provided descriptions of phrases commonly used by patients that require clarification on the part of the nurse. These included referring to "they," using the phrase "you know," and overgeneralizing responses to situations. The nurse clarifies who "they" are, responds that she or he does not know and needs further information, and assists patients to be more specific as they describe their experiences (Forchuk, 1993).

Phases of the Nurse–Patient Relationship

Peplau (1952) introduced the phases of the nurse–patient relationship in her interpersonal relations theory. This time-limited relationship is interpersonal in nature and has a starting point, proceeds through identifiable phases, and ends. Initially, Peplau (1952) included four phases in the relationship: orientation, identification, exploitation, and resolution. In 1991, Forchuk, a Canadian researcher who has tested and refined some of Peplau's work, proposed three phases: orientation, working, and resolution (Peplau, 1992). Forchuk's recommendation of a three-phase nurse–patient relationship resolves the lack of easy differentiation between the identification and exploitation stages. These two phases were collapsed into the working phase. By renaming these two phases the working phase, a more accurate reflection of what actually occurs in this important aspect of the nurse–patient relationship is provided. Although the nurse–patient relationship is time limited in nature, much of this relationship is spent "working."

Orientation Phase

The relationship begins with the orientation phase (Peplau, 1952). This phase is particularly important because it sets the stage for the development of the relationship. During the orientation period, the nurse and patient's relationship is still new and unfamiliar. Nurse and patient get to know each other as people; their expectations and roles are understood. During this first phase, the patient expresses a "felt need" and seeks professional assistance from the nurse. In reaction to this need, the nurse helps the individual by recognizing and assessing his or her situation. It is during the assessment that the patient's needs are evaluated by the patient and nurse working together as a team. Through this process, trust develops between the patient and the nurse. Also, the parameters for the relationship are clarified. Nursing diagnoses, goals, and outcomes for the patient are created based on the assessment information. Nursing interventions are implemented, and the evaluations of the patient's goals are also incorporated (Peplau, 1992).

Working Phase

The working phase incorporates identification and exploitation. The focus of the working phase is twofold: first is the patient, who "exploits" resources to improve health; second is the nurse, who enacts the roles of "resource person, counselor, surrogate, and teacher in facilitating . . . development toward well-being" (Fitzpatrick & Wallace, 2005, p. 460). This phase of the relationship is meant to be flexible so that the patient is able to function "dependently, independently, or interdependently with the nurse, based on . . . developmental capacity, level of anxiety, self-awareness, and needs" (Fitzpatrick & Wallace, 2005, p. 460). A balance between independence and dependence must exist here, and it is the nurse who must aid the patient in its development (Lakeman, 1999).

During the exploitation phase of the working phase, the client assumes an active role on the health team by taking advantage of available services and determining the degree to which they are used (Erci, 2008). Within this phase, the client begins to develop responsibility and independence, becoming better able to face new challenges in the future (Erci, 2008). Peplau (1992) wrote that "[e]xploiting what a situation offers gives rise to new differentiations of the problem and the development and improvement of skill in interpersonal relations" (pp. 41–42).

Resolution Phase

The resolution phase is the last phase and involves the patient's continual movement from dependence to independence, based on both a distancing from the nurse and a strengthening of individual's ability to manage care (Peplau, 1952). According to Peplau, resolution can take place only when the patient has gained the ability to be free from nursing assistance and act independently (Lloyd, Hancock, & Campbell, 2007). At this point, old needs are abandoned, and new goals are adopted (Lakeman, 1999). The completion of the resolution phase results in the mutual termination of the nurse–patient relationship and involves planning for future sources of support (Peplau, 1952). Completion of this final phase "is one measure of the success of . . . all the other phases" (Lloyd et al., 2007, p. 50).

Applications of the Theory

Almost all of the research that has tested Peplau's nurse–patient relationship has been conducted by Forchuk (1994, 1995) and colleagues (Forchuk & Brown, 1989; Forchuk et al., 1998; Forchuk et al., 1998). Much of Forchuk's work has focused on the orientation phase. Forchuk and Brown (1989) emphasized the importance of being able to identify the orientation phase and not rush movement into the working phase. To assist in this, they developed a one-page instrument, the Relationship Form, which they have used to determine the current phase of the relationship and overall progression from phase to phase.[2]

Peplau first wrote about the nurse–patient relationship in 1952. She hoped that through this work, nurses would change how they interacted with their patients. She wanted nurses to "do with" clients rather than "do to" (Forschuk, 1993). The majority of the work that has tested Peplau's nurse–patient relationship has been conducted with individuals with severe mental illness, many of them in psychiatric hospitals. In these studies, patients did move through the phases of the nurse–patient relationship.

As psychiatric nurses have changed the location of their practice from hospital to community, they have carried Peplau's work to this new arena. Unfortunately, there has been limited testing of the nurse–patient relationship in community settings. Parrish, Peden, and

---

[2]For additional information, please visit DavisPlus at http://davisplus.fadavis.com.

Staten (2008) explored strategies used by advanced practice psychiatric nurses treating individuals with depression. All the participants in this study practiced in community settings. When describing the strategies used, the nurse–patient relationship was the primary vehicle by which strategies were delivered. These strategies included active listening, partnering with the client, and a holistic view of the client. This work supports the integration of Peplau's nurse–patient relationship into the work of the psychiatric nurse.

Moving beyond application of Peplau's theory in psychiatric settings with psychiatric patients, Merritt and Proctor (2010) used Peplau's four phases of the nurse–patient relationship to guide their practice as mental health consultation liaison nurses. Working with patients experiencing psychiatric symptoms but who did not have a psychiatric disorder, these practitioners were guided by Peplau's four phases of the nurse–patient relationship. This clinical application led to better engagement with patients, provided patients with the tools needed to address life changes that precipitated their illness, and finally resulted in movement toward health that included meaningful, productive living. They concluded that Peplau's work provided a model to ensure successful engagement with patients requiring consultation liaison nursing interventions.

Peplau's theoretical work on the nurse–patient relationship continues to be essential to nursing practice. To increase patient satisfaction with care received in health-care settings, relationship-based care has become an important component in the delivery of nursing care. Large institutions are educating their workforce on the importance of having a relationship, a connection with those with whom the nurse interacts and to whom he or she provides care. The premise is that by putting the patient and his or her family at the center of care, patient satisfaction and outcomes will improve. In response to this and other changes in health care, Jones (2012) wrote a thoughtful editorial encouraging nurse leaders and educators to reclaim the structure of the nurse–patient relationship as defined by Peplau. He

raised the question: Isn't relationship-based care what Peplau described as early as the 1950s? One such institution, St. Mary's located in Evansville, Indiana, has developed a model of relationship-based care. It is defined as "healthcare achieved through collaborative relationships. Relationship-Based Care takes place in a caring, competent and healing environment organized around the needs and priorities of the patients and their families who are at the center of the care team" (www.stmarys.org/relationshipbasedcare; retrieved February 5, 2013). Some of the principles of this type of care include developing a therapeutic relationship, being knowledgeable of self, experiencing change that occurs over time, and believing that everyone has a valuable contribution to make. As literature describing relationship-based care is reviewed (Campbell, 2009; Small & Small, 2011), citations of Peplau's work are notably lacking. Their absence may be attributed to how thoroughly Peplau's writings have become integral to nursing practice—as if they belong to nursing, are a part of nursing's language and culture, and are no longer recognizable as being separate from what is nursing.

Not only is nursing practice enhanced when Peplau's work is reviewed and applied, it also may provide guidance in maintaining professional roles. In a more informal society with its consequent easing of professional behaviors in registered nurses, boundary violations reported to boards of nursing are increasing (Jones, Fitzpatrick, & Drake, 2008). A return to the structure of the nurse–patient relationship and revisiting the roles as defined by Peplau may be needed (Jones, 2012). Peplau clearly articulated the roles of the nurse. At the time when she was writing about this, nursing was moving from hospital-based educational systems into university settings. The focus of nursing was on becoming a profession. With this movement, more autonomy in nursing practice was needed. To provide a framework for this, Peplau developed, primarily for psychiatric-mental health nurses, six roles that were integral in the nurse–patient relationship. These were described earlier in this chapter.

The stranger role has particular relevance to establishing professional boundaries. All nurse–patient relationships begin with meeting the patient. The nurse enters into this relationship as a nurse, not as a friend. The nurse is respectful of the patient and values his or her privacy. When a nurse moves from professional to friend, boundary issues have been violated. If this is not recognized or even raised as a concern, nursing care deteriorates. If every interaction is therapeutic, as described by Peplau, then in the nurse–patient relationship there is no time for social chit-chat or developing friendships. The work of nursing is to engage the patient in therapeutic relationships that move them toward greater health. This was as vital to nursing in the 1950s as it is today.

Practice Exemplar

Karen Thomas is a 49-year-old married woman who has a scheduled appointment with an advanced practice psychiatric nurse (APPN). She appears anxious and uncomfortable in the encounter with the APPN. In an effort to help Ms. Thomas feel more comfortable, the APPN offers her a glass of water or cup of coffee. Ms. Thomas announces that she has not eaten all day and would like something to drink. The APPN provides a cup of water and several crackers for Ms. Thomas to eat. Once they are both seated, the APPN asks Ms. Thomas about the reason for the appointment (what brought her here today). Ms. Thomas replies that she does not know; her husband made the appointment for her. To more fully understand the reason for her husband making the appointment, the APPN asks Ms. Thomas to tell her what aspects of her behavior were viewed by her husband as calling for attention. Once again, Ms. Thomas shares that she does not know. Continuing to focus on getting acquainted and enhancing Ms. Thomas's comfort in this beginning relationship, the APPN asks Ms. Thomas to tell her about herself. Ms. Thomas shares that she has been depressed in the past and was treated by a psychiatric nurse practitioner, who prescribed an antidepressant medication. Becoming tearful, she also shares that she left her husband several days ago and has moved in with her oldest son, stating that she "just needs some time to think." For the next 15 minutes, Ms. Thomas talks about her marriage, her love for her husband, and her lack of trust in him. She also shares symptoms of depression that are present. Ms. Thomas speaks tangentially and is a poor historian when recalling events in the marriage that have caused her pain. Her responses are guarded as she alludes to marital infidelity on the part of her husband. Interspersed throughout the conversation are statements about her dislike of medications. The APPN then begins to ask more pointed assessment questions related to depressive symptoms. Ms. Thomas shares that she has very poor sleep, cannot concentrate, is isolating herself, has difficulties making decisions, and feels hopeless about her future. At this point, Ms. Thomas also shares that she had never taken the antidepressant prescribed for her. By sharing this, Ms. Thomas indicates the beginning of a trusting relationship with the APPN. Once the initial assessment is complete, a preliminary diagnosis is determined, and client and nurse are ready to move into the working phase.

The working phase is initiated with problem identification. For Ms. Thomas, the primary problem is major depression with a secondary problem, partner-relational issues. The APPN, acting as a resource person, provides education about the illness, major depression. Included is information about the biological causes of the illness, genetic predisposition, and explanations about the symptoms. A partnership is formed as the APPN and Ms. Thomas discuss treatment options. Although Ms. Thomas shares that she does not like to take medications, she agrees to an appointment with a psychiatric nurse practitioner, who will conduct a medication evaluation. That appointment is scheduled later in the week. Ms. Thomas also shares that she really wants to talk about her relationship with her husband and come to some decision about the future of their marriage. Marital counseling is mentioned as a possible treatment option, but the APPN suggests that this be delayed until

Continued

Practice Exemplar cont.

Ms. Thomas's depressive symptoms have decreased. The first session ends with both client and nurse committed to working to decrease Ms. Thomas's depressive symptoms. Ms. Thomas is reminded about her appointment for a medication evaluation, and a second therapy appointment is made with the APPN.

At the second visit, Ms. Thomas reports that she has started taking an antidepressant but as of yet has not seen any relief of her symptoms. The APPN provides information about the usual length of time required for results to occur. Although Ms. Thomas does not see noticeable results from the medication, the APPN shares that Ms. Thomas looks more relaxed and seems less anxious. Ms. Thomas states that she would like to spend this session talking about her relationship with her husband. She describes what was once a very happy marriage. The APPN listens, asks for clarification when needed, and encourages Ms. Thomas to share her perceptions of her marriage. The APPN asks Ms. Thomas again to talk about what might have caused her husband to call and make the therapy appointment for her. Ms. Thomas shares that her husband does not want their marriage to end; however, she is not sure yet about their future. Her perception is that her husband thinks she is the one with the problem and once she is "fixed" that their marriage will return to its former state of happiness. The session ends with the APPN asking Ms. Thomas to focus on her own physical and mental health. Possible interventions include beginning an exercise program, practicing stress reduction strategies, and reconnecting with individuals who have been supportive in the past.

At the next session, Ms. Thomas is noticeably improved. She states that she is sleeping, not crying as much, concentrating better, and feeling more hopeful about her marriage. She also shares that she and her husband have met for dinner several times and that he is willing to come with her for marital counseling. However, she shares that she is not yet ready for this, preferring to spend time focusing on her own mental health. Over the course of several months, Ms. Thomas and the APPN meet. In these sessions, Ms. Thomas explores her childhood, talks about the recent death of her mother, decides to begin a new exercise program, and reconnects with childhood friends. Through this work, Ms. Thomas grows more secure in who she is and in how she wants to live. During this same time period, she continues to meet her husband regularly for dinner and sometimes a movie.

At their final session, Ms. Thomas shares that she is ready to go with her husband to marital counseling. As a result of antidepressant medication and therapy, the problem of major depression has been resolved. However, the focus of this last session returns to depression. This is done to help Ms. Thomas recognize the early symptoms of depression to prevent a relapse. Ms. Thomas shares that her first symptoms were not sleeping well and withdrawing from friends and family. The APPN emphasizes the importance of monitoring this and calling for an appointment if these early symptoms occur. The focus now is on the secondary problem of partner-relationship issues. With this, the APPN makes a referral to a marital and family therapist.

■ Summary

Peplau is considered the first modern-day nurse theorist. Her clinical work provided direction for the practice of psychiatric-mental health nursing. This occurred at a time when there were few innovations in the care of the mentally ill. She valued education, believing that attaining advanced degrees would move the nursing profession forward. She also believed that nursing research should be grounded in clinical problems. She worked tirelessly to advance the profession of nursing, as both an educator and a leader at the national and international levels. Her contributions continue to have an influence today.

References

Campbell, M. P. (2009). Relationship based Care is here! *The Journal of Lancaster General Hospital, 4* (3), 87–89.

Erci, B. (2008). Nursing theories applied to vulnerable populations: Examples from Turkey. In: M. de Chesney & B. A. Anderson (Eds.), Caring for the vulnerable: Perspectives in nursing theory, practice and research (2nd ed., pp. 45–60). Sudbury, MA: Jones and Bartlett.

Fitzpatrick, J. J., & Wallace, M. (2005). Encyclopedia of nursing research. New York: Springer.

Forchuk, C. (1991). Peplau's theory: Concepts and their relations. *Nursing Science Quarterly, 4*(2), 64–80. doi: 10.1177/089431849100400205

Forchuk, C. (1993). Hildegard E. Peplau: Interpersonal nursing. Newbury Park, CA: Sage.

Forchuk, C. (1994). The orientation phase of the nurse–client relationship: Testing Peplau's theory. *Journal of Advanced Nursing, 20*(3), 532–537.

Forchuk, C. (1995). Development of nurse-client relationship: What helps? *Journal of the American Psychiatric Nurses Association, 1,* 146–151.

Forchuk, C., & Brown, B. (1989). Establishing a nurse–client relationship. *Journal of Psychosocial Nursing, 27*(2), 30–34.

Forchuk, C., Jewell, J., Schofield, R., Sircelj, M., & Valledor, T. (1998). From hospital to community: Bridging therapeutic relationships. *Journal of Psychiatric and Mental Health Nursing, 5,* 197–202.

Forchuk, C., Westwell, J., Martin, A., Azzapardi, W. B., Kosterewa-Tolman, D., & Hux, M. (1998). Factors influencing movement of chronic psychiatric patients from the orientation to the working phase of the nurse-client relationship on an inpatient unit. *Perspectives in Psychiatric Care, 34,* 36–44.

Jones, J. (2012). Has anybody seen my old friend Peplau? The absence of interpersonal curricula in programs of nursing? *Archives of Psychiatric Nursing, 26,* 167–168.

Jones, J., Fitzpatrick, J.J., & Drake, V. (2008). Frequency of post-licensure registered nurse boundary violations with patients in the State of Ohio: A comparison based on type of pre-licensure registered nurse

education. *Archives of Psychiatric Nursing, 22,* 356–363.

Lakeman, R. (1999). Remembering Hildegard Peplau. *Vision, 5*(8), 29–31.

Lloyd, H., Hancock, H., & Campbell, S. (2007). *Principles of care.* London: Blackwell.

Merritt, M.K. & Procter, N. (2010). Conceptualising the functional role of mental health consultation-liaison nursing in multi-morbidity using Peplau's nursing theory. *Contemporary Nurse, 34,* 158–166.

Parrish, E., Peden, A. R., & Staten, R. R. (2008). Strategies used by advanced practice psychiatric nurses in treating adults with depression. *Perspectives in Psychiatric Care, 44,* 232–240.

Peplau, H. E. (1952). *Interpersonal relations in nursing.* New York: G. P. Putnam's Sons. (English edition reissued as a paperback in 1988 by Macmillan Education, London.)

Peplau, H. E. (1960). Talking with patients. *American Journal of Nursing, 60,* 964–967.

Peplau, H. E. (1962). The crux of psychiatric nursing. *American Journal of Nursing, 62,* 50–54.

Peplau, H. E. (1987). Tomorrow's world. *Nursing Times, 83,* 29–33.

Peplau, H. E. (1988). The art and science of nursing: Similarities, differences and relations. *Nursing Science Quarterly, 1,* 8–15.

Peplau, H. E. (1989). Clinical supervision of staff nurses. In A. O'Toole, & S. R. Welt (Eds.), *Interpersonal theory in nursing practice: Selected works of Hildegard Peplau* (pp. 164–167). New York: Springer.

Peplau, H. E. (1992). Interpersonal relations: A theoretical framework for application in nursing practice. *Nursing Science Quarterly, 5*(1), 13–18.

Peplau, H. E. (1998). Life of an angel: Interview with Hildegard Peplau (1998). Hatherleigh Co. Audiotape available from the American Psychiatric Nurses Association: www.apna.org/items.htm

Small, D. C., & Small, R.M. (2011). Patients first! Engaging the hearts and minds of nurses with a patient-centered practice model. *Online Journal of Issues in Nursing, 16* (2), 1091–3734.

Introducing the Theorist

Joyce Travelbee (1926–1973) practiced psychiatric/mental health nursing for more than 30 years in both the clinical setting and as a nurse educator. She is best known for her human-to-human relationship model, a middle-range theory that guides the nurse–patient interaction with emphasis on helping the patient find hope and meaning in the illness experience (Travelbee, 1971). The human-to-human relationship model provided an early framework for delivering patient-centered care, as promoted today by the Agency for Healthcare Research and Quality with the U.S. Department of Health and Human Services and as noted in the Institute of Medicine's (2001) report, "Crossing the Quality Chasm: A New Health System for the 21st Century."

Travelbee graduated from the diploma nursing program at Charity Hospital School of Nursing in New Orleans, Louisiana, in 1943. Her early clinical practice at Charity Hospital, combined with her faith, spirituality, and religious background, influenced her view on nursing and later the development of her theoretical model. She received her bachelor of science degree in nursing from Louisiana State University in 1956 and later her master of science degree in nursing with a focus on psychiatric/mental health nursing in 1959 from Yale University. Travelbee taught psychiatric and mental health nursing at Louisiana State University, New Orleans; the Department of Nursing Education at New York University; the University of Mississippi School of Nursing in Jackson; and at the Hotel Dieu School of Nursing in New Orleans, Louisiana (Meleis, 1997; Travelbee, 1971). As a clinical instructor and later a professor of nursing, Travelbee (1972) incorporated her philosophy of caring into her teaching methods, challenging students to learn not only from their textbooks and nursing colleagues but rather from the patients and their relatives themselves. She later served as a nursing consultant for the Veteran's Administration Hospital in MS and

was enrolled in doctoral study at the time of her death at age 47. Travelbee was Director of Graduate Education at the Louisiana State University School of Nursing when she died.

Travelbee's first book, *Interpersonal Aspects of Nursing* (1966), identified the purpose of nursing and the roles of the nurse in achieving this purpose. The delicate balance between scientific knowledge and the ability to apply evidence-based interventions with the therapeutic use of self in effecting change was described and the ultimate goal of helping the patient find hope and meaning in the illness experience was identified. In Travelbee's second book, *Intervention in Psychiatric Nursing: Process in the One-to-One Relationship* (1969), the role of the psychiatric nurse in patient care is described, the concept of communication in the human-to-human relationship is examined, and the process of establishing, maintaining, and terminating a relationship is described.

Overview of Travelbee's Conceptualization

Travelbee's human-to-human relationship model was based on the work of nurse theorists Hildegard Peplau and Ida Jean Orlando (Tomey & Alligood, 2006). Viktor E. Frankl's *logotherapy* guided Travelbee's (1971) concept of nursing intervention and the role of the nurse in helping patients and their families find meaning in the illness experience.

Caring, in the human-to-human relationship model, involves the dynamic, reciprocal, interpersonal connection between the nurse and patient, developed through communication and the mutual commitment to perceive self and other as unique and valued. Through the therapeutic use of self and the integration of evidence-based knowledge, the nurse provides quality patient care that can foster the patient's trust and confidence in the nurse (Travelbee, 1971). The meaning of the illness experience becomes self-actualizing for the patient as the nurse helps the patient find meaning in the experience. The purpose of the nurse is to "enable (the individual) to help themselves . . . in prevention of illness and promotion of health, and in assisting those who are incapable, or unable, to help themselves" (Travelbee, 1969, p. 7).

The human-to-human relationship "refers to an experience or series of experiences between the human being who is nurse and an ill person," culminating in the nurse meeting the ill person's unique needs (Travelbee, 1971, pp. 16–17). The term *patient* is not used in Travelbee's model, because *patient* refers to a label or category of people, rather than a unique individual in need of nursing care. The purpose of nursing, according to Travelbee (1971), is "to assist an individual, family or community to prevent or cope with the experience of illness and suffering and, if necessary, to find meaning in these experiences" (p. 16). Simply caring about an individual is not sufficient for providing quality care but rather the integration of a broad knowledge base with the therapeutic use of self is needed. To effect change in the human relationship, the nurse must transcend her sense of self to focus on the recipient of care (Travelbee, 1969).

Transcendence of the traditional titles of *nurse* and *patient* is necessary to prevent dehumanization of the ill person. With the rapid expansion of health technology, combined with financial constraints leading to restructuring of nurse–patient ratios, competing demands are placed on the nurse's time and attention. An emotional detachment between the nurse and ill person is created when the nurse views the ill person as simply "patient," rather than as a unique individual with his own understanding of the illness experience. By performing nursing tasks without an emotional investment in the nurse–patient relationship, the ill person's physical needs are met. However, the ill person recognizes the lack of caring in the transaction and is left alone to suffer with the symptoms of illness. Dehumanization occurs when the ill person is left alone to find meaning in his illness experience.

Many ill persons and their family members may ask questions such as "why me?" or "why my loved one?" By inquiring into the individual's perception of his illness and how he has derived meaning from his illness experience, the nurse can assess his coping ability and provide nursing interventions to prevent suffering

and despair. Hope and motivation are important nursing tasks in caring for an ill person in despair. However, the nurse "cannot 'give' hope to another person; she can, however, strive to provide some ways and means for an ill person to experience hope" (Travelbee, 1971, p. 83).

All human beings endure suffering, although the experience of suffering differs from one individual to another (Travelbee, 1971). Suffering may be inevitable, but one's attitude toward it affects how an individual copes with any illness. If the patient's needs are not met in his suffering, he may develop "despairful not-caring," in which he does not care if he dies or recovers, or "apathetic indifference," in which he has "lost the will to live" (Travelbee, 1971, pp. 180–181). Hope helps the suffering person to cope, and it is an assumption of Travelbee's (1971) that "the role of the nurse . . . [is] to assist the ill person [to] experience hope in order to cope with the stress of illness and suffering" (p. 77).

To relieve the patient's suffering and to foster hope, the nurse provides care based on the individual's unique needs. Nursing care, according to Travelbee (1971), is delivered through five stages: observation, interpretation, decision making, action (or nursing intervention), and appraisal (or evaluation). The nursing intervention is designed to achieve the purpose of nursing and is communicated to the patient. The goals of communication in the nursing process are "to know (the) person, (to) ascertain and meet the nursing needs of ill persons, and (to) fulfill the purpose of nursing" (Travelbee, 1971, p. 96).

In the observation stage of nursing care, the nurse "does not observe signs of illness" but rather collects sensory data to identify a problem or need (Travelbee, 1971, p. 99). The nurse validates her interpretation of the problem or need with the ill person and decides whether or not to act upon her interpretation. A nursing intervention is developed in alignment with the purpose of nursing, and requires the nurse to "assist ill persons to find meaning in the experience of illness, suffering, and pain" (Travelbee, 1971, p. 158). However, the nurse may not assume she understands the meaning of the illness experience to the ill person without first inquiring into this meaning. To do so would communicate to the ill person that his or her experience is not of value to the nurse, resulting in dehumanization. The nurse evaluates the outcomes of her nursing intervention based on objectives developed before the phase of appraisal.

In meeting the ill person's needs through the human-to-human relationship, the nurse employs a disciplined intellectual approach or a logical approach consistent with nursing standards and clinical practice guidelines to identify, manage, and evaluate the ill person's problem (Travelbee, 1971). Each stage in the nursing process may be employed without the establishment of a human-to-human relationship. An acute medical need may be met, but the patient's deeper spiritual and emotional needs are neglected. These spiritual and emotional needs are addressed in the human-to-human relationship in the progression through five phases: the original encounter, emerging identities, empathy, sympathy, and rapport.

In the phase of the original encounter, the nurse and ill person form judgments about each other that will guide and shape future nurse–person interactions. Past experiences, the media, and stereotypes may influence one's perception of another, blocking the development of a human-to-human relationship. In the phase of emerging identities, a bond begins to form between nurse and person as each individual begins to "appreciate the uniqueness of the other" (Travelbee, 1971, p. 132). The bond is created and shaped through each nurse–person interaction and is facilitated by the therapeutic use of self, combined with nursing knowledge. The nurse must recognize how she perceives the person to create a foundation of empathy.

In the phase of empathy, the nurse begins to see the individual "beyond outward behavior and sense accurately another's inner experience at a given point in time" (Travelbee, 1971, p. 136). Empathy enables the nurse to predict what the person is experiencing and requires acceptance because empathy involves the "intellectual and . . . emotional comprehension of another person" (Travelbee, 1964). Empathy is the precursor to sympathy, or the "desire, almost an urge, to help or aid an individual in order to relieve his distress" (Travelbee, 1964). Sympathy is not pity, but rather a demonstration to the person that he is not carrying the burden of illness alone. Trust develops between the nurse and person in the phase of sympathy, and the person's distress is diminished.

Rapport is essential in the nurse–patient relationship. Travelbee (1971) defined rapport as "a process, a happening, and experience, or series of experiences, undergone simultaneously by nurse and the recipient of her care" (p. 150). Rapport "is composed of a cluster of interrelated thoughts and feelings: interest in and concern for, others; empathy, compassion, and sympathy; a non-judgmental attitude, and respect for each individual as a unique human being" (Travelbee, 1963). Through the establishment of rapport, the nurse is able to foster a meaningful relationship with the ill person during multiple points of contact in the care setting. Rapport is not established in every nurse–person encounter; however, emotional involvement is required from the nurse. To establish this emotional bond with one's patient, the nurse must first ensure her own emotional needs are met.

In Travelbee's second book, *Intervention in Psychiatric Nursing,* implementation of the human-to-human relationship model is explained through the stages of selecting and establishing a patient relationship, the process of maintaining the relationship, and ultimate termination of the relationship. Patients in the acute care facility are typically assigned to a nurse based on acuity, skill level and experience of the nurse. However, nurses can select a patient to develop a one-on-one relationship with based on availability and willingness of the nurse and patient.

During the preinteraction phase, the nurse and patient relationship is chosen or assigned. The nurse may have preconceived thoughts and feelings toward the patient she is entering the relationship with and must identify these prejudices before the next phase of their relationship.

Goals and objectives for the interaction are established before the first meeting and may evolve over time (Travelbee, 1969, p. 143). Once the nurse and patient are acquainted, both the nurse and patient begin to assess each other and make an assumption about the other. The nurse should clarify to the patient that she is not there simply to collect data but rather to get to "know" the patient (p. 151). Data should be collected in a manner that is sensitive to the patient's privacy and comfort level. The nurse's own thoughts and feelings of the interaction must be considered following a one-on-one interaction to determine whether her own behavior may have affected the patient interaction (Travelbee, 1969, p. 132). Likewise, the nurse must evaluate whether the interaction met previously established objectives and set goals for future interactions. The nurse and patient affect each other's thoughts and feelings during each encounter, based on "the nurse's knowledge and her ability to use it, the ill person's willingness or capacity to respond to the nurse's effort, and the kind of problem experienced by the ill person" (Travelbee, 1969, p. 139).

The phase of emerging identities occurs when the nurse and the patient have overcome their own anxieties about the interaction, stereotypes, and past experiences. The nurse and patient come to see each other as unique, and the nurse works to transcend her view of the situation. The nurse helps the patient to identify problems and helps the patient change his own behaviors. During this stage of development, the nurse helps the patient find meaning in the illness experience "whether this suffering be predominately mental, physical, or spiritual in origin" (Travelbee, 1969, p 157). Eventually, the relationship is terminated, and preparation for termination of the relationship should begin early in the Phase of Emerging Identities. Patients may feel abandoned or angry regarding the termination if remaining in the facility. In some cases, the nurse may be able to elicit their thoughts and feelings. Those to be discharged from the facility should be encouraged to express their fears and be assisted in problem-solving solutions.

Practice Applications

Cook (1989) used Travelbee's nursing concepts to design a support group for nurses facing organizational restructuring at a New York hospital. The purpose of the support group was to help nurses develop more meaningful perceptions of their roles during a nursing shortage created during a financial crisis that resulted in a restructuring of patient care delivery and nurse/patient ratios. Group morale was low in the beginning, and nurses were frustrated with higher nurse/patient ratios. The support group met over 2 weeks, and the group intervention was designed by incorporating Hoff's theory on crisis intervention with Travelbee's phases of observation and communication. Travelbee's human-to-human relationship was used to guide supportive discussions and problem-solving as nurses struggled to regain a sense of meaning and purpose related to their professional identity.

Participants shared their perceptions of their work environment during the initial encounter. Support group members discussed the similarities and differences in their work perceptions during the phase of emerging identities. Empathy and trust developed as nurses became more accepting and nonjudgmental of each other's perceptions, culminating in the establishment of rapport as group members were able to "recapture" the meaning of nursing (Cook, 1989).

Cook (1989) found that nurses who had threatened to quit earlier had remained in the system by the end of the support group. Nurse productivity had increased over time, and the number of sick days taken by the nurses had diminished over the 6-month period after program cessation. Nurses regained a sense of meaning of their work and reported increased job satisfaction after completion of the program. Travelbee's ideas hold potential as an effective nursing intervention for improving nurse retention rates. However, further research is necessary because the exact number of nurses recruited into the support group and the actual number of nurses who completed the program are unknown.

Practice Exemplar

Luciana came into nurse practitioner Janice's office for her annual well-woman examination. A 53-year-old mother of three without insurance, Luciana had delayed her visit for several months due to lack of money. Despite a nagging feeling that the pain in her breasts might be serious, Luciana waited until she could no longer tolerate the pain and the redness and swelling of the breasts that had since developed.

When Janice explained to Luciana that she was a nurse practitioner and would be performing her examination today and addressing any concerns she may have. Luciana sat silently, looking slightly below Janice's eyes as she spoke. She avoided eye contact until asked if something was wrong. Unable to wait for Janice to complete the history, Luciana lifted her shirt and showed the nurse practitioner her erythematous, swollen breasts. The most significant swelling noted was located in the upper left quadrant, where Janice's own mother-in-law had experienced her most significant swelling and lesions from her breast cancer 5 years earlier—a cancer she hid from her family until it was too late to intervene.

"What do you think this means?" Luciana asked. Stunned by her bluntness, Janice took a closer look at the swelling and warm, red skin across Luciana's chest. Dread filled quickly inside Janice. "Do you think this is cancer?" she asked. Trying to think back to what she had been taught to say in her nursing education, her mind drew a blank and honesty was the only thought to come to mind. "Yes," Janice replied softly. "I do." Tears began to fall from Luciana's calm face, as though she knew she had breast cancer all along. Janice gave her a big hug and whispered softly into her left ear, "It will be alright. I am going to help you." Luciana explained that she did not work and did not have either health insurance or Medicaid. Janice explained that programs were available to help provide financial assistance and that she would help her contact a representative from a state-run breast cancer program. Janice carefully finished performing her physical examination, taking care to document the extent of her swelling and the size, shape, smoothness, mobility, and location of any lumps palpated during the clinical breast examination.

Once the examination was finished, Janice excused herself and sought out the office manager. She pulled Sophia aside in private and explained the situation. They contacted their local representative from the health department in charge of a grant that allocated money for diagnostic mammography and arranged for the patient to obtain the mammography through the program. Janice returned to the examination room with the referral form, prescription for the diagnostic imaging, and contact information for the program representative. The patient began to cry softly as she expressed concern for her three children and wondered who would take care of them? Janice hugged Luciana as she cried and shared her story of working as a stay-at-home mom while her husband worked for low wages. She felt lonely and missed her family who lived abroad. She had not shared her breast pain with any one, wanting to protect her family from worrying about her. Tears began to fall from Janice's own eyes, as she remembered her mother-in-law lying in a hospice bed when she finally shared the gaping wounds where her own breast cancer had eaten away at her skin. Dread had filled inside Janice then, too, as she knew she was powerless to help her. As Janice hugged Luciana, a shimmer of hope radiated from somewhere in that examination room as she realized she could actually do something to help Luciana. Even though she did not have a background in oncology, Janice knew how to connect her with providers that could further evaluate and manage her breast cancer. Janice showed Luciana the documents that she had carried into the examination room and explained how she could obtain the mammogram at no charge. Janice described the program being offered through the health department and gave her the name of the woman who would now help facilitate the care she needed.

Practice Exemplar cont.

Luciana looked her in the eyes, hopefully empowered by the information Janice had given her, and said "thank you."

Several days later, Janice received the radiologist's report from Luciana's diagnostic mammography. The report confirmed that Luciana did indeed have breast cancer. Fortunately, Sophia, the assistant office manager, had spoken with Jan at the health department and learned Luciana had received Medicaid and was now under the care of an oncologist with experience in treating breast cancer. Luciana returned to the clinic a couple weeks later and expressed her gratitude for their help in getting her the health care she needed. She had started chemotherapy treatment and her mother had come to stay with her to help take care of her children.

Travelbee's concepts are evident in this exemplar. Janice, the nurse practitioner, collected the preliminary patient history and examination findings needed to formulate a diagnosis during the Stage of Observation. However, Janice's interpretation of nonspoken cues and body language led her to the purpose of Luciana's visit and to identify Luciana's fear related to the breast cancer. By identifying barriers to care and existing sources of support for the patient (Concept of Decision-Making), Janice developed a care plan that involved a referral to the health department for access to a state grant available to fund Luciana's mammogram and to a representative with the state Medicaid program for financial assistance with breast cancer treatment (Concept of Action, or Nursing Intervention). By caring for her as a person, Luciana was able to express her story freely and let go of her feelings of powerlessness and fear that had built up inside her since she first noticed her breast pain. The barrier between Janice-as-clinician and Luciana-as-patient blurred as they connected in that examination room, their stories intertwining as they came together as woman-to-woman each affected by breast cancer differently and yet somehow the same (concept of appraisal).

■ Summary

Travelbee's conceptualizations of the human-to-human relationship guide the nurse–patient interaction with an emphasis on helping the patient find hope and meaning in the illness experience. Scientific knowledge and clinical competence are incorporated into Travelbee's concept of therapeutic use of self to effect change in patient-centered care. Patients are viewed as unique, and nursing care is delivered over five stages: observation, interpretation, decision making, action (or nursing intervention), and appraisal (or evaluation).

References

Cook, L. (1989). Nurses in crisis: A support group based on Travelbee's nursing theory. *Nursing and Health Care, 10*(4), 203–205.

Institute of Medicine. (2001). Crossing the quality chasm: A new health system for the 21st Century. Available at: www.iom.edu/Reports/2001/Crossing-the-Quality-Chasm-A-New-Health-System-for-the-21st-Century.aspx

Meleis, A. I. (1997). *Theoretical nursing: Development & progress* (3rd ed.). New York: Lippincott.

Tomey, A. M., & Alligood, M. R. (2006). *Nursing theorists and their work* (6th ed.). St. Louis, MO: Mosby Elsevier.

Travelbee, J. (1963). What do we mean by rapport? *American Journal of Nursing, 63*(2), 70–72.

Travelbee, J. (1964). What's wrong with sympathy? *American Journal of Nursing, 64*(1), 68–71.

Travelbee, J. (1966). *Interpersonal aspects of nursing.* Philadelphia, PA: F. A. Davis.

Travelbee, J. (1969). *Intervention in psychiatric nursing: Process in the one-to-one relationship.* Philadelphia: F.A. Davis.

Travelbee, J. (1971). *Interpersonal aspects of nursing* (2nd ed.). Philadelphia: F. A. Davis.

Travelbee, J. (1972). Speaking out: To find meaning in illness. *Nursing, 2*(12), 6–8.

Introducing the Theorist

Ida Jean Orlando was born in 1926 in New York. Her nursing education began at New York Medical College School of Nursing where she received a diploma in nursing. In 1951, she received a bachelor of science degree in public health nursing from St. John's University in Brooklyn, New York, and in 1954, she completed a master's degree in nursing from Columbia University. Orlando's early nursing practice experience included obstetrics, medicine, and emergency room nursing. Her first book, *The Dynamic Nurse–Patient Relationship: Function, Process and Principles* (1961/1990), was based on her research and blended nursing practice, psychiatric–mental health nursing, and nursing education. It was published when she was director of the graduate program in mental health and psychiatric nursing at Yale University School of Nursing. Ida Jean Orlando passed away November 28, 2007.

Orlando's theoretical work is both practice and research based. She received funding from the National Institute of Mental Health to improve education of nurses about interpersonal relationships. As a consultant at McLean Hospital in Belmont, Massachusetts, Orlando continued to study nursing practice and developed an educational program and nursing service department based on her theory. From evaluation of this program, she published her second book, *The Discipline and Teaching of Nursing Process* (Orlando, 1972; Rittman, 1991).

Overview of Orlando's Theory of the Dynamic Nurse–Patient Relationship

Nursing is responsive to individuals who suffer or anticipate a sense of helplessness; it is focused on the process of care in an immediate experience; it is concerned with providing direct assistance to individuals in whatever setting they are found for the purpose of avoiding, relieving, diminishing or curing the individual's sense of helplessness (Orlando, 1972).

The essence of Orlando's theory, the dynamic nurse–patient relationship, reflects her beliefs that practice should be based on needs of the patient and that communication with the patient is essential to understanding needs and providing effective nursing care. Following is an overview of the major components of Orlando's work:

1. *The nursing process* includes identifying the needs of patients, responses of the nurse, and nursing action. The nursing process, as envisioned and practiced by Orlando, is not the linear model often taught today but is more reflexive and circular and occurs during encounters with patients.
2. *Understanding the meaning* of patient behavior is influenced by the nurse's perceptions, thoughts, and feelings. It may be validated through communication between the nurse and the patient. Patients experience distress when they cannot cope with unmet needs. Nurses use direct and indirect observations of patient behavior to discover distress and meaning.
3. *Nurse–patient interactions* are unique, complex, and dynamic processes. Nurses help patients express and understand the meaning of behavior. The basis for nursing action is the distress experienced and expressed by the patient.
4. *Professional nurses* function in an independent role from physicians and other healthcare providers.

Practice Applications

Orlando's theoretical work was based on analysis of thousands of nurse–patient interactions to describe major attributes of the relationship. Based on this work, her later book provided direction for understanding and using the nursing process (Orlando, 1972). This has been known as the first theory of nursing process and has been widely used in nursing education and practice in the United States and across the globe. Orlando considered her overall work to be a theoretical framework for the practice of professional nursing, emphasizing the essentiality of the nurse–patient relationship. Orlando's theoretical work reveals and bears witness to the essence of nursing as a practice discipline.

Orlando's work has been used as a foundation for master's theses (Grove, 2008; Hendren, 2012). Reinforcing Orlando's theory as a practice and conceptual framework continues to be relevant and applicable to nursing situations in today's healthcare environment.

Laurent (2000) proposed a dynamic leader–follower relationship model using Orlando's dynamic nurse–patient relationship. The dynamic leader-follower relationship model refocuses the nature of "control" through shared responsibility and meaning making, thereby granting the employee or patient the ability to actively engage in resolving the issue or problem at hand. The emphasis is on recognizing in both patient care and management that the person who knows most about the situation is the person himself or herself. To be truly effective in resolving a problem or situation involves engaging in a dynamic relationship of shared responsibility and active participation on the part of both parties (i.e., nurse–patient/nurse manager–employee) without which the true nature of the issue at hand may go unresolved. Laurant (2000) suggested that engaging in a dynamic relationship with the other provides a means by which management of care and/or employees becomes a process of providing direction rather than control, thereby generating nursing leaders in roles of authority rather than just nurse managers of care.

Aponte (2009) employed Orlando's Dynamic Nurse–Patient Relationship as a conceptual framework for the Influenza Initiative in New York City to address the linguistic disparities within communities. A needs survey identified unmet linguistic needs and gaps existing within the city; nursing students, many of whom were bilingual, served as translators for non-English speaking Spanish, Chinese, Russian, and Ukraine residents. Orlando's

theoretical framework was used to describe the communication among the nursing students, homecare nurses, and city residents (Aponte, 2009, p. 326). Dufault et al. (2010) developed a cost-effective, easy-to-use, best practice protocol for nurse-to-nurse shift handoffs at Newport Hospital, using specific components of Orlando's theory of deliberative nursing process. Abraham (2011) proposed addressing fall risk in hospitals using Orlando's conceptualizations. The author asserts that three elements (patient's behavior, nurse's reaction, and anything the nurse does to alleviate the distress) can effectively act as a roadmap for decreasing fall risk.

The New Hampshire Hospital, a university-affiliated psychiatric facility, adopted Orlando's framework for nursing practice (Potter, Vitale-Nolen, & Dawson, 2005; Potter, Williams, & Constanzo, 2004). Two nursing interventions stemmed directly from the adoption of Orlando's ideas. Potter, Williams, and Constanzo (2004) developed a structured group curriculum for nurse-led psychoeducational groups in an inpatient setting. Both nurses and patients demonstrated improved comfort, active involvement and learning from combining Orlando's dynamic nurse–patient relationship and a psychoeducational curriculum with training in group leadership.

Potter, Vitale-Nolen, and Dawson (2005) conducted a quasi-experimental study to determine the effectiveness of implementing a safety agreement tool among patients who threaten self-harm. Orlando's concepts were used to guide the creation of the safety agreement. Results demonstrated that RNs perceived the safety agreements as promoting a more positive and effective nurse–patient relationship related to the risk of self-harm and believed the safety agreements increased their comfort in helping patients at risk for self-harm. The nurses were divided, however, about whether the safety agreements enhanced their relationships with patients, and the majority did not feel the safety agreements decreased self-harming incidents. The rate of self-harm incidents was not statistically significant but the authors report the findings as clinically significant citing no increase in self-harming rates despite higher acuity levels and shorter hospital stays during post implementation stages.

Sheldon and Ellington (2008) conducted a pilot study to expand Orlando's process into sequential steps that further define the deliberative nursing process. The authors used cognitive interviews with a convenience sample of five experienced nurses to gain insight into the process of nurse communication with patients and the strategies nurses use when responding to patient concerns.

Practice Exemplar

Krystal, a 23-year-old woman with a history of asthma, presents to the emergency department with her boyfriend. She states, "I just can't seem to catch my breath, I just can't seem to relax"; appearing extremely agitated. Avoiding eye contact, Krystal fearfully explains to the nurse that she has not been able to obtain any of her regular medications for approximately 4 months. The nurse obtains vital signs including a blood pressure of 113/68; pulse of 98; respiratory rate of 22; an oral temperature of 37.0 degrees Celsius; and an oxygen saturation of 95% on room air. Assessment reveals no increased work of breathing with slight, bilateral, expiratory wheezing. The nurse, employing standing orders, places the patient on 2L of oxygen per nasal cannula and initiates a respiratory treatment.

Seeking privacy with the patient, the nurse kindly asks the boyfriend to wait in the patient lounge. He becomes argumentative and reluctant to leave, the nurse calmly states that she simply needs to complete her assessment with the patient and again asks again for him to wait in the lounge; this time he complies. Further investigation by the nurse reveals that Krystal normally uses albuterol and Advair to control her asthma, but she has been unable to obtain her medications over the past 4 months because of "personal problems."

In this example, the nurse formulates an immediate hypothesis based on direct and indirect observations and attempts to validate this hypothesis by collecting additional data (questioning the patient about her normal medications, observing the boyfriend's reluctance to leave the room, assessing the patient's agitated state and refusal to make eye contact, and obtaining vital signs). From the patient data, the nurse formulates several additional hypotheses about the patient. The nurse may hypothesize that Krystal needs financial assistance in obtaining her medications and additional education about asthma and the role of medications in managing the disease. A nurse not using Orlando's theory might administer the necessary asthma medications; provide asthma education and resources for obtaining free or low cost medications. A nurse using Orlando's theoretical framework, however, understands that no nursing action should be taken without first validating each hypothesis with the patient as a means of determining the patient's immediate needs. The nurse in this situation validates with the patient the source of her anxiety and inability to catch her breath. In doing so, the nurse learns that the patient's concern now is not with her wheezing or obtaining her asthma medication but rather with her boyfriend.

The nurse hypothesizes that Krystal is a victim of intimate partner violence. Again, the nurse seeks to validate this with the patient, asking Krystal if her boyfriend is physically or emotionally harming her. Krystal continues to look fearfully at the door and states, "He is going to kill me if I tell you anything." The nurse assures Krystal that she is in a safe place right now, that she is not alone and that there are safety measures that can be taken to remove the boyfriend from the premises if that would make Krystal feel safer. Krystal requests the nurse to do this and begins crying, telling the nurse she had a fight with her boyfriend today and he hit her. "He always makes sure to hit me where people can't see, and he is always sorry." The nurse asks if Krystal is injured in any way right now. Krystal pulls up her shirt to reveal extensive bruising at various stages of healing to her torso and what looks like several

Practice Exemplar cont.

fresh cigarette burns to both her breasts. The nurse asks Krystal if it would be okay to perform some additional assessments to ensure no further internal injury has occurred. Krystal nods her head yes, and the nurse asks if this has happened before. Krystal tells the nurse that these days it happens almost daily but that she deserves it because she doesn't have a job and he is the only one who loves her. "I want to leave. I really do, but I am afraid he will kill me, and I don't have anywhere else to go." The nurse acknowledges Krystal's distress, clarifying that Krystal does not deserve this type of treatment and that she fears for her safety, emphasizing abuse is a crime and only worsens over time.

At this point, the nurse discusses how the patient wishes to address this concern ensuring there is a dynamic interaction occurring between the patient and the nurse. Offering the patient the resources and opportunity to express and understand the meaning of her own behavior inspires Krystal to find meaning in the experience and ownership in the choices needed to address these concerns. Using her nursing knowledge of domestic abuse, the nurse engages Krystal in a conversation about the cycle of violence and empowers Krystal by providing her with choices and resources to address her current situation. After the nurse–patient interaction, Krystal decides to go to a local domestic abuse shelter for women (the nurse makes arrangements by calling the shelter and providing transportation), to file a police report (the nurse arranges for an officer to come to the hospital), and allow for photos and documentation of her injuries to be charted (documentation follows the guidelines needed to be admissible in a court of law if necessary). The nurse also provides Krystal with the number for the National Resource Center on Domestic Violence, and with two websites one for Violence Against Women Network (www.vawnet.org) and the Florida Coalition Against Domestic Violence (www.fcadv.org). The nurse calls the shelter a few days later to check that Krystal is safe and learns that Krystal will be remaining at the shelter and has not had any further correspondence with her boyfriend.

Through mutual engagement, the patient and nurse were able to create a dynamic environment that fostered effective communication and the ability to address the immediate needs of the patient. Providing asthma education and financial resources would not have addressed Krystal's need for physical safety related to domestic abuse because the plan would have been based on an invalid hypothesis. The nurse in this situation used her perception and knowledge of the nursing situation to explore the meaning of Krystal's behavior. Through communication and validation with the patient of the nurses' hypotheses, perceptions and supporting data, the nurse was able to elicit the nature of the patient's problem and mutually engage the patient in identifying what help was needed. After mutual decision making, the nurse took deliberative nursing actions to meet Krystal's immediate needs including initiating safety protocols, providing resources, gathering additional data, and creating a supportive and encouraging environment for the patient.

Summary

The most important contribution of Orlando's theoretical work is the primacy of the nurse–client relationship. Inherent in this theory is a strong statement: What transpires between the patient and the nurse is of the highest value. The true worth of her ideas is that it clearly states what nursing is or should be today. Regardless of the changes in the health-care system, the human transaction between the nurse and the patient in any setting holds the greatest value —not only for nursing, but also for society at large. Orlando's writings can serve as a philosophy as well as a theory, because it is the foundation on which our profession has been built. With all of the benefits that modern technology and modern health care bring—and there are many—we need to pause and ask the question, What is at risk in health care today? The answer to that question may lead to reconsideration of the value of Orlando's theory as perhaps the critical link for enhancing relationships between nursing and patient today (Rittman, 1991).

References

Abraham, S. (2011). Fall prevention conceptual framework. *The Health Care Manager, 30*(2), 179–184. doi: 10.1097/HCM.0b013e31826fb74

Aponte, J. (2009). Meeting the linguistic needs of urban communities. *Home Health Nurse, 27*(5), 324–329.

Dufault, M., Duquette, C. E., Ehmann, J., Hehl, R., Lavin, M., Martin, V., Moore, M. A., Sargent, S., Stout, P., Willey, C. (2010). Translating an evidence-based protocol for nurse-to-nurse shift handoffs. *Worldviews on Evidence-Based Nursing, 7*(2), 59–75.

Grove, C. (2008). *Staff intervention to improve patient satisfaction* (master's thesis). Retrieved from ProQuest Dissertations and Theses database. (UMI 1454183)

Hendren, D. W. (2012). *Emergency departments and STEMI care, are the guidelines being followed?* (master's thesis). Retrieved from ProQuest Dissertations and Theses database. (UMI 1520156)

Laurent, C. L. (2000). A nursing theory of nursing leadership. *Journal of Nursing Management, 8,* 83–87.

Orlando, I. J. (1990). *The dynamic nurse–patient relationship: Function, process and principles.* New York: National League for Nursing New York: G. P. Putnam's Sons. (Original work published 1961)

Orlando, I. J. (1972). *The discipline and teaching of nursing process: An evaluative study.* New York: G. P. Putnam's Sons.

Potter, M. L., Vitale-Nolen, R., & Dawson, A. M. (2005). Implementation of safety agreements in an acute psychiatric facility. *Journal of the American Psychiatric Nurses Association, 11*(3), 144–155. doi: 10.1177/1078390305277443

Potter, M. L., Williams, R. B. & Costanzo, R. (2004). Using nursing theory and structured psychoeducational curriculum with inpatient groups. *Journal of the American Psychiatric Nurses Association, 10*(3), 122–128. doi: 10.1177/1078390304265212

Rittman, M. R. (1991). Ida Jean Orlando (Pelletier)—the dynamic nurse–patient relationship. In: M. Parker (Ed.), *Nursing theories and nursing practice* (pp. 125–130). Philadelphia: F. A. Davis.

Sheldon, L. K., & Ellington, L. (2008). Application of a model of social information processing to nursing theory: How nurses respond to patients. *Journal of Advanced Nursing 64*(4), 388–398. doi: 10.111/j.1365-2648.2008.04795.x

III

Conceptual Models/Grand Theories in the Integrative-Interactive Paradigm

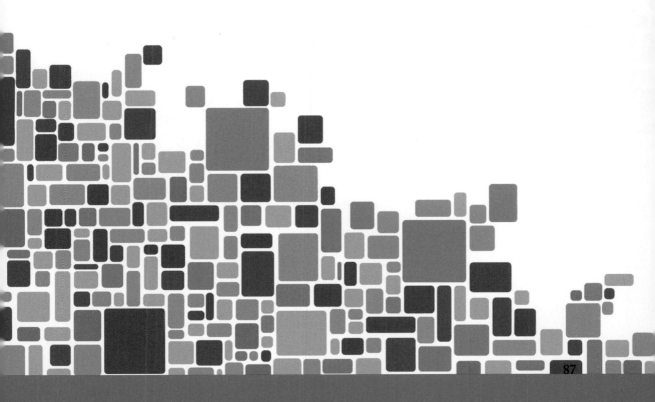

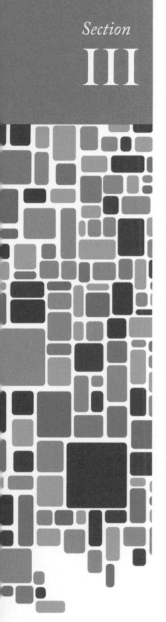

Section

III

Section III includes seven chapters on the conceptual models or grand theories situated in the integrative-interactive nursing paradigm. These chapters are written by either the theorist or an author designated as an authority on the theory by the theorist or the community of scholars advancing that theory. Theories in the integrative-interactive paradigm view persons[1] as integrated wholes or integrated systems interacting with the larger environmental system. The integrated dimensions of the person are influenced by environmental factors leading to some change that impacts health or well-being. The subjectivity of the person and the multidimensional nature of any outcome are considered. Most of the theories are based explicitly on a systems perspective.

In Chapter 7, Johnson's behavioral systems model is described. It includes principles of wholeness and order, stabilization, reorganization, hierarchic interaction, and dialectic contradiction. The person is viewed as a compilation of subsystems. According to Johnson, the goal of nursing is to restore, maintain, or attain behavioral system balance and stability at the highest possible level.

Chapter 8 features Orem's self-care deficit nursing theory, a conceptual model with four interrelated theories associated with it: theory of nursing systems, theory of self-care deficit, and the theory of self-care and theory of dependent care. According to Orem, when requirements for self-care exceed capacity for self-care, self-care deficits occur. Nursing systems are designed to address these self-care deficits.

King's theory of goal attainment presented in Chapter 9 offers a view that the goal of nursing is to help persons maintain health or regain health. This is accomplished through a transaction, setting a mutually agreed-upon goal with the patient.

In Chapter 10, Pamela Senesac and Sr. Callista Roy describe the Roy adaptation model and its applications. In this model, the person is viewed as a holistic adaptive system with coping processes to maintain adaptation and promote person–environment transformations. The adaptive system can be integrated, compensatory, or compromised depending on the level of adaptation. Nurses promote coping and adaptation within health and illness.

Lois White Lowry and Patricia Deal Aylward authored Chapter 12 on Neuman's systems model. The model includes the client–client system with a basic structure protected from stressors by lines of defense and resistance. The concern of nursing is to keep the client stable by assessing the actual or potential effects of stressors and assisting client adjustments for optimal wellness.

In Chapter 13, Erickson, Tomlin, and Swain's modeling and role modeling theory is presented by Helen Erickson. Modeling and role modeling theory provides a guide for the practice or process of nursing. The theory integrates a holistic philosophy with concepts from a variety of theoretical perspectives such as adaptation, need status, and developmental task resolution.

The final chapter in this section is Dossey's theory of integral nursing, a relatively new grand theory that posits an integral worldview and body–mind–spirit connectedness. The theory is informed by a variety of ideas including Nightingale's tenets, holism, multidimensionality, spiral dynamics, chaos theory, and complexity. It includes the major concepts of healing, the metaparadigm of nursing, patterns of knowing, and Wilber's integral theory and Wilber's all quadrants, all levels, all lines.

---

[1] Person refers to individuals, families, groups or communities.

Chapter 7

Dorothy Johnson's Behavioral System Model and Its Applications

BONNIE HOLADAY

Introducing the Theorist
Overview of Johnson's Behavioral
System Model
Applications of the Model
Practice Exemplar by Kelly White
Summary
References

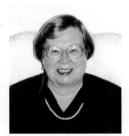

Dorothy Johnson

Introducing the Theorist

Dorothy Johnson's earliest publications pertained to the knowledge base nurses needed for nursing care (Johnson, 1959, 1961). Throughout her career, Johnson (1919–1999) stressed that nursing had a unique, independent contribution to health care that was distinct from "delegated medical care." Johnson was one of the first "grand theorists" to present her views as a conceptual model. Her model was the first to provide a guide to both understanding and action. These two ideas—understanding seen first as a holistic, behavioral system process mediated by a complex framework and second as an active process of encounter and response—are central to the work of other theorists who followed her lead and developed conceptual models for nursing practice.

Dorothy Johnson received her associate of arts degree from Armstrong Junior College in Savannah, Georgia, in 1938 and her bachelor of science in nursing degree from Vanderbilt University in 1942. She practiced briefly as a staff nurse at the Chatham-Savannah Health Council before attending Harvard University, where she received her master of public health in 1948. She began her academic career at Vanderbilt University School of Nursing. A call from Lulu Hassenplug, Dean of the School of Nursing, enticed her to the University of California at Los Angeles in 1949. She served there as an assistant, associate, and professor of pediatric nursing until her retirement in 1978. Johnson is recognized as one of the founders of modern systems-based nursing theory (Glennister, 2011; Meleis, 2011).

89

During her academic career, Dorothy Johnson addressed issues related to nursing practice, education, and science. While she was a pediatric nursing advisor at the Christian Medical College School of Nursing in Vellare, South India, she wrote a series of clinical articles for the *Nursing Journal of India* (Johnson, 1956, 1957). She worked with the California Nurses' Association, the National League for Nursing, and the American Nurses' Association to examine the role of the clinical nurse specialist, the scope of nursing practice, and the need for nursing research. She also completed a Public Health Service–funded research project ("Crying as a Physiologic State in the Newborn Infant") in 1963 (Johnson & Smith, 1963). The foundations of her model and her beliefs about nursing are clearly evident in these early publications.

Overview of Johnson's Behavioral System Model

Johnson noted that her theory, the Johnson behavioral system model (JBSM), evolved from philosophical ideas, theory, and research; her clinical background; and many years of thought, discussions, and writing (Johnson, 1968). She cited a number of sources for her theory. From Florence Nightingale came the belief that nursing's concern is a focus on the person rather than the disease. Systems theorists (Buckley, 1968; Chin, 1961; Parsons & Shils, 1951; Rapoport, 1968; Von Bertalanffy, 1968) were all sources for her model. Johnson's background as a pediatric nurse is also evident in the development of her model. In her papers, Johnson cited developmental literature to support the validity of a behavioral system model (Ainsworth, 1964; Crandal, 1963; Gerwitz, 1972; Kagan, 1964; Sears, Maccoby, & Levin, 1954). Johnson also noted that a number of her subsystems had biological underpinnings.

Johnson's theory and her related writings reflect her knowledge about both development and general systems theories. The combination of nursing, development, and general systems introduces some of the specifics into the rhetoric about nursing theory development that make it possible to test hypotheses and conduct critical experiments.

Five Core Principles

Johnson's model incorporates five core principles of system thinking: wholeness and order, stabilization, reorganization, hierarchic interaction, and dialectical contradiction. Each of these general systems principles has analogs in developmental theories that Johnson used to verify the validity of her model (Johnson, 1980, 1990). Wholeness and order provide the basis for continuity and identity, stabilization for development, reorganization for growth and/or change, hierarchic interaction for discontinuity, and dialectical contradiction for motivation. Johnson conceptualized a person as an open system with organized, interrelated, and interdependent subsystems. By virtue of subsystem interaction and independence, the whole of the human organism (system) is greater than the sum of its parts (subsystems). Wholes and their parts create a system with dual constraints: Neither has continuity and identity without the other.

The overall representation of the model can also be viewed as a behavioral system within an environment. The behavioral system and the environment are linked by interactions and transactions. We define the person (behavioral system) as comprising subsystems and the environment as comprising physical, interpersonal (e.g., father, friend, mother, sibling), and sociocultural (e.g., rules and mores of home, school, country, and other cultural contexts) components that supply the sustenal imperatives (Grubbs, 1980; Holaday, 1997; Johnson, 1990; Meleis, 2011). Sustenal imperatives are the necessary prerequisites for the optimal functioning of the behavioral system. The environment must supply the sustenal imperatives of protection, nurturance, and stimulation to all subsystems to allow them to develop and to maintain stability. Some examples of conditions that protect, stimulate, and nurture related to achievement would include encouragement from parents and peers; enriched, stimulating environments, awards and recognition; and increased autonomy and responsibility.

Wholeness and Order

The developmental analogy of wholeness and order is continuity and identity. Given the behavioral system's potential for plasticity, a basic feature of the system is that both continuity and change can exist across the life span. The presence of or potentiality for at least some plasticity means that the key way of casting the issue of continuity is not a matter of deciding what exists for a given process or function of a subsystem. Instead, the issue should be cast in terms of determining patterns of interactions among levels of the behavioral system that may promote continuity for a particular subsystem at a given point in time. Johnson's work implies that continuity is in the relationship of the parts rather than in their individuality. Johnson (1990) noted that at the psychological level, attachment (affiliation) and dependency are examples of important specific behaviors that change over time, although the representation (meaning) may remain the same. Johnson stated: "[D]evelopmentally, dependence behavior in the socially optimum case evolves from almost total dependence on others to a greater degree of dependence on self, with a certain amount of interdependence essential to the survival of social groups" (1990, p. 28). In terms of behavioral system balance, this pattern of dependence to independence may be repeated as the behavioral system engages in new situations during the course of a lifetime.

Stabilization

Stabilization or behavioral system balance is another core principle of the JBSM. Dynamic systems respond to contextual changes by either a homeostatic or homeorhetic process. Systems have a set point (like a thermostat) that they try to maintain by altering internal conditions to compensate for changes in external conditions. Human thermoregulation is an example of a homeostatic process that is primarily biological but is also behavioral (turning on the heater). The use of attribution of ability or effort is a behavioral homeostatic process we use to interpret activities so that they are consistent with our mental organization.

From a behavioral system perspective, homeorhesis is a more important stabilizing process than is homeostasis. In homeorhesis, the system stabilizes around a trajectory rather than a set point. A toddler placed in a body cast may show motor lags when the cast is removed but soon show age-appropriate motor skills. An adult newly diagnosed with asthma who does not receive proper education until a year after diagnosis can successfully incorporate the material into her daily activities. These are examples of homeorhetic processes or self-righting tendencies that can occur over time.

What nurses observe as development or adaptation of the behavioral system is a product of stabilization. When a person is ill or threatened with illness, he or she is subject to biopsychosocial perturbations. The nurse, according to Johnson (1980, 1990), acts as the external regulator and monitors patient response, looking for successful adaptation to occur. If behavioral system balance returns, there is no need for intervention. If not, the nurse intervenes to help the patient restore behavioral system balance. It is hoped that the patient matures and with additional hospitalizations, the previous patterns of response have been assimilated, and there are few disturbances.

Reorganization

Adaptive reorganization occurs when the behavioral system encounters new experiences in the environment that cannot be balanced by existing system mechanisms. Adaptation is defined as change that permits the behavioral system to maintain its set points best in new situations. To the extent that the behavioral system cannot assimilate the new conditions with existing regulatory mechanisms, accommodation must occur either as a new relationship between subsystems or by the establishment of a higher order or different cognitive schema (set, choice). The nurse acts to provide conditions or resources essential to help the accommodation process, may impose regulatory or control mechanisms to stimulate or reinforce certain behaviors, or may attempt to repair structural components (Johnson, 1980). If the focus is on a structural part of the subsystem, then the nurse will focus on the goal, set, choice, or action of a specific subsystem. The nurse might provide an educational intervention to alter the client's set and broaden the range of choices available.

The difference between stabilization and reorganization is that the latter involves change or evolution. A behavioral system is embedded in an environment, but it is capable of operating independently of environmental constraints through the process of adaptation. The diagnosis of a chronic illness, the birth of a child, or the development of a healthy lifestyle regimen to prevent problems in later years are all examples in which accommodation not only promotes behavioral system balance but also involves a developmental process that results in the establishment of a higher order or more complex behavioral system.

Hierarchic Interaction

Each behavioral system exists in a context of hierarchical relationships and environmental relationships. From the perspective of general systems theory, a behavioral system that has the properties of wholeness and order, stabilization, and reorganization will also demonstrate a hierarchic structure (Buckley, 1968). Hierarchies, or a pattern of relying on particular subsystems, lead to a degree of stability. A disruption or failure will not destroy the whole system but instead will lead to decomposition to the next level of stability.

The judgment that a discontinuity has occurred is typically based on a lack of correlation between assessments at two points of time. For example, one's lifestyle before surgery is not a good fit postoperatively. These discontinuities can provide opportunities for reorganization and development.

Dialectical Contradiction

The last core principle is the motivational force for behavioral change. Johnson (1980) described these as drives and noted that these responses are developed and modified over time through maturation, experience, and learning. A person's activities in the environment lead to knowledge and development. However, by acting on the world, each person is constantly changing it and his or her goals, and therefore changing what he or she needs to know. The number of environmental domains that the person is responding to includes the biological, psychological, cultural, familial, social, and physical setting. The person needs to resolve (maintain behavioral system balance of) a cascade of contradictions between goals related to physical status, social roles, and cognitive status when faced with illness or the threat of illness. Nurses' interventions during these periods can make a significant difference in the lives of the persons involved because the nurse can help clients compare opposing propositions and make decisions. Dealing with these contradictions can be viewed as the "driving force" of development as resolution brings about a higher level of understanding of the issue at hand. This may also alter the persons set, choice and action. Behavioral system balance is restored and a new level of development is attained.

Johnson's model is unique in part because it takes from both general systems and developmental theories. One may analyze the patient's response in terms of behavioral system balance and, from a developmental perspective, ask, "Where did this come from, and where is it going?" The developmental component necessitates that we identify and understand the processes of stabilization and sources of disturbances that lead to reorganization. These need to be evaluated by age, gender, and culture. The combination of systems theory and development identifies "nursing's unique social mission and our special realm of original responsibility in patient care" (Johnson, 1990, p. 32).

Major Concepts of the Model

Next, we review the model as a behavioral system within an environment.

Person

Johnson conceptualized a nursing client as a behavioral system. The behavioral system is orderly, repetitive, and organized with interrelated and interdependent biological and behavioral subsystems. **The client is seen as a collection of behavioral subsystems that interrelate to form the behavioral system.** The system may be defined as "those complex, overt actions or responses to a variety of stimuli present in the surrounding environment that are purposeful and functional" (Auger, 1976, p. 22). These ways of behaving form an organized and integrated functional unit that determines

Table 7 · 1 The Subsystems of Behavior

Achievement Subsystem

Goal	Mastery or control of self or the environment
Function	To set appropriate goals
	To direct behaviors toward achieving a desired goal
	To perceive recognition from others
	To differentiate between immediate goals and long-term goals
	To interpret feedback (input received) to evaluate the achievement of goals

Affiliative Subsystem

Goal	To relate or belong to someone or something other than oneself; to achieve intimacy and inclusion
Function	To form cooperative and interdependent role relationships within human social systems
	To develop and use interpersonal skills to achieve intimacy and inclusion
	To share
	To be related to another in a definite way
	To use narcissistic feelings in an appropriate way

Aggressive/Protective Subsystem

Goal	To protect self or others from real or imagined threatening objects, persons, or ideas; to achieve self-protection and self-assertion
Function	To recognize biological, environmental, or health systems that are potential threats to self or others
	To mobilize resources to respond to challenges identified as threats
	To use resources or feedback mechanisms to alter biological, environmental, or health input or human responses in order to diminish threats to self or others
	To protect one's achievement goals
	To protect one's beliefs
	To protect one's identity or self-concept

Dependency Subsystem

Goal	To obtain focused attention, approval, nurturance, and physical assistance; to maintain the environmental resources needed for assistance; to gain trust and reliance
Function	To obtain approval, reassurance about self
	To make others aware of self
	To induce others to care for physical needs
	To evolve from a state of total dependence on others to a state of increased dependence on the self
	To recognize and accept situations requiring reversal of self-dependence (dependence on others)
	To focus on another or oneself in relation to social, psychological, and cultural needs and desires

Eliminative Subsystem

Goal	To expel biological wastes; to externalize the internal biological environment
Function	To recognize and interpret input from the biological system that signals readiness for waste excretion
	To maintain physiological homeostasis through excretion
	To adjust to alterations in biological capabilities related to waste excretion while maintaining a sense of control over waste excretion
	To relieve feelings of tension in the self
	To express one's feelings, emotions, and ideas verbally or nonverbally

Continued

Table 7 · 1 **The Subsystems of Behavior—cont'd**

Ingestive Subsystem

Goal	To take in needed resources from the environment to maintain the integrity of the organism or to achieve a state of pleasure; to internalize the external environment
Function	To sustain life through nutritive intake To alter ineffective patterns of nutritive intake To relieve pain or other psychophysiological subsystems To obtain knowledge or information useful to the self To obtain physical and/or emotional pleasure from intake of nutritive or nonnutritive substances

Restorative Subsystem

Goal	To relieve fatigue and/or achieve a state of equilibrium by reestablishing or replenishing the energy distribution among the other subsystems; to redistribute energy
Function	To maintain and/or return to physiological homeostasis To produce relaxation of the self system

Sexual Subsystem

Goal	To procreate, to gratify or attract; to fulfill expectations associated with one's gender; to care for others and to be cared about by them
Function	To develop a self-concept or self-identity based on gender To project an image of oneself as a sexual being To recognize and interpret biological system input related to sexual gratification and/or procreation To establish meaningful relationships in which sexual gratification and/or procreation may be obtained

Sources: Based on J. Grubbs (1980). An interpretation of the Johnson behavioral system model. In J. P. Riehl & C. Roy (Eds.), *Conceptual models for nursing practice* (2nd ed., pp. 217–254). New York: Appleton-Century-Crofts; D. E. Johnson (1980). The behavioral system model for nursing. In J. P. Riehl & C. Roy (Eds.), *Conceptual models for nursing practice* (2nd ed., pp. 207–216). New York: Appleton-Century-Crofts; D. Wilkie (1987). *Operationalization of the JBSM.* Unpublished paper, University of California, San Francisco; and B. Holaday (1972). *Operationalization of the JBSM.* Unpublished paper, University of California, Los Angeles.

and limits the interaction between the person and environment and establishes the relationship of the person to the objects, events, and situations in the environment. Johnson (1980, p. 209) considered such "behavior to be orderly, purposeful and predictable; that is, it is functionally efficient and effective most of the time, and is sufficiently stable and recurrent to be amenable to description and exploration."

Subsystems

The parts of the behavioral system are called subsystems. They carry out specialized tasks or functions needed to maintain the integrity of the whole behavioral system and manage its relationship to the environment. Each of these subsystems has a set of behavioral responses that is developed and modified through motivation, experience, and learning.

Johnson identified seven subsystems. However, in this author's operationalization of the model, as in Grubbs (1980), I have included eight subsystems. These eight subsystems and their goals and functions are described in Table 7-1. Johnson noted that these subsystems are found cross-culturally and across a broad range of the phylogenetic scale. She also noted the significance of social and cultural factors involved in the development of the subsystems. She did not consider the seven subsystems as complete, because "the ultimate group of response systems to be identified in the behavioral system will undoubtedly change as research reveals new subsystems or indicated changes in the structure, functions, or behavioral groupings in the original set" (Johnson, 1980, p. 214).

Each subsystem has functions that serve to meet the conceptual goal. Functional behaviors are the activities carried out to meet these goals. These behaviors may vary with each individual, depending on the person's age, sex, motives, cultural values, social norms, and self-concepts. For the subsystem goals to be accomplished, behavioral system structural components must meet functional requirements of the behavioral system.

Each subsystem is composed of at least four structural components that interact in a specific pattern: goal, set, choice, and action. The goal of a subsystem is defined as the desired result or consequence of the behavior. The basis for the goal is a universal drive that can be shown to exist through scientific research. In general, the drive of each subsystem is the same for all people, but there are variations among individuals (and within individuals over time) in the specific objects or events that are drive-fulfilling, in the value placed on goal attainment, and in drive strength. With drives as the impetus for the behavior, goals can be identified and are considered universal.

The behavioral set is a predisposition to act in a certain way in a given situation. The behavioral set represents a relatively stable and habitual behavioral pattern of responses to particular drives or stimuli. It is learned behavior and is influenced by knowledge, attitudes, and beliefs. The set contains two components: perseveration and preparation. The perseveratory set refers to a consistent tendency to react to certain stimuli with the same pattern of behavior. The preparatory set is contingent on the function of the perseveratory set. The preparatory set functions to establish priorities for attending or not attending to various stimuli.

The conceptual set is an additional component to the model (Holaday, 1982). It is a process of ordering that serves as the mediating link between stimuli from the preparatory and perseveratory sets. Here attitudes, beliefs, information, and knowledge are examined before a choice is made. There are three levels of processing—an inadequate conceptual set, a developing conceptual set, and a sophisticated conceptual set.

The third and fourth components of each subsystem are choice and action. Choice refers to the individual's repertoire of alternative

behaviors in a situation that will best meet the goal and attain the desired outcome. The larger the behavioral repertoire of alternative behaviors in a situation, the more adaptable is the individual. The fourth structural component of each subsystem is the observable action of the individual. The concern is with the efficiency and effectiveness of the behavior in goal attainment. Actions are any observable responses to stimuli.

For the eight subsystems to develop and maintain stability, each must have a constant supply of functional requirements (sustenal imperatives). The concept of functional requirements tends to be confined to conditions of the system's survival, and it includes biological as well as psychosocial needs. The problems are related to establishing the types of functional requirements (universal vs. highly specific) and finding procedures for validating the assumptions of these requirements. It also suggests a classification of the various states or processes on the basis of some principle and perhaps the establishment of a hierarchy among them. The Johnson model proposes that for the behavior to be maintained, it must be protected, nurtured, and stimulated: It requires protection from noxious stimuli that threaten the survival of the behavioral system; nurturance, which provides adequate input to sustain behavior; and stimulation, which contributes to continued growth of the behavior and counteracts stagnation. A deficiency in any or all of these functional requirements threatens the behavioral system as a whole, or the effective functioning of the particular subsystem with which it is directly involved.

Environment

In systems theory, the term *environment* is defined as the set of all objects for which a change in attributes will affect the system as well as those objects whose attributes are changed by the behavior of the system (von Bertalanffy, 1968). Johnson referred to the internal and external environment of the system. She also referred to the interaction between the person and the environment and to the objects, events, and situations in the environment. She further noted that there are forces in the environment that impinge on the person and to which the person adjusts. Thus, the JBSM environment consists of all elements that are not a part of the individual's behavioral system but that influence the system and can also serve as a source of sustenal imperatives. Some of these elements can be manipulated by the nurse to achieve health (behavioral system balance or stability) for the patient. Johnson provided no other specific definition of the environment, nor did she identify what she considered internal versus external environment. But much can be inferred from her writings, and system theory also provides additional insights into the environment component of the model.

The external environment may include people, objects, and phenomena that can potentially permeate the boundary of the behavioral system. This external stimulus forms an organized or meaningful pattern that elicits a response from the individual. The behavioral system attempts to maintain equilibrium in response to environmental factors by assimilating and accommodating to the forces that impinge on it. Areas of external environment of interest to nurses include the physical settings, people, objects, phenomena, and psychosocial–cultural attributes of an environment.

Johnson provided detailed information about the internal structure and how it functions. She also noted that "[i]llness or other sudden internal or external environmental change is most frequently responsible for system malfunction" (Johnson, 1980, p. 212). Such factors as physiology; temperament; ego; age; and related developmental capacities, attitudes, and self-concept are general regulators that may be viewed as a class of internalized intervening variables that influence set, choice, and action. They are key areas for nursing assessment. For example, a nurse attempting to respond to the needs of an acutely ill hospitalized 6-year-old would need to know something about the developmental capacities of a 6-year-old and about self-concept and ego development to understand the child's behavior.

Health

Johnson viewed health as efficient and effective functioning of the system and as behavioral

system balance and stability. Behavioral system balance and stability are demonstrated by observed behavior that is purposeful, orderly, and predictable. Such behavior is maintained when it is efficient and effective in managing the person's relationship to the environment.

Behavior changes when efficiency and effectiveness are no longer evident or when a more optimal level of functioning is perceived. Individuals are said to achieve efficient and effective behavioral functioning when their behavior is commensurate with social demands, when they are able to modify their behavior in ways that support biological imperatives, when they are able to benefit to the fullest extent during illness from the physician's knowledge and skill, and when their behavior does not reveal unnecessary trauma as a consequence of illness (Johnson, 1980, p. 207).

Behavior system imbalance and instability are not described explicitly but can be inferred from the following statement to be a malfunction of the behavioral system:

The subsystems and the system as a whole tend to be self-maintaining and self-perpetuating so long as conditions in the internal and external environment of the system remain orderly and predictable, the conditions and resources necessary to their functional requirements are met, and the interrelationships among the subsystems are harmonious. If these conditions are not met, malfunction becomes apparent in behavior that is in part disorganized, erratic, and dysfunctional. Illness or other sudden internal or external environmental change is most frequently responsible for such malfunctions. (Johnson, 1980, p. 212)

Thus, Johnson equated behavioral system imbalance and instability with illness. However, as Meleis (2011) has pointed out, we must consider that illness may be separate from behavioral system functioning. Johnson also referred to physical and social health but did not specifically define wellness. Just as the inference about illness may be made, it may be inferred that wellness is behavioral system balance and stability, as well as efficient and effective behavioral functioning.

Nursing and Nursing Therapeutics

Nursing is viewed as "a service that is complementary to that of medicine and other health professions, but which makes its own distinctive contribution to the health and well-being of people" (Johnson, 1980, p. 207). She distinguished nursing from medicine by noting that nursing views the patient as a behavioral system, and medicine views the patient as a biological system. In her view, the specific goal of nursing action is "to restore, maintain, or attain behavioral system balance and stability at the highest possible level for the individual" (Johnson, 1980, p. 214). This goal may be expanded to include helping the person achieve an optimal level of balance and functioning when this is possible and desired.

The goal of the system's action is behavioral system balance. For the nurse, the area of concern is a behavioral system threatened by the loss of order and predictability through illness or the threat of illness. The goal of a nurse's action is to maintain or restore the individual's behavioral system balance and stability or to help the individual achieve a more optimal level of balance and functioning.

Johnson did not specify the steps of the nursing process but clearly identified the role of the nurse as an external regulatory force. She also identified questions to be asked when analyzing system functioning, and she provided diagnostic classifications to delineate disturbances and guidelines for interventions.

Johnson (1980) expected the nurse to base judgments about behavioral system balance and stability on knowledge and an explicit value system. One important point she made about the value system is that

> given that the person has been provided with an adequate understanding of the potential for and means to obtain a more optimal level of behavioral functioning than is evident at the present time, the final judgment of the desired level of functioning is the right of the individual. (Johnson, 1980, p. 215)

The source of difficulty arises from structural and functional stresses. Structural and functional problems develop when the system is unable to meet its own functional requirements. As a result of the inability to meet functional requirements, structural impairments may take place. In addition, functional stress may be found as a result of structural damage or from the dysfunctional consequences of the behavior. Other problems develop when the system's control and regulatory mechanisms fail to develop or become defective.

Four diagnostic classifications to delineate these disturbances are differentiated in the model. A disorder originating within any one subsystem is classified as either an insufficiency, which exists when a subsystem is not functioning or developed to its fullest capacity due to inadequacy of functional requirements, or as a discrepancy, which exists when a behavior does not meet the intended conceptual goal. Disorders found between more than one subsystem are classified either as an incompatibility, which exists when the behaviors of two or more subsystems in the same situation conflict with each other to the detriment of the individual, or as dominance, which exists when the behavior of one subsystem is used more than any other, regardless of the situation or to the detriment of the other subsystems. This is also an area where Johnson believed additional diagnostic classifications would be developed. Nursing therapeutics address these three areas.

The next critical element is the nature of the interventions the nurse would use to respond to the behavioral system imbalance. The first step is a thorough assessment to find the source of the difficulty or the origin of the problem. There are at least three types of interventions that the nurse can use to bring about change. The nurse may attempt to repair damaged structural units by altering the individual's set and choice. The second would be for the nurse to impose regulatory and control measures. The nurse acts outside the patient environment to provide the conditions, resources, and controls necessary to restore behavioral system balance. The nurse also acts within and upon the external environment and the internal interactions of the subsystem to create change and restore stability. The third, and most common, treatment modality is to supply or to help the client find his or her own supplies of essential functional requirements. The nurse may provide nurturance (resources and conditions necessary for survival and growth; the nurse may train the client to cope with new stimuli and encourage effective behaviors), stimulation (provision of stimuli that brings forth new behaviors or increases behaviors, provides motivation for a particular behavior, and provides opportunities for appropriate behaviors), and protection (safeguarding from noxious stimuli, defending from unnecessary threats, and coping with a threat on the individual's behalf). The nurse and the client negotiate the treatment plan.

Applications of the Model

Fundamental to any professional discipline is the development of a scientific body of knowledge that can be used to guide its practice. JBSM has served as a means for identifying, labeling, and classifying phenomena important to the nursing discipline. Nurses have used the JBSM model since the early 1970s, and the model has demonstrated its ability to provide a medium for theoretical growth; organization for nurses' thinking, observations, and interpretations of what was observed; a systematic structure and rationale for activities; direction to the search for relevant research questions; solutions for patient care problems; and, finally, criteria to determine whether a problem has been solved.

Practice-Focused Research

Stevenson and Woods (1986) stated: "Nursing science is the domain of knowledge concerned with the adaptation of individuals and groups to actual or potential health problems, the environments that influence health in humans and the therapeutic interventions that promote health and affect the consequences of illness" (1986, p. 6). This position focuses efforts in nursing science on the expansion of knowledge about clients' health problems and nursing therapeutics. Nurse researchers have demonstrated the usefulness of Johnson's model in a

clinical practice in a variety of ways. The majority of the research focuses on clients' functioning in terms of maintaining or restoring behavioral system balance, understanding the system and/or subsystems by focusing on the basic sciences, or focusing on the nurse as an agent of action who uses the JBSM to gather diagnostic data or to provide care that influences behavioral system balance.

Derdiarian (1990, 1991) examined the nurse as an action agent within the practice domain. She focused on the nurses' assessment of the patient using the JBSM and the effect of using this instrument on the quality of care (Derdiarian, 1990, 1991). This approach expanded the view of nursing knowledge from exclusively client-based to knowledge about the context and practice of nursing that is model-based. The results of these studies found a significant increase in patient and nurse satisfaction when the JBSM was used. Derdiarian (1983, 1988; Derdiarian & Forsythe, 1983) also found that a model-based, valid, and reliable instrument could improve the comprehensiveness and the quality of assessment data; the method of assessment; and the quality of nursing diagnosis, interventions, and outcome. Derdiarian's body of work reflects the complexity of nursing's knowledge as well as the strategic problem-solving capabilities of the JBSM. Her 1991 article in *Nursing Administration Quarterly* demonstrated the clear relationship between Johnson's theory and nursing practice.

Others have demonstrated the utility of Johnson's model for clinical practice. Tamilarasi and Kanimozhi (2009) used the JBSM to develop interventions to improve the quality of life of breast cancer survivors. Oyedele (2010) used the JBSM to develop and test nursing interventions to prevent teen pregnancy in South African teens. Box 7-1 highlights other JBSM research. Talerico (1999) found that the JBSM demonstrated utility in accounting for differences in the expression of aggressive behavioral actions in elders with dementia in a way that the biomedical model has proved unable. Wang and Palmer (2010) used the JBSM to gain a better understanding of women's toileting behavior, and Colling, Owen, McCreedy,

Box 7-1	**Bonnie Holaday's Research Highlighted**

My program of research has examined normal and atypical patterns of behavior of children with a chronic illness and the behavior of their parents and the interrelationship between the children and the environment. My goal was to determine the causes of instability within and between subsystems (e.g., breakdown in internal regulatory or control mechanisms) and to identify the source of problems in behavioral system balance.

and Newman (2003) used it to study the effectiveness of a continence program for frail elders. Poster, Dee, and Randell (1997) found the JBSM was an effective framework to evaluate patient outcomes.

Education

Johnson's model was used as the basis for undergraduate education at the UCLA School of Nursing. The curriculum was developed by the faculty; however, no published material is available that describes this process. Texts by Wu (1973) and Auger (1976) extended Johnson's model and provided some idea of the content of that curriculum. Later, in the 1980s, Harris (1986) described the use of Johnson's theory as a framework for UCLA's curriculum. The Universities of Hawaii, Alaska, and Colorado also used the JBSM as a basis for their undergraduate curricula.

Loveland-Cherry and Wilkerson (1983) analyzed Johnson's model and concluded that the model could be used to develop a curriculum. The primary focus of the program would be the study of the person as a behavioral system. The student would need a background in systems theory and in the biological, psychological, sociological sciences, and genetics. The mapping of the human genome and clinical exome and genome sequencing has provided evidence that genes serve as general regulators of behavioral system activity.

Nursing Practice and Administration

Johnson has influenced nursing practice because she enabled nurses to make statements about the links between nursing input and health outcomes for clients. The model has been useful in practice because it identifies an end product (behavioral system balance), which is nursing's goal. **Nursing's specific objective is to maintain or restore the person's behavioral system balance and stability, or to help the person achieve a more optimum level of functioning.** The model provides a means for identifying the source of the problem in the system. Nursing is seen as the external regulatory force that acts to restore balance (Johnson, 1980).

One of the best examples of the model's use in practice has been at the University of California, Los Angeles, Neuropsychiatric Institute. Auger and Dee (1983) designed a patient classification system using the JBSM. Each subsystem of behavior was operationalized in terms of critical adaptive and maladaptive behaviors. The behavioral statements were designed to be measurable, relevant to the clinical setting, observable, and specific to the subsystem. The use of the model has had a major effect on all phases of the nursing process, including a more systematic assessment process, identification of patient strengths and problem areas, and an objective means for evaluating the quality of nursing care (Dee & Auger, 1983).

The early works of Dee and Auger led to further refinement in the patient classification system. Behavioral indices for each subsystem have been further operationalized in terms of critical adaptive and maladaptive behaviors. Behavioral data is gathered to determine the effectiveness of each subsystem (Dee, 1990; Dee & Randell, 1989).

The scores serve as an acuity rating system and provide a basis for allocating resources. These resources are allocated based on the assigned levels of nursing intervention, and resource needs are calculated based on the total number of patients assigned according to levels of nursing interventions and the hours of nursing care associated with each of the levels (Dee & Randell, 1989). The development of this system has provided nursing administration with the ability to identify the levels of staff needed to provide care (licensed vocational nurse vs. registered nurse), bill patients for actual nursing care services, and identify nursing services that are absolutely necessary in times of budgetary restraint. Recent research has demonstrated the importance of a model-based nursing database in medical records (Poster et al., 1997) and the effectiveness of using a model to identify the characteristics of a large hospital's managed behavioral health population in relation to observed nursing care needs, level of patient functioning on admission and discharge, and length of stay (Dee, Van Servellen, & Brecht, 1998).[1]

The work of Vivien Dee and her colleagues has demonstrated the validity and usefulness of the JBSM as a basis for clinical practice within a health care setting. From the findings of their work, it is clear that the JBSM established a systematic framework for patient assessment and nursing interventions, provided a common frame of reference for all practitioners in the clinical setting, provided a framework for the integration of staff knowledge about the clients, and promoted continuity in the delivery of care. These findings should be generalizable to a variety of clinical settings.

---

[1] For additional information please see the bonus chapter content available at http://davisplus.fadavis.com

Practice Exemplar

Provided by Kelly White

During the change-of-shift report that morning, I was told that a new patient had just been wheeled onto the floor at 7:00 a.m. As a result, it was my responsibility to complete the admission paperwork and organize the patient's day. He was a 49-year-old man who was admitted through the emergency department to our oncology floor for fever and neutropenia secondary to recent chemotherapy for lung cancer.

Immediately after my initial rounds, to ensure all my patients were stable and comfortable, I rolled the computer on wheels into his room to begin the nursing admission process. Jim explained to me that he was diagnosed with small cell lung carcinoma 2 months earlier after he was admitted to another hospital for coughing, chest pain, and shortness of breath. He went on to explain that a recent magnetic resonance imaging scan showed metastasis to the liver and brain.

His past health history revealed that he irregularly visited his primary health care provider. He is 6 feet 3 inches tall and weighs 168 pounds (76.4 kg). He states that he has lost 67 pounds in the past 6 months. His appetite has significantly diminished because "everything tastes like metal." He has a history of smoking three packs per day of cigarettes for 30 years. He states he quit when he began his chemotherapy.

Jim, a high school graduate, is married to his high school sweetheart, Ellen. He lives with his wife and three children in their home. He and his wife are currently unemployed secondary to recent layoffs at the factory where they both worked. He explained that Ellen has been emotionally pushing him away and occasionally disappears from the home for hours at a time without explaining her whereabouts. He informs me that before his diagnosis, they were the best of friends and inseparable.

He has tolerated his treatments well until now, except for having frequent, burning, uncontrolled diarrhea for days at a time after his chemotherapy treatments. These episodes have caused raw, tender patches of skin around his rectal area that become increasingly more painful and irritated with each bowel movement.

Jim is exceptionally tearful this morning as he expresses concerns about his own future and the future of his family. He informs me that Ellen's mother is flying in from out of state to care for the children while he is hospitalized.

Practice Exemplar cont.

Assessment

Johnson's behavioral systems model guided the assessment process. The significant behavioral data are as follows:

Achievement subsystem

Jim is losing control of his life and of the relationships that matter most to him as a person—his family.

He is a high school graduate.

Affiliative protective subsystem

Jim is married but states that his wife is distancing herself from him. He feels he is losing his "best friend" at a time when he really needs this support.

Aggressive protective subsystem

Jim is protective of his health now (he quit smoking when he began chemotherapy) but has a long history of neglecting it (smoking for 30 years, unexplained weight loss for 4 months, irregular visits to his primary health-care provider).

Dependency subsystem

Jim is realizing his ability to care for self and family is diminishing and will continue to diminish as his health deteriorates. He questions who he can depend on because his wife is not emotionally available to him.

Eliminative subsystem

Jim is experiencing frequent, burning, uncontrolled diarrhea for days at a time after his chemotherapy treatments. These episodes have caused raw, tender patches of skin around his rectal area that become increasingly more painful and irritated with each bowel movement.

Ingestive subsystem

Jim has lost 67 pounds in 6 months and has decreased appetite secondary to the chemotherapy side effects.

Restorative subsystem

Jim currently experiences shortness of breath, pain, and fatigue.

Sexual subsystem

Jim has shortness of breath and possible pain on exertion, which may be leading to concerns about his sexual abilities.

Jim's wife, Ellen, is distant these days, which would have an effect on the couple's intimacy.

The environmental assessment is as follows:

Internal/external

After the admission process was completed, I had several concerns for my new patient. I recognized that Jim was a middle-aged man whose developmental stage was compromised regarding his productivity with family and career due to his illness. Mental and physical abilities could be impaired as this disease process advances. In addition, this may create further strain on his relationship with his wife, as she attempts to deal with her own feelings about his diagnosis. Family support would be essential as Jim's journey continued. Lastly, Jim needed to be educated on the expectations of his diagnosis, participate in a plan for treatment during his hospital stay, and assist in the development of goals for his future.

Diagnostic Analysis

Jim is likely uncertain about his future as a husband, father, employee, and friend. Realizing this, I encouraged Jim to verbalize his concerns regarding these four areas of his life while I completed my physical assessment and assisted him in settling into his new environment. At first he was hesitant to speak about his family concerns but soon opened up to me after I sat down in a chair at his bedside and simply made him my complete focus for 5 minutes. As a result of this brief interaction, together we were able to develop short-term goals related to his hospitalization and home life throughout the rest of my shift with him that day. In addition, he acquiesced and allowed me to order a social work consult, recognizing that he would no longer be able to adequately meet his family's needs independently at this time.

We also addressed the skin impairment issues in his rectal area. I was able to offer him ideas on how to keep the area from experiencing further breakdown. Lastly, the wound care nurse was consulted.

Continued

Practice Exemplar cont.

Evaluation

During his 10-day hospitalization, Jim and his wife agreed to speak to a counselor regarding their thoughts on Jim's diagnosis and prognosis upon his discharge. Jim's rectal area healed because he did not receive any chemotherapy/radiation during his stay. He received tips on how to prevent breakdown in that area from the wound care nurse who took care of him on a daily basis. Jim gained 3 pounds during his stay and maintained that he would continue drinking nutrition supplements daily, regardless of his appetite changes during his cancer treatment. Jim's stamina and thirst for life grew stronger as his body grew physically stronger. As he was being discharged, he whispered to me that he was thankful for the care he had received while on our floor, and he believed that the nurses had brought him and his wife closer than they had been in months. He stated that they were talking about the future and that Ellen had acknowledged her fears to him the previous evening. Jim was wheeled out of the hospital because he continued to have shortness of breath on extended exertion. As his wife drove away from the hospital, Jim waved to me with a genuine smile and a sparkle in his eye.

Epilogue

Jim passed away peacefully 3 months later at home, with his wife and children at his side. His wife contacted me soon afterward to let me know that the nursing care Jim received during his first stay on our unit opened the doors to allow them both to recognize that they needed to modify their approach to the course of his disease. In the end, they flourished as a couple and a family, creating a supportive transition for Jim and the entire family.

■ Summary

The Johnson Behavioral System Model captures the richness and complexity of nursing. It also addresses the interdependent functional biological, psychological, and sociological components within the behavioral system and locates this within a larger social system. The JBSM focuses on the person as a whole, as well as on the complex interrelationships among its constituent parts. Once the diagnosis has been made, the nurse can proceed inward to the subsystem and outward to the environment. It also asks nurses to be systems thinkers as they formulate their assessment plan, make their diagnosis of the problem, and plan interventions. The JBSM provides nurses with a clear conception of their goal and of their mission as an integral part of the health-care team.

Johnson expected the theory's further development in the future and that it would uncover and shape significant research problems that have both theoretical and practical value to the discipline. Some examples include examining the levels of integration (biological, psychological, and sociocultural) within and between the subsystems. For example, a study could examine the way a person deals with the transition from health to illness with the onset of asthma. There is concern with the relations between one's biological system (e.g., unstable, problems breathing), one's psychological self (e.g., achievement goals, need for assistance, self-concept), self in relation to the physical environment (e.g., allergens, being away from home), and transactions related to the sociocultural context (e.g., attitudes and values about the sick). The study of transitions (e.g., the onset of puberty, menopause, death of a spouse, onset of acute illness) also represents a treasury of open problems for research with the JBSM. Findings obtained from these studies will provide not only an opportunity to revise and advance the theoretical conceptualization of the JBSM, but also information about nursing interventions. The JBSM approach leads us to seek common organizational parameters in every scientific explanation and does so using a shared language about nursing and nursing care.

References

Ainsworth, M. (1964). Patterns of attachment behavior shown by the infant in interactions with mother. *Merrill-Palmer Quarterly, 10,* 51–58.

Auger, J. (1976). *Behavioral systems and nursing.* Englewood Cliffs, NJ: Prentice-Hall.

Auger, J., & Dee, V. (1983). A patient classification system based on the behavioral systems model of nursing: Part 1. *Journal of Nursing Administration, 13*(4), 38–43.

Buckley, W. (Ed.). (1968). *Modern systems research for the behavioral scientist.* Chicago: Aldine.

Chin, R. (1961). The utility of system models and developmental models for practitioners. In K. Benne, W. Bennis, & R. Chin (Eds.), *The planning of change.* New York: Holt.

Colling, J., Owen, T. R., McCreedy, M., & Newman, D. (2003). The effects of a continence program on frail community-dwelling elderly persons. *Urologic Nursing, 23*(2), 117–131.

Crandal, V. (1963). Achievement. In H. W. Stevenson (Ed.), *Child psychology.* Chicago: University of Chicago Press.

Dee, V. (1990). Implementation of the Johnson model: One hospital's experience. In: M. Parker (Ed.), *Nursing theories in practice* (pp. 33–63). New York: National League for Nursing.

Dee, V., & Auger, J. (1983). A patient classification system based on the Behavioral System Model of Nursing: Part 2. *Journal of Nursing Administration, 13*(5), 18–23.

Dee, V., & Randell, B. P. (1989). *NPH patient classification system: A theory based nursing practice model for staffing.* Paper presented at the UCLA Neuropsychiatric Institute, Los Angeles, CA.

Dee, V., Van Servellen, G., & Brecht, M. (1998). Managed behavioral health care patients and their nursing care problems, level of functioning and impairment on discharge. *Journal of the American Psychiatric Nurses Association, 4*(2), 57–66.

Derdiarian, A. K. (1983). An instrument for theory and research development using the behavioral systems model for nursing: The cancer patient. *Nursing Research, 32,* 196–201.

Derdiarian, A. K. (1988). Sensitivity of the Derdiarian Behavioral Systems Model Instrument to age, site and type of cancer: A preliminary validation study. *Scholarly Inquiring for Nursing Practice, 2,* 103–121.

Derdiarian, A. K. (1990). The relationships among the subsystems of Johnson's behavioral system model. *Image, 22,* 219–225.

Derdiarian, A. K. (1991). Effects of using a nursing model-based instrument on the quality of nursing care. *Nursing Administration Quarterly, 15*(3), 1–16.

Derdiarian, A. K., & Forsythe, A. B. (1983). An instrument for theory and research development using the behavioral systems model for nursing: The cancer patient. Part II. *Nursing Research, 3,* 260–266.

Gerwitz, J. (Ed.). (1972). *Attachment and dependency.* Englewood Cliffs, NJ: Prentice-Hall.

Glennister, D. (2011). Towards a general systems theory of nursing: A literature review. *Proceedings of the 55th Annual Meetings of the ISSS (International Society for Systems Sciences).* Retrieved February 20, 2013, at www.journals.isss.org/index.php/proceedings55th/article/view1717/569

Grubbs, J. (1980). An interpretation of the Johnson behavioral system model. In J. P. Riehl & C. Roy (Eds.), *Conceptual models for nursing practice* (pp. 217–254). New York: Appleton-Century-Crofts.

Harris, R. B. (1986). Introduction of a conceptual model into a fundamental baccalaureate course. *Journal of Nursing Education, 25,* 66–69.

Holaday, B. (1972). Unpublished operationalization of the Johnson Model. University of California, Los Angeles.

Holaday, B. (1981). Maternal response to their chronically ill infants' attachment behavior of crying. *Nursing Research, 30,* 343–348.

Holaday, B. (1982). Maternal conceptual set development: Identifying patterns of maternal response to chronically ill infant crying. *Maternal Child Nursing Journal, 11,* 47–59.

Holaday, B. (1987). Patterns of interaction between mothers and their chronically ill infants. *Maternal Child Nursing Journal, 16,* 29–45.

Holaday, B. (1997). Johnson's behavioral system model in nursing practice. In M. Alligood & A. Marriner-Tomey (Eds.), *Nursing theory: Utilization and application* (pp. 49–70). St. Louis, MO: Mosby-Year Book.

Holaday, B., Turner-Henson, A., & Swan, J. (1997). The Johnson behavioral system model: Explaining activities of chronically ill children. In P. Hinton-Walker & B. Newman (Eds.), *Blueprint for use of nursing models: Education, research, practice, and administration* (pp. 33–63). New York: National League for Nursing.

Johnson, D. E. (1956). A story of three children. *The Nursing Journal of India, XLVII*(9), 313–322.

Johnson, D. E. (1957). Nursing care of the ill child. *The Nursing Journal of India, XLVIII*(1), 12–14.

Johnson, D. E. (1959). The nature and science of nursing. *Nursing Outlook, 7,* 291–294.

Johnson, D. E. (1961). The significance of nursing care. *American Journal of Nursing, 61,* 63–66.

Johnson, D. E. (1968). *One conceptual model of nursing.* Unpublished lecture. Vanderbilt University.

Johnson, D. E. (1980). The behavioral system model for nursing. In J. P. Riehl & C. Roy (Eds.), *Conceptual models for nursing practice* (2nd ed., pp. 207–216). New York: Appleton-Century-Crofts.

Johnson, D. E. (1990). The behavioral system model for nursing. In M. E. Parker (Ed.), *Nursing theories in practice* (pp. 23–32). New York: National League for Nursing.

Johnson, D. E., & Smith, M. M. (1963). *Crying as a physiologic state in the newborn infant.* Unpublished research report, PHS Grant NV-00055-01 (formerly GS–9768).

Kagan, J. (1964). Acquisition and significance of sex role identity. In R. Hoffman & G. Hoffman (Eds.), *Review of child development research.* New York: Russell Sage Foundation.

Loveland-Cherry, C., & Wilkerson, S. (1983). Dorothy Johnson's behavioral system model. In J. Fitzpatrick & A. Whall (Eds.), *Conceptual models of nursing: Analysis and application.* Bowie, MD: Robert J. Brady.

Meleis, A. I. (2011). *Theoretical nursing: Development and progress* (5th ed.). Philadelphia: Lippincott, Williams & Wilkins.

Oyedele, O.A. (2010). *Guidelines to prevent teenage pregnancy based on the Johnson Behavioural Systems Model.* Doctoral dissertation from the Adelaide Tambo School of Nursing Science, Tshwane University of Technology, South Africa.

Parsons, T., & Shils, E. A. (Eds.). (1951). *Toward a general theory of action: Theoretical foundations for the social sciences.* New York: Harper & Row.

Poster, E. C., Dee, V., & Randell, B. P. (1997). The Johnson behavioral systems model as a framework for patient outcome evaluation. *Journal of the American Psychiatric Nurses Association, 3*(3), 73–80.

Rapoport, A. (1968). Forward to modern systems research for the behavior scientist. In W. Buckley (Ed.), *Modern systems research for the behavioral scientist.* Chicago: Aldine.

Sears, R., Maccoby, E., & Levin, H. (1954). *Patterns of child rearing.* White Plains, NY: Row & Peterson.

Stevenson, J. S., & Woods, N. F. (1986). Nursing science and contemporary science: Emerging paradigms. In *Setting the agenda for year 2000: Knowledge development in nursing* (pp. 6–20). Kansas City, MO: American Academy of Nursing.

Talerico, K. A. (1999). *Correlates of aggressive behavioral actions of older adults with dementia.* Doctoral dissertation, School of Nursing, University of Pennsylvania.

Tamilarasi, B., & Kanimozhi, M. (2009). Improving quality of life in breast cancer survivors: Theoretical approach. *The Nursing Journal of India, C*(12). Retrieved Feburary 20, 2013, from http://www.tnaionline.org/dec-09/7.htm

von Bertalanffy, L. (1968). *General systems theory: Foundations, development, application.* New York: George Braziller.

Wang, K., & Palmer, M. H. (2010). Women's toileting behaviour related to urinary elimination: Concept analysis. *Journal of Advanced Nursing, 66*(8), 1874–1884.

Wilkie, D. (1987). Unpublished operationalization of the Johnson model. University of California, San Francisco.

Wu, R. (1973). *Behavior and illness.* Englewood Cliffs, NJ: Prentice-Hall.

Chapter 8

Dorothea Orem's Self-Care Deficit Nursing Theory

DONNA L. HARTWEG

Introducing the Theorist
Overview of the Theory
Applications of the Theory
Practice Applications
Practice Exemplar by Laureen Fleck
Summary
References

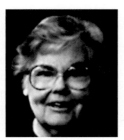

Dorothea E. Orem

Introducing the Theorist

Dorothea E. Orem (1914–2007) dedicated her life to creating and developing a theoretical structure to improve nursing practice. As a voracious reader and extraordinary thinker, she framed her ideas in both theoretical and the practical terms. She viewed nursing knowledge as theoretical, with conceptual structure and elements as exemplified in her self-care deficit nursing theory (SCDNT), and as "practically practical," with knowledge, rules, and defined roles for practice situations (Orem, 2001).

Orem's personal life experiences, formal education, employment, and her reading of philosophers such as Aristotle, Aquinas, Harre (1970), and Wallace (1983) directed her thinking (Orem, 2006). She sought to understand the phenomena she observed, creating conceptualizations of nursing education, disciplinary knowledge, and finally, a general theory of nursing or SCDNT.

Orem worked independently and then collaboratively until her death at age 93. For a lifetime of contributions to nursing science and practice, Orem received honors from organizations such as Sigma Theta Tau, the American Academy of Nursing, the National League for Nursing, and Catholic University of America as well as four honorary doctorates.

Orem received her initial nursing education at Providence Hospital School of Nursing in Washington, DC. After her 1934 graduation, Orem quickly moved into hospital staff/supervisory positions in operating and emergency areas. Her BSN Ed from Catholic University of America (1939) led to a faculty position there. After completing her MSN Ed at Catholic University (1946), Orem became

Director of Nursing Service and Education at Provident Hospital School of Nursing in Detroit (Taylor, 2007).

Orem's early formulations on the nature of nursing occurred while she was working for the Indiana State Board of Health between 1949 and 1957 (Hartweg, 1991). She became aware of nurses' ability to "do nursing," but their inability to "describe nursing." Without this understanding, Orem believed nurses could not improve practice. She made an initial effort to define nursing in a report titled "The Art of Nursing in Hospital Service: An Analysis" (Orem, 1956). The language of the patient doing-for-self or the nurse helping to-do-for-self appears in the report as antecedent language for the concept of self-care.

During her tenure at the Office of Education, Vocational Section in Washington, DC, Orem generated a simple yet important question: Why do people need nursing? In *Guides for Developing Curriculum for the Education of Practical Nurses* (Orem, 1959), she expanded the question to what she termed "the proper object of nursing": "What condition exists in a person when judgments are made that a nurse(s) should be brought into the situation?" (Orem, 2001, p. 20). Her answer was *the inability of persons to provide continuously for themselves the amount and quality of required self-care because of situations of personal health.*

Although Orem worked independently, two groups contributed to the theory's early development (Taylor, 2007). The first group was the Nursing Model Committee at Catholic University of America. In 1968, the Nursing Development Conference Group (NDCG) was formed and continued the work of the Nursing Model committee. The collaborative process and outcomes were published in *Concept Formalization: Process and Product* (NDCG, 1973, 1979), edited by Orem. Concurrent with group work, Orem published the first of six editions of *Nursing: Concepts of Practice* (1971), which has been translated into many languages.

By 1989, the global impact of Orem's work was evident when the First International self-care deficit nursing theory Conference was held in Kansas City (Hartweg, 1991). These conferences encouraged international collaboration among institutions.

In 1991, the International Orem Society (IOS) for Nursing Science and Scholarship was founded by a group of international scholars. The IOS's mission is "To disseminate information related to development of nursing science and its articulation with the science of self-care" (www.scdnt.com). This mission has been realized through the publication of newsletters (1993–2001) and a peer-reviewed journal, *Self-Care, Dependent Care & Nursing* begun in 2002 (www.scdnt.com/ja/jarchive.html). Twelve biennial Orem congresses have been held throughout the world (Berbiglia, Hohmann, & Bekel, 2012; www.ioscongress2012.lu).

In 1995, Orem convened the Orem Study Group. This international group of scholars met regularly at her home in Savannah, GA, for immersion in areas of SCDNT needing further development. Several publications resulted from this group work (Denyes, Orem, & Bekel, 2001; Taylor, Renpenning, Geden, Neuman, & Hart, 2001). Work groups continue today to refine or develop concepts such as the universal requisite of normalcy (personal communication, Taylor & Renpenning, January, 20, 2014).

Many of Orem's original papers are published in *Self-Care Theory in Nursing: Selected Papers of Dorothea Orem* (Renpenning & Taylor, 2003) and are also available in the Mason Chesney Archives of the Johns Hopkins Medical Institutions for the Orem Collection (www.medicalarchives.jhmi.edu/papers/orem.html) and in the archives of the IOS website. Audios and videos of the theorist's lectures are available through the Helene Fuld Health Trust (1988) and the National League for Nursing (1987). *Self-Care Science, Nursing Theory, and Evidence-based Practice* (Taylor & Renpenning, 2011) is the most recent theory development and practice publication. Orem's 50-year influence on nursing science and practice is also summarized in recent works by Clarke, Allison, Berbiglia, and Taylor (2009) and by Taylor (2011).[1]

---

[1]For additional information please see the bonus chapter content available at http://davisplus.fadavis.com

Overview of the Theory

As noted earlier, Orem's general theory of nursing is correctly referred to as self-care deficit nursing theory. Orem believed a general model or theory created for a practical science such as nursing encompasses not only the What and Why, but also the Who and How (Orem, 2006). This action theory therefore includes clear specifications for nurse and patient roles. The grand theory originally comprised three interrelated theories: the theory of self-care, the theory of self-care deficit, and the theory of nursing systems. A fourth, the theory of dependent care, emerged over time to address the complexity not only of the individual in need of care but also of the caregivers whose requisites and capabilities influence the design of the nursing system (Taylor & Renpenning, 2011). The building blocks of these theories are six major concepts, with parallel concepts from the theory of dependent care, and one peripheral concept. The following is a brief overview of each theory and concept. Readers are encouraged to study relevant sections in Orem's *Concepts of Practice* (2001) or other citations to enhance understanding.

Foundational to learning any theory is exploration of its underlying assumptions, the key to conceptual understanding. Many principles emerged from Orem's independent work as well as from discussions within the Nursing Development Conference Group and the Nursing Study Group. Five general assumptions/principles about humans provided guidance to Orem's conceptualizations (Orem, 2001, p. 140). When thinking about humans within the context of the theory, Orem viewed two types: those who need nursing care and those who produce it (Orem, 2006). In the simplest terms, this is the patient and the nurse, respectively. These assumptions also reveal human powers and properties necessary for self-care. Consistent with most Orem writings, the term *patient* is used to refer to the recipient of care.

Four Constituent Theories Within Self-Care Deficit Nursing Theory

Each theory includes a central idea, presuppositions, and propositions. The central idea presents the general focus of the theory, the presuppositions are assumptions specific to this theory, and the propositions are statements about the concepts and their interrelationships. The propositions have changed over time with SCDNT refinement. These occurred in part through theory testing that validated or invalidated hypotheses generated from the relationships. As Orem used terminology at various levels of abstraction within constituent theories, the reader is advised to thoroughly study SCDNT concepts, including the synonyms. For example, agency is also called capability, ability and/or power.

1. Theory of Self-Care (TSC)

The central idea describes self-care in contrast to other forms of care. Self-care, or care for oneself, must be learned and be deliberately performed for life, human functioning, and well-being. Six presuppositions articulate Orem's notions about necessary resources, capabilities for learning, and motivation for self-care. However, there are situational variations that affect self-care such as culture.

Orem (2001) expanded two sets of propositions from previous writings. She introduced requirements necessary for life, health, and well-being and explained the complexity of a self-care system. A person performing self-care must first *estimate or investigate what can and should be done*. This is a complex action of knowing and seeking information on specific care measures. The self-care sequence continues by *deciding what can be done* and finally *producing the care* (see Orem, 2001, pp. 143–145).

2. Theory of Dependent Care

Taylor and others (2001) formalized the theory of dependent care as a corollary theory to the theory of self-care. Concepts within the theory of dependent care (TDC) parallel those in the theory of self-care. Assumptions relate to the nature of interpersonal action systems and social dependency. Within a particular social unit such as a family, the self-care agent (the patient) is in a socially dependent relationship with the person or persons providing care, such as a parent (the dependent-care agent). The presence of a self-care deficit of the dependent also gives rise to the need for nursing (Taylor & Renpenning, 2011; Taylor, Renpenning, Geden, Neuman, & Hart, 2001).

3. Theory of Self-Care Deficit

The central idea describes *why people need nursing* (Orem, 2001, pp. 146–147). Requirements for nursing are health-related limitations for knowing, deciding, and producing care to self. Orem presents two sets of presuppositions that articulate this theory with the theory of self-care and what she calls the idea of *social dependency*. To engage in self-care, persons must have values and capabilities to learn (to know), to decide, and to manage self (to produce and regulate care). The second set presents the context of nursing as a health service when people are in a state of social dependency.

The theory of self-care deficit (TSCD) includes nine propositions called principles or guides for future development and theory testing. These statements are essential ideas of the larger, SCDNT. Orem describes the situations that affect *legitimate nursing*. Nursing is legitimate or needed when the individual's self-care capabilities and care demands are *equal to, less than, or more than* at a point in time. With the existence of this inequity, a self-care deficit exists, and nursing is needed. In a dependent-care system, a self-care deficit exists in the patient as well as a dependent-care deficit in a caregiver. The latter is an inequity between the dependent-care demand and agency (abilities) to care for the person in need of health care. Legitimate nursing also occurs when a future deficit relationship is predicted such as an upcoming surgery.

4. Theory of Nursing Systems

The fourth theory, the theory of nursing systems (TNS), encompasses the three others. The central focus is the product of nursing, establishing both structure and content for nursing practice as well as the nursing role (see Orem, 2001, pp. 111, 147–149). The four presuppositions direct the nurse to major complexities of nursing practice. For example, Orem stated that "*Nursing has results-achieving operations that must be articulated with the interpersonal and societal features of nursing*"

(Orem, 2001, p. 147). Although much of the theory relates to diagnosis, actions, and outcomes based on a deficit relationship between self-care capabilities and self-care demand, Orem also presents theoretical work related to the interpersonal relationship between nurse and person(s) receiving nursing and a social contract between the nurse and patient(s) (Orem, 2001, pp. 314–317). These components are often overlooked when studying the SCDNT and are important antecedents and concurrent actions in the process of nursing.

The theory of nursing systems includes seven propositions related to most SCDNT concepts but adds nursing agency (capabilities of the nurse) and nursing systems (complex actions). Nursing agency and nursing systems are linked to the concepts of the person receiving care or dependent care, such as self-care capabilities (agency), self-care demands (therapeutic self-care demand), and limitations (deficits) for self-care. Through this, the general theory or SCDNT becomes concrete to the practicing nurse. Although the language is implicit, Orem proposes that nursing systems are determined by the person's (or dependent-care agent's) self-care limitations (capabilities in relationship to health-related self-care or dependent-care demand). Nursing systems therefore vary by the amount of care the nurse must provide, such as a total care system, or wholly compensatory system (e.g., unconscious critical care patient); partial care, or partially compensatory system (e.g., patient in rehabilitation); or supportive-educative system (e.g., patient needing teaching).

Theoretical development by Orem scholars and others continues as nursing practice evolves. The addition of the theory of dependent care is a major example and extends basic concepts, such as adding "dependent-care system" (Taylor & Renpenning, 2011). Other concepts such as self-care and self-care requisites, their processes and core operations, continue to be explicated (Denyes, Orem & Bekel, 2001). Some researchers or theorists develop the subconcepts of basic concepts such as self-care agency through exploration of congruent theories. For example, Pickens (2012) proposed exploration of motivation, a foundational capability and power component of self-care agency, through examination of several theories including self-determination theory (Ryan, Patrick, Deci, & Williams, 2008). Others create new concepts, such as spiritual self-care (White, Peters, & Schim, 2011) or extend general concepts such as environment (Banfield, 2011).

Concepts

SCDNT is constructed from six basic concepts and a peripheral concept. Four concepts are patient related: self-care/dependent care, self-care agency/dependent-care agency, therapeutic self-care demand/dependent-care demand, and self-care deficit/dependent-care deficit. Two concepts relate to the nurse: nursing agency and nursing system. Basic conditioning factors, the peripheral concept, is related to both the self-care agent (person receiving care)/dependent-care agent (family member/friend providing care) and also to the nurse (nurse agent). Orem defines agent as the *person who engages in a course of action or has the power to do so* (Orem, 2001, p. 514). Hence there is a self-care agent, a dependent-care agent, and a nurse agent. The unit of service is a person(s), whether that is the individual (self-care agent) or another on whom the person is socially dependent (dependent-care agent). Orem also addresses multiperson situations and multiperson units such as entire families, groups, or communities.

Each concept is defined and presented with levels of abstraction. Varied constructs within each concept allow theoretical testing at the level of middle-range theory or at the practice application level whether with the individual or multiperson situations. All constructs and concepts build on decades of Orem's independent and collaborative work. A "kite-like" model provides a visual guide for the six concepts and their interrelationships (Fig. 8-1). For a model of concepts and relationships of dependent care, the reader is referred to Taylor and Renpenning (2011, p. 112). For a model of multiperson structure, the reader is referred to Taylor and Renpenning (2001).

Basic Conditioning Factors

A peripheral concept, basic conditioning factors (BCFs), is related to three major concepts. For simplicity, only the patient component is presented rather than the parallel dependent-care components. In general, basic conditioning factors relate to the patient concepts (self-care agency and therapeutic self-care demand) and

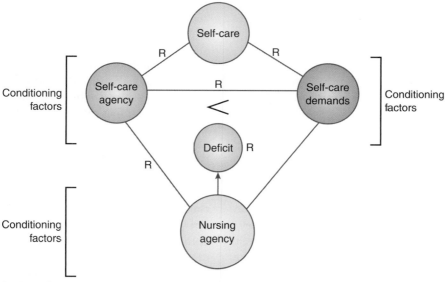

Fig 8 • 1 Structure of SCDNT.

one nurse concept (nursing agency). These conditioning factors are values that affect the constructs: age, gender, developmental state, health state, sociocultural orientation, health-care system factors, family system factors, pattern of living, environmental factors, and resource availability and adequacy (Orem, 2001, p. 245). For example, the family system factor such as living alone or with others may affect the person's ability (self-care agency) to care for self after hospital discharge. The self-care demand (care requirements) of a person taking insulin for type 2 diabetes will vary based on availability of resources and health system services (e.g., access to medications and care services). These same BCFs apply to nursing agency, such as health state. A nurse with recent back surgery may have limitations in nursing capabilities (nurse agency) in relationship to specific care demands of the patient.

These BCF categories have many subfactors that have not been explicitly defined and continue in development. For example, sociocultural orientation refers to culture with its various components such as values and practices. Sociocultural includes economic conditions as well as others. The BCFs related to nursing agency include those such as age but expand to include nursing experience and education. A clinical specialist in diabetes usually has more capabilities in caring for the self-care agent with type 2 diabetes than one without such credentials. All these affect the parameters of the nurse's capability to provide care.

Self-Care (Dependent Care)

Orem (2001) defined self-care as the *practice of activities that individuals initiate and perform on their own behalf in maintaining life, health, and well-being* (p. 43). Self-care is purposeful action performed in sequence and with a pattern. Although engagement in purposeful self-care may not improve health or well-being, a positive outcome is assumed. Dependent care is performed by mature, responsible persons on behalf of socially dependent individuals or self-care agents such as an infant, child, or cognitively impaired person. The purpose is to meet the person's health-related demands (dependent-care demand) and/or to develop their self-care

capabilities (self-care agency; Taylor et al., 2001; Taylor & Renpenning, 2011).

Although the practice of maintaining life is self-explanatory, Orem (2001) viewed outcomes of health and well-being as related but different. Health is a state of physical–psychological, structural–functional soundness and wholeness. In contrast, well-being is conceived as *experiences of contentment, pleasure, and kinds of happiness; by spiritual experiences; by movement toward fulfilment of one's self-ideal; and by continuing personalization* (Orem, 2001, p. 186). Self-care performed deliberately for well-being versus structural–functional health was conceptualized and developed as health promotion self-care by Hartweg (1990, 1993) and Hartweg and Berbiglia (1996). Exploration of the relationship between self-care and well-being was later conducted by Matchim, Armer, and Stewart (2008).

Key to understanding self-care and dependent care is the concept of deliberate action, a voluntary behavior to achieve a goal. Deliberate action is preceded by investigating and deciding what choice to make (Orem, 2001). In practice, the nurse's understanding of each of these phases of investigating, deciding, and producing self-care is essential for positive health outcomes. Take two situations: A pregnant woman avoids alcohol for her fetus's health and a woman with breast cancer requires chemotherapy for life and health. Each woman must first know and understand the relationship of self-care to life, health, and well-being. Decision making follows, such as deciding to avoid alcohol or choosing to engage in chemotherapy. Finally, the individual must take action, such as not drinking when offered alcohol or accepting chemotherapy treatment. Without each phase, self-care does not occur. The pregnant woman may know the dangers to her fetus and decide not to drink but engage in drinking when pressured to do so. The woman with cancer may understand the health outcome without treatment, decide to have treatment, then not follow through because transportation to chemotherapy sessions disrupts her husband's employment. Because each phase of the action sequence has many components, nurses often provide partial support to patients and self-care action does not occur. If skills related to the operation to avoid alcohol when pressured or the operations necessary for transportation to a cancer center are not anticipated by the nurse for these patients, the self-care action sequences may not be completed. Then outcomes related to life, health, and well-being are affected.

Self-Care Agency (Dependent Care Agency)

Orem (2001) defined self-care agency (SCA) as *complex acquired capability to meet one's continuing requirements for care of self that regulates life processes, maintains or promotes integrity of human structure and functioning [health] and human development, and promotes well-being* (p. 254). Capability, ability, and power are all terms used to express *agency*. Self-care agency is therefore the mature or maturing individual's capability for deliberate action to care for self. Dependent care agency is *a complex acquired ability of mature or maturing persons to know and meet some or all of the self-care requisites of persons who have health-derived or health associated limitations of self-care agency, which places them in socially dependent relationships for care* (Taylor & Renpenning, 2011, p. 108). Viewed as the *summation of all human capabilities needed for performing self-care*, these range from a very basic ability, such as memory, to capability for a specific action in a sequence to meet a specific self-care demand or requirement. At this concrete level, the capabilities of knowing, deciding, and acting or producing self-care are necessary. If these capabilities do not exist, then the abilities of others are necessary, such as the family member or the nurse. A three-part, hierarchical model of self-care agency provides a visualization of this structure (Fig. 8-2). Understanding these elements is necessary to determine the self-care agent role, dependent-care agent role, and the nurse role.

Foundational Capabilities and Dispositions

Foundational capabilities and dispositions are at the most basic level (Orem, 2001, pp. 262–263). These are capabilities for all types of *deliberate action*, not just self-care. Included

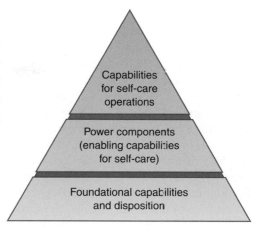

Fig 8 • 2 Structure of self-care agency.

are abilities related to perception, memory, and orientation. One example is the deliberate act of repairing a car. One must have perception of the concept of the car and its parts, memory of methods of repair, and orientation of self to the equipment and vehicle. If these foundational abilities are not present, then actions cannot occur.

Power Components

At the midlevel of the hierarchy are the power components, or 10 powers or types of abilities necessary for *self-care*. Examples are the valuing of health, ability to acquire knowledge about self-care resources, and physical energy for self-care. At a very general level, these capabilities relate to knowledge, motivation, and skills to produce self-care. If a mature person becomes comatose, the abilities to maintain attention, to reason, to make decisions, to physically carry out the actions are not functioning. The self-care actions necessary for life, health, and well-being must then be performed by the dependent-care agent or the nurse agent.

Capabilities for Estimative, Transitional, and Productive Operations

The most concrete level of self-care agency is one specific to the individual's detailed components of self-care demand or requirements. Capabilities related to estimative operations are those necessary to determine what self-care actions are needed in a specific nursing situation at one point in time—in other words, capabilities of investigating and estimating what needs to be done. This includes capabilities of learning in situations related to health and well-being. For example, does the person newly diagnosed with asthma have the capability to learn about regular exercise activities and rescue medication? Does the person know how to obtain the necessary resources? Transitional operations relate to abilities necessary for decision making, such as reflecting on the course of action and making an appropriate decision. The patient may have the capabilities to learn and obtain resources but not the ability to make the decision. The asthma patient has the capability to learn about exercise and medication but not the capability to make the decision to follow through on directions. Capabilities for productive operations are those necessary for preparing the self for the action, carrying out the action, monitoring the effects, and evaluating the action's effectiveness. If the person decides to use the inhaler, does the person have the ability to take time to engage in the necessary self-care, to physically push the device, to monitor the changes, and determine the effectiveness of the action? Just as the action sequence is important in the self-care concept, these types of capabilities reveal the complexity of human capability.

At the concrete practice level, self-care agency also varies by development and operability. For example, the nurse must determine whether capabilities for learning are fully developed at the level necessary to understand and retain information about the required actions. For example, a mature adult with late stage Alzheimer's disease is not able to retain new information. The self-care agency is therefore *developed but declining*, creating the possible need for dependent-care agency or nursing agency. A second determination is the operability of agency. Is agency not operative, partially operative, or fully operative? A comatose patient may have fully developed capabilities before a motor vehicle accident, but the trauma results in inoperable cognitive functioning. SCA is therefore *developed, but not operative* at that moment in time. In this situation, the nurse agent must provide care. Similar variations of development and operability occur with dependent-care agency and must be considered by the nurse when developing the self-care or dependent-care system.

Therapeutic Self-Care Demand (Dependent-Care Demand)

Therapeutic self-care demand (TSCD) is a complex theoretical concept that summarizes all actions that should be performed over time for life, health, and well-being. When first developed, the concept was referred to as *action demand* or *self-care demand* (Orem, 2001). Readers will therefore see these terms used in Orem's writings and in the literature. Dependent care demand is the summation of all care actions *for meeting the dependent caregiver's therapeutic self-care demand when his or her agency is not adequate or operational* (Taylor & Renpenning, 2011, p. 108).

The word *therapeutic* is essential to one's understanding of the concept. Consideration is always on a therapeutic outcome of life, health, and well-being. A Haitian mother in a remote village may expect to apply horse or cow dung to the severed umbilical cord to facilitate drying, a culturally adjusted self-care measure for a newborn. With horse/cow dung as the major carrier of *Clostridium tetanus*, this dependent-care action may lead to disease and infant death, not a *therapeutic* outcome.

Constructing or calculating a TSCD requires extensive nursing knowledge of evidenced-based practice, communication, and interpersonal skills. Both scientific nursing knowledge and knowledge of the person and environment are merged to formulate *what needs to be done* in a particular nursing situation (NDCG, 1979). The process of calculating the TSCD includes adjusting values by the basic conditioning factors. For example, a mental health patient will have different needs based on the type of mental health condition (health state), family system factors, and health-care resources.

Self-Care Requisites

To provide the framework for determining the TSCD, Orem developed three types of self-care requisites (or requirements): universal, developmental, and health deviation. These are the *purposes or goals* for which actions are performed for life, health, and well-being. The individual sleeps once each day and engages in daily activities to meet the requisite or goal of *maintaining a balance of activity and rest.* Without rest, a human cannot survive. Therefore, these are general statements within a three-part framework that provide a level of abstraction similar to the power components of self-care agency. Denyes et al. (2001) explicated the self-care requisite *to maintain an adequate intake of water.* Their work demonstrates the complexity of actions necessary to meet a basic human need. Without consideration of this complexity, analysis and diagnosis of patient requirements is not complete. This scholarly contribution by Denyes and others (2001) can serve as a model for structuring information regarding all other requisites (personal communication, Dr. Susan G. Taylor, March 12, 2013).

Universal Self-Care Requisites

The eight universal self-care requisites (USCR) are necessary for all human beings of all ages and in all conditions, such as air, food, activity and rest, solitude, and social interaction. The BCFs influence the quality and quantity of the action necessary to achieve the purpose. Actions to be performed over time that meet the requisite, *prevention of hazards to human life, human functioning, and human well-being (the purpose),* will vary for an infant (e.g., keeping crib rails up) versus an adult (e.g., ambulation safety). Some requisites are very general yet provide important concepts necessary for all humans. One example is the concept of normalcy, the eighth USCR. The goal is *promotion of human functioning and development within social groups in accord with human potential, human limitations, and the human desire to be normal* (Orem, 2001, p. 225). Practice examples in the literature have emerged, such as the importance of normalcy to individuals with learning disabilities (Horan, 2004). These two requisites, prevention of hazards and promotion of normalcy, also relate to the other six USCRs. For example, when maintaining a sufficient intake of food, one must consider hazards to ingestion of food such as avoiding pesticides.

Developmental Self-Care Requisites

Orem (2001) identified three types of developmental self-care requisites (DSCRs). The first refers to actions necessary for general human developmental processes throughout the life span. These requisites are often met by dependent-care agents when caring for developing infants and children or when disaster and serious physical or mental illness affects adults. Engagement in self-development, the second DSCR, refers to demands for action by individuals in positive roles and in positive mental health. Examples include self-reflection, goal-setting, and responsibility in one's roles. The third DSCR, interferences with development, expresses goals achieved by actions that are necessary in situational crises such as loss of friends and relatives, loss of job, or terminal illness. Originally subsumed under USCRs, Orem created the developmental self-care requisite category to indicate the importance of human development to life, health, and well-being.

Health Deviation Self-Care Requisites

Health deviation self-care requisites (HDSCR) are situation-specific requisites or goals when people have disease, injuries, or are under professional medical care. These six requisites guide actions when pathology exists or when medical interventions are prescribed. The first HDSCR refers in part to a patient purpose: *to seek and secure appropriate medical assistance for genetic, physiological, or psychological conditions known to produce or be associated with human pathology* (Orem, 2001, p. 235). For a person with history of breast cancer, seeking regular diagnostic tests is a goal to preserve life, health, and well-being. A teenager in treatment for severe acne takes action to meet HDSCR 5: to modify *the self-concept (and self-image) in accepting oneself as being in a particular state of health and in need of a specific form of health care* (Orem, p. 235).

Each TSCD, through the three types of self-care requisites, is individualized and adjusted by the basic conditioning factors (BCFs) such as age, health state, and sociocultural orientation. Once adjusted to the specific patient in a unique situation, the purposes are specific for the patient or type of patient. These are called "particularized self-care requisites." Dennis and Jesek-Hale (2003) proposed a list of particularized self-care requisites for a nursing population of newborns. Although created for nursery newborns, a group particularized by age, the individual patient adjustments are then made. For example, a newborn's sucking needs may vary, necessitating variation in feeding methods. More recent nursing literature continues to expand the types of requisites varied by specific diseases or illnesses that provide a basis for application to specific patients and caregivers.

Self-Care Deficit (Dependent-Care Deficit)

As a theoretical concept, self-care deficit expresses the value of the relationship between two other concepts: self-care agency and therapeutic self-care demand (Orem, 2001). When the person's self-care agency is not adequate to meet all self-care requisites (TSCD), a self-care deficit exists. This qualitative and quantitative relationship at the conceptual level of abstraction is expressed as "equal to," "more than," or "less than" (see Fig. 8-1). A deficit relationship is also described as complete or partial; a complete deficit suggests no capability to engage in self-care or dependent care. An example of a complete deficit may exist in a premature infant in a neonatal intensive care unit. A partial self-care deficit may exist in a patient recovering from a routine bowel resection 1 day after surgery. This person is able to provide some self-care.

Understanding self-care deficit is necessary to appreciate Orem's concept of *legitimate nursing*. If a nurse determines a patient has self-care agency (estimative, transitional, and productive capabilities) to carry out a sequence of actions to meet the self-care requisites, then nursing is not necessary. A self-care deficit or anticipated self-care deficit must exist before a nursing system is designed and implemented. The nurse reflects with the patient: Is self-care agency (and/or dependent-care agency) adequate to meet the therapeutic self-care demand? If adequate, there is no need for nursing.

A dependent-care deficit is a statement of the relationship between the dependent-care demand and the powers and capabilities of the dependent-care agent to meet the self-care deficit of the socially dependent person, the self-care agent (Taylor & Renpenning, 2011). When this deficit occurs, then a need for nursing exists. When a parent has the capabilities to meet all health-related self-care requisites of an ill child, then no nursing is needed.

When an existing or potential self-care deficit is identified and legitimate nursing is needed, an analysis by the nurse/patient/dependent-care agents results in identification of types of limitations in relationship to the particularized self-care requisites. These are generally described as limitations of knowing, limitations or restrictions of decision-making, and limitations in ability to engage in result-achieving courses of action. Orem classified these into sets of limitations (Orem, 2001, pp. 279–282).

Nursing System (Dependent-Care System)

Orem describes a nursing system as an "action system," an action or a sequence of actions performed for a purpose. This is a composite of all the nurse's concrete actions completed or to be completed for or with a self-care agent to promote life, health, and well-being. The composite of actions and their sequence produced by the dependent-care agent to meet the therapeutic dependent self-care demand is termed a dependent-care system (Taylor et al., 2001). These actions relate to three types of subsystems: interpersonal, social/contractual, and professional-technological.

The interpersonal subsystem includes all necessary actions or operations such as entering into and maintaining effective relationships with the patient and/or family or others involved in care. The social/contractual subsystem relates to all nursing actions/operations to reach agreements with the patient and others related to information necessary to determine the therapeutic self-care demand and self-care agency of an individual and caregivers. Within this subsystem, the nurse, in collaboration with the patient or dependent-caregiver, determines roles for all care participants (Orem, 2001). These are based on social norms and other variables such as basic conditioning factors. Although other nursing theories emphasize interpersonal interactions, Orem's general theory clearly specifies details of interpersonal and contractual operations as necessary antecedents and concurrent components of care. This element of Orem's model is often overlooked and clarifies the decision-making process and collaborative relationship within the nurse–patient–family/multiperson roles.

The professional–technological subsystem comprises actions/operations that are diagnostic, prescriptive, regulatory, evaluative, and case management. The latter involves placing all operations within a system that uses resources effectively and efficiently with a positive patient outcome. Orem views the professional–technological subsystem as the process of nursing, a nonlinear one that integrates all operations of this subsystem with those of the interpersonal and the social–contractual. This involves collecting data to determine existing and projected universal, developmental, and health-deviation self-care requisites, and methods to meet these requisites as adjusted by the basic conditioning factors. Using the interpersonal and social–contractual subsystems, the nurse incorporates modifications of her or his diagnosis and prescriptions in collaboration with the patient and family on *what is possible.* The nurse also identifies the patient's usual self-care practices and assesses the person's estimative, transitional, and productive capabilities for knowledge, skills, and motivation in relationship to the known self-care requisites. That is, are the capabilities (self-care agency/dependent-care agency) needed to meet the self-care requisites developed, operable, and adequate? Are there limitations in knowing, deciding, or producing self-care? If no limitations exist, then there is no need for nursing and no nursing system is developed. If there is a self-care deficit or dependent-care deficit, then the nurse and patient or caregivers reach agreement about the patient's role, the family's role, and/or the nurse's role. Orem (2001) charted the progression of these steps by subsystems (pp. 311, 314–317).

With determination of a real or potential self-care deficit or dependent-care deficit, the nurse develops one of three types of nursing systems: wholly compensatory, partly compensatory, or supportive-educative (developmental). The nurse then continues the query: *Who can or should perform actions that require movement in space and controlled manipulation?* (Orem, 2001, p. 350). If the answer is only the nurse, then a wholly compensatory system is designed. If the patient has some capabilities to perform operations or actions, then the nurse and patient share responsibilities. If the patient can perform all actions that control movement in space and controlled manipulation, but nurse actions are required for support (physical or psychological), then the system is supportive–educative. Note, in all systems, the self-care deficit is the necessary element that leads to the design of a nursing system. Using the interpersonal and social–contractual operations, the nurse first enters into an interpersonal relationship and an agreement to determine a real or potential self-care deficit, prescribe roles, and implement productive operations of self-care and/or dependent care. Regulation or treatment operations are designed or planned and then produced or performed. Control operations are used to appraise and evaluate the effectiveness of nursing actions and to determine whether adjustments should be made. These appraisals emphasize validity of operations or actions in relationship to standards. Selecting valid operations in the plan and in evaluation incorporate evidence-based practices. These processes, including diagnosis, prescription, designing, planning, regulating, and controlling, can be viewed as elements of Orem's steps in the process of nursing (Fig. 8-3).

Orem's language of the nursing process varies from the standard language of assessment, diagnosis, planning, implementation, and evaluation. The interaction of the three aforementioned subsystems creates a model for true collaboration with the recipient of care or the caregiver.

The three steps of Orem's process of nursing are as follows: (1) diagnosis and prescription, (2) design and plan, and (3) produce and

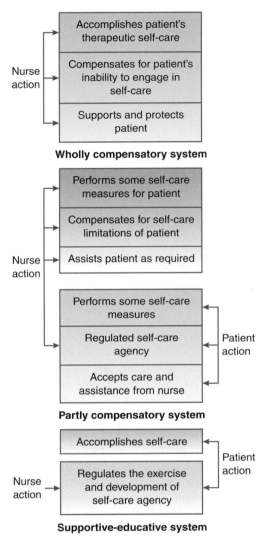

Fig 8 • 3   Basic nursing system.

control. For example, Orem considers the term "assessment" too limiting. Within Orem's process, assessments are made throughout the iterative social–contractual and professional-technological operations. During the first step of diagnosis, data are collected on the basic conditioning factors and a determination is made about their relationship to the self-care requisites and to self-care agency. How does health state (e.g., type 2 diabetes) affect the individual's universal, developmental, and health-deviation self-care requirements? How does the basic conditioning factor, or health state, affect the individual's self-care agency

(capabilities)? What, if any, are limitations for deliberate action related to the estimative (investigative–knowing), transitional (decision making), and productive (performing) phases of self-care? (Orem, 2001, p. 312). The nurse collects information, analyses it, and makes judgments about the information within the limits of nursing agency (capabilities of the nurse, such as expertise).

Orem describes nursing as a specialized helping service and identifies five helping methods to overcome self-care limitations or regulate functioning and development of patients or their dependents. Nurses employ one or more of these methods throughout the process of nursing, including acting for or doing for another, guiding another, supporting another, providing for a developmental environment, and teaching another (Orem, 2001, pp. 56–60). Acting for or doing for another includes physical assistance such as positioning the patient. Assuming self-care agency that is developed and operable, the nurse replaces this method with others that focus on cognitive development, such as guiding and teaching. These methods are not unique to nursing, but are used by most health professionals. Through their unique role functions, nurses perform a specific sequence of actions in relationship to the identified patient and/or dependent-care agent's self-care limitations in combination with other health professionals to meet the self-care requirements.

Although comparisons are made between these steps and those of the general nursing process, Orem's complexity is unique in addressing an integration of interpersonal, social–contractual, and professional–technological subsystems. The intricacy of her steps is also evident in the complexity of the diagnostic and prescriptive components. The practice exemplar in this chapter provides one simplified example of this process.

Nursing Agency

Nursing agency is the power or ability to nurse. The agency or capabilities are necessary to *know and meet patients' therapeutic self-care demands and to protect and to regulate the exercise of development of patient's self-care agency* (Orem, 2001,

p. 290). Nursing agency is analogous to self-care agency but with capabilities performed on behalf of "legitimate patients." Similar to self-care agency, nursing agency is affected by basic conditioning factors. The nurse's family system, as well as nursing education and experience, may affect his or her ability to nurse.

Orem categorizes nursing capabilities (agency) as interpersonal, social–contractual, and professional-technological. That is, the nurse must have capabilities within each of the subsystems described in the nursing system. Capabilities that result in desirable interpersonal nurse characteristics include effective communication skills and ability to form relationships with patients and significant others. Social–contractual characteristics require the ability to apply knowledge of variations in patients to nursing situations and to form contracts with patients and others for clear role boundaries. Desirable professional-technologic characteristics require the ability to perform techniques related to the process of nursing: diagnosis of therapeutic self-care demand of an assigned patient with consideration of all self-care requisites (universal, developmental, and health deviation) and a concomitant diagnosis of a patient's self-care agency. Other desired nurse characteristics include the ability to prescribe roles: Assuming a self-care deficit (and therefore a legitimate patient), what are the roles and related responsibilities of the nurse, the patient, the aide, and the family? Nurses must also have the ability to know and apply care measures such as general helping techniques (teaching, guiding) and specialized interventions and technologies such as those identified with evidence-based practice. These necessary nursing capabilities also have implications for nursing education and nursing administration. Knowledge of all components of nursing agency will direct nursing curricula for successful development of nursing abilities. Likewise, knowledge related to nursing administration is critical to operability of nursing agency (Banfield, 2011).

Multiperson Situations and Units

Taylor and Renpenning (2001) extended application of Orem's concepts to families,

groups, and communities, where the recipient of nursing care is more than a single individual with a self-care deficit. They distinguished among types of multiperson units, such as community groups and family or residential group units. These authors present categories of multiperson care systems, create family and community as basic conditioning factors, and present a model of community as aggregate. This model appropriately incorporates additional basic conditioning factors such as public policy, health-care system changes, and community development. Other frameworks such as a community participation model have been developed (Isaramalai, 2002).

Community groups have a selected number of common self-care requisites and/or limitations of knowledge, decision making, and producing care. These can be based on requirements of entire communities, groups within the communities, or to other situations when groups have common needs. For example, the focus of a student health nurse at a university may be a group of first-year students and the self-care requisite, prevention of the hazards of alcohol poisoning. The self-care limitations of the group may be knowledge of binge drinking outcomes and the skills to resist peer pressure at parties. This environment and situation, the college milieu and new independence, creates the common set of self-care requisites. The action system designed by the college health nurse is to develop the knowledge, decision-making, and result-producing skills of new students collectively so life, health, and well-being are enhanced for the group, as well as the college community.

Family or others in a communal living arrangement are another type of multiperson unit of service. Because of the interrelationship of the individuals in the living unit, the purpose of nursing varies from that for a community group. In this situation, the focus is often an individual, as well as the family as a unit. The health-related requirements of one individual trigger the need for nursing but also affect the unit as a whole. In one situation, an elderly parent moves into the family home. Not only is the therapeutic self-care demand of the parent involved, but also the needs of family members as it affects their self-care requisites. The health of the unit is therefore established and maintained by meeting the therapeutic self-care demands of all members and facilitating the development and exercise of self-care agency for each group member (Taylor & Renpenning, 2011).

Applications of the Theory
Nursing Education Applications

Many educational programs used Orem's conceptualizations to frame the curriculum and to guide nursing practice (Hartweg, 2001; Ransom, 2008). Taylor and Hartweg (2002) found Orem's conceptualization was the most frequently used nursing theory in U.S. programs. Examples of Orem-based schools included Morris Harvey College in Charleston, West Virginia, Georgetown University, the University of Missouri—Columbia, and Illinois Wesleyan University (Taylor, 2007). Current application of Orem's theory in nursing education ranges from application to pedagogy in a hybrid RN-BSN course in the United States (Davidson, 2012) to use as a general framework for nursing education in Germany (Hintze, 2011).

Research Applications

The use of SCDNT as a framework for research continues to increase with application to specific populations and conditions. Studies range from those with general reference to Orem's theory to more sophisticated exploration of concepts and their relationships. Early Orem studies concentrated on theory development and testing, including creation of theory-derived research instruments (Gast et al., 1989), a necessary process in theory building. Examples of widely used concept-based instruments include those by Denyes (1981, 1988) on self-care practices and self-care agency. The Appraisal of Self-care Agency (ASA scale) was an early tool used in international research (van Achterberg et al., 1991) and later modified for specific populations (West & Isenberg, 1997). More recent instruments derive from structural components of SCDNT but are applicable in more specific situations: Self-Care for Adults on Dialysis Tool (Costantini, Beanlands, & Horsburgh, 2011); Spanish Version of the Child and Adolescent Self-Care Performance Questionnaire (Jaimovich, Campos, Campos & Moore, 2009); The Nutrition Self-Care Inventory (Fleck, 2012); and Self-Care Outcomes (Valente, Saunders, & Uman, 2011).

A few Orem scholars continue with development of theoretical elements through well-designed programs of research with specific populations. For example, Armer et al. (2009) studied select power components (elements of self-care agency) to describe those important in developing supportive-educative nursing systems with postmastectomy breast cancer patients. A secondary analysis of this study contributed to identification of the types of self-care limitations experienced by this population. The results have potential to promote effective nursing interventions (Armer, Brooks, & Steward, 2011). Research is needed on actions and methods to meet health deviation self-care requisites in a variety of specific health situations (Casida, Peters, Peters, & Magnan, 2009).

Many studies use SCDNT as a framework for research and reference select concepts but with limited application (Lundberg & Thrakul, 2011). For example, Carthron and others (2010) used Orem's SCDNT to guide research related to specific concepts such as therapeutic self-care demand and self-care agency. However, a family system factor (the primary care role of grand-mothering) on type 2 diabetes self-management was the primary emphasis within the study. Other studies combine elements from SCDNT with other theories without consideration of the congruence of underlying assumptions. For example, Singleton, Bienemy, Hutchinson, Dellinger, and Rami (2011) framed their study in part within Orem's theory of self-care as well as in the health belief model and the concept of self-efficacy. This combination of concepts and theories in research studies is common. Further, Klainin and Ounnapiruk (2010) summarized research findings from 20 studies of Thai elderly guided by Orem's SCDNT. Although their analysis revealed two of six major concepts and one peripheral concept were evident in the research, many studies explored other non–SCDNT-specific concepts such as self-concept, self-efficacy, and locus of control. The authors suggest that SCDNT should be revisited to include additional concepts to strengthen the theory.

Table 8-1 provides examples of domestic and international theory development and practice-related research conducted in the past 5 years at the time of this writing.

Table 8 · 1 Examples of Research Applications

Author (Year), Country	Purpose	Population/ Settings	SCDNT Concept(s)	Methods	Results
Armer, Brooks, & Steward (2011), USA	To examine patient perceptions of SC limitations to meet TSCD to reduce lymphedema	Breast cancer survivors, postsurgery (N = 14)	SCA, especially estimative, transitional, and productive phases of self-care necessary to decrease risk of lymphedema; supportive-educative nursing system	Secondary analysis of qualitative data from pilot study (Armer et al., 2009)	Identified types of self-care limitations in relationship to sets of limitations, e.g., "knowing." Most limitations were not related to lack of knowledge but to energy, patterns of living, etc. Emphasized the "supportive" element in this nursing system.
Arvidsson, Bergman, Arvidsson, Fridlund, & Tops (2011), Sweden	To describe the meaning of health-promoting SC in patients with rheumatic diseases	Rheumatic disease patients (N = 12)	Health-promoting SC	Phenomenology	Perspectives revealed that SC requires dialogues with the body and environment, power struggles with the disease, and making choices to fight the disease. SC was viewed as a way of life.
Burdette (2012), USA	To examine relationship among SCA, SC, and obesity	Rural midlife women (N = 224)	BCFs, SCA, and SC practices; complemented with rural nursing theory	Predictive correlational design was used.	SCA predicted SC. Education, employment, and health status facilitated SC practices; smoking and chronic conditions were barriers.
Carthron, Johnson, Hubbart, Strickland, & Nance (2010), USA	To compare diabetes self-management activities of primary caregiving grandmothers (GM)	African American GMs with type 2 diabetes (N = 68, 34 per group)	BCF (family system factor of grandmother role; patterns of	Nonexperimental, comparative design	Before and after beginning caregiving: GMs were statistically different with fewer days of eating

Continued

Table 8 · 1   **Examples of Research Applications—cont'd**

Author (Year), Country	Purpose	Population/ Settings	SCDNT Concept(s)	Methods	Results
	before and after beginning caregiving activities; to compare these GMs' self-management activities with those of GMs not providing primary care		living); TSCD; SCA, especially power components		a healthy diet and fewer performed self-management blood glucose tests. Fewer self-management blood glucose tests and fewer eye examinations were performed by GMs providing primary care to grandchildren.
Kim (2011), Korea	To determine effectiveness of a program to develop SCA based on SC needs specific to prostatectomy	Prostate cancer patients (N = 69)	SCA; quality of life	Quasi-experimental; nonequivalent control group using pre–post test design	Significant difference was found between self-care agency and quality of life in treatment group vs control group at 8 weeks after prostatectomy.
Lundberg & Thrakul (2011), Sweden & Thailand	To explore Thai Muslim women's self-management of type 2 diabetes	Thai Muslim women living in Bangkok (N = 29)	Orem's SCDNT was used as framework	Ethnographic study using participant observation	Four themes emerged on self-management: daily life practices (dietary, exercise, medicine, doctor follow-up, blood sugar self-monitoring, use of herbal remedies), affect of illness, family support and need for everyday life as before diagnosis (e.g., maintaining religious practices during Ramadan).
Ovayolu, Ovayolu, & Karadag (2011), Turkey	To explore relationship among SCA, disability levels, and other factors	Turkish patients with rheumatoid arthritis (RA) (N = 467)	SCA; Factors related to healthcare, such as pain and disability level.	Cross-sectional; descriptive–correlational	For patients with RA, patients with higher disability and pain had lower self-care agency. The potential for development of

Table 8 · 1	**Examples of Research Applications—cont'd**				
Author (Year), Country	**Purpose**	**Population/ Settings**	**SCDNT Concept(s)**	**Methods**	**Results**
					knowledge, skills, and resources necessary for SC were identified.
Rujiwatthanakorn, Panpakdee, Malathum, & Tanomsup (2011), Thailand	To examine effectiveness of a SC management program	Thais with essential hypertension (N = 96)	SC demands, self-care ability and blood pressure control	Quasi-experimental	Patients in treatment group had higher knowledge of self-care demands and self-care ability regarding medication, dietary, physical activity, self-monitoring. Both systolic and diastolic readings of treatment group were lower than control group.
Surucu & Kizilci (2012), Turkey	To explore the use of SCDNT in diabetes self-management education	Type 2 diabetes patients	TSCD, HDSCR, SCA	Descriptive case study	Demonstrated improvement in health indicators after design of a nursing system directed at deficits in SCA related to HDSCR.
Thi (2012), South Vietnam	To describe levels of SC knowledge in patients	Hepatitis B inpatients and outpatients (N = 230)	SCA (SC knowledge), SCR, BCFs	Descriptive/ comparative	51% of patients had the required hepatitis B SC knowledge, especially need for exercise, rest, and methods of prevention of transmission through sexual activity. There was a knowledge deficit related to diet and management/ monitoring of disease. Level of education, type of occupation, previous health education, and

Continued

Table 8 · 1 **Examples of Research Applications—cont'd**

Author (Year), Country	Purpose	Population/ Settings	SCDNT Concept(s)	Methods	Results
Wilson, Mood, Nordstrom (2012), USA	To determine whether reading low literacy pamphlets on radiation side effects affect patient knowledge	Urban radiation oncology clinic patients, (N = 47)	SCA: SC knowledge of radiation side effects	Nonexperimental, exploratory	health-care setting affected levels of SC knowledge. Knowledge about radiation side effect management varied by literacy level despite low literacy level of pamphlets. Supported premise that foundational capacities for self-care include skills for reading, writing, communication perception and reasoning.

Note. BCF = basic conditioning factors; HDSCR = health deviation self-care requisites; SC = self-care or self-care practices; SCA = self-care agency; SCDNT = self-care deficit nursing theory; SCR = self-care requisites; TSCD = therapeutic self-care demand.

Practice Applications

Nursing practice has informed development of SCDNT as SCDNT has guided nursing practice and research. Biggs (2008) conducted a review of nursing literature from 1999 to 2007. The results revealed more than 400 articles, including those in *International Orem Society Newsletters* and *Self-Care, Dependent-Care, and Nursing,* the official journal of the International Orem Society. Although Biggs noted a tremendous increase in publications during that period, the author observed that SCDNT research has not always contributed to theory progression and development or to nursing practice. She identified deficient areas such as those related to concepts such as therapeutic self-care demand, self-care deficit, nursing systems, and the methods of helping or assisting. Recent publications on Orem based practice address areas identified by Biggs.

Table 8-2 provides examples of specific practice applications in the past 5 years at the time of this writing.

One theoretical application to nursing practice exemplifies the continued scholarly work necessary for practice models and addresses one deficit area noted by Biggs (2008). Casida and colleagues (2009) applied Orem's general theoretical framework to formulate and develop the health-deviation self-care requisites of patients with left ventricular assist devices. This article specifies not only the self-care requisites for this population but also the necessary subsystems unique to practice applications. This work illustrates the complexity of SCDNT and also the utility of SCDNT for patients with all types of technology assisted living.

One change in the past few years has been an emphasis on self-management rather than or in conjunction with self-care (Ryan, Aloe, &

Table 8 · 2   Examples of Practice Applications

Author (Year), Country	Health or Illness Focus	Settings	SCDNT Concept(s)	Patient or Practice Focus (Selected Examples)	Other
Alspach (2011), USA	Hypertension/heart failure in elderly	Critical care unit	SC	Development of checklist tool to measure SC at home after critical care discharge	Editorial demonstrating use of theoretical framework to design a brief checklist
Casida, Peters, Peters, & Magnan (2009), USA	Left-ventricular assist devices (LVAD)	Acute care	HDSCR, including SC systems	Reformulation of HDSCR common to patients with LVAD using five guidelines described by Orem (2001) to validate form and adequacy	An exemplar for the six HDSCRs specific health situation and model for developing other conditions using multifaceted technological care
Green (2012), USA	Children with special needs	School setting	SCR; SCD; BCF; SCA; DCA; SCS	Demonstration of utility of SCDNT through two case studies: wholly compensatory system for child with cerebral palsy; partly compensatory for child with asthma; and supportive-educative system for diabetic.	An example of types of nursing systems
Hohdorf (2010), Germany	Hospitalized patients	Acute care settings	SCDNT	Exemplified change of focus to theory-based nursing practice	One hospital's goal to improve quality care and decrease length of stay by moving to theory based practice
Hudson & Macdonald (2010), Canada	Adults with hemodialysis arteriovenous fistula self-cannulation	Community dialysis unit	SCDNT as framework; all concepts including NA	Demonstration of SCDNT as guide to develop and update patient-teaching resources in preparation for home care; assisted nurses with role clarification	An example of application or SCDNT to arteriovenous fistula SC

Continued

Table 8 · 2 **Examples of Practice Applications—cont'd**

Author (Year), Country	Health or Illness Focus	Settings	SCDNT Concept(s)	Patient or Practice Focus (Selected Examples)	Other
Pickens (2012), USA	Adults with schizophrenia	Psychiatric nursing care	SCA: motivation component	Explored various theories of motivation to develop SCDNT's foundational capability and power component of motivation	Theoretical paper incorporating elements of other theories to expand supportive-developmental technologies in patients with serious mental illness
Seed & Torkelson (2012), USA	Acute psychiatric care	Recovery principles	SCDNT concepts in alignment with recovery can be used to structure interventions and research in acute psychiatric settings	SCDNT provided a comprehensive framework for delivering interventions that empower individuals to make choices in care and treatment through partnerships and education	Demonstrates use of SCDNT toward partner-based relationships for recovery from mental illness
Surucu & Kizilci, (2012), Turkey	Use of SCDNT in type 2 diabetes self-management education	University setting; diabetes education center	BCFs; SCA; SCD; TSCD, with emphasis on HDSCR	Implemented steps of general nursing process using Orem-specific concepts	This case study provides an exemplar for self-management of type 2 diabetes
Swanson & Tidwell (2011), USA	Integration model of shared governance using magnet components to promote patient safety	Orem's self-care deficit theory as general practice framework	SCA; SCD; helping methods	Demonstrates incorporation of SCDNT as the theoretical guide to professional practice at one institution and its combination shared governance to enhance patient safety	SCDNT as component of health system practice model
Wanchai, Armer, & Stewart (2010), USA, Canada, Germany	Breast cancer survivors	Multiple settings based on review of 11 studies from 1990 through 2009	SCA	SC agency enhancement through use of complementary or alternative therapies to meet HDSCR, specifically to	

Table 8 · 2   Examples of Practice Applications—cont'd

Author (Year), Country	Health or Illness Focus	Settings	SCDNT Concept(s)	Patient or Practice Focus (Selected Examples)	Other
				maintain physical and emotional well-being and to manage side effects of treatment	

BCFs = basic conditioning factors; DCA = dependent-care agency; HDSCR = health deviation self-care requisites; NA = nursing agency; SC = self-care; SCA = self-care agency; SCD = self-care deficit; SCR = self-care requisites; SCS = self-care systems; TSCD = therapeutic self-care demand.

Mason-Johnson, 2009; Sürücu & Kizilci, 2012; Swanlund, Scherck, Metcalfe, & Jesek-Hale, 2008; Wilson, Mood, & Nordstrom, 2012). Orem (2001) introduced the term *self-management* in her final book, defining the concept as the *ability to manage self in stable or changing environments and ability to manage one's personal affairs* (p. 111). This definition relates to continuity of contacts and interactions one would expect over time with nursing, especially when caring for people with chronic conditions such as diabetes. By nature, chronic disease variations over time are collaboratively managed by the self-care agent, dependent-care agent, the nurse agent, and others. The dependent-care theory enhances the self-management component, a uniqueness of SCDNT (Casida et al., 2009). With increases in chronic illness and treatment, especially in relationship to allocation of health-care dollars, countries such as Thailand now emphasize self-management versus self-care in health policy decisions (personal communication, Prof. Dr. Somchit Hanucharurnkul, January 15, 2013). Taylor and Renpenning (2011) presented diverse perspectives on self-management, describing it first as a subset of self-care with emphasis on creating a sense of order in life using all available resources, social and other. Another perspective relates to controlling and directing actions in a particular situation at a particular time. This includes incorporating standardized models for self-management in specific health situations such as diabetes.

In addition to creating models for specific health-care conditions, Orem's SCDNT is also used as a general framework for nursing practice in health care institutions. For example, Cedars Sinai Medical Center in Los Angeles, California, integrates SCDNT with its shared governance model to promote patient safety (Swanson & Tidwell, 2011). However, most practice applications use the general theory or elements of the theory with specific populations. Table 8-2 includes diverse examples from English publications. However, the reader is also directed to non-English publications including examples from practitioners or researchers in Brazil (Herculano, De Souse, Galvão, Caetano, & Damasceno, 2011) and China (Su & Jueng, 2011).

To further develop the sciences of self-care related to specific self-care systems and to nursing systems for diverse populations around the globe, collaboration will be necessary between reflective practitioners and scholars (Taylor & Renpenning, 2011). Orem's wise approach to theory development, combining independent work with formal collaboration among practitioners, administrators, educators, and researchers will determine the future of self-care deficit nursing theory. The International Orem Society for Nursing Science and Scholarship continues as an important avenue for collaborative work among expert and novice SCDNT scholars around the globe.

Practice Exemplar

Provided by Laureen M. Fleck, PhD, FNP-BC, CDE

Marion W. presents to a primary care office seeking care for recent fatigue. She is assigned to the nurse practitioner. The nurse explains the need for information to determine what needs to be done and by whom to promote Marion's life, health, and well-being. Information regarding Marion is gathered in part using Orem's conceptualizations as a guide. First, the nurse introduces herself and then describes the information she will seek to help her with the health situation. Marion agrees to provide information to the best of her knowledge. As the nurse and Marion have entered into a professional relationship and agreed to the roles of nurse and patient, the nurse initiates the three steps of Orem's process of nursing:

Step 1: Diagnosis and Prescription
I. Basic Conditioning Factors

As basic conditioning factors affect the value of therapeutic self-care demand and self-care agency, the nurse seeks information regarding the following: age, gender, developmental state, patterns of living, family system factors, sociocultural factors, health state, health-care system factors, availability and adequacy of resources, and external environmental factors such as the physical or biological.

Marion is 42, female, in a developmental stage of adulthood where she carries out tasks of family and work responsibilities as a productive member of society. The history related to patterns of living and family system reveals employment as a school crossing guard, a role that allows time after school with her children, ages 5, 7, and 9. Her husband works for "the city" but recently had hours cut to 4 days per week. Therefore, money is tight. They pay bills on time, but no money remains at the end of the month. She has learned to stretch their money by shopping at the local discount store for clothes and food and cooking "one-pot meals" so that they have leftovers to stretch throughout the week. As an African American, she worships in a community-based black church, a source of spiritual strength and social support. Marion has a high school education.

Questions about health state and health system reveal Marion has type 2 diabetes that was diagnosed more than 5 years ago. Except for periodic fatigue, she believes she has managed this chronic condition by following the treatment plan, faithfully taking oral medication, and checking blood sugar once per day. The morning reading was 230 mg/dL. Although the family has no health insurance, Marion has access to the community health care clinic and free oral medications. There is a small co-pay for her blood glucose testing strips, which is now a concern. The children receive health care through the State Children's Health Insurance Program. The neighborhood Marion lives in has a safe, outdoor environment. The latter has been a comfort because she works as a crossing guard and walks her children to school. Although she enjoys this exercise, her increasing fatigue discourages additional exercise.

When asked about her perception of her current condition, Marion expressed concern for her weight and considers this a partial explanation for the fatigue. She desires to lose weight but admits she has no willpower, snacks late at night, and finds "healthy foods" too expensive. At 205 lbs (93 kg) and 5 feet 3 inches (1.6 m), Marion is classified as obese with a body mass index of 38 kg/m^2.

II. Calculating the Therapeutic Self-Care Demand

With Marion, the nurse identifies many actions that should be performed to meet the universal, developmental, and health deviation self-care requisites. Her health state and health system factors (including previous treatment modalities) are major conditioners of two universal self-care requisites: maintain a sufficient intake of food and maintain a balance between activity and rest. Throughout the interview, the nurse determines that Marion is clear about her chronic condition and has accepted herself in need of continued monitoring and care, including quarterly

Practice Exemplar cont.

hemoglobin A1C and lipid blood tests (American Diabetes Association [ADA], 2013)

Two health deviation self-care requisites also emerge as the primary focus for seeking helping services: being aware and attending to effects and results of pathological conditions; and effectively carrying out medically prescribed diagnostic and therapeutic measures. Without additional self-care actions beyond the prescribed medication, short walks, and daily blood glucose testing, the risks of uncontrolled diabetes may lead to diabetic retinopathy, nephropathy, neuropathy, and cardiovascular disease (ADA, 2013).

One particularized self-care requisite (PSCRs) is presented as an example, with the related actions Marion should perform to improve her health and well-being. Once the actions to be performed and concomitant methods are identified, then the nurse determines Marion's self-care agency: the capabilities of knowing (estimative operations), deciding (transitional operations), and performing these actions (productive operations).

PSCR: Reduce and maintain blood glucose level within normal parameters through increased blood glucose monitoring, appropriate healthy food choices, and increased activity. If this PSCR is achieved, Marion's weight will be decreased, a related purpose that provides motivation to engage in self-care. The methods to achieve the PSCR include detailed actions:

A. Increase blood glucose monitoring to twice per day; set goals for 100–110 mg/dL fasting and <140 mg/dL at 2 hours after a main meal.

1. Obtain discounted glucose monitoring strips from ABC drug company.
2. Obtain assistance from community clinic for monthly replacement request to ABC drug company.
3. Monitor glucose level through testing two times per day, with one test before breakfast and one test 2 hours after a main meal. Add more testing when needed for symptoms of high or low blood sugar (ADA, 2013).

4. Seek assistance from health professional when levels are below 60 mg/dL and not responsive to sugar intake or higher than 300 mg/dL with feelings of fatigue, thirst, or visual disturbances.
5. Adjust activity and meal planning/portion sizes when levels are not within parameters.

B. Make healthy food choices.

6. Seek knowledge of healthy food choices for family meal planning from dietitian at clinic.
7. Review family expenses with health professional to adjust grocery budget to purchase affordable but healthy foods.
8. Eat three balanced meals per day including midmorning, afternoon, and evening snack as desired. These meals and snacks will have portion sizes established between Marion and the nurse.
9. All meals will have a selection of protein, fats, and carbohydrates, and the snacks will be limited to 15 grams of carbohydrate or less (ADA, 2013).

C. Increase physical activity to 150 minutes/week of moderate intensity exercise (ADA, 2013).

10. Gain knowledge regarding step-walking program to increase activity. Discuss community options for safe walking areas.
11. Explore budget to include properly fitting footwear. Tennis shoes with socks are to be worn for each walk. Obtain free pedometer from clinic to measure performance of steps and walking.
12. Review pedometer measures three times a week. Increase steps by 10% each week if natural increase in steps has not occurred. For example, if walking 2000 steps/walk increase next walk by 200 steps as a goal. Maintain goals until 10,000 step/day is achieved (ADA, 2013).

III. Determining Self-Care Agency

The nurse and Marion then seek information about self-care agency or the capabilities related to knowledge, decision making, and

Continued

performance necessary to meet this PSCR. This includes the ability to seek and obtain required resources important to each action. What capabilities are necessary to increase blood glucose testing? Does Marion have the knowledge about access to drug company resources (testing strips) available to persons with their income level? Does she have the communication skills to seek resources from the community center? Does she have the knowledge regarding blood glucose parameters and methods to adjust exercise and diet to maintain the levels? The nurse and Marion together determine capabilities for each of these components of each action necessary to meet her particularized self-care requisite.

After collecting and analyzing data about her abilities in relationship to the required actions, the nurse determines the absence or existence of a self-care deficit—that is, is self-agency adequate to meet the therapeutic self-care demand? The nurse quickly determines throughout the data collection period that Marion's foundational and disposition capabilities (necessary for any deliberate action) and the power components (necessary for self-care) are developed and operable. The question is the adequacy of self-care agency in relationship to this PSCR.

1. Blood glucose monitoring: The nurse learns that Marion possesses necessary capabilities of knowing, deciding, and performing to obtain additional testing strips from ABC drug company and to increase her blood glucose testing to two times per day. After questioning, the nurse determines Marion is aware of norms and in general the effect of food and exercise. In addition to verbalizing available time for testing, Marion also recalls that the school nurse where she works agreed to be a resource if blood glucose readings are not within the required range. She agreed to seek out this resource if adjustment in exercise or food intake is needed. The nurse practitioner concludes Marion's self-care capabilities of knowing, deciding, and

performing the necessary actions is intact to meet the particularized self-care requisite, maintain blood glucose level at 100–110 mg/dL fasting and <140 mg/dL at 2 hours after a main meal.

2. Dietary practices: The nurse seeks information from Marion on her knowledge of effective dietary practices and healthy foods, including flexibility in the family budget, shopping practices, and family cultural practices that may influence her food purchases. The nurse learns Marion has misinformation about her selected foods and is aware of resources, such as the local health department that offers free classes by a registered dietitian. However, transportation to dietary classes is not possible because her husband uses the only car to drive to work. Although Marion understands the relationship of her high blood glucose levels to the resulting fatigue, she seems to focus on losing weight, a possible motivational asset. Marion maintains the ability to shop, cook, use the stove safely, and ingest all food types.

3. The nurse assesses that Marion enjoys walking and generally feels safe in the surrounding environment. She also has time while the children are at school to take walks. The nurse discovers that Marion is not aware of proper foot care or the step program for increasing exercise. Marion does not believe the family budget can manage both changes in food purchases as well as the purchase of good walking shoes.

IV. Self-Care Limitations

Marion has self-care limitations in the area of knowledge and decision making about required dietary actions. The limitations of knowing are related to healthy dietary practices. This includes the use of carbohydrate counting. She lacks knowledge about purchasing options for healthier foods and methods to incorporate these into her meal effort. Although interested, she is unable to enroll in dietary classes at the health department due to transportation issues. Marion has knowledge

Practice Exemplar cont.

and decision-making authority for managing the family budget but has no experience incorporating healthier foods into the planning. Marion also has self-care limitations in relationship to knowledge of the step program, proper footwear, and related foot care. No resources exist to purchase the necessary walking shoes. Major capabilities include Marion's ability to learn, availability of time, and her motivation to lose weight, and hence have less fatigue. If Marion decides to make healthier food choices that are affordable and also increase her general activity, she will need monitoring, counseling, and support from a health professional related to the blood glucose levels, access to resources for classes, budgeting, and purchase of equipment.

With analysis of self-care agency in relationship to the particularized self-care requisite, the nurse and patient establish the presence of a self-care deficit. Now that legitimate nursing has been established, a nursing system is designed.

Step 2: Design and Plan of Nursing System

Now that the self-care limitations of knowing are identified, the nurse will use helping methods of guiding and supporting by designing a supportive-educative nursing system. The design involves planning Marion's activities to meet the particularized self-care requisite with nurse guidance and monitoring and also to establishing the nurse's role. Together they agree on communication methods to work together to monitor progress as Marion attends classes to learn healthy dietary practices and increase activity. Marion agrees to share information related to blood glucose testing with the school nurse and the pharmacist at the community clinic when refilling medication and supplies.

The nurse agrees to seek out resources for transportation to the health department for dietary classes, purchase of footwear, assistance to fill out forms, and also to meet with Marion every 2 weeks to review food consumption and activity records. Although the goal is to maintain blood glucose levels at 100–110 mg/dL fasting and <140 mg/dL at 2 hours after a main meal, the priority actions relate to dietary changes, followed by slow, incremental changes in activity. The nurse expects it will take 1 month to obtain the necessary footwear. Objectives will be reviewed at 1 month. Marion knows that weight loss is her objective, but she must start changes in dietary practices. The goal for weight loss will be set at the first month's meeting after attendance at the dietary sessions and initial experience with changing the family's food purchases and meal planning. Marion and the nurse practitioner begin implementing their roles as prescribed.

Step 3: Treatment, Regulation, Case Management, Control/Evaluation

Marion and the nurse begin implementing their agreed-on actions as they collaborate within the nursing system. The nurse practitioner maintains contact via phone with Marion as she completes actions, such as seeking resources for the dietary classes and footwear. Marion contacts the school nurse where she works to see if she will be a resource for weekly reports on blood glucose levels. She also seeks out additional testing strips and calls the clinic to obtain the routine forms for monthly renewal requests. They proceed through each of these actions as agreed on as social–contractual operations. Throughout this step, the interpersonal operations are essential as the nurse evaluates Marion's progress and new roles are determined and agreed on. This continues over time, with continued review of the design, the role prescriptions, until Marion's therapeutic self-care demand is decreased or self-care agency is developed so no self-care deficit exists, and nursing is no longer required.

Throughout the process, nursing agency was evident. The capabilities related to interpersonal, social–contractual, and professional–technological operations were evident.

■ Summary

This chapter provided an overview of Orem's self-care deficit nursing theory. Orem created this general theory of nursing to address the proper objective of nursing through the question, *What condition exists in a person when judgments are made that a nurse(s) should be brought into the situation* (i.e., that a person should be under nursing care; Orem, 2001, p. 20)? The grand theory comprises four interrelated theories: the theory of self-care, theory of dependent care, theory of self-care deficit, and theory of nursing systems. The building blocks of these theories are six major concepts and one peripheral concept. Orem's SCDNT has been applied extensively in nursing practice throughout the United States and internationally in diverse settings and with diverse populations. SCDNT continues to be used as a framework for research with specific patient populations throughout the world. Collaboration among scholars, researchers, and practitioners is necessary to provide the science of self-care useful to improve nursing practice into the future (Taylor & Renpenning, 2011).

References

Alspach, J. (2011). Editorial: The patient's capacity for self-care: Advocating for pre-discharge assessment. *Critical Care Nurse, 31*(2), 10–14. doi:10.4037/ccn2011419

American Diabetes Association. (2013). Clinical practice recommendations 2013. *Diabetes Care 36*(1), s12–s66.

Armer, J. M., Brooks, C. W., & Stewart, B. R. (2011). Limitations of self-care in reducing the risk of lymphedema: Supportive–educative systems. *Nursing Science Quarterly, 24*(1), 57–63.

Armer, J. M., Shook, R. P., Schneider, M. K., Brooks, C. W., Peterson, J., & Stewart, B. R. (2009). Enhancing supportive-educative nursing systems to reduce risk of post-breast cancer lymphedema. *Self-Care, Dependent-Care, & Nursing, 17*(1), 6–17.

Arvidsson, S., Bergman, S., Arvidsson, B., Fridlund, B., & Tops, A. B. (2011). Experiences of health-promoting self-care in people living with rheumatic diseases. *Journal of Advanced Nursing, 67*(6), 1264–1272.

Banfield, B. E. (2011). Environment: A perspective of the self-care deficit nursing theory. *Nursing Science Quarterly, 24*(2), 96–100.

Berbiglia, V. A., Hohmann, J., & Bekel, G. (Eds.). (2012). *World Congress on Future Nursing Systems: New approaches, new evidence for 2020. Bulletin luxembourgeios des questions sociales* (Vol. 29). Luxembourg: ALOSS.

Biggs, A. J. (2008). Orem's self-care deficit nursing theory: Update on the state of the art and science. *Nursing Science Quarterly, 21*(3), 200–206.

Burdette, L. (2012). Relationship between self-care agency, self-care practices, and obesity among rural midlife women. In V. Berbiglia, J. Hohmann, & G. Bekel (Eds.), *World Congress on Future Nursing Systems: New approaches, new evidence for 2020. Bulletin luxembourgeois des questions sociales* (Vol. 29, pp. 111–130). Luxembourg: ALOSS.

Carthron, D. L., Johnson, T. M., Hubbart, T. D., Strickland, C., & Nance, K. (2010). "Give me some sugar!" The diabetes self-management activities of African-American primary caregiving grandmothers. *Journal of Nursing Scholarship, 42*(3), 330–337.

Casida, J. M., Peters, R. M., & Magnan, M. A. (2009). Self-care demands of persons living with an implantable left-ventricular assist device. *Research and Theory in Nursing Practice: An International Journal, 23*(4), 279–293.

Clark, P. N., Allison, S. E., Berbiglia, V. A., & Taylor, S. G. (2009). The impact of Dorothea E. Orem's life and work: An interview with Orem scholars. *Nursing Science Quarterly, 22*, 41–46.

Costantini, L., Beanlands, H., & Horsburgh, M. E. (2011). Development of the Self-Care for Adults on Dialysis Tool (SCAD). *The CANNT Journal, 21*(2), 38–43.

Davidson, S. (2012). Challenging RN-BSN students to apply Orem's Theory to practice. In V. Berbiglia, J. Hohmann, & G. Bekel (Eds.), *World Congress on Future Nursing Systems New Approaches, New Evidence for 2020: Bulletin luxembourgeois des questions sociales* (Vol. 29, pp. 131–138). Luxembourg: ALOSS.

Dennis, C. M., & Jesek-Hale, S. M. (2003). Calculating the therapeutic self-care demand for a nursing population of nursery newborns' particularized self-care requisites. *Self-Care, Dependent-Care, & Nursing, 11*(1), 3–10.

Denyes, M. J. (1981). *Development of an instrument to measure self-care agency in adolescents.* Doctoral dissertation, University of Michigan, 1980. *Dissertation Abstract International, 41,* 1716B.

Denyes, M. J. (1988). Orem's model used for health promotion: Directions from research. *Advances in Nursing Science, 11,* p. 13.

Denyes, M. J., Orem, D. E., & Bekel, G. (2001). Self-care: A foundational science. *Nursing Science Quarterly, 14*(2), 48–54.

Fleck, L. M. (2012). The Nutrition Self Care Inventory. In V. A. Berbiglia, J. Hohmann, J., & G. Bekel (Eds.), *World Congress on Future Nursing Systems: New approaches, new evidence for 2020. Bulletin luxembourgeios des questions sociales* (Vol. 29, pp. 139–154). Luxembourg: ALOSS.

Gast, H., Denyes, M. J., Campbell, J. C., Hartweg, D. L., Schott-Baer, D., & Isenberg, M. (1989). Self-care agency: Conceptualizations and operationalizations. *Advances in Nursing Science, 12*(1), 26–38.

Green, R. (2012). Application of the self-care deficit nursing theory to the care of children with special health care needs in the school setting. *Self-Care, Dependent-Care, & Nursing, 19*(1), 35–40.

Harre, R. (1970). *The principles of scientific thinking.* Chicago: University of Chicago Press.

Hartweg, D. L. (1990). Health promotion self-care within Orem's general theory of nursing. *Journal of Advanced Nursing, 15*(1), 35–41.

Hartweg, D. L. (1991). *Dorothea Orem: Self-care deficit nursing theory.* Newbury Park, CA: Sage.

Hartweg, D. L. (1993). Self-care actions of healthy, middle-aged women to promote well-being. *Nursing Research, 42*(4), 221–227.

Hartweg, D. L. (2001). Use of Orem's conceptualizations in a baccalaureate nursing program (1980–2000). *International Orem Society Newsletter, 8*(1), 5–7.

Hartweg, D. L., & Berbiglia, V. A. (1996). Determining the adequacy of a health promotion self-care interview guide with healthy, middle-aged Mexican-American women: A pilot study. *Health Care for Women International, 17*(1), 57–68.

Helene Fuld Health Trust. (1988). *The nurse theorists: Portraits of excellence: Dorothea Orem.* Oakland, CA: Studio III.

Herculano, M. M. S., de Sousa, V. E. C., Galvão, M. R. G., Caetano, J.A., & Damasceno, A. K. C. (2011). Nursing process application in a patient with gestational hypertension based in Orem. *Revista de Rede de Enfermagem do Nordeste, 12*(2), 401–408.

Hintze, A. (2011). Orem-based nursing education in Germany. *Nursing Science Quarterly, 24*(1), 66–70.

Hohdorf, M. (2010). Self-care deficit nursing theory in Ingolstadt—An approach to practice development in nursing care. *Self-Care, Dependent-Care, and Nursing, 18*(1), 19–25.

Horan, P. (2004). Exploring Orem's self-care deficit nursing theory in learning disability nursing: Philosophical parity paper, part 1. *Learning Disability Practice, 7*(4), 28–33.

Hudson, S., & MacDonald, M. (2010). Hemodialysis arteriovenous fistula self-cannulation: Moving theory to practice in developing patient-teaching resources. *Clinical Nursing Specialist, 24*(6), 304–312.

Isaramalai, S. (2002). *Developing a cross-cultural measure of the self-as-career inventory questionnaire for the Thai population.* Unpublished doctoral dissertation, University of Missouri.

Jaimovich, S., Campos, M. S., Campos, M. C., & Moore, J. B. (2009). Spanish version of the Child and Adolescent Self-Care Performance Questionnaire: Psychometric Testing. *Pediatric Nursing, 35*(2), 109–114.

Kim, H. S. (2011). Development and evaluation of self-care agency promoting programme for prostatectomy patients. *International Journal of Urological Nursing, 5*(1), 34–44.

Klainin, P., & Ounnapiruk, L. (2010). A meta-analysis of self-care behaviour research on elders in Thailand: An update. *Nursing Science Quarterly, 23*(2), 156–163.

Lundberg, P. C., & Thrakul, S. (2011). Diabetes type 2 self-management among Thai Muslim women. *Nursing and Healthcare in Chronic Illness, 3*, 52-60 doi: 10.1111/j.1752-9824.2011.01079.x

Matchim, Y. M., Armer, J. M., & Stewart, B. R. (2008). A qualitative study of participants' perceptions of effect of mindfulness meditation practice on self-care and overall well-being. *Self-Care, Dependent-Care, & Nursing, 16*(2), 45–53.

National League for Nursing. (1987). *Nursing theory: A circle of knowledge.* New York: Author.

Nursing Development Conference Group. (1973). *Concept formalization: Process and product.* Boston: Little, Brown.

Nursing Development Conference Group. (1979). *Concept formalization: Process and product* (2nd Ed.). Boston: Little, Brown.

Orem, D. E. (1956). The art of nursing in hospital nursing service: An analysis. In K. M. Renpenning & S. G. Taylor (Eds.), *Self-Care Theory in Nursing: Selected Papers of Dorothea Orem.* New York: Springer.

Orem, D. E. (1959). *Guides for developing curricular for the education of practical nurses.* Washington, DC: U.S. Government Printing Office.

Orem, D. E. (1971). *Nursing: Concept of practice.* New York: McGraw-Hill.

Orem, D. E. (2001). *Nursing: Concept of practice* (6th ed.). St. Louis, MO: Mosby.

Orem, D. E. (2006). Dorothea E. Orem's self-care nursing theory. In M. E. Parker (Ed.), *Nursing theories and nursing practice* (2nd ed., pp. 141–149). Philadelphia: F. A Davis.

Ovayolu, O. U., Ovayolu, N., & Karadag, G. (2011). The relationship between self-care agency, disability levels, and factors regarding situations among patients with rheumatoid arthritis. *Journal of Clinical Nursing, 21*, 101–110.

Pickens, J. (2012). Development of self-care agency through enhancement of motivation in people with schizophrenia. In V. Berbiglia, J. Hohmann, & G. Bekel (Eds.), *World Congress on Future Nursing Systems. New approaches, new evidence for 2020. Bulletin luxembourgeois des questions sociales* (Vol. 29, pp. 237–248). Luxembourg: ALOSS.

Ransom, J. E. (2008). Facilitating emerging nursing agency in undergraduate nursing students. *Self-Care, Dependent Care, & Nursing, 16*(2), 39–45.

Renpenning, K. Mc., & Taylor, S. G. (Eds.). (2003). *Self-care theory in nursing: Selected papers of Dorothea Orem.* New York: Springer.

Ryan, M., Aloe, K., & Mason-Johnson, J. (2009). Improving self-management and reducing hospital readmission in heart failure patients. *Clinical Nurse Specialist, 23*(4), 216–221.

Ryan, R. M., Patrick, H., Deci, E. L., & Williams, G. C. (2008). Facilitating health behaviour change and its maintenance: Interventions based on self-determination theory. *The European Health Psychologist, 10,* 2–5.

Rujiwatthanakorn, D., Panpakdee, O., Malathum, P., & Tanomsup. S. (2011). Thais with essential hypertension. *Pacific Rim Int J Nurs Res, 15*(2), 97–110.

Singleton, E. K., Bienemy, C., Hutchinson, S. W., Dellinger, A., & Rami, J. S. (2011, Fall). A pilot study: A descriptive correctional study of factors associated with weight in college nursing students. *The ABNF Journal,* 89–95

Sürücü, H. A., & Kizilci, S. (2012). Use of Orem's self-care deficit nursing theory in the self-management education of patients with type 2 diabetes: A case study. *Self-Care, Dependent Care, and Nursing, 19*(1), 53–59.

Su, H., & Jueng, R. (2011). A nursing experience of applying Orem's theory to the care of an acute pancreatitis patient [in Chinese]. *Tzu Chi Nursing Journal, 10*(4), 1.

Swanlund, S. L., Scherck, K. A., Metcalfe, S. A., & Jesek-Hale, S. R. (2008). Keys to successful self-management of medications. *Nursing Science Quarterly, 21*(3), 238–246.

Swanson, J. W. & Tidwell, C. A. (2011). Improving the culture of patient safety through the Magnet journey. *OJIN: The Online Journal of Issues in Nursing 16*(3). doi:10.3912/OJIN.Vol16No03Man01

Taylor, S. G. (2001). Orem's general theory of nursing and families. *Nursing Science Quarterly, 14*(1), 7–9.

Taylor, S. G. (2007). The development of self-care deficit nursing theory: A historical analysis. *Self-Care, Dependent Care, & Nursing, 15*(1), 22–25.

Taylor, S. G. (2011). Dorothea Orem's legacy. *Nursing Science Quarterly, 24*(5), 5–6. doi: 10.1177/0894318410389064.

Taylor, S. G., & Hartweg, D. L. (2002). Nursing theory use in baccalaureate programs in the United States (#27). Proceedings of the Seventh International Self-Care Deficit Nursing Theory Conference: The Practice of Nursing: Using and Extending self-care deficit nursing theory, Atlanta, Georgia.

Taylor, S. G., & Renpenning, K. Mc. (2001). The practice of nursing in multiperson situations, family and community. In D. E. Orem (Ed.), *Nursing: Concepts of practice* (6th ed., pp. 394–433). St. Louis, MO: C. V. Mosby.

Taylor, S. G., & Renpenning, K. (2011). *Self-care science, nursing theory and evidence-based practice.* New York: Springer.

Taylor, S. G., Renpenning, K. Mc., Geden, E. A., Neuman, B. M., & Hart, M. A. (2001). A theory of dependent-care: A corollary theory to Orem's theory of self-care. *Nursing Science Quarterly, 14*(1), 39–47.

Thi, T. L. (2012). An analysis of self-care knowledge of hepatitis B patients. In V. Berbiglia, J. Hohmann, & G. Bekel (Eds.), *World Congress on Future Nursing Systems. New approaches, new evidence for 2020. Bulletin luxembourgeois des questions sociales* (Vol. 29, pp. 224–236). Luxembourg: ALOSS.

Valente, S. M., Saunders, J. M., & Uman, G. (2011, Dec.). Self-care outcomes: Instrument development. *Journal of Chi Eta Phi Sorority.*

van Achterberg, T., Lorensen, M., Isenberg, M. A., Evers, G., Levin, E., & Philipsen, H. (1991). The Norwegian, Danish and Dutch version of the Appraisal of Self-care Agency scale; Comparing reliability aspects. *Scandinavian Journal of Caring Sciences, 5*(2), 101–108.

Wallace, W. A. (1983). *From a realist point of view: Essays on the philosophy of science.* Washington, DC: University Press of America.

Wanchai, A., Armer, J. M., & Stewart, B. R. (2010). Self-care agency using complementary and alternative medicine (CAM) among breast cancer survivors. *Self-Care, Dependent-Care, & Nursing, 18*(01), 8–18.

West, P., & Isenberg, M. (1997). Instrument development: The Mental Health-Related Self-Care Agency Scale. *Archives of Psychiatric Nursing, 11*(3), 126–132.

White, M. L. Peters, R., & Schim, S. M. (2011). Spirituality and spiritual self-care: Expanding self-care deficit nursing theory. *Nursing Science Quarterly, 24*(1), 48–56.

Wilson, F. L., Mood, D., & Nordstrom, C. K. (2010). The influence of easy-to read pamphlets about self-care management of radiation side effects on patients' knowledge. *Oncology Nursing Forum, 37*(6), 774–781.

Imogene King's Theory of Goal Attainment

Chapter 9

CHRISTINA L. SIELOFF AND
MAUREEN A. FREY

Introducing the Theorist
Overview of the Conceptual System
(King's Conceptual System and Theory of
Goal Attainment)
Applications of the Theory In Practice
Practice Exemplar by Mary B. Killeen
Summary
References

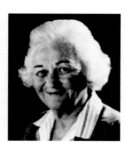

Imogene M. King

Introducing the Theorist

Imogene M. King was born on January 30, 1923, in West Point, Iowa. She received a diploma in nursing from St. John's Hospital School of Nursing, St. Louis, Missouri (1945); a bachelor of science in nursing education (1948); a master of science in nursing from St. Louis University (1957); and a doctor of education (EdD) from Teachers College, Columbia University, New York (1961). She held educational, administrative, and leadership positions at St. John's Hospital School of Nursing, the Ohio State University, Loyola University, the Division of Nursing in the U.S. Department of Health, Education, and Welfare, and the University of South Florida. King's hallmark theory publications include: "A Conceptual Frame of Reference for Nursing" (1968), *Towards a Theory for Nursing: General Concepts of Human Behaviour* (1971), and *A Theory for Nursing: Systems, Concepts, Process* (1981). Since 1981, King has clarified and expanded her conceptual system, her middle-range theory of goal attainment, and the transaction process model in multiple book chapters, articles in professional journals, and presentations. After retiring as professor emerita from the University of South Florida in 1990, King remained an active contributor to nursing's theoretical development and worked with individuals and groups in developing additional middle range theories, applying her theoretical formulations to various populations and settings and implementing the theory of goal attainment in clinical practice. King received recognition and numerous awards for her distinguished career in nursing from the American Nurses Association, the Florida Nurses Association, the American Academy of Nursing, and Sigma Theta Tau International. King died in December 2007. Her theoretical formulations for nursing continue to be taught at all levels of nursing education and applied and extended by national and international scholars.[1]

Overview of the Conceptual System (King's Conceptual System and Theory of Goal Attainment)

Theoretical Evolution in King's Own Words

My first theory publication pronounced the problems and prospect of knowledge development in nursing (King, 1964). More than 30 years ago, the problems were identified as (1) lack of a professional nursing language, (2) a theoretical nursing phenomena, and (3) limited concept development. Today, theories and conceptual frameworks have identified theoretical approaches to knowledge development and utilization of knowledge in practice. Concept development is a continuous process in the nursing science movement (King, 1988).

My rationale for developing a schematic representation of nursing phenomena was influenced by the Howland systems model (Howland, 1976) and the Howland and McDowell conceptual framework (Howland & McDowell, 1964). The levels of interaction in those works influenced my ideas relative to organizing a conceptual frame of reference for nursing. Because concepts offer one approach to structure knowledge for nursing, a thorough review of nursing literature provided me with ideas to identify five comprehensive concepts as a basis for a conceptual system for nursing. The overall concept is a human being, commonly referred to as an "individual" or a "person." Initially, I selected abstract concepts of perception, communication, interpersonal relations, health, and social institutions (King, 1968). These ideas forced me to review my knowledge of philosophy relative to the nature of human beings (ontology) and to the nature of knowledge (epistemology).

Philosophical Foundation

In the late 1960s, while auditing a series of courses in systems research, I was introduced to a philosophy of science called general system theory (von Bertalanffy, 1968). This philosophy of science gained momentum in the 1950s, although its roots date to an earlier period. This philosophy refuted logical positivism and reductionism and proposed the idea of isomorphism and perspectivism in knowledge development. Von Bertalanffy, credited with originating the idea of general system theory, defined this philosophy of science movement as a "general science of wholeness: systems of elements in mutual interaction" (von Bertalanffy, 1968, p. 37).

My philosophical position is rooted in general system theory, which guides the study of organized complexity as whole systems. This philosophy gave me the impetus to focus on knowledge development as an information-processing, goal-seeking, and decision-making system. General system theory provides a holistic approach to study nursing phenomena as an open system and frees one's thinking from the parts-versus-whole dilemma. In any discussion of the nature of nursing, the central ideas revolve around the nature of human beings and their interaction with internal and external environments. During this journey, I began to conceptualize a theory for nursing. However, because a manuscript was due in the publisher's office, I organized my ideas into a conceptual system (formerly called a "conceptual framework"), and the result was the publication of a book titled *Toward a Theory of Nursing* (King, 1971).

For additional information about the theorist, publications and research using King's conceptual model and the theory of goal attainment (Tables 9-1 to 9-15), please go to bonus chapter content available at http://davisplus.fadavis.com. Some tables are specifically referenced throughout the text to further guide the reader.

Design of a Conceptual System

A conceptual system provides structure for organizing multiple ideas into meaningful wholes. From my initial set of ideas in 1968 and 1971, my conceptual framework was refined to show some unity and relationships among the concepts. The conceptual system consists of individual systems, interpersonal systems, and social systems and concepts that are important for understanding the interactions within and between the systems (Fig. 9-1).

The next step in this process was to review the research literature in the discipline in which the concepts had been studied. For example, the concept of perception has been studied in psychology for many years. The literature indicated that most of the early studies dealt with sensory perception. Around the 1950s, psychologists began to study interpersonal perception, which related to my ideas about interactions. From this research literature, I identified the characteristics of perception and defined the concept for my framework. I continued searching literature for knowledge of each of the concepts in my framework. An update on my conceptual system was published in 1995 (King, 1995).

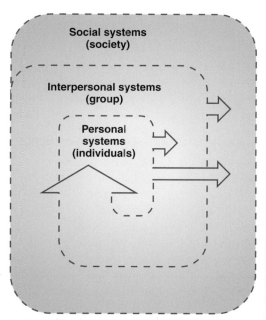

Fig 9 • 1 King's conceptual system.

Process for Development of Concepts

"Searching for scientific knowledge in nursing is an ongoing dynamic process of continuous identification, development, and validation of relevant concepts" (King, 1975, p. 25). What is a concept? A concept is an organization of reference points. Words are the verbal symbols used to explain events and things in our environment and relationships to past experiences. Northrop (1969) noted: "[C]oncepts fall into different types according to the different sources of their meaning. . . . A concept is a term to which meaning has been assigned." Concepts are the categories in a theory.

The concept development and validation process is as follows:

1. Review, analyze, and synthesize research literature related to the concept.
2. From the review, identify the characteristics (attributes) of the concept.
3. From the characteristics, write a conceptual definition.
4. Review literature to select an instrument or develop an instrument.
5. Design a study to measure the characteristics of the concept.
6. Select the population to be sampled.
7. Collect data.
8. Analyze and interpret data.
9. Write results of findings and conclusions.
10. State implications for adding to nursing knowledge.

Concepts that represent phenomena in nursing are structured within a framework and theory to show relationships.

Multiple concepts were identified from my analysis of nursing literature (King, 1981). The concepts that provided substantive knowledge about human beings (self, body image, perception, growth and development, learning, time, and personal space) were placed within the personal system, those related to small groups (interaction, communication, role, transactions, and stress) were placed within the interpersonal system, and those related to large groups that make up a society (decision making, organization, power, status, and authority) were placed within the social system (King, 1995). However, knowledge from all of the concepts is used in nurses' interactions with individuals and groups within social organizations, such as the family, the educational system, and the political system. Knowledge of these concepts came from my synthesis of research in many disciplines. Concepts, when defined from research literature, give nurses knowledge that can be applied in the concrete world of nursing. The concepts represent basic knowledge that nurses use in their role and functions either in practice, education, or administration. In addition, the concepts provide ideas for research in nursing.

One of my goals was to identify what I call the essence of nursing. That brought me back to the question: What is the nature of human beings? A vicious circle? Not really! Because nurses are first and foremost human beings who give nursing care to other human beings, my philosophy of the nature of human beings has been presented along with assumptions I have made about individuals (King, 1989a). Recognizing that a conceptual system represents structure for a discipline, the next step in the process of knowledge development was to derive one or more theories from this structure.

Lo and behold, a theory of goal attainment was developed (King, 1981, 1992). More recently, others have derived theories from my conceptual system (Frey & Sieloff, 1995).

Theory of Goal Attainment

Generally speaking, nursing care's goal is to help individuals maintain health or regain health (King, 1990). Concepts are essential elements in theories. When a theory is derived from a conceptual system, concepts are selected from that system. Remember my question: What is the essence of nursing? The concepts of self, perception, communication, interaction, transaction, role, growth and development, stress, time, and personal space were selected for the theory of goal attainment.

Transaction Process Model

A transaction model, shown in Figure 9-2, was developed that represented the process in which individuals interact to set goals that result in goal attainment (King, 1981, 1995).

The model is a human process that can be observed in many situations when two or more people interact, such as in the family and in

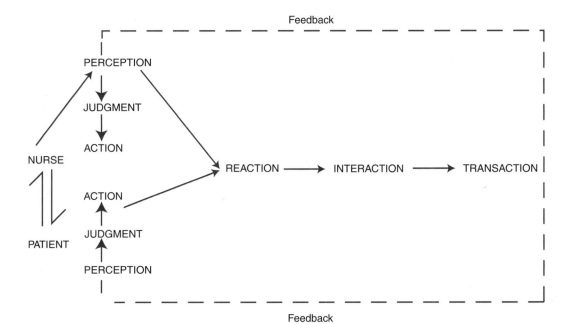

Fig 9 • 2 Transaction process model. *(From King, I. M. [1981]. A theory for nursing: Systems, concepts, process [p. 145]. New York: Wiley.)*

social events (King, 1996). As nurses, we bring knowledge and skills that influence our perceptions, communications, and interactions in performing the functions of the role. In your role as a nurse, after interacting with a patient, sit down and write a description of your behavior and that of the patient. It is my belief that you can identify your perceptions, mental judgments, mental action, and reaction (negative or positive). Did you make a transaction? That is, did you exchange information and set a goal with the patient? Did you explore the means for the patient to use to achieve the goal? Was the goal achieved? If not, why? It is my opinion that most nurses use this process but are not aware that it is based in a nursing theory. With knowledge of the concepts and of the process, nurses have a scientific base for practice that can be clearly articulated and documented to show quality care. How can a nurse document this transaction model in practice?

Documentation System

A documentation system was designed to implement the transaction process that leads to goal attainment (King, 1984). Most nurses use the nursing process to assess, diagnose, plan, implement, and evaluate, which I call a method. My transaction process provides the theoretical knowledge base to implement this method. For example, as one assesses the patient and the environment and makes a nursing diagnosis, the concepts of perception, communication, and interaction represent knowledge the nurse uses to gather information and make a judgment. A transaction is made when the nurse and patient decide mutually on the goals to be attained, agree on the means to attain goals that represent the plan of care, and then implement the plan. Evaluation determines whether or not goals were attained. If not, you ask why, and the process begins again. The documentation is recorded directly in the patient's chart. The patient's record indicates the process used to achieve goals. On discharge, the summary indicates goals set and goals achieved. One does not need multiple forms when this documentation system is in place, and the quality of nursing care is recorded. Why do nurses insist on designing critical paths, various care plans, and other types of forms when, with knowledge of this system, the nurse documents nursing care directly on the patient's chart? Why do we use multiple forms to complicate a process that is knowledge-based and also provides essential data to demonstrate outcomes and to evaluate quality nursing care?

Federal laws have been passed that indicate that patients must be involved in decisions about their care and about dying. This transaction process provides a scientifically based process to help nurses implement federal laws such as the Patient Self-Determination Act (Federal Register, 1995).

Goal Attainment Scale

Analysis of nursing research literature in the 1970s revealed that few instruments were designed for nursing research. In the late 1980s, the faculty at the University of Maryland, experts in measurement and evaluation, applied for and received a grant to conduct conferences to teach nurses to design reliable and valid instruments. I had the privilege of participating in this 2-year continuing education conference, where I developed a Goal Attainment Scale (King, 1989b). This instrument may be used to measure goal attainment. It may also be used as an assessment tool to provide patient data to plan and implement nursing care.

Vision for the Future

My vision for the future of nursing is that nursing will provide access to health care for all citizens. The United States' health-care system will be structured using my conceptual system. Entry into the system will be via nurses' assessment so that individuals are directed to the right place in the system for nursing care, medical care, social services information, health teaching, or rehabilitation. My transaction process will be used by every practicing nurse so that goals can be achieved to demonstrate quality care that is cost-effective. My conceptual system, theory of goal attainment, and transaction process model will continue to serve a useful purpose in delivering professional nursing care. The relevance of evidence-based practice, using my theory, joins the art of nursing of the 20th century to the science of nursing in the 21st century.

Concepts and Middle-Range Theory Development Within King's Conceptual System or the Theory of Goal Attainment

Concept development within a conceptual framework is particularly valuable, as it often explicates concepts more clearly than a theorist may have done in his or her original work. Concept development may also demonstrate how other concepts of interest to nursing can be examined through a nursing lens. Such explication further assists the development of nursing knowledge by enabling the nurse to better understand the application of the concept within specific practice situations. Examples of concepts developed from within King's work include the following: collaborative alliance relationship (Hernandez, 2007); decision making (Ehrenberger, Alligood, Thomas, Wallace, & Licavoli, 2007), empathy (May, 2007), holistic nursing (Li, Li, & Xu, 2010), managerial coaching (Batson & Yoder, 2012), patient satisfaction with nursing care (Killeen, 2007), sibling closeness (Lehna, 2009), and whole person care (Joseph, Laughon, & Bogue, 2011).[2]

Applications of the Theory in Practice

Since the first publication of King's work (1971), nursing's interest in the application of her work to practice has grown. The fact that she was one of the few theorists who generated both a framework and a middle range theory further expanded her work. Today, new publications related to King's work are a frequent occurrence. Additional middle-range theories have been generated and tested, and applications to practice have expanded. After her retirement, King continued to publish and examine new applications of the theory. The

purpose of this part of the chapter is to provide an updated review of the state of the art in terms of the application of King's conceptual system (KCS) and middle-range theory in a variety of areas: practice, administration, education, and research. Publications, identified from a review of the literature, are summarized and briefly discussed. Finally, recommendations are made for future knowledge development in relation to KCS and middle-range theory, particularly in relation to the importance of their application within an evidence-based practice environment.

In conducting the literature review, the authors began with the broadest category of application—application within KCS to nursing care situations. Because a conceptual framework is, by nature, very broad and abstract, it can serve only to guide, rather than to prescriptively direct, nursing practice.

Development of middle-range theories is a natural extension of a conceptual framework. Middle-range theories, clearly developed from within a conceptual framework, accomplish two goals: (1) Such theories can be directly applied to nursing situations, whereas a conceptual framework is usually too abstract for such direct application, and (2) validation of middle-range theories, clearly developed within a particular conceptual framework, lends validation to the conceptual framework itself. King (1981) stated that individuals act to maintain their own health. Although not explicitly stated, the converse is probably true as well: Individuals often do things that are not good for their health. Accordingly, it is not surprising that the KCS and related middle-range theory are often directed toward patient and group behaviors that influence health.

In addition to the middle-range theory of goal attainment (King, 1981), several other middle-range theories have been developed from within King's interacting systems framework. In terms of the personal system, Brooks and Thomas (1997) used King's framework to derive a theory of perceptual awareness. The focus was to develop the concepts of judgment and action as core concepts in the personal system. Other concepts in the theory included communication, perception, and decision making.

---

[2]See Table 9-2 in the bonus chapter content available at http://davisplus.fadavis.com.

In relation to the interpersonal system, several middle-range theories have been developed regarding families. Doornbos (2007), using her family health theory, addressed family health in terms of families of adults with persistent mental illness. Thomason and Lagowski (2008) used concepts from King along with other nursing theorists to develop a model for collaboration through reciprocation in health-care organizations. In relation to social systems, Sieloff and Bularzik (2011) revised the "theory of group power within organizations" to the "theory of group empowerment within organizations" to assist in explaining the ability of groups to empower themselves within organizations.[3]

Review of the literature identified instruments specifically designed within King's framework. King (1988) developed the Health Goal Attainment instrument, designed to detail the level of attainment of health goals by individual clients. The Nurse Performance Goal Attainment (NPGA) was developed by Kameoka, Funashima, and Sugimori (2007).

Applications in Nursing Practice

There have been many applications of King's middle-range theory to nursing practice because the theory focuses on concepts relevant to all nursing situations—the attainment of client goals. The application of the middle-range theory of goal attainment (King, 1981) is documented in several categories: (1) general application of the theory, (2) exploring a particular concept within the context of the theory of goal attainment, (3) exploring a particular concept related to the theory of goal attainment, and (4) application of the theory in nonclinical nursing situations. For example, King (1997) described the use of the theory of goal attainment in nursing practice. Short-term group psychotherapy was the focus of theory application for Laben, Sneed, and Seidel (1995). D'Souza, Somayaji, and Subrahmanya (2011) used the theory to "examine determinants of

reproductive health and related quality of life among Indian women in mining communities" (p. 1963).

Nursing Process and Nursing Terminologies, Including Standardized Nursing Languages

Within the nursing profession, the nursing process has consistently been used as the basis for nursing practice. King's framework and middle-range theory of goal attainment (1981) have been clearly linked to the process of nursing. Although many published applications have broad reference to the nursing process, several deserve special recognition. First, King herself (1981) clearly linked the theory of goal attainment to nursing process as theory and to nursing process as method. Application of King's work to nursing curricula further strengthened this link.

In addition, the steps of the nursing process have long been integrated within the KCS and the middle-range theory of goal attainment (Daubenmire & King, 1973; D'Souza, Somayaji, & Suybrahmanya, 2011; Woods, 1994). In these process applications, assessment, diagnosis, and goal-setting occur, followed by actions based on the nurse–client goals. The evaluation component of the nursing process consistently refers back to the original goal statement(s). In related research, Frey and Norris (1997) also drew parallels between the processes of critical thinking, nursing, and transaction.

Over time, nursing has developed nursing terminologies that are used to assist the profession to improve communication both within, and external to, the profession. These terminologies include the nursing diagnoses, nursing interventions, and nursing outcomes. With the use of these standardized nursing languages (SNLs), the nursing process is further refined. Standardized terms for diagnoses, interventions, and outcomes also potentially improve communication among nurses.

Using SNLs also enables the development of middle-range theory by building on concepts unique to nursing, such as those concepts of King that can be directly applied to the nursing process: action, reaction, interaction,

---

See Table 9-5 in the bonus chapter content available at http://davisplus.fadavis.com.

transaction, goal setting, and goal attainment. Biegen and Tripp-Reimer (1997) suggested middle-range theories be constructed from the concepts in the taxonomies of the nursing languages focusing on outcomes. Alternatively, King's framework and theory may be used as a theoretical basis for these phenomena and may assist in knowledge development in nursing in the future.

With the advent of SNLs, "outcome identification" is identified as a step in the nursing process after assessment and diagnosis (McFarland & McFarland, 1997, p. 3). King's (1981) concept of mutual goal setting is analogous to the outcomes identification step, because King's concept of goal attainment is congruent with the evaluation of client outcomes.

In addition, King's concept of perception (1981) lends itself well to the definition of client outcomes. Moorhead, Johnson, and Maas (2013) define a nursing-sensitive patient outcome as "an individual, family or community state, behaviour or perception that is measured along a continuum in response to nursing intervention(s)" (p. 2). This is fortuitous because the development of nursing knowledge requires the use of client outcome measurement. The use of standardized client outcomes as study variables increases the ease with which research findings can be compared across settings and contributes to knowledge development. Therefore, King's concept of mutually set goals may be studied as "expected outcomes." Also, by using SNLs, King's (1981) middle-range theory of goal attainment can be conceptualized as the "attainment of expected outcomes" as the evaluation step in the application of the nursing process.

In summary, although these terminologies, including SNLs, were developed after many of the original nursing theorists had completed their works, nursing frameworks such as the KCS (1981) can still find application and use within the terminologies. In addition, it is this type of application that further demonstrates the framework's utility across time. For example, Chaves and Araujo (2006), Ferreira De Sourza, Figueiredo De Martino, and Daena De Morais Lopes (2006), Goyatá, Rossi, and Dalri (2006), and Palmer (2006) implemented nursing diagnoses within the context of King's framework.[4]

Applications in Client Systems

KCS and middle-range theory of goal attainment have a long history of application with large groups or social systems (organizations, communities). The earliest applications involved the use of the framework and theory to guide continuing education (Brown & Lee, 1980) and nursing curricula (Daubenmire, 1989; Gulitz & King, 1988). More contemporary applications address a variety of organizational settings. For example, the framework served as the basis for the development of a middle-range theory relating to practice in a nursing home (Zurakowski, 2007). Nwinee (2011) used King's work, along with Peplau's, to develop the sociobehavioral self-care management nursing model (p. 91). In addition, the theory of goal attainment has been proposed as the practice model for case management (Hampton, 1994; Tritsch, 1996). These latter applications are especially important because they may be the first use of the framework by other disciplines.

Applicable to administration and management in a variety of settings, a middle-range theory of group power within organizations has been developed and revised to the theory of group empowerment within organizations (Sieloff, 1995, 2003, 2007; Sieloff & Dunn, 2008; Sieloff & Bularzik, 2011). Educational settings, also considered as social systems, have been the focus of application of King's work (George, Roach, & Andfrade, 2011; Greef, Strydom, Wessels, & Schutte, 2009; Ritter, 2008).[5]

Multidisciplinary Applications

Because of King's emphasis on the attainment of goals and the relevancy of goal attainment to many disciplines, both within and external to health care, it is reasonable to expect that

---

[4]See Table 9-4 in the bonus chapter content available at http://davisplus.fadavis.com.
[5]See Table 9-8 in the bonus chapter content available at http://davisplus.fadavis.com.

King's work can find application beyond nursing-specific situations. Two specific examples of this include the application of King's work to case management (Hampton, 1994; Sowell & Lowenstein, 1994) and to managed care (Hampton, 1994). Both case management and managed care incorporate multiple disciplines as they work to improve the overall quality and cost-efficiency of the health care provided. These applications also address the continuum of care, a priority in today's health-care environment. Specific researchers (Fewster-Thuente & Velsor-Friedrich, 2008; Khowaja, 2006) detailed their research related to multidisciplinary activities and interdisciplinary collaborations, respectively.[6]

Multicultural Applications

Multicultural applications of KCS and related theories are many. Such applications are particularly critical because many theoretical formulations are limited by their culture-bound nature. Several authors specifically addressed the utility of King's framework and theory for transcultural nursing. Spratlen (1976) drew heavily from King's framework and theory to integrate ethnic cultural factors into nursing curricula and to develop a culturally oriented model for mental health care. Key elements derived from King's work were the focus on perceptions and communication patterns that motivate action, reaction, interaction, and transaction. Rooda (1992) derived propositions from the midrange theory of goal attainment as the framework for a conceptual model for multicultural nursing.

Cultural relevance has also been demonstrated in reviews by Frey, Rooke, Sieloff, Messmer, and Kameoka (1995) and Husting (1997). Although Husting identified that cultural issues were implicit variables throughout King's framework, particular attention was given to the concept of health, which, according to King (1990), acquires meaning from cultural values and social norms.

Undoubtedly, the strongest evidence for the cultural utility of King's conceptual framework and midrange theory of goal attainment (1981) is the extent of work that has been done in other cultures. Applications of the framework and related theories have been documented in the following countries beyond the United States: Brazil (Firmino, Cavalcante, & Celia, 2010), Canada (Plummer & Molzahn, 2009), China (Li, Li, & Xu, 2010), India (D'Souza, Somayaji, & Subrahmanya, 2011; George et al., 2011), Japan (Kameoka et al., 2007), Portugal (Chaves & Araujo, 2006; Goyatá et al., 2006; Pelloso & Tavares, 2006), Slovenia (Harih & Pajnkihar, 2009), Sweden (Rooke, 1995a, 1995b), and West Africa (Nwinee, 2011). In Japan, a culture very different from the United States with regard to communication style, Kameoka (1995) used the classification system of nurse–patient interactions identified within the theory of goal attainment (King, 1981) to analyze nurse–patient interactions. In addition to research and publications regarding the application of King's work to nursing practice internationally, publications by and about King have been translated into other languages, including Japanese (King, 1976, 1985; Kobayashi, 1970). Therefore, perception and the influence of culture on perception were identified as strengths of King's theory.

Research Applications in Varied Settings and Populations

KCS has been used to guide nursing practice and research in multiple settings and with multiple populations. For example, Harih and Pajnkihar (2009) applied King's model in treating elderly diabetes patients. Joseph et al. (2011) examined the implementation of whole-person care.[7] As stated previously, diseases or diagnoses are often identified as the focus for the application of nursing knowledge. Maloni (2007) and Nwinee (2011) conducted research with patients with diabetes, and women with breast cancer were the focus of the work of Funghetto, Terra, and Wolff (2003). In addition, clients with chronic

---

[6]See Table 9-14 in the bonus chapter content available at http://davisplus.fadavis.com.

[7]See Table 9-11 in the bonus chapter content available at http://davisplus.fadavis.com.

obstructive pulmonary disease were involved in research by Wicks, Rice, and Talley (2007). Clients experiencing a variety of psychiatric concerns have also been the focus of work, using King's conceptualizations (Murray & Baier, 1996; Schreiber, 1991). Clients' concerns ranged from psychotic symptoms (Kemppainen, 1990) to families experiencing chronic mental illness (Doornbos, 2007), to clients in short-term group psychotherapy (Laben, Sneed, & Seidel, 1995).[8] The theory has also been applied in nonclinical nursing situations. Secrest, Iorio, and Martz (2005) used the theory in examining the empowerment of nursing assistants. Li et al. (2010) explored the "development of the concept of holistic nursing" (p. 33).[9]

Research Applications with Clients Across the Life Span

Additional evidence of the scope and usefulness of King's framework and theory is its use with clients across the life span. Several applications have targeted high-risk infants (Frey & Norris, 1997; Syzmanski, 1991). Frey (1993, 1995, 1996) developed and tested relationships among multiple systems with children, youth, and young adults. Lehna (2009) explicated the concept of sibling closeness in a study of siblings experiencing a major burn trauma. Interestingly, these studies considered personal systems (infants), interpersonal systems (parents, families), and social systems (the nursing staff and hospital environment). Clearly, a strength of King's framework and theory is its utility in encompassing complex settings and situations.

KCS and the midrange theory of goal attainment have also been used to guide practice with adults (young adults, adults, mature adults) with a broad range of concerns. Goyatá et al. (2006) used King's work in their study of adults experiencing burns. Additional examples of applications focusing on adults include individuals with hypertension (Firmino et al., 2010) and perceptions of students toward

obesity (Ongoco, 2012). Gender-specific work included Sharts-Hopko's (2007) use of a middle-range theory of health perception to study the health status of women during menopause transition and Martin's (1990) application of the framework toward cancer awareness among males.

Several of the applications with adults have targeted the mature adult, thus demonstrating contributions to the nursing specialty of gerontology. Reed (2007) used a middle-range theory to examine the relationship of social support and health in older adults. Harih and Pajnkihar (2009) applied "King's model in the treatment of elderly diabetes patients" (p. 201). Clearly, these applications, and others, show how the complexity of King's framework and midrange theory increases its usefulness for nursing.[10]

Research Applications to Client Systems

In addition to discussing client populations across the life span, client populations can be identified by focus of care (client system) and/or focus of health problem (phenomenon of concern). The focus of care, or interest, can be an individual (personal system) or group (interpersonal or social system). Thus, application of King's work, across client systems, can be divided into the three systems identified within the KCS (1981): personal (the individual), interpersonal (small groups), and social (large groups/society).

Use with personal systems has included both patients and nurses. LaMar (2008) examined nurses in a tertiary acute care organization as the personal system of interest. Nursing students as personal systems were the focus of Lockhart and Goodfellow's research (2009). When the focus of interest moves from an individual to include interaction between two people, the interpersonal system is involved. Interpersonal systems often include clients and nurses. An example of an application to a nurse–client dyad is Langford's (2008) study of the perceptions of transactions with nurse practitioners and obese adolescents. In relation

---

[8]See Table 9-8 and 9-11 in the bonus chapter content available at http://davisplus.fadavis.com.

[9]See Table 9-3 in the bonus chapter content available at http://davisplus.fadavis.com.

[10] See Table 9-7 in the bonus chapter content available at http://davisplus.fadavis.com.

to interpersonal systems, or small groups, many publications focus on the family. Frey and Norris (1997) used both KCS and the theory of goal attainment in planning care with families of premature infants. Alligood (2010) described "family health care with King's theory of goal attainment" (p. 99).

Research Applications Focusing on Phenomena of Concern to Clients

Within King's work, it is critically important for the nurse to focus on, and address, the phenomenon of concern to the client. Without this emphasis on the client's perspective, mutual goal setting cannot occur. Hence, a client's phenomenon of concern was selected as neutral terminology that clearly demonstrated the broad application of King's work to a wide variety of practice situations. A topic that frequently divides nurses is their area of specialty. However, by using a consistent framework across specialties, nurses may be able to focus more clearly on their commonalities, rather than highlighting their differences.[11] A review of the literature clearly demonstrates that King's framework and related theories have application within a variety of nursing specialties.[12] This application is evident whether one is reviewing a "traditional" specialty, such as surgical nursing (Bruns, Norwood, Bosworth, & Gill, 2009; Lockhart & Goodfellow, 2009; Sivaramalingam, 2008), or the nontraditional specialties of forensic nursing (Laben et al., 1991) and/or nursing administration (Gianfermi & Buchholz, 2011; Joseph et al., 2011).

Health is one area that certainly binds clients and nurses. Improved health is clearly the desired end point, or outcome, of nursing care and something to which clients aspire. Review of the outcome of nursing care, as addressed in published applications, tends to support the goal of improved health directly and/or indirectly, as the result of the application of King's work. Health status is explicitly

the outcome of concern in practice applications by Smith (1988). Several applications used health-related terms. For example, DeHowitt (1992) studied well-being, and D'Souza et al. (2011) examined the determinants of health.

Health promotion has also been an emphasis for the application of King's ideas. Sexual counseling was the focus of work by Villeneuve and Ozolins (1991). Health behaviors were Hanna's (1995) focus of study, and Plummer and Molzahn (2009) explored the "quality of life in contemporary nursing theory" (p. 134). Frey (1996, 1997) examined both health behaviors and illness management behaviors in several groups of children with chronic conditions as well as risky behaviors (1996). Recently, researchers have explored weight loss and obesity (Langford, 2008; Ongoco, 2012).

Research Applications in Varied Work Settings

An additional potential source of division within the nursing profession is the work sites where nursing is practiced and care is delivered. As the delivery of health care moves from the acute care hospital to community-based agencies and clients' homes, it is important to highlight commonalities across these settings, and it is important to identify that King's framework and middle-range theory of goal attainment continue to be applicable. Although many applications tend to be with nurses and clients in traditional settings, successful applications have been shown across other, including newer and nontraditional settings. From hospitals (Bogue, Jospeh, & Sieloff, 2009; Firmino et al., 2010; Kameoka et al., 2007) to nursing homes (Zurakowski, 2007), King's framework and related theories provide a foundation on which nurses can build their practice interventions. In addition, the use of the KCS and related theories are evident within quality improvement projects (Anderson & Mangino, 2006; Durston, 2006; Khowaja, 2006).[13] Nurses also use the theory

---

[11]See Table 9-9 in the bonus chapter content available at http://davisplus.fadavis.com.

[12]See Table 9-10 in the bonus chapter content available at http://davisplus.fadavis.com.

[13]See Table 9-11 in the bonus chapter content available at http://davisplus.fadavis.com.

of goal attainment (King, 1981) to examine concepts related to the theory. This application was demonstrated by Smith (2003), by Jones and Bugge (2006), by Sivaramalingam (2008) in a study of patients' perceptions of nurses' roles and responsibilities, and by Mardis (2012) in a study of patients' perceptions of minimal lift equipment.

Relationship to Evidence-Based Practice

From an evidence-based practice and King perspective, the profession must implement three strategies to apply theory-based research findings effectively. First, nursing as a discipline must agree on rules of evidence in evaluation of quality research that reflect the unique contribution of nursing to health care. Second, the nursing rules of evidence must include heavier weight for research that is derived from, or adds to, nursing theory. Third, the nursing rules of evidence must reflect higher scores when nursing's central beliefs are affirmed in the choice of variables. This third strategy, for the use of concepts central to nursing, has clear relevance for evidence-based practice when using King's (1981) concepts as reformulated within interventions or outcomes. Outcomes, as in King's concept of goal attainment, provide data for evidence-based practice.

Currently, safety and quality initiatives in organizations, with evidence-based practice as the innovation, use many concepts initially defined by King and found in middle-range theories (Sieloff & Frey, 2007). King's (1981) work on the concepts of client and nurse perceptions, and the achievement of mutual goals has been assimilated and accepted as core beliefs of the discipline of nursing. Research conducted with a King theoretical base is well positioned for application by nurse caregivers (Bruns et al.,

2009; Gemmill et al., 2011; Mardis, 2011), nurse administrators (Sieloff & Bularzik, 2011), and client-consumers (Killeen, 2007) as part of evolving evidence-based nursing practice.[14]

Recommendations for Future Applications Related to King's Framework and Theory

Obviously, new nursing knowledge has resulted from applications of King's framework and theory. However, nursing is evolving as a science. Additional work continues to be needed. On the basis of a review of the applications previously discussed, recommendations for future applications continue to focus on (1) the need for evidence-based nursing practice that is theoretically derived; (2) the integration of King's work in evidence-based nursing practice; (3) the integration of King's concepts within SNLs; (4) analysis of the future effect of managed care, continuous quality improvement, and technology on King's concepts; (5) identification, or development and implementation, of additional relevant instruments; and (6) clarification of effective nursing interventions, including identification of relevant Nursing Interventions Classifications, based on King's work.

As part of its mission, the King International Nursing Group (KING) (www.kingnursing.org) continuously monitors the latest publications and research based on King's work and related theories, providing updates to members. To further assist in the dissemination of such research, KING also conducts a biannual research conference. The following Exemplar illustrates the application of the theory of goal attainment to an interdisciplinary team, quality improvement, and evidence-based practice.

---

[14]See Table 9-12 in the bonus chapter content available at http://davisplus.fadavis.com.

Practice Exemplar

Provided by Mary B. Killeen, PhD, RN, NEA-BC

Claire Smith, RN, BSN, is a recent nursing graduate in her first position on a medical intensive care unit in a suburban community hospital. Claire's manager suggests that she should join the unit's interdisciplinary quality improvement committee to develop her leadership skills. The goal of the committee is to improve patient care by using the best available evidence to develop and implement practice protocols.

At the first meeting, Claire was asked if she had any burning clinical questions as a new graduate. She stated that she was taught to avoid use of normal saline for tracheal suctioning. However, she noticed many respiratory therapists and some nurses routinely using normal saline with suctioning. When asked about this practice, she was told that normal saline was useful to break up secretions and aid in their removal. The committee affirmed Claire's observation of contradictory practices between what is taught and what is done in practice. After discussion, the group formulated the following clinical question: Does instilling normal saline decrease favorable patient outcomes among patients with endotracheal tubes or tracheostomies?

Claire suggests to the committee that King's theory of goal attainment might be useful as a theoretical guide for this project because the question is focused on patient outcomes, or according to King's theory, goals. The nursing members are familiar with King's theory, and all members value using theory to guide practice. Claire's proposal is accepted. Claire experienced working on EBP group projects as a student, so she feels comfortable volunteering to develop a draft of the theoretical foundation for the project. Two other committee members agree to work on the plan and present it at the next meeting.

The following are the questions and the conclusions that Claire and her colleagues discussed:

1. *How does King's theory of goal attainment help the unit's quality improvement (QI) committee?*

   Goal attainment theory is derived from KCS, which includes personal, interpersonal, and social systems. The QI committee is a type of interpersonal system. An interpersonal system encompasses individuals in groups interacting to achieve goals. The QI committee is engaged in the committee's goal attainment for the benefit of patients. "Role expectations and role performance of nurses and clients influence transactions" (King, 1981, p. 147). When used in interdisciplinary teams, the transaction process in King's theory facilitates mutual goal setting with nurses, and ultimately patients, based on each member of the team's specific knowledge and functions.

   Multidisciplinary care conferences, an example of a situation where goal-setting among professionals occurs, is a label for an indirect nursing intervention within the Nursing Interventions Classification (NIC; Bulechek, Butcher, & Dochterman, 2008). Some of the activities listed under this NIC reflect King's (1981) concepts: "establish mutually agreeable goals; solicit input for patient care planning; revise patient care plan, as necessary; discuss progress toward goals; and provide data to facilitate evaluation of patient care plan" (p. 501).

2. *How does King define goals and goal attainment and how are these related to quality patient outcomes?*

   According to King's theory of goal attainment (1981), goals are mutually agreed upon, and through a transaction process, are attained. Goals are similar to outcomes that are achieved after agreement on the definitions and measurement of the outcomes. Quality improvement has shown agreement that evaluation of care must include process and outcomes. Outcomes are

Continued

the results of interventions or processes. The term "outcome" assumes that a process is central to effective care. An outcome is defined as a change in a patient's health status. Effectiveness of care can be measured by whether the patient goals (i.e., outcomes) have been attained. The QI Committee engages in goal attainment through communication by setting goals, exploring means, and agreeing on means to achieve goals. In this example, members will gather information, examine data and evidence, interpret the information, and participate in developing a protocol for patients to achieve quality patient outcomes, that is, goals.

3. *How does King's theory of goal attainment provide a theoretical foundation for the clinical problem of using normal saline with suctioning?*

First, the use of King's theory will help guide the literature search to include studies that address interventions or processes that lead to favorable patient outcomes or goals among patients similar to the population on the unit. Claire's subgroup enlisted the help of the hospital librarian in searching the literature using the elements of the clinical

question and the theoretical concepts as key words. Second, the theoretical formulation of the study helps organize the implementation and evaluation plans so they are attainable.

4. *What key words would you use for the search considering the clinical question and King's theory?*

Key words used are *endotracheal tubes, tracheostomies, normal saline, suctioning, outcomes, King's theory of goal attainment,* and *goal attainment.*

5. *How does a theoretical foundation, such as King's theory of goal attainment, apply to a quality improvement or EBP project?*

Claire used these criteria from her nursing program to develop a theoretical foundation for the project.

The theoretical foundation for the project was presented to the committee and accepted (Fig. 9–3).

6. *What were the results of the committee's work?*

The search strategy included MEDLINE, CINAHL, Cochrane Library, Joanna Briggs Institute, and TRIP databases. All types of evidence (nonexperimental, experimental, qualitative studies, systematic reviews) were

Clinical Problem Elements	King's Concepts	Application to the Project
Population: *patients with endotracheal tubes or tracheostomies*	Clients and nurses	Members of the Interdisciplinary Committee
Intervention: normal saline with suctioning	Transaction process: Disturbance	Clinical problem formulated and relevance to unit discussed.
Outcomes	Goals explored	Evidence sought and examined to select measurable goals/outcomes.
Outcomes	Explore means to achieve goals	Implementation plan devised.
Outcomes	Agree on means to achieve goals	Implementation plan accepted by members.

Fig 9 • 3 Theoretical foundation for a quality improvement project using Imogene King's theory of goal attainment derived from King's conceptual system (1981).

Practice Exemplar cont.

included. The evidence was evaluated by the QI committee and included physiological and psychological effects of instillation of normal saline. The collective evidence, relevant to their unit's practice problem, did not support the routine use of normal saline with suctioning (similar to Halm & Kriski-Hagel, 2008). From the evidence, the committee selected the specific outcomes to track for the project: sputum recovery, oxygenation, and subjective symptoms of pain, anxiety, and dyspnea. Owing to anticipated

small samples, hemodynamic alterations and infections were not selected as outcomes. The committee devised a theory-based implementation plan to discontinue normal saline for suctioning using the five Ws (who, what, where, when, why) and how as the outline for the plan. Change processes were employed in the plan. Evaluation of the attainment of outcomes will address the effectiveness of the plan using the measurable outcomes and the degree to which they were attained.

■ Summary

An essential component in the analysis of conceptual frameworks and theories is the consideration of their adequacy (Ellis, 1968). Adequacy depends on the three interrelated characteristics of scope, usefulness, and complexity. Conceptual frameworks are broad in scope and sufficiently complex to be useful for many situations. Theories, on the other hand, are narrower in scope, usually addressing less abstract concepts, and are more specific in terms of the nature and direction of relationships and focus.

King fully intended her conceptual system for nursing to be useful in all nursing situations. Likewise, the middle-range theory of goal attainment (King, 1981) has broad scope

because interaction is a part of every nursing encounter. Although previous evaluations of the scope of King's framework and middle-range theory have resulted in mixed reviews (Austin & Champion, 1983; Carter & Dufour, 1994; Frey, 1996; Jonas, 1987; Meleis, 2012), the nursing profession has clearly recognized their scope and usefulness. In addition, the variety of practice applications evident in the literature clearly attests to the complexity of King's work. As researchers continue to integrate King's theory and framework with the dynamic health-care environment, future applications involving evidence-based practice will continue to demonstrate the adequacy of King's work in nursing practice.

References

Alligood, M. (2010). Family healthcare with King's theory of goal attainment. *Nursing Science Quarterly, 23*(2), 99–104. doi:10.1177/0894318410362553

Anderson, C. D., & Mangino, R. R. (2006). Nurse shift report: Who says you can't talk in front of the patient? *Nursing Administration Quarterly, 30*(2), 112–122.

Austin, J. K., & Champion, V. L. (1983). King's theory for nursing: Explication and evaluation. In P. L. Chinn (Ed.), *Advances in nursing theory development* (pp. 49–61). Rockville, MD: Aspen.

Batson, V. D., & Yoder, L. H. (2012). Managerial coaching: A concept analysis. *Journal of Advanced Nursing, 68*(7), 1658–1669. doi:10.1111/j.1365-2648.2011.05840.x

Biegen, M. A., & Tripp-Reimer, T. (1997). Implications of nursing taxonomies for middle-range theory development. *Advances in Nursing Science, 19*(3), 37–49.

Bogue, R., Joseph, M., & Sieloff, C. (2009). Shared governance as vertical alignment of nursing group power and nurse practice council effectiveness. *Journal of Nursing Management, 17*(1), 4–14.

Brooks, E. M., & Thomas, S. (1997). The perception and judgment of senior baccalaureate student nurses in clinical decision making. *Advances in Nursing Science, 19*(3), 50–69.

Brown, S. T., & Lee, B. T. (1980). Imogene King's conceptual framework: A proposed model for continuing nursing education. *Journal of Advanced Nursing, 5*, 467–473.

Bruns, A., Norwood, B., Bosworth, G., & Hill, L. (2009). The cerebral oximeter: What is the efficacy? *AANA Journal, 77*(2), 137–144.

Bulechek, G. M., Butcher, H. K., & Dochterman, J. M. (2008). *Nursing interventions classification (NIC)* (5th ed.). St. Louis, MO: C. V. Mosby.

Carter, K. F., & Dufour, L. T. (1994). King's theory: A critique of the critiques. *Nursing Science Quarterly, 7*(3), 128–133.

Chaves, E. S., & Araujo, T. L. (2006). Nursing care for an adolescent with cardiovascular risk [in Portuguese]. *Ciencia Cuidado e Saude, 5*(1), 82–87.

Daubenmire, M. J. (1989). A baccalaureate nursing curriculum based on King's conceptual framework. In J. P. Riehl-Sisca (Ed.), *Conceptual models for nursing practice* (3rd ed., pp. 167–178). Norwalk, CT: Appleton & Lange.

Daubenmire, M. J., & King, I. M. (1973). Nursing process models: A systems approach. *Nursing Outlook, 21,* 512–517.

DeHowitt, M. C. (1992). King's conceptual model and individual psychotherapy. *Perspectives in Psychiatric Care, 28*(4), 11–14.

Doornbos, M. M. (2007). King's conceptual system and family health theory in the families of adults with persistent mental illness—An evolving conceptualization. In C. L. Sieloff & M. A. Frey (Eds.), *Middle range theory development using King's conceptual system* (pp. 31–49). New York: Springer.

D'Souza, M., Somayaji, G., & Subrahmanya, N. K. (2011). Determinants of reproductive health and related quality of life among Indian women in mining communities. *Journal of Advanced Nursing, 67*(9), 1963–1975. doi:10.1111/j.1365-2648.2011.05641.x

Durston, P. (2006, April). Partners in caring: A partnership for healing. *Nursing Administration Quarterly, 30*(2), 105–111. Retrieved August 22, 2008, from CINAHL with Full Text database.

Ehrenberger, H. E., Alligood, M. R., Thomas, S. P., Wallace, D. C., & Licavoli, C. M. (2007). Testing a theory of decision making derived from King's systems framework in women eligible for a cancer clinical trial. In C. L. Sieloff & M. A. Frey (Eds.), *Middle range theory development using King's conceptual system* (pp. 75–91). New York: Springer.

Ellis, R. (1968). Characteristics of significant theories. *Nursing Research, 17,* 217–222.

Fawcett, J. (2008). The added value of nursing conceptual model-based research. *Journal of Advanced Nursing, 61*(6), 583.

Federal Register. (1995). Final Revisions: 60(123), Tuesday. June 27, 1995, p. 33294 forward.

Ferreira De Souza, E., Figueiredo De Martino, M. M., & Daena De Morais Lopes, M. H. (2006, January–March). Analyzing nursing diagnoses in chronic renal clients using Imogene King's conceptual system. *International Journal of Nursing Terminologies & Classifications, 17*(1), 53–54.

Fewster-Thuente, L., & Velsor-Friedrich, B. (2008). Interdisciplinary collaboration for healthcare professionals. *Nursing Administration Quarterly, 32*(1), 40–48.

Firmino, de Fatima, L., Cavalcante, & Celia. (2010). Perceptions of people about hypertension and concepts of Imogene King [Portuguese]. *Revista Gaucha De Enfermagem, 31*(3), 499–507. doi:10.1590/S1983-14472010000300013

Frey, M. A. (1993). A theoretical perspective of family and child health derived from King's conceptual framework of nursing: A deductive approach to theory building. In S. L. Feetham, S. B. Meister, J. M. Bell, & C. L. Gillis (Eds.), *The nursing of families: Theory/research/education/practice* (pp. 30–37). Newbury Park, CA: Sage.

Frey, M. A. (1995). Toward a theory of families, children, and chronic illness. In M. A. Frey & C. L. Sieloff (Eds.), *Advancing King's systems framework and theory of nursing* (pp. 109–125). Thousand Oaks, CA: Sage.

Frey, M. A. (1996). Behavioral correlates of health and illness in youths with chronic illness. *Advanced Nursing Research, 9*(4), 167–176.

Frey, M. A. (1997). Health promotion in youth with chronic illness: Are we on the right track? *Quality Nursing, 3*(5), 13–18.

Frey, M. A., & Norris, D. M. (1997). King's systems framework and theory in nursing practice. In A. Marriner-Tomey (Ed.), *Nursing theory utilization and application* (pp. 71–88). St. Louis, MO: C. V. Mosby.

Frey, M. A., Rooke, L., Sieloff, C. L., Messmer, P., & Kameoka, T. (1995). King's framework and theory in Japan, Sweden, and the United States. *Image: Journal of Nursing Scholarship, 27*(2), 127–130.

Frey, M. A., & Sieloff, C. L. (1995). *Advancing King's systems framework and theory of nursing.* Thousand Oaks, CA: Sage.

Funghetto, S. S., Terra, M. G., & Wolff, L. R. (2003). Woman [sic] with breast cancer: Perception about the disease, family and society [in Portuguese]. *Revista Brasileira de Enfermagem, 56*(5), 528–532.

Gemmill, R., Kravits, K., Ortiz, M., Anderson, C., Lai, L., & Grant, M. (2011). What do surgical oncology staff nurses know about colorectal cancer ostomy care? *Journal of Continuing Education In Nursing, 42*(2), 81–88. doi:10.3928/00220124-20101101-04

George, A., Roach, E., & Andrade, M. (2011). Nursing education: Opportunities and challenges [online]. *Nursing Journal of India, 102*(6). http://tnaionline.org/thenursing.htm

Gianfermi, R. E., & Buchholz, S. W. (2011). Exploring the relationship between job satisfaction nursing group outcome attainment capability in nurse administrators. *Journal of Nursing Management, 19*(8), 1012–1019. doi:10.1111/j.1365-2834.2011.01328.x

Goyatá, S., Rossi, L., & Dalri, M. (2006, January–February). Nursing diagnoses for family members of adult burned patients near hospital discharge [in Portuguese]. *Revista Latino-Americana de Enfermagem, 14*(1), 102–109.

Greeff, M., E, E., Strydom, C., Wessels, C., & Schutte, P. (2009, March). Students' community health service delivery: Experiences of involved parties. *Curatinis, 32*(1), 33–44.

Gulitz, E. A., & King, I. M. (1988). King's general systems model: Application to curriculum development. *Nursing Science Quarterly, 1,* 128–132.

Halm, M. A., & Kriski-Hagel, K. (2008). Instilling normal saline with suctioning: Beneficial technique or potentially harmful sacred cow? *American Journal of Critical Care, 17*(5), 469–472.

Hampton, D. C. (1994). King's theory of goal attainment as a framework for managed care implementation in a hospital setting. *Nursing Science Quarterly, 7*(4), 170–173.

Hanna, K. M. (1995). Use of King's theory of goal attainment to promote adolescents' health behavior. In M. A. Frey & C. L. Sieloff (Eds.), *Advancing King's systems framework and theory of nursing* (pp. 239–250). Thousand Oaks, CA: Sage.

Harih, M., & Pajnkihar, M. (2009). Application of Imogene M. King's nursing model in the treatment of elderly diabetes patients. *Slovenian Nursing Review: Journal of the Nurses and Midwives Association of Slovenia, 43*(3), 201–208.

Hernandez, C. A. (2007). The theory of integration: Congruency with King's conceptual system. In C. L. Sieloff & M. A. Frey (Eds.), *Middle range theory development using King's conceptual system* (pp. 105–124). New York: Springer.

Howland, D., & McDowell, W. (1964). A measurement of patient care: A conceptual framework. *Nursing Research, 13*(4), 320–324.

Husting, P. M. (1997). A transcultural critique of Imogene King's theory of goal attainment. *Journal of Multicultural Nursing & Health, 3*(3), 15–20.

Jonas, C. M. (1987). King's goal attainment theory: Use in gerontological nursing practice. *Perspectives: Journal of the Gerontological Nursing Association, 11*(4), 9–12.

Joseph, M., Laughon, D., & Bogue, R. J. (2011). An examination of the sustainable adoption of whole-person care (WPC). *Journal of Nursing Management, 19*(8), 989–997. doi:10.1111/j.1365-2834.2011.01317.x

Kameoka, T. (1995). Analyzing nurse-patient interactions in Japan. In M. A. Frey & C. L. Sieloff (Eds.), *Advancing King's systems framework and theory of goal attainment* (pp. 251–260). Thousand Oaks, CA: Sage.

Kameoka, T., Funashima, N., & Sugimori, M. (2007). If goals are attained, satisfaction will occur in nurse-patient interaction: An empirical test. In C. L. Sieloff & M. A. Frey (Eds.), *Middle range theory development using King's conceptual system* (pp. 261–272). New York: Springer.

Kemppainen, J. K. (1990). Imogene King's theory: A nursing case study of a psychotic client with human immunodeficiency virus infection. *Archives of Psychiatric Nursing, 4*(6), 384–388.

Khowaja, D. (2006). Utilization of King's interacting systems framework and theory of goal attainment with new multidisciplinary model: Clinical pathway. *Australian Journal of Advanced Nursing, 24*(2), 44–50.

Killeen, M. B. (2007). Development and initial testing of a theory of patient satisfaction with nursing care. In C. L. Sieloff & M. A. Frey (Eds.), *Middle range theory development using King's conceptual system* (pp. 138–163). New York: Springer.

King, I. M. (1964). Nursing theory: Problems and prospect. *Nursing Science, 2*(5), 294.

King, I. M. (1968). A conceptual frame of reference for nursing. *Nursing Research, 17,* 27–31.

King, I. M. (1971). *Toward a theory for nursing: General concepts of human behavior.* New York: Wiley.

King, I. M. (1975). A process for developing concepts for nursing through research. In P. J. Verhonick (Ed.), *Nursing research* (p. 25). Boston: Little, Brown.

King, I. M. (1976). *Toward a theory of nursing: General concepts of human behavior* (M. Sugimori, trans.). Tokyo: Igaku-Shoin.

King, I. M. (1981). *A theory of goal attainment: Systems, concepts, process.* New York: Wiley.

King, I. M. (1984). Effectiveness of nursing care: Use of a goal oriented nursing record in end stage renal disease. *American Association of Nephrology Nurses and Technicians Journal, 11*(2), 11–17, 60.

King, I. M. (1985). *A theory for nursing: Systems, concepts, process* (M. Sugimori, trans.). Tokyo: Igaku-Shoin.

King, I. M. (1988). Concepts: Essential elements of theories. *Nursing Science Quarterly, 1*(1), 22–24.

King, I. M. (1989a). King's general systems framework and theory. In J. P. Riehl-Sisca (Ed.), *Conceptual models for nursing practice* (pp. 149–158). Norwalk, CT: Appleton & Lang.

King, I. M. (1989b). King's systems framework for nursing administration. In B. Henry (Ed.), *Dimensions of nursing administration: Theory, research, education* (p. 35). Cambridge, England: Blackwell Scientific.

King, I. M. (1990). Health as a goal for nursing. *Nursing Science Quarterly, 3,* 123–128.

King, I. M. (1992). King's theory of goal attainment. *Nursing Science Quarterly, 5,* 19–26.

King, I. M. (1995). The theory of goal attainment. In M. A. Frey & C. L. Sieloff (Eds.), *Advancing King's systems framework and theory of goal attainment* (pp. 23–32). Thousand Oaks, CA: Sage.

King, I. M. (1996). The theory of goal attainment in research and practice. *Nursing Science Quarterly, 9,* 61–66.

King, I. M. (1997). King's theory of goal attainment in practice. *Nursing Science Quarterly, 10*(4), 180–185.

Kobayashi, F. T. (1970). A conceptual frame of reference for nursing. *Japanese Journal of Nursing Research, 3*(3), 199–204.

Laben, J. K., Dodd, D., & Sneed, L. (1991). King's theory of goal attainment applied in group therapy for inpatient juvenile offenders, maximum security state offenders, and community parolees, using visual aids. *Issues in Mental Health Nursing, 12*(1), 51–64.

Laben, J. K., Sneed, L. D., & Seidel, S. L. (1995). Goal attainment in short-term group psychotherapy settings: Clinical implications for practice. In M. A. Frey & C. L. Sieloff (Eds.), *Advancing King's systems framework and theory of nursing* (pp. 261–277). Thousand Oaks, CA: Sage.

LaMar, K. (2008). Compass: the direction for professional nursing development at a tertiary care facility. *Journal for Nurses in Staff Development, 24*(4), 155–161.

Langford, R. (2008). Perceptions of transactions with nurse practitioners and weight loss in obese adolescents. *Southern Online Journal of Nursing Research, 8*(2). http://www.resourcenter.net/images/SNRS/Files/SOJNR_articles2/Vol08Num02Main.html

Lehna, C. (2009). "Sibling closeness," a concept explication using the hybrid model, in siblings experiencing a major burn trauma. *Southern Online Journal Of Nursing Research,* 9(4).

Li, H., Li, C., & Xu, C. (2010). Review of the development of the concept of holistic nursing. *Yi Shi Za Zhi ,* 40(1), 33-37.

Lockhart, J., & Goodfellow, L. (2009). The effect of a 5-week head & neck surgical oncology on nursing students' perceptions of facial disfigurement: Part I. *ORL-Head & Neck Nursing, 27*(3), 7–12.

Maloni, H. W. (2007). *An intervention to effect hypertension, glycemic control, diabetes self-management, self-efficacy, and satisfaction with care in type 2 diabetic VA health care users with inadequate functional health literacy skills.* Doctoral dissertation, the Catholic University of America, Washington, DC. ProQuest Dissertations and Theses, 258-n/a. Retrieved from http://search.proquest.com/docview/304885625?accountid=28148. (304885625)

Mardis, S. (2010). *Patients' perceptions of minimal lift equipment.* Doctoral dissertation, Northern Kentucky University, Highland Heights. ProQuest Dissertations and Theses, 61. Retrieved from http://search.proquest.com/docview/251125913?accountid=28148. (251125913)

Martin, J. P. (1990). Male cancer awareness: Impact of an employee education program. *Oncology Nursing Forum, 17,* 59–64.

May, B. A. (2007). Relationships among basic empathy, self-awareness, and learning styles of baccalaureate prenursing students within King's personal system. In C. L. Sieloff & M. A. Frey (Eds.), *Middle range theory development using King's conceptual system* (pp. 164–177). New York: Springer.

McFarland, G. K., & McFarland, E. A. (1997). *Nursing diagnosis and intervention: Planning for patient care.* St. Louis, MO: Mosby-Year Book.

Meleis, A. (2012). *Theoretical nursing: Developments and progress* (5th ed.). Philadelphia: Wolters/Kluwer Health/Lippincott Williams & Wilkins.

Moorhead, S., Johnson, M., & Maas, M. L. (2013). *Nursing outcomes classification: Measurement of health outcomes* (5th ed.). St. Louis, MO: Mosby.

Murray, R. L. E., & Baier, M. (1996). King's conceptual framework applied to a transitional living program. *Perspectives in Psychiatric Care, 32*(1), 15–19.

Northrop, F. C. S. (1969). *The logic of the sciences and the humanities.* Cleveland, OH: Meridian.

Nwinee, J. (2011). Nwinee Socio-Behavioural Self-Care Management Nursing Model. *West African Journal of Nursing, 22*(1), 91–98.

Ongoco, E. K. P. (2012). *Comparison of attitudes and beliefs toward obesity of student nurse and non-nursing students.* Doctoral dissertation, California State University, Long Beach). ProQuest Dissertations and Theses. Retrieved from http://search.proquest.com/docview/1011639370?accountid=28148

Palmer, J. A. (2006). Nursing implications for older adult patient education. *Plastic Surgical Nursing, 26*(4), 189–194.

Pelloso, S. M., & Tavares, M. S. G. (2006). Family problems and mother's death [in Portuguese]. *Ciencia Cuidado e Saude, 5*(Suppl.), 19–25.

Plummer, M., & Molzahn, A. (2009, April). Quality of life in contemporary nursing theory: A concept analysis. *Nursing Science Quarterly, 22*(2), 134–140.

Reed, J. E. F. (2007). Social support and health of older adults. In C. L. Sieloff & M. A. Frey (Eds.), *Middle range theory development using King's conceptual system* (pp. 92–104). New York: Springer.

Ritter, K. W. (2008). *The benefits of a peer-based mentor/tutor program for undergraduate students in a four-year traditional baccalaureate in nursing program.* Northern Kentucky University, Highland Heights). ProQuest Dissertations and Theses, 56. Retrieved from http://search.proquest.com/docview/304829420?accountid=28148 (304829420)

Rooda, L. A. (1992). The development of a conceptual model for multicultural nursing. *Journal of Holistic Nursing, 10*(4), 337–347.

Rooke, L. (1995a). The concept of space in King's systems framework: Its implications for nursing. In M. A. Frey & C. L. Sieloff (Eds.), *Advancing King's systems framework and theory of nursing* (pp. 79–96). Thousand Oaks, CA: Sage.

Rooke, L. (1995b). Focusing on King's theory and systems framework in education by using an experiential learning model: A challenge to improve the quality of nursing care. In M. A. Frey & C. L. Sieloff (Eds.), *Advancing King's systems framework and theory of nursing* (pp. 278–293). Thousand Oaks, CA: Sage.

Schreiber, R. (1991). Psychiatric assessment—"A la King." *Nursing Management, 22*(5), 90, 92, 94.

Secrest, J., Iorio, D. H., & Martz, W. (2005). The meaning of work for nursing assistants who stay in long-term care. *International Journal of Older People Nursing, 14*(8b), 90–97.

Sharts-Hopko, N. C. (2007). A theory of health perception: Understanding the menopause transition. In C. L. Sieloff & M. A. Frey (Eds.), *Middle range theory development using King's conceptual system* (pp. 178–195). New York: Springer.

Sieloff, C. L. (1995). Development of a theory of departmental power. In M. A. Frey & C. L. Sieloff

(Eds.), *Advancing King's systems framework and theory of nursing* (pp. 46–65). Thousand Oaks, CA: Sage.

Sieloff, C. L. (2003). Measuring nursing power within organizations. *Journal of Nursing Scholarship, 35*(2), 183–187.

Sieloff, C. L. (2007). The theory of group power within organizations—Evolving conceptualization within King's conceptual system. In C. L. Sieloff & M. A. Frey (Eds.), *Middle range theory development using King's conceptual system* (pp. 196–214). New York: Springer.

Sieloff, C. L., & Bularzik, A. M. (2011). Group power through the lens of the 21st century and beyond: further validation of the Sieloff-King Assessment of Group Power within Organizations. *Journal Of Nursing Management, 19*(8), 1020–1027. doi:10.1111/j.1365-2834.2011.01314.x

Sieloff, C., & Dunn, K. (2008, September). Factor validation of an instrument measuring group power. *Journal of Nursing Measurement, 16*(2), 113–124.

Sieloff, C. L., & Frey, M. (2007). *Middle range theories for nursing practice using King's interacting systems framework.* New York: Springer.

Sivaramalingam, S. (2008). Surgical patients' perceptions of nurse's roles and responsibilities. Doctoral dissertation, D'Youville College, Buffalo, NY. ProQuest Dissertations and Theses, 85. Retrieved from http://search.proquest.com/docview/304324687?accountid=28148. (304324687)

Smith, M. C. (1988). King's theory in practice. *Nursing Science Quarterly, 1,* 145–146.

Sowell, R. L., & Lowenstein, A. (1994). King's theory: A framework for quality; linking theory to practice. *Nursing Connections, 7*(2), 19–31.

Spratlen, L. P. (1976). Introducing ethnic-cultural factors in models of nursing: Some mental health care applications. *Journal of Nursing Education, 15*(2), 23–29.

Syzmanski, M. E. (1991). Use of nursing theories in the care of families with high-risk infants: Challenges for the future. *Journal of Perinatal and Neonatal Nursing, 4*(4), 71–77.

Thomason, D., & Lagowski, L. (2008, December). Business and leadership. Sustaining a healthy work force in the 21st century—a model for collaborating through reciprocation. *AAOHN Journal, 56*(12), 503–513.

Tritsch, J. M. (1996). Application of King's theory of goal attainment and the Carondelet St. Mary's case management model. *Nursing Science Quarterly, 11*(2), 69–73.

Villeneuve, M. J., & Ozolins, P. H. (1991). Sexual counselling in the neuroscience setting: Theory and practical tips for nurses. *AXON, 12*(3), 63–67.

Von Bertalanffy, L. (1968). *General system theory.* New York: Braziller.

Wicks, M. N., Rice, M. C., & Talley, C. H. (2007). Further exploration of family health within the context of chronic obstructive pulmonary disease. In C. L. Sieloff & M. A. Frey (Eds.), *Middle range theory development using King's conceptual system* (pp. 215–236). New York: Springer.

Woods, E. C. (1994). King's theory in practice with elders. *Nursing Science Quarterly, 7*(2), 65–69.

Zurakowski, T. L. (2007). Theory of social and interpersonal influences on health. In C. L. Sieloff & M. A. Frey (Eds.), *Middle range theory development using King's conceptual system* (pp. 237–257). New York: Springer.

Chapter 10

Sister Callista Roy's Adaptation Model

PAMELA SENESAC AND
SISTER CALLISTA ROY

Introducing the Theorist
Overview of the Roy Adaptation Model
Applications of the Theory
Practice Exemplar
Summary
References

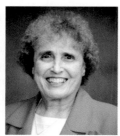

Sister Callista Roy

Introducing the Theorist

Sister Callista Roy is a highly respected nurse theorist, writer, lecturer, researcher, and teacher. She is currently Professor and Nurse Theorist at the Connell School of Nursing at Boston College. Roy holds concurrent appointments as Research Professor in Nursing at her alma mater, Mt. Saint Mary's College, Los Angeles, CA, and as Faculty Senior Scientist, Yvonne L. Munn Center for Nursing Research, Massachusetts General Hospital, Boston, MA. Roy has been a member of the Sisters of St. Joseph of Carondolet for more than 50 years.

Roy is recognized worldwide in the field of nursing and considered to be among nursing's great living thinkers. As a theorist, Roy often emphasizes her primary commitment to define and develop nursing knowledge and regards her work with the Roy adaptation model as a rich source of knowledge for improving nursing practice for individuals and for groups. In the first decade of the 21st century, Roy provided an expanded, values-based concept of adaptation based on insights related to the place of the person in the universe and in society. A prolific thinker, educator, and writer, she has welcomed the contributions of others in the development of the work; she notes that her best work is yet to come and likely will be done by one of her students.

Roy credits the major influences of her family, her religious commitment, and her teachers and mentors in her personal and professional growth. Born in Los Angeles, California, in 1939, Roy is the oldest daughter of a family of seven boys and seven girls. A deep spirit of faith, hope, love, commitment to God, and

153

service to others was central in the family. Her mother was a licensed vocational nurse and instilled the values of always seeking to know more about people and their care and of selfless giving as a nurse.

Roy was awarded a bachelor of arts degree with a major in nursing from Mount St. Mary's College, Los Angeles; a master's degree in pediatric nursing and a master's degree and a PhD in sociology from the University of California, Los Angeles. Roy completed a 2-year postdoctoral program as a clinical nurse scholar in neuroscience nursing at the University of California, San Francisco. She was a Senior Fulbright Scholar in Australia. Important mentors in her life have included Dorothy E. Johnson, Ruth Wu, Connie Robinson, and Barbara Smith Moran.

Roy is best known for developing and continually updating the Roy adaptation model as a framework for theory, practice, and research in nursing. Books on the model have been translated into many languages, including French, Italian, Spanish, Finnish, Chinese, Korean, and Japanese. Two publications that Roy considers significant are *The Roy Adaptation Model* (Roy, 2009) and *Nursing Knowledge Development and Clinical Practice* (Roy & Jones, 2007). Another important work is a two-part project analyzing research based on the Roy adaptation model and using the findings for knowledge development. The first was a critical analysis of 25 years of model-based literature, which included 163 studies published in 46 English-speaking journals, as well as dissertations and theses. It was published as a research monograph by Sigma Theta Tau International and entitled *The Roy Adaptation Model-based Research: Twenty-five Years of Contributions to Nursing Science* (Boston-Based Adaptation Research in Nursing Society, 1999). The research literature of the next 15 years was analyzed and used to create middle range theories as evidence for practice. Including 172 studies and currently in press, this work is entitled *Generating Middle Range Theory: Evidence for Practice* (Buckner & Hayden, in press).

Roy was honored as a Living Legend by the American Academy of Nursing and the Massachusetts Association of Registered Nurses.

She has received many other awards, including the National League for Nursing Martha Rogers Award for advancing nursing science; the Sigma Theta Tau International Founders Award for contributions to professional practice; and four honorary doctorates. Sigma Theta Tau International, Honor Society of Nursing included Roy as an inaugural inductee to the Nurse Researcher Hall of Fame.[1]

Overview of the Roy Adaption Model

The Roy adaptation model (Roy, 1970, 1984, 1988a, 1988b, 2009, 2011a, 2011b, 2014; Roy & Andrews, 1991, 1999; Roy & Roberts, 1981; Roy, Whetzell & Fredrickson, 2009) has been in use for more than 40 years, providing direction for nursing practice, education, and research. Extensive implementation efforts around the world and continuing philosophical and scientific developments by the theorist have contributed to model-based knowledge for nursing practice. The purpose of this chapter is to describe the model as the foundation for knowledge-based practice. The developments of the model, including assumptions and major concepts are described. The reader is introduced to the knowledge that the model provides as the basis for planning nursing care along with applications in practice and three practice exemplars.

Historical Development

Under the mentorship of Dorothy E. Johnson, Roy first developed a description of the adaptation model while a master's student at the University of California at Los Angeles. The first publication on the model appeared in 1970 (Roy, 1970) while Roy was on the faculty of the baccalaureate nursing program of a small liberal arts college. There, she had the opportunity to lead the implementation of this model of nursing as the basis of the nursing curriculum. During the next decade, more than 1500 faculty and students at Mount St. Mary's College

---

[1]For additional information please see the bonus chapter content available at http://davisplus.fadavis.com

helped to clarify, refine, and develop this approach to nursing. The constant influence of practice was important during this development. One example of data from practice used in model development was the derivation of four adaptive modes from 500 samples of patient behaviors described by nursing students.

The mid-1970s to the mid-1980s saw the expansion of the use of the model in nursing education. Roy and the faculty at her home institution consulted on curriculum in more than 30 schools across the United States and Canada. By 1987, it was estimated that more than 100,000 students had graduated from curricula based on the Roy model. Theory development was also a focus during this time, and 91 propositions based on the model were identified. These described relationships between and among concepts of the regulator and the cognator and the four adaptive modes (Roy & Roberts, 1981). In the 1980s, Roy also was influenced by postdoctoral work in neuroscience nursing and an increasing number of commitments in other countries. Roy focused on contemporary movements in nursing knowledge and the continued integration of spirituality with an understanding of nursing's role in promoting adaptation. The first decade of the 21st century included a greater focus on philosophy, knowledge for practice, and global concerns.

Philosophical, Scientific, and Cultural Assumptions

Assumptions provide the beliefs, values, and accepted knowledge that form the basis for the work. For the Roy adaptation model, the concept of adaptation rests on scientific and philosophic assumptions that Roy has developed over time. The scientific assumptions initially reflected von Bertalanffy's (1968) general systems theory and Helson's (1964) adaptation-level theory. Later beliefs about the unity and meaningfulness of the created universe were included (Young, 1986). Early identification of the philosophic assumptions for the model named humanism and veritivity. In 1988, Roy introduced the concept of veritivity as an option to total relativity. Veritivity was a term coined by Roy, based on the Latin word *veritas*. For Roy, the word offered the notion of the rootedness of all knowledge being one. Veritivity is the principle within the Roy Adaptation Model of human nature that affirms a common purposefulness of human existence. Veritivity is the affirmation that human beings are viewed in the context of the purposefulness of their existence, unity of purpose of humankind, activity and creativity for the common good, and the value and meaning of life.

Currently, Roy views the 21st century as a time of transition, transformation, and need for spiritual vision. The further development of the philosophic assumptions focuses on people's mutuality with others, the world, and a God-figure. The development and expansion of the major concepts of the model show the influence of the theorist's scientific and philosophic background and global experiences. For nursing in the 21st century, Roy (1997) provided a redefinition of adaptation and a restatement of the assumptions that are foundational to the model, which led to expanded philosophical and scientific assumptions in contemporary society and to adding cultural assumptions. These assumptions are listed in Table 10-1 and further described in the basic work on the model (Roy, 2009). Roy also uses the idea of cosmic unity that stresses her vision for the future and emphasizes the principle that people and Earth have common patterns and integral relationships. Rather than the system acting to maintain itself, the emphasis shifts to the purposefulness of human existence in a creative universe.

Model Concepts

The underlying assumptions of the Roy adaptation model are the basis for and are evident in the specific description of the major concepts of the model. The major concepts include people as adaptive systems (both individuals and groups), the environment, health, and the goal of nursing.

People as Adaptive Systems

Roy describes people, both individually and in groups, as holistic adaptive systems, complete with coping processes acting to maintain adaptation and to promote person and environment

Table 10 · 1	Assumptions of the Roy Adaptation Model for the 21st Century

Philosophic Assumptions

Persons have mutual relationships with the world and the God-figure.
Human meaning is rooted in an omega point convergence of the universe.
God is intimately revealed in the diversity of creation and is the common destiny of creation.
Persons use human creative abilities of awareness, enlightenment, and faith.
Persons are accountable for entering the process of deriving, sustaining, and transforming the universe.

Scientific Assumptions

Systems of matter and energy progress to higher levels of complex self-organization.
Consciousness and meaning are consistent of person and environment integration.
Awareness of self and environment is rooted in thinking and feeling.
Human decisions are accountable for the integration of creative processes.
Thinking and feeling mediate human action.
System relationships include acceptance, protection, and fostering interdependence.
Persons and the Earth have common patterns and integral relations.
Person and environment transformations created human consciousness.
Integration of human and environment meanings result in adaptation.

Cultural Assumptions

Experiences within a specific culture will influence how each element of the Roy adaptation model is expressed.
Within a culture, there may be a concept that is central to the culture and will influence some or all of the elements of the Roy adaptation model to a greater or lesser extent.
Cultural expressions of the elements of the Roy adaptation model may lead to changes in practice activities such as nursing assessment.
As Roy adaptation model elements evolve within a cultural perspective, implications for education and research may differ from experience in the original culture.

transformations. As with any type of system, people have internal processes that act to maintain the integrity of the individual or group. These processes have been broadly categorized as a *regulator* subsystem and a *cognator* subsystem for the person related to a *stabilizer* subsystem and an *innovator* subsystem for the group. The *regulator* uses physiological processes such as chemical, neurological, and endocrine responses to cope with the changing environment. For example, when an individual sees a sudden threat, such as an oncoming car approaching when stepping off the curb, an increase of adrenal hormones provides immediate energy enabling him or her to escape harm. The *cognator* subsystem involves the cognitive and emotional processes that interact with the environment. In the example of the individual who escapes from an oncoming car, the *cognator* acts to process the emotion of fear. The person also processes perceptions of the situation and comes to a new decision about where and how to cross the street safely.

The coping processes for the group relate to stability and change. The *stabilizer* subsystem has structures, values, and daily activities to accomplish the primary purpose of the group. Thus a family group is structured to earn a living and to provide for the nurturance and education of children. Family values also influence how the members respond to the environment to fulfill their responsibilities to maintain the family. Groups also have processes to respond to the environment with innovation and change by way of the *innovator* subsystem. For example, organizations use strategic planning activities and team-building sessions. When the *innovator* is functioning well, the group creates new goals and growth, achieving new mastery and transformation. Nurses can use *innovator* subsystems to create organizational change in practice.

Both the *cognator-regulator* and *stabilizer-innovator* coping processes are manifested in four particular ways of adapting in each individual and in groups of people. These four ways of categorizing the effects of coping activity are called *adaptive modes*. These four modes, initially developed for human systems as individuals, were expanded to encompass groups. These are termed the *physiological–physical, self-concept–group identity, role function*, and *interdependence modes*. These four major categories describe responses to and interaction with the environment and are how adaptation can be observed.

For individuals, the *physiological mode* in the Roy adaptation model is associated with the way people as individuals interact as physical beings with the environment. Behavior in this mode is the manifestation of the physiological activities of all the cells, tissues, organs, and systems comprising the human body. The *physiological mode* has nine components: the five basic needs of oxygenation, nutrition, elimination, activity and rest, and protection and four complex processes that are involved in physiological adaptation, including the senses; fluid, electrolyte, and acid–base balance; neurological function; and endocrine function. The underlying need for the *physiological mode* is physiological integrity.

The category of behavior related to the personal aspects of individuals is termed the *self-concept*. The basic need underlying the *self-concept mode* has been identified as psychic and spiritual integrity; one needs to know who one is to be or exist with a sense of unity. Self-concept is defined as the composite of beliefs and feelings that a person holds about him- or herself at a given time. Formed from internal perceptions and perceptions of others, self-concept directs one's behavior. Components of the *self-concept mode* are the physical self, including body sensation and body image; and the personal self, including self-consistency, self-ideal, and moral–ethical–spiritual self. Processes in the mode are the developing self, perceiving self, and focusing self.

Behavior relating to positions in society is termed the *role function mode* for both the individual and the group. From the perspective of the individual, the *role function mode* focuses on the roles that the individual occupies in society. A role, as the functioning unit of society, is defined as a set of expectations about how a person occupying one position behaves toward a person occupying another position. The basic need underlying the *role function mode* for the individual has been identified as social integrity, the need to know who one is in relation to others in order to act. The underlying processes include developing roles and role taking.

Behavior related to interdependent relationships of individuals and groups is the *interdependence mode*, the final adaptive mode Roy describes. For the individual, the mode focuses on interactions related to the giving and receiving of love, respect, and value. The basic need of this mode is termed *relational integrity*, the feeling of security in nurturing relationships. Two specific relationships are the focus within the *interdependence mode* for the individual: significant others, persons who are the most important to the individual, and support systems, others contributing to meeting interdependence needs. Interdependence processes include affectional adequacy and developmental adequacy.

For people in groups it is more appropriate to use the term *physical* in referring to the first adaptive mode. At the group level, this mode relates to the manner in which the human adaptive system of the group manifests adaptation relative to basic operating resources, that is, participants, physical facilities, and fiscal resources. The basic need associated with the *physical mode* for the group is resource adequacy, or wholeness achieved by adapting to change in physical resource needs. Processes in this mode for groups include resource management and strategic planning.

Group identity is the relevant term used for the second mode related to groups. Identity integrity is the need underlying this group adaptive mode. The mode comprises interpersonal relationships, group self-image, social milieu, and culture.

A nurse can have a self-concept of seeing self as physically capable of the work involved. In addition, the nurse feels comfortable meeting self-expectations of being a caring professional. In a social system, such as a nursing care unit, an associated culture can be described. There is a social environment experienced by the nurses, administrators, and other staff that is reflected by those who are part of the nursing care group. The group feels shared values and counts on each other. As such, the *self-concept–group identity mode* can reflect adaptive or ineffective behaviors associated with an individual nurse or the nursing care unit as an adaptive system. As we note later in the chapter, two processes identified in this mode are group shared identity and family coherence.

Roles within a group are the vehicles through which the goals of the social system are actually accomplished. They are the action components associated with group infrastructure. Roles are designed to contribute to the accomplishment of the group's mission, or the tasks or functions associated with the group. The *role function mode* includes the functions of administrators and staff, the management of information, and systems for decision making and maintaining order. The basic need associated with the *group role function mode* is termed *role clarity*, the need to understand and commit to fulfil expected tasks, to achieve common goals. Processes involve socializing for role expectations, reciprocating roles, and integrating roles.

For groups, the *interdependence mode* pertains to the social context in which the group operates. It involves private and public contacts both within the group and with those outside the group. The components of group interdependence include context, infrastructure, and resources. The processes for group interdependence include relational integrity, developmental adequacy, and resource adequacy.

The four adaptive modes are interrelated, which can be illustrated by drawing the modes as overlapping circles. The *physiological–physical mode* is intersected by each of the other three modes. Behavior in the *physiological–physical mode* can have an effect on or act as a stimulus for one or all of the other modes. In addition, a given stimulus can affect more than one mode, or a particular behavior can be indicative of adaptation in more than one mode. Such complex relationships among modes further demonstrate the holistic nature of humans as adaptive systems. The adaptive modes and coping processes for individuals and groups of individuals are described by the Roy adaptation model (Roy, 2009).

Environment

The Roy adaptation model defines environment as all the conditions, circumstances, and influences surrounding and affecting the development and behavior of individuals and groups. Given the model's view of the place of the person in the evolving universe, environment is a biophysical community of beings with complex patterns of interaction, feedback, growth, and decline, constituting periodic and long-term rhythms. Individual and environmental interactions are input for the individual or group as adaptive systems. This input involves both internal and external factors. Roy used the work of Helson (1964), a physiological psychologist, to categorize these factors as focal, contextual, and residual stimuli.

The *focal* is the stimulus most immediately confronting the individual and holding the focus of attention; *contextual* stimuli are those factors also acting in the situation; and *residual* are possible factors that as yet have an unknown affect. A specific internal input stimulus is an adaptation level that represents the individual's or group's coping capacities. This changing level of ability has an internal effect on adaptive behaviors. Roy defined three levels of adaptation: integrated, compensatory, and compromised. *Integrated adaptation* occurs when the structures and functions of the adaptive modes are working as a whole to meet human needs. The *compensatory adaptation* level occurs when the *cognator* and *regulator* or stabilizer and *innovator* are activated by a challenge. *Compromised adaptation* occurs when integrated and compensatory processes are inadequate, creating an adaptation problem.

Health

Roy's concept of health is related to the concept of adaptation and the idea that adaptive responses promote integrity. Individuals and groups are viewed as adaptive systems that interact with the environment and grow, change, develop, and flourish. Health is the reflection of personal and environmental interactions that are adaptive. According to the Roy adaptation model, health is defined as (1) a process, (2) a state of being, and (3) becoming whole and integrated in a way that reflects individual and environment mutuality.

Goal of Nursing

When Roy began her theoretical work, the goal of nursing was the first major concept of her nursing model to be described. She began by attempting to identify the unique function of nursing in promoting health. As a number of health-care workers have the goal of promoting health, it seemed important to identify a unique goal for nursing. While she was working as a staff nurse in pediatric settings, Roy noted the great resiliency of children in responding to major physiological and psychological changes. Yet nursing intervention was needed to support and promote this positive coping. It seemed, then, that the concept of adaptation, or positive coping, might be used to describe the goal or function of nursing. From this initial notion, Roy developed a description of the goal of nursing: the promotion of adaptation for individuals and groups in each of the four adaptive modes, thus contributing to health, quality of life, and dying with dignity.

Basis for Practice—Theory and Process

The assumptions and concepts of the model provide the basis for theory building for nursing practice, as well as a specific approach to the nursing process. As early as the 1970s, human life processes and patterns were identified as the common focus of nursing knowledge (Donaldson & Crowley, 1978). In a more recent article, a central unifying focus of nursing has extended this view to include nursing concepts categorized as facilitating humanization, meaning, choice, quality of life, and healing, living, and dying (Willis, Grace, & Roy, 2008). Adaptation is a significant life process that leads to these ideals.

Theory Development for Practice

To lead to middle-range theories within the model, Roy identified the major life processes within each adaptive mode. For example, in the physiological mode, there are processes and patterns for the need for oxygenation that include ventilation, patterns of gas exchange, transport of gases, and compensation for inadequate oxygenation. Similarly, the *self-concept mode* has three processes identified to meet the person's need for psychic and spiritual integrity: the developing self, the perceiving self, and the focusing self. On the group level, two examples of processes identified to meet the need for a shared self-image are group shared identity and family coherence. The *group identity mode* reflects how people in groups perceive themselves based on environmental feedback about the group. Persons in a group have perceptions about their shared relations, goals, and values. The social milieu and the culture provide feedback for the group. The *social milieu* refers to the human-made environment in which the group is embedded, including economic, political, religious, and family structures. Ethnicity and socioeconomic status in particular make up the social culture, a specific part of the milieu or environment of the group.

The belief systems of the milieu and social culture act as stimuli for the group and also affect other groups with which the group interacts. The family is most often the first group with which a person identifies. The group self-image and shared responsibility for goal achievement is central to group identity. Identity integrity is the basic need underlying the *group identity mode*. Nursing care uses the understanding of these processes to evaluate the adaptation level and to provide care to promote integrated processes at the highest level of adaptation possible.

To develop knowledge for practice from the grand theory, Roy described a five-step process for developing middle or practice level theory and nursing knowledge:

1. Select a life process.
2. Study the life process in the literature and in people.
3. Develop an intervention strategy to enhance the life process.

4. Derive a proposition for practice.
5. Test the proposition in research.

Processes can also be identified by using qualitative research to identify and describe human experiences.

Nursing Process for Care

The nursing process based on the model stems from the assumptions and concepts of the model. First-level assessment of behavior involves gathering data about the behavior of the person or group as an adaptive system in each of the adaptive modes. Second-level assessment is the assessment of stimuli, that is, the identification of internal and external stimuli that influence the adaptive behaviors. Stimuli are classified as focal, contextual, and residual. The nurse uses the first- and second-level assessment to make a nursing judgment called a nursing diagnosis. In collaboration with the person or group, the data are interpreted in statements about the adaptation status of the person, including behavior and most relevant stimuli. The adaptation level is then classified as integrated, compensatory, or compromised.

Also, in collaboration with the person or group, the nurse sets goals, establishing clear statements of the behavioral outcomes for nursing care. Interventions then involve the determination of how best to assist the person in attaining the established goals. These may involve changing stimuli or strengthening coping ability. The aim is to promote an integrated adaptation level. Evaluation involves judging the effectiveness of the nursing intervention in relation to the resulting behavior in comparison with the goal established. The steps of the nursing process have been given in sequential order; however, the process is ongoing and the steps can be simultaneous. For example, the nurse may be intervening in one adaptive mode and assessing in another at the same time.

Applications of the Theory

Senesac (2003) reviewed published projects that have implemented the Roy adaptation model in institutional practice settings and identified seven distinct projects ranging from an ideology basis for a single unit to hospital-wide projects. In some cases the published project developed from a unit implementation to a full agency implementation, as in one of the early projects reported by Mastal et al. (1982). Gray (1991) discussed involvement in five projects. She reported that not all implementation projects were completed due to changes in hospital management, philosophy, or direction.

Gray's initial work was at a 132-bed acute care, not-for-profit children's hospital. Other projects varied from a 100-bed proprietary hospital to a 248-bed nonprofit, community-owned hospital. The main focus of the implementation projects was to improve patient care through quality nursing care plans and in some cases to develop performance standards. Two implementation projects in Colombia were reported on by Moreno-Ferguson and Alvarado-Garcia (2009). One project was in an ambulatory rehabilitation service (Moreno-Ferguson, 2001) and the other a pediatric intensive care unit of a cardiology institute (Monroy, 2003). As hospitals in the United States work toward certification of Magnet Status, more nursing groups are requesting information about application of the Roy adaptation model in institutional health-care settings.

Practice Exemplar

Family coherence is an indicator of positive adaptation and refers to a state of unity or a consistent sequence of thought that connects family members who share group identity, goals, and values (Roy, 2009). When interacting with families of other cultures, health-care providers need to assess cultural norms and beliefs that determine patterns of interaction with the health and social services system, health-care decision making, the availability of social support for caregivers, and may have implications for the psychosocial experience of family caregivers and the clients. Roy's group identity mode provides a useful conceptual framework that guides health-care providers working with families of diverse ethnic backgrounds.

Practice Exemplar cont.

Introduction to the Practice Exemplar—the Wang Family

The Wang family includes David Wang; his wife, Teresa Wang; their 7-year old daughter, Vivian Wang; and extended family including David's mother, Uncle Frank Wang; his daughter Lisa Wang, 32; and her husband and their 5-year-old son (Zhan, 2003). David's parents immigrated to the United States when he was ten years old. The Wang family opened a small Chinese restaurant, which David has managed since his father's retirement. David's parents participate regularly in activities organized by Chinatown's Council on Aging.

David and his parents have a *shared self-image* as Chinese immigrants and a shared *group identity* as the Wang family. The Wang family shares a strong cultural commitment to the value of *filial piety*. To family members, this means to be good to one's parents and take care of them; to engage in good conduct and bring a good name to parents and ancestors; to perform one's job well to support parents and carry out sacrifices to the ancestors; and to show love, respect, and support. The term *filial* denotes the respect and obedience that a child, primarily a son, should show to his parents, especially to his father.

David's father suffered a stroke and died at the age of 78. His mother began to show decline in memory, experiencing difficulty finding her way in familiar places, misplacing objects, becoming disoriented and easily irritated. David took his mother for a physical examination; she was diagnosed as having dementia and referred to a specialist. Recognizing that his mother was unable to live independently, David arranged for her to live with his family. David and his wife took on the family caregiver role while trying to keep their respective jobs. David's cousin visited them regularly and helped with household chores. David was glad that he was able to keep the family together despite the passing of his father and the cognitive impairment of his mother.

David provides primary financial support for his family. As his mother's cognitive function deteriorated, David became overwhelmed by caring for his mother while being responsible for managing the restaurant. His wife quit her job to attend to her mother-in-law's care. When David and his wife tried to find someone in the Chinese community to provide respite care for their mother, they heard some strong negative reactions. Some considered his mother's dementia as "insanity" or "a mental disorder." Some talked about dementia as contagious or believed his mother's dementia was being caused by bad *Feng Shui*, an ancient Chinese belief in which *Feng* (the force of wind) and *Shui* (the flow of water) are viewed as living energies that flow around one's home and affect one's life and well-being. If *Feng Shui* flows gently and peacefully, it brings happiness and health to one's family. If *Feng Shui* stagnates, one can be ill, poor, and unfortunate (Beattie, 2000). The perception of dementia triggered a strong negative response from the Chinese community, and his mother's friends stopped visiting her. David's daughter began to miss school, and her grades were declining. Both David and his wife were feeling overwhelmed and depressed.

Analysis of the Practice Exemplar

In the case of the Wang family, the focus of nursing practice is on the relational system of the family. To begin planning nursing care, the family is addressed as an adaptive system.

Assessment of behaviors

The nurse met with David and Teresa to assess family structure, function, relationships, and consistency, and their employment status, living arrangements, and the division of family caregiving responsibilities. The nurse assessed how decisions are made in the family, from small daily decisions to larger, health-care-related decisions. The nurse observed that David and his wife show love, respect, and loyalty to David's mother and to each other. Although the mother's needs for care are met, individual needs of both David and his wife,

Continued

Teresa are unmet. Alternating care for David's mother, maintaining their jobs, and attending to Vivian's schoolwork and growth needs is challenging. The nurse finds out that the Wang family holds a strong Chinese tradition of *filial piety* and that they feel a moral obligation to take care of their mother. The strong stigma attached to dementia in the Chinese community takes an emotional toll on them.

Assessment of stimuli

The nurse conducts a second level of assessment by meeting with the extended Wang family to identify influencing factors, or stimuli, related to group identity and family coherence. The major stimuli are the demands they face and the problems posed for them to solve. David's mother requires medical and personal care. David needs to work to ensure health insurance for his family and to secure income to pay for the cost of personal care. Finding Chinese-speaking home health aides is challenging. The social stigma toward dementia is strong in the Chinese community, bringing shame to the Wang family and isolating David's mother from her ethnic community. The Wang family agrees that the stigma and reaction from the external social environment have become stressors to family caregiving.

Nursing diagnosis

The nurse identifies three *tentative* diagnoses. First, the Wang family has a strong ethnic heritage related to the group's responsibility to maintain values and goals. Second, family conflict exists as the demands of family caregiving for the mother increase. Third, strong stigma attached to dementia in the Chinese community creates prejudice against the Wang family and causes some family members to feel distressed and ambivalent.

The nurse continues to assess behaviors of shared identity and cohesion in the Wang family, looking for common perceptions, feelings, and experiences of caregiving for the loved one with dementia. The nurse learns that David, as the only son, has a moral responsibility to care for his mother and considers himself solely responsible. The nurse asks each member of the Wang family to find common

orientations by sharing their thinking and feelings. David and his wife openly share their feelings and frustrations. Lisa and her father express their willingness to share responsibility and help out.

Goal setting

At the next meeting, the nurse helps the Wang family set up attainable short-term goals based on shared cognitive and emotional orientations and common values. Attaining goals requires shared responsibilities and some division of labor. Their goals include (1) working together with home health aides; (2) supporting each other through shared feelings and thoughts and the shared responsibilities of caregiving based on each individual's desire, skill, and availability; and (3) communicating with the Chinese community about the stigma toward dementia and finding ways to demystify dementia.

The Wang family decides to have Lisa Chang, a social worker in a community hospital, lead the search for home health aides. David Wang convenes family meetings as needed, and Frank Wang leads the talk with key players in the Chinese community. Despite the stressors they have encountered, family members feel a sense of unity through compensatory adaptation process.

Intervention

Nursing intervention involves focusing on the stimuli affecting the behavior and managing the stimuli by altering, increasing, or decreasing, removing, or maintaining stimuli. The nurse (1) assesses the Wang family with respect to shared values, shared goals, shared relations, group identify, and social environment and stimuli; (2) works with the Wang family to write down shared goals, values, and expectations; and (3) encourages the family to explore additional resources. The nurse also helps the Wang family to use effective coping strategies to strengthen compensatory processes by acknowledging that the family is transcending the crisis, identifying additional resources in support of family caregiving, and by reinforcing their shared goals, values, relations, and group identity.

Practice Exemplar cont.

Evaluation

The nurse evaluates the effectiveness of the nursing intervention. Lisa Chang called her social work network and found appropriate home health aides to provide personal care to David's mother. This allows David to attend to his work and allows his wife to spend more time with their daughter, attending to her schoolwork and personal needs. Vivian has not been absent from school again.

David Wang hired a manager to help operate the restaurant so that he has time to take his mother to appointments and to maintain a stable income. David's mother's old friend visited her briefly. Frank Wang, an activist in the Chinese community, began to talk with other Chinese about dementia.

The strong stigma attached to dementia in the Chinese community influenced the adaptation problem experienced by the Wang family. Social stigma can be pervasive, distorting the perceptions of individuals, affecting the perception of a disease and how a dementia diagnosis and services are sought,

and how caregiving is supported. To reduce stigma in promotion of effective adaptation of family caregivers and health-care providers, families and the community need to work together toward better understanding of dementia, its diagnosis, treatment, and care options. Educational and service outreach is the first step to reduce the stigma in the Chinese community. Educational materials and service need to be linguistically appropriate and adaptable to Chinese patients and their families. Elderly Chinese immigrants often read Chinese newspapers to connect themselves to their culture and people. Publishing dementia information and related educational articles in widely circulated Chinese newspapers is a way to reach out to Chinese families. Bilingual professional staff and linguistically appropriate oral and written instructions on dementia are helpful (Valle, 1998).

Reprinted from: Roy, C. & Zhan, l. (2010). Sister Callista Roy's Adaptation Model. In Nursing Theories and Nursing Practice (3rd. Ed.).

■ Summary

This chapter focused on the Roy adaptation model as a foundation for knowledge-based practice. The background of the theorist and the historical development of the model were presented briefly. Roy's most recent theoretical developments were the main focus of the description of the model assumptions and major concepts (. The process for theory becoming the basis for developing knowledge for practice was introduced by outlining how to develop

middle- and practice-level theory that is tested in research. In particular, the effects of the Roy adaptation model on practice were articulated from a general summary of major practice projects and through a practice exemplar. The exemplar illustrates the use of the self-identity adaptive mode as an example of using theory-based knowledge to provide care for a Chinese family dealing with a parent diagnosed with dementia.

References

Beattie, A. (2000). *Using Feng Shui.* Vancouver: Raincoast Books.

Boston-Based Adaptation Research in Nursing Society. (1999). *Roy adaptation model-based research: 25 years of contributions to nursing science.* Indianapolis, IN: Centre Nursing Press.

Buckner, E. B., & Hayden, S. (2014). Synthesis of middle range theory of adapting in chronic health conditions. In C. Roy with the Roy Adaptation Association, *Generating middle range theory: Evidence for practice* (pp. 277–308). New York, NY: Springer Publishing Company.

Donaldson, S. K., & Crowley, D. (1978). The discipline of nursing. *Nursing Outlook, 26,* 113–120.

Gray, J. (1991). The Roy adaptation model in nursing practice. In C. Roy & H. A. Andrews (Eds.), *The Roy adaptation model: The definitive statement* (pp. 429–443). Norwalk, CT: Appleton & Lange.

Helson, H. (1964). *Adaptation level theory.* New York: Harper & Row.

Mastal, M. F., Hammond, H., & Roberts, M. P. (1982). Theory into hospital practice: A pilot implementation. *The Journal of Nursing Administration, 12,* 9–15.

Monroy, P. (2003). Aproximación a la experiencia de aplicación del Modelo de Callista Roy en la Unidad de cuidado intensivo pediátrico. *Enfermería Hoy, 1*(1), 17–20.

Moreno-Ferguson, M. E. (2001). Aplicacion del modelo de adaptacion en un servicio de rehabilitacion ambulatoria, *Aquichan, 1*(1), 14–17.

Moreno-Ferguson, M. E., & Alvarado-Garcia, A. M. (2009). Aplicacion del modelo de adaptacion de Callista Roy en Latinoamerica: Revision de la literatura. *Aquichan, 9*(1), 62–72.

Roy, C. (1970). Adaptation: A conceptual framework for nursing. *Nursing Outlook, 18,* 42–45.

Roy, C. (1984). *Introduction to nursing: An adaptation model* (2nd ed.). Englewood Cliffs, NJ: Prentice-Hall.

Roy, C. (1988a). Altered cognition: An information processing approach. In P. H. Mitchell, L. C. Hodges, M. Muwaswes, & C. A. Walleck (Eds.), *AANN's neuroscience nursing, phenomenon and practice: Human responses to neurological health problems* (pp. 185–211). Norwalk, CT: Appleton & Lange.

Roy, C. (1988b). Human information processing. In J. J. Fitzpatrick, R. L. Taunton, & J. Q. Benoliel (Eds.), *Annual review of nursing research* (pp. 237–261). New York: Springer.

Roy, C. (1997). *Knowledge as universal cosmic imperative. Proceedings of nursing knowledge impact conference 1996* (pp. 95–118). Chestnut Hill, MA: Boston College Press.

Roy, C. (2009). *The Roy adaptation model* (3rd ed.). Upper Saddle River, NJ: Prentice-Hall Health.

Roy, S. C. (2011a). Extending the Roy adaptation model to meet changing global needs. *Nursing Science Quarterly, 24*(4), 345–351. nsq.sagepub.com

Roy, S. C. (2011b). Research based on the Roy adaptation model: Last 25 years. *Nursing Science Quarterly, 24*(4), 312–320. nsq.sagepub.com

Roy, C.with the RAA. (Ed.). (2014). *Generating middle range theory: Evidence for practice.* New York, NY: Springer Publishing Company.

Roy, C., & Andrews, H. A. (1991). *The Roy adaptation model: The definitive statement.* East Norwalk, CT: Appleton & Lange.

Roy, C., & Andrews, H. A. (1999). *The Roy adaptation model* (2nd ed.). Stamford, CT: Appleton & Lange.

Roy, C., & Jones, D. (Eds.). (2007). *Nursing knowledge development and clinical practice.* New York: Springer.

Roy, C., & Roberts, S. (1981). *Theory construction in nursing: An adaptation model.* Englewood Cliffs, NJ: Prentice-Hall.

Roy, C., Whetsell, M.V., & Frederickson, K. (2009).The Roy adaptation model and research: Global Perspective *Nursing Science Quarterly, 22*(3), 209–211.

Senesac, P. (2003). Implementing the Roy adaptation model: From theory to practice. *Roy Adaptation Association Review, 4*(2), 5.

Valle, R. (1998). *Caregiving across cultures: Working with dementing illness and ethnically diverse populations.* Boca Raton, FL: Taylor & Francis.

von Bertalanffy, L. (1968). *General system theory: Foundations, development, applications.* New York: George Braziller.

Willis, D., Grace, P., & Roy, C. (2008). A central unifying focus for the discipline: Facilitating humanization, meaning, choice, quality of life and healing in living and dying. *Advances in Nursing Science, 31*(1), E28–40. Retrieved from www.advancesinnursingscience.com

Young, L. B. (1986). *The unfinished universe.* New York: Simon & Schuster.

Zhan, L. (2003). *Asian Americans: Vulnerable population, model intervention, and clarifying agendas.* Sudbury, MA: Jones and Bartlett.

Betty Neuman's Systems Model

LOIS WHITE LOWRY AND
PATRICIA DEAL AYLWARD

Introducing the Theorist
Overview of the Neuman Systems Model
Applications of the Theory
Practice Exemplar
Summary
References

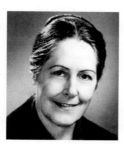

Betty Neuman

Introducing the Theorist

Betty Neuman developed the Neuman systems model (NSM) in 1970 to "provide unity, or a focal point, for student learning" (Neuman, 2002b, p. 327) at the School of Nursing, University of California at Los Angeles (UCLA). Neuman recognized the need for educators and practitioners to have a framework to view nursing comprehensively within various contexts. Although she developed the model strictly as a teaching aid, it is now used globally as a nursing conceptual model to guide curriculum development, research studies, and clinical practice in the full array of health-care disciplines.

Neuman's autobiography, touched on briefly here, is presented more fully in the latest edition of her book focusing on the model (Neuman & Fawcett, 2011). Neuman was born in southeastern Ohio on a 100-acre family farm on September 11, 1924. Her father died at age 37 when she was 11, and she, her mother, and two brothers worked hard to keep the farm.

Neuman idealized nursing because her father had praised nurses during his 6 years of intermittent hospitalizations. In gratitude, she developed a strong commitment to become an excellent bedside nurse. She also attributed her decisions about her life's work to the important influence of her mother's charity experiences as a self-taught rural midwife.

Betty Neuman graduated from high school soon after the onset of World War II. Although she had dreamed of attending nearby Marietta College, she lacked the financial means and instead became an aircraft instrument repair technician. After the Cadet Nurse

Corps Program became available, she entered the 3-year diploma nurse program at People Hospital, Akron, Ohio (currently General Hospital Medical Center).

She completed her baccalaureate degree in nursing and earned a master's degree, with a major in public health nursing, from UCLA. During her master's program, she worked on special projects, as a relief psychiatric head nurse and as a volunteer crisis counselor. Because of these experiences, Neuman became one of the first California Nurse Licensed Clinical Fellows of the American Association of Marriage and Family Therapy.

In 1967, Neuman became a faculty member at UCLA and assumed the role of chair of the program from which she had graduated. She expanded the master's program, focusing on interdisciplinary practice in community mental health.

In 1970, she developed the NSM as a guide for graduate nursing students. The model was first published in the May–June 1972 issue of *Nursing Research*. Since 1980, several important changes have enhanced the model. A nursing process format was designed, and in 1989, Neuman introduced the concepts of the created environment and the spiritual variable. In collaboration with Dr. Audrey Koertvelyessy, Neuman developed a theory of client system stability. Along with the Neuman Systems Trustees Group, she continues to clarify concepts and components of the model.

Neuman completed a doctoral degree in clinical psychology in 1985 from Pacific Western University. She received honorary doctorates from Neumann College in Aston, Pennsylvania, and Grand Valley State University in Allendale, Michigan. She is an honorary fellow in the American Academy of Nursing.

Overview of the Neuman Systems Model

The philosophic base of the Neuman Systems Model encompasses wholism, a wellness orientation, client perception and motivation, and a dynamic systems perspective of energy and variable interaction with the environment to mitigate possible harm from internal and external stressors, while caregivers and clients form a partnership relationship to negotiated desired outcome goals for optimal health retention, restoration, and maintenance. This philosophic base pervades all aspects of the model.
—BETTY NEUMAN (2002c, p. 12)

As its name suggests, the Neuman systems model is classified as a systems model or a systems category of knowledge. Neuman (1995) defined *system* as a pervasive order that holds together its parts. With this definition in mind, she writes that nursing can be readily conceptualized as a complete whole, with identifiable smaller wholes or parts. The complete whole structure is maintained by interrelationships among identifiable smaller wholes or parts through regulations that evolve out of the dynamics of the open system. In the system there is dynamic energy exchange, moving either toward or away from stability. Energy moves toward negentropy, or evolution, as a system absorbs energy to increase its organization, complexity, and development when it moves toward a steady or wellness state. An open system of energy exchange is never at rest. The open system tends to move cyclically toward differentiation and elaboration for further growth and survival of the organism. With the dynamic energy exchange, the system can also move away from stability. Energy can move toward extinction (entropy) by gradual disorganization, increasing randomness, and energy dissipation.

The NSM illustrates a client–client system and presents nursing as a discipline concerned primarily with defining appropriate nursing actions in stressor-related situations or in possible reactions of the client–client system. The client and environment may be positively or negatively affected by each other. There is a tendency within any system to maintain a steady state or balance among the various disruptive forces operating within or upon it. Neuman has identified these forces as stressors and suggests that possible reactions and actual reactions with identifiable signs or symptoms may be mitigated through appropriate early interventions (Neuman, 1995).

Unique Perspectives of the Neuman Systems Model

Neuman (2002c, p. 14; 2011a, p. 14) has identified 10 unique perspectives inherent within her model. They describe, define, and connect concepts essential to understanding the conceptual model that is presented in the next section of this chapter.

1. Each individual client or group as a client system is unique; each system is a composite of common known factors or innate characteristics within a normal, given range of response contained within a basic structure.
2. The client as a system is in a dynamic, constant energy exchange with the environment.
3. Many known, unknown, and universal environmental stressors exist. Each differs in its potential for disturbing a client's usual stability level, or normal line of defense. The particular interrelationships of client variables—physiological, psychological, sociocultural, developmental, and spiritual—at any point in time can affect the degree to which a client is protected by the flexible line of defense against possible reaction to a single stressor or a combination of stressors.
4. Each individual client–client system has evolved a normal range of response to the environment that is referred to as a normal line of defense, or usual wellness/stability state. It represents change over time through coping with diverse stress encounters. The normal line of defense can be used as a standard from which to measure health deviation.
5. When the cushioning, accordion-like effect of the flexible line of defense is no longer capable of protecting the client–client system against an environmental stressor, the stressor breaks through the normal line of defense. The interrelationships of variables—physiological, psychological, sociocultural, developmental, and spiritual—determine the nature and degree of system reaction or possible reaction to the stressor.
6. The client, whether in a state of wellness or illness, is a dynamic composite of the interrelationships of variables—physiological, psychological, sociocultural, developmental, and spiritual. Wellness is on a continuum of available energy to support the system in an optimal state of system stability.
7. Implicit within each client system are internal resistance factors known as lines of resistance, which function to stabilize and return the client to the usual wellness state (normal line of defense) or possibly to a higher level of stability after an environmental stressor reaction.
8. Primary prevention relates to general knowledge that is applied in client assessment and intervention in identification and reduction or mitigation of possible or actual risk factors associated with environmental stressors to prevent possible reaction. The goal of health promotion is included in primary prevention.
9. Secondary prevention relates to symptomatology after a reaction to stressors, appropriate ranking of intervention priorities, and treatment to reduce their noxious effects.
10. Tertiary prevention relates to the adaptive processes taking place as reconstitution begins and maintenance factors move the client back in a circular manner toward primary prevention.

The Conceptual Model

Neuman's original diagram of her model is illustrated in Figure 11-1. The conceptual model was developed to explain the client–client system as an individual person for the discipline of nursing. Neuman chose the term *client* to show respect for collaborative relationships that exist between the client and the caregiver in Neuman's model, as well as the wellness perspective of the model. The model can be applied to an individual, a group, a community, or a social issue and is appropriate for nursing and other health disciplines (Neuman, 1995, 2002c, 2011a, p.15).

The NSM provides a way of looking at the domain of nursing: humans, environment, health, and nursing.

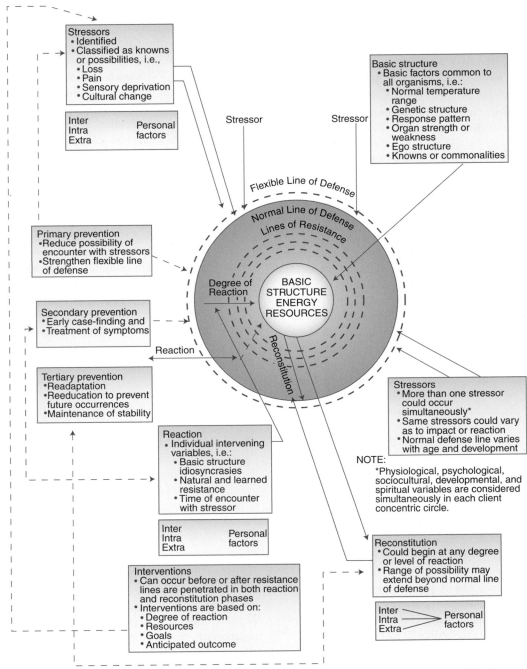

Fig 11 • 1 The Neuman systems model. (Original diagram copyright 1970 by Betty Neuman. A holistic view of a dynamic open client–client system interacting with environmental stressors, along with client and caregiver collaborative participation in promoting an optimum state of wellness.) *(From Neuman, 1995, p. 17, with permission.)*

Client–Client System

The client–client system (see Fig. 11-1) consists of the flexible line of defense, the normal line of defense, lines of resistance, and the basic structure energy resources (shown at the core of the concentric circles in Fig. 11-2). Five client variables—physiological, psychological, sociocultural, developmental, and spiritual—occur and are considered simultaneously in each concentric circle that makes up the client–client system (Neuman, 1995, 2002c, 2011a).

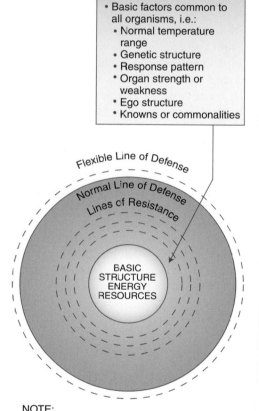

Basic structure
• Basic factors common to all organisms, i.e.:
  • Normal temperature range
  • Genetic structure
  • Response pattern
  • Organ strength or weakness
  • Ego structure
  • Knowns or commonalities

Flexible Line of Defense
Normal Line of Defense
Lines of Resistance

BASIC STRUCTURE ENERGY RESOURCES

NOTE:
Physiological, psychological, sociocultural, developmental, and spiritual variables occur and are considered simultaneously in each client concentric circle.

Fig 11 • 2 Client–client system. The structure of the client-client system, including the five variables that are occurring simultaneously in each client concentric circle. *(From Neuman, 1995, p. 26, with permission.)*

Flexible Line of Defense

Stressors must penetrate the flexible line of defense before they are capable of penetrating the rest of the client system. Neuman described this line of defense as accordion-like in function. The flexible line of defense acts like a protective buffer system to help prevent stressor invasion of the client system and protects the normal line of defense. The client has more protection from stressors when the flexible line expands away from the normal line of defense. The opposite is true when the flexible line moves closer to the normal line of defense. The effectiveness of the buffer system can be reduced by single or multiple stressors. The flexible line of defense can be rapidly altered over a relatively short time period by states of emergency, or short-term conditions, such as loss of sleep, poor nutrition, or dehydration (Neuman, 1995, 2002c; 2011a, p. 17). Consider the latter examples. What are the effects of short-term loss of sleep, poor nutrition, or dehydration on a client's normal state of wellness? Will these situations increase the possibility for stressor penetration? The answer is that the possibility for stressor penetration may be increased. The actual response depends on the accordion-like function previously described, along with the other components of the client system.

Normal Line of Defense

The normal line of defense represents what the client has become over time, or the usual state of wellness. The nurse should determine the client's usual level of wellness to recognize a change. The normal line of defense is considered dynamic because it can expand or contract over time. The usual wellness level or system stability can decrease, remain the same, or improve after treatment of a stressor reaction. The normal line of defense is dynamic because of its ability to become and remain stabilized with life stressors over time, protecting the basic structure and system integrity (Neuman, 1995, 2002c, 2011, p. 18).

Lines of Resistance

Neuman identified the series of concentric broken circles that surround the basic structure as lines of resistance for the client. When the normal line of defense is penetrated by environmental stressors, a degree of reaction, or signs and/or symptoms, will occur. Each line of resistance contains known and unknown internal and external resource factors. These factors support the client's basic structure and the normal line of defense, resulting in protection of system integrity. Examples of the factors that support the basic structure and normal line of defense include the body's mobilization of white blood cells and activation of the immune system mechanisms. There is a decrease in the signs or symptoms, or a reversal of the reaction to stressors, when the lines of resistance are effective. The system reconstitutes itself, and system stability is returned. The level of wellness may be higher or lower than it was before the stressor penetration. When the lines of resistance are ineffective, energy depletion and death may occur (Neuman, 1995, 2002c, 2011a, p. 18).

Basic Structure

The basic structure or central core consists of factors that are common to the human species. Neuman offered the following examples of basic survival factors: temperature range, genetic structure, response pattern, organ strength or weakness, ego structure, and knowns or commonalities (Neuman, 1995, 2002c, 2011a, p. 16).

Five Client Variables

Neuman (1995, p. 28; 2002c, p. 17; 2011a, p. 16) identified five variables that are contained in all client systems: physiological, psychological, sociocultural, developmental, and spiritual. These variables are considered simultaneously in each client concentric circle. They are present in varying degrees of development and in a wide range of interactive styles and potential. Neuman offers the following definitions for each variable:

Physiological: Refers to bodily structure and function
Psychological: Refers to mental processes and relationships
Sociocultural: Refers to combined social and cultural functions
Developmental: Refers to life-developmental processes
Spiritual: Refers to spiritual beliefs and influence

Neuman elaborated that the spiritual variable is an innate component of the basic structure. Although it may or may not be acknowledged or developed by the client or client system, Neuman views the spiritual variable as being on a continuum of development that penetrates all other client system variables and supports the client's optimal wellness. The client–client system can have a complete lack of awareness of the spiritual variable's presence and potential, deny its presence, or have a conscious and highly developed spiritual understanding that supports the client's optimal wellness.

Neuman explained that the spirit controls the mind, and the mind consciously or unconsciously controls the body. She used an analogy of a seed to clarify this idea.

It is assumed that each person is born with a spiritual energy force, or "seed," within the spiritual variable, as identified in the basic structure of the client system. The seed or human spirit with its enormous energy potential lies on a continuum of dormant, unacceptable, or undeveloped to recognition, development, and positive system influence. Traditionally, a seed must have environmental catalysts, such as timing, warmth, moisture, and nutrients, to burst forth with the energy that transforms into a living form that then, in turn, as it becomes further nourished and develops, offers itself as sustenance, generating power as long as its own source of nurture exists (Neuman, 2002c, p. 16; 2011, Box 1-1, p. 17).

The spiritual variable affects or is affected by a condition and interacts with other variables in a positive or negative way. Neuman gave the example of grief or loss (psychological state), which may inactivate, decrease, initiate, or increase spirituality. There can be movement in either direction of a continuum (Neuman, 1995, 2002c, 2011a, p. 17). Neuman believes that spiritual variable considerations are necessary for a truly holistic perspective and for a truly caring concern for the client–client system.

Fulton (1995) has studied the spiritual variable in depth. She elaborated on research studies that extend our understanding of the following aspects of spirituality: spiritual well-being, spiritual needs, spiritual distress, and spiritual care. She suggested that spiritual needs include (1) the need for meaning and purpose in life, (2) the need to receive love and give love, (3) the need for hope and creativity, and (4) the need for forgiving, trusting relationships with self, others, and God or a deity or a guiding philosophy.

Environment

A second concept identified by Neuman is the environment, as illustrated in Figure 11-3. She defined *environment* broadly as "all internal and external factors or influences surrounding the identified client or client system" (Neuman, 1995, p. 30; 2002c, p. 18; 2011, pp. 20–21), including:

- Internal environment: intrapersonal factors
- External environment: Inter- and extrapersonal factors

- Created environment: Intra-, inter-, and extrapersonal factors (Neuman, 1995, p. 31; 2002c, pp. 18–19; 2011a, pp. 20–21)

The internal environment consists of all forces or interactive influences contained within the boundaries of the client–client system. Examples of intrapersonal forces are presented for each variable.

- Physiological variable: autoimmune response, degree of mobility, range of body function
- Psychological and sociocultural variables: attitudes, values, expectations, behavior patterns, coping patterns, conditioned responses
- Developmental variable: age, degree of normalcy, factors related to the present situation
- Spiritual variable: hope, sustaining forces (Neuman, 1995; 2002c; 2011, p. 17)

The external environment consists of all forces or interactive influences existing outside the client–client system. Interpersonal factors in the environment are forces between

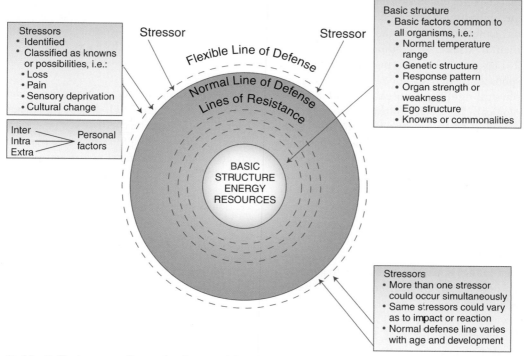

Fig 11 • 3 Environment. Internal and external factors surrounding the client–client system. *(From Neuman, 1995, p. 27, with permission.)*

people or client systems. These factors include the relationships and resources of family, friends, or caregivers. Extrapersonal factors include education, finances, employment, and other resources (Neuman, 1995, 2002c).

Neuman (1995, 2002c, 2011a, pp. 20–21) identified a third environment as the "created environment." The client unconsciously mobilizes all system variables, including the basic structure of energy factors, toward system integration, stability, and integrity to create a safe environment. This safe, created environment offers a protective perceptive coping shield that helps the client to function. A major objective of this environment is to stimulate the client's health. Neuman pointed out that what was originally created to safeguard the health of the system may have a negative effect because of the binding of available energy. This environment represents an open system that exchanges energy with the internal and external environments. The created environment supersedes or goes beyond the internal and external environments while encompassing both; it provides an insulating effect to change the response or possible response of the client to environmental stressors. Neuman (1995, 2002c, 2011) gave the following examples of responses: use of denial or envy (psychological), physical rigidity or muscle constraint (physiological), life-cycle continuation of survival patterns (developmental), required social space range (sociocultural), and sustaining hope (spiritual).

Neuman believes the caregiver, through assessment, will need to determine (1) what has been created (nature of the created environment), (2) the outcome of the created environment (extent of its use and client value), and (3) the ideal that has yet to be created (the protection that is needed or possible, to a lesser or greater degree). This assessment is necessary to best understand and support the client's created environment (Neuman, 1995, 2002c, 2011a). Neuman suggested that further research is needed to understand the client's awareness of the created environment and its relationship to health. She believes that as the caregiver

recognizes the value of the client-created environment and purposefully intervenes, the interpersonal relationship can become one of important mutual exchange (Neuman, 1995, 2002c, 2011a). de Kuiper (2011) added her perspective of the created environment and guidelines for nursing practice.

Health

Health is a third concept in Neuman's model. She believes that health (or wellness) and illness are on opposite ends of the continuum. *Health* is equated with optimal system stability (the best possible wellness state at any given time). Client movement toward wellness exists when more energy is built and stored than expended. Client movement toward illness and death exists when more energy is needed than is available to support life. The degree of wellness depends on the amount of energy required to return to and maintain system stability. The system is stable when more energy is available than is being used. Health is seen as varying levels within a normal range, rising and falling throughout the life span. These changes are in response to basic structure factors and reflect satisfactory or unsatisfactory adjustment by the client system to environmental stressors (Neuman, 1995, 2002c, 2011a, p. 23).

Nursing

Nursing is a fourth concept in Neuman's model and is depicted in Figure 11-4. Nursing's major concern is to keep the client system stable by (1) accurately assessing the effects and possible effects of environmental stressors and (2) assisting client adjustments required for optimal wellness. Nursing actions, which are called prevention as intervention, are initiated to keep the system stable. Neuman created a typology for her prevention as intervention nursing actions that includes primary prevention as intervention, secondary prevention as intervention, and tertiary prevention as intervention. All of these actions are initiated to best retain, attain, and maintain optimal client health or wellness. Neuman (1995, 2002c) believes the nurse creates a linkage among the client, the environment, health, and nursing in the process of keeping the system stable.

Primary prevention
• Reduce possibility of
  encounter with stressors
• Strengthen flexible line
  of defense

Secondary prevention
• Early case-finding and
• Treatment of symptoms

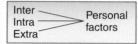

Tertiary prevention
• Readaptation
• Reeducation to prevent
  future occurrences
• Maintenance of stability

Interventions
• Can occur before or after resistance
  lines are penetrated in both reaction
  and reconstitution phases
• Interventions are based on:
  • Degree of reaction
  • Resources
  • Goals
  • Anticipated outcome

Fig 11 • 4 Nursing. Accurately assessing the effects and possible effects of environmental stressors (inter-, intra-, and extrapersonal factors) and using appropriate prevention by interventions to assist with client adjustments for an optimal level of wellness. *(From Neuman, 1995, p. 29, with permission.)*

Prevention as Intervention

The nurse collaborates with the client to establish relevant goals. These goals are derived only after validating with the client and synthesizing comprehensive client data and relevant theory to determine an appropriate nursing diagnostic statement. With the nursing diagnostic statement and goals in mind, appropriate interventions can be planned and implemented (Neuman, 1995, 2002c, 2011a, pp. 25–29).

Primary prevention as intervention involves the nurse's actions that promote client wellness by stress prevention and reduction of risk factors. These interventions can begin at any point a stressor is suspected or identified, before a reaction has occurred. They protect the normal line of defense by reducing the possibility of an encounter with a stressor and strengthening the flexible lines of defense. Health promotion is a significant intervention. The goal of primary prevention as intervention is to *retain* optimal stability or wellness. Ideally, the nurse should consider primary prevention along with secondary and tertiary preventions as interventions when actual client problems exist.

Once a reaction from a stressor occurs, the nurse can use secondary prevention as intervention to treat the symptoms within the nurse's scope of practice, reduce the degree of reaction to the stressors, and protect the basic structure by strengthening the lines of resistance. The goal of secondary prevention as intervention is to *attain* optimal client system stability or wellness and energy conservation. The nurse uses as much of the client's existing internal and external resources (lines of resistance) as possible to stabilize the system.

Reconstitution represents the return and maintenance of system stability after nursing intervention for stressor reaction. The state of wellness may be higher, the same, or lower than the state of wellness before the system was stabilized. Death occurs when secondary prevention as intervention fails to protect the basic structure and thus fails to reconstitute the client (Neuman, 1995, 2002c).

Tertiary prevention as intervention can begin at any point in the client's reconstitution. This includes interventions that promote (1) readaptation, (2) reeducation to prevent further occurrences, and (3) maintenance of stability. These actions are designed to *maintain* an optimal wellness level by supporting existing strengths and conserving client system energy. Tertiary prevention tends to lead back toward primary prevention in a circular fashion. Neuman pointed out that one or all three of these prevention modalities give direction to, or may be used simultaneously for, nursing actions with possible synergistic benefits (Neuman, 1995, 2002, 2011, pp. 28–29).

Nursing Tools for Model Implementation

Neuman designed the NSM nursing process format and the NSM Assessment and Intervention Tool: Client Assessment and Nursing Diagnosis to facilitate implementation of the Neuman model. These tools are presented in all the editions of *The Neuman Systems Model* (Neuman, 1982, 1989, 1995, 2002c; 2011a; Neuman & Lowry, 2011).

The NSM nursing process format reflects a process that guides information processing and goal-directed activities. Neuman uses the nursing process within three categories: nursing diagnosis, nursing goals, and nursing outcomes. In 1982, doctoral students validated the Neuman nursing process format. The format's validity and social utility have been supported in a wide variety of nursing education and practice areas.

The Neuman Systems Model Assessment and Intervention Tool

The Client Assessment and Nursing Diagnosis tool is used to guide the nursing process. The nurse collects holistic, comprehensive data to determine the effect or possible effect of environmental stressors on the client system then validates the data with the client before formulating a nursing diagnosis. Selected nursing diagnoses are prioritized and related to relevant knowledge. Nursing goals are determined mutually with the caregiver–client–client system, along with mutually agreed on prevention as intervention strategies. Mutually agreed on goals and interventions are consistent with current mandates within the health-care system for client rights related to health-care issues.

The Client Assessment and Nursing Diagnosis tool with primary, secondary, and tertiary prevention as intervention was developed to convey appropriate nursing actions with each typology of prevention. There are clear instructions for writing appropriate nursing actions (Neuman, 2002a, p. 354; 2011b, pp. 343–350), which students are encouraged to review before writing these nursing actions. Keep in mind that the nature of stressors and their threat to the client–client system are first determined for each type of prevention before any other nursing actions are initiated. The same stressors could produce variable effects or reactions. Nursing outcomes are determined by the accomplishment of the interventions and evaluation of goals after intervention.

Applications of the Theory

Because the model is flexible and adaptable to a wide range of groups and situations, people have used it globally for more than three decades. Neuman's first book, *The Neuman Systems Model: Application to Nursing Education and Practice,* was published in 1982 as a response to requests for data and support in applying the model in practice settings and as a guide for entire nursing curricula. The second and third editions (1989, 1995) present examples of the use of the model in practice and education, primarily. The fourth edition (2002c) includes integrative reviews of practice, educational, and research literature and discussions of practice and educational tools. The fifth edition (Neuman & Fawcett, 2011) continues the tradition of including contributions that reflect the broad applicability of the model. Guidelines and available tools for NSM-based practice, educational programs, and research are summarized.

Application of the Neuman Systems Model to Nursing Practice

"The function of a conceptual model in nursing practice is to provide a distinctive frame of reference that guides approaches to patient care" (Amaya, 2002, p. 43). There is a critical need for meaningful definitions and conceptual frames of reference for nursing practice if the profession is to be established as a science (Neuman, 2002c).

The NSM is being used in diverse practice settings globally such as critical care nursing, psychiatric mental health nursing, gerontological nursing, perinatal nursing, community nursing, occupational health nursing, rehabilitation, and advanced nursing practice (Amaya, 2002; Bueno & Sengin, 1995; Chiverton & Flannery, 1995; McGee, 1995; Peirce & Fulmer, 1995; Groesbeck, 2011; Merks, van Tilburg, & Lowry, 2011; Russell, Hileman, & Grant, 1995; Stuart & Wright, 1995; Trepanier, Dunn, & Sprague, 1995; Ware & Shannahan, 1995).

The model is used to guide practice in clients with acute and chronic health-care problems (e.g., hypertension, chronic obstructive pulmonary disease, renal disease, cardiac surgery, cognitive impairment, mental illness, multiple sclerosis, pain, grief, pediatric cancers, perinatal stressors); to meet family needs of clients in critical care; to provide stable support groups for parents with infants in neonatal intensive care units; and to meet the needs of home caregivers, with emphasis on clients with cancer, HIV/AIDS, and head trauma (Beddome, 1995; Beynon, 1995; Craig, 1995; Damant, 1995; Davies & Proctor, 1995; Engberg, Bjalming, & Bertilson, 1995; Felix, Hinds, Wolfe, & Martin, 1995; Vaughan & Gough, 1995; Verberk, 1995). An excellent example of how the comprehensive NSM can be used to gather and analyze individual client system data is found in Tarko and Helewka (2011, pp. 37–69). Ume-Nwangbo, DeWan, and Lowry (2006) provided two examples of using the model to provide care: first, for an individual client; second, for a family client. "Nurses who conduct their practice from a nursing theory base, while assisting individuals and families to meet their health needs, are more likely to provide comprehensive, individualized care that exemplifies best practices" (p. 31).

Application of the Neuman Systems Model to Nursing Education

Neuman originally designed the model "as a focal point for student learning" (2011, p. 332) because it considered four variables of human experience: physiological, psychological, sociocultural and developmental. Before

long, the potential of using the model for curriculum development was recognized at all levels of nursing education in the United States, Canada, and globally. The NSM was selected because it is a systems approach, comprehensive, and holistic and focuses on health and prevention. Programs adopting the model in the 1980s used it in its entirety. Through the years, some programs moved to a more eclectic approach that combines the model concepts of stress, systems, and primary prevention with concepts from other models. Appendix F in Neuman and Fawcett (2011) summarizes 28 programs currently using the NSM at the time of publication. Two baccalaureate programs at Newberry College, Newberry, SC, and Cedar Crest College, Allentown, PA, adopted the model in 2007 and 2009, respectively. The department of Psychiatric Nursing at Douglas College, British Columbia, Canada, follows a Neuman-based curriculum for advanced practice psychiatric nurses (Tarko & Helewka, pp. 216–220). MacEwan University in Edmonton, Alberta, Canada, is planning for the adoption of the model for their curriculum in fall of 2011 (personal communication, Betty Neuman, January, 2013).

Educators have developed tools with NSM terminology to guide student learning and examine student progress in courses within Neuman-based nursing programs (Newman et al., 2011). The Lowry-Jopp Neuman Model Evaluation Instrument (LJNMEI) has been used by two associate-degree nursing programs, one at Cecil Community College and the other at Indiana University—Ft. Wayne. The objective of the evaluation instrument is to assess the efficacy of being educated within a Neuman-based curriculum. Participants were assessed at graduation and 7 months after graduation. Findings indicate that graduates internalized the Neuman concepts well and continued to practice from the model perspective if they were encouraged by their colleagues. Graduates who were employed in institutions that did not encourage use of the model for assessments often did not continue to use it (Beckman, Boxley-Harges, Bruick-Sorge, & Eichenauer, 1998; Lowry, 1998).

The LJNMEI instrument was adapted for use by the practicing nurses at the Emergis Psychiatric Institute in Zeeland, Holland, in 2002. Data have been collected for a decade to track the efficacy of using the NSM for delivering quality patient care within this psychiatric health-care system. Other disciplines in the institution became interested in using the model as well with no significant difference for knowledge of the NSM among nurses, psychiatrists, and psychologists. Having all disciplines practicing from one theoretical perspective enables an integrated approach to motivate and stimulate clients to reach their levels of optimum stability (Merks et al., 2011).

Application of the Neuman Systems Model to Nursing Administration and Management

Although there is less evidence of the use of the NSM in administration compared with practice and education, the available literature is increasing and emphasizes how complex systems are greatly benefitted by using a systems approach as a guide to management (Pew Health Professions Commission, 1995; Sanders & Kelley, 2002). For example, the purpose of the Magnet recognition program is to promote quality patient care within a culture that supports professional nursing practice (McClure, 2005). This is the gold standard for work environments in health care. One of the attributes of Magnet status is practicing from a professional model of care. Nurses and administrators with knowledge of the NSM are poised to assume leadership roles within these hospital systems. The model emphasizes comprehensive patient care to facilitate the delivery of primary, secondary and tertiary interventions, within a culture supporting professional nursing practice. Some examples of magnet hospitals using the NSM are Allegiance Health, Michigan (Burnett & Johnson-Crisanti, 2011); Riverside Methodist Hospital, Ohio (Kinder, Napier, Rupertino, Surace, & Burkholder, 2011); Abingdon Memorial Hospital, Philadelphia (Breckenridge, 2011); and the South Jersey Healthcare System (Boxer, 2008). These exemplars describe how nurses combine their professional model of care (the NSM) with the

other Magnet criteria to achieve quality health care and national recognition. Nursing research in these institutions is reported in publications and at the Biennial International Neuman Systems Model Symposia.

Application of the Neuman Systems Model to Nursing Research

Each edition of *The Neuman Systems Model* from the second to the fifth (1989–2011) provides a chapter that summarizes the research based on the model completed in the years between the editions. Through the years, the growth of Neuman-based research is evident. In the early years, most of the research was descriptive, focusing on one concept from the model, such as stressor reactions or primary prevention interventions. Many of the early studies were completed by master's and doctoral students as fulfillment of their advanced degrees (Fawcett, 2011, pp. 393–404). To date there are 132 master's theses, 110 doctoral dissertations, and 109 Neuman-based studies completed by researchers.

Neuman-based research has progressed developmentally through the decades as researchers become more sophisticated and informed about processes that lead to sound conceptual model-based studies. Conceptual models provide the broad framework for organizing the phenomena to be studied through research and are critical because they are precursors for theory development. The models provide the concepts and propositions (connecting statements) that explain the model. For example, the NSM provides the context and structure for research. Because the concepts are abstract, the model cannot be tested in a single research study. Thus, midrange theories must be derived from the NSM concepts, and these theories can then be tested in individual studies.

Fawcett (1989) developed a structure that is used by researchers when developing a research study from a conceptual model. This conceptual-theoretical-empirical (CTE) framework presents the model concepts to be studied at the upper level, then the more observable concepts being studied at the second level, and the instruments that will be used to collect data about the second level concepts at the third level. This CTE diagram shows explicit vertical linkages. Then a narrative explanation is necessary to clarify the concepts and propositions displayed in the CTE diagram. Examples of studies developed from CTE frameworks can be found in research chapters in two editions of Neuman and Fawcett (2002, 2011).

A second major contribution of Fawcett to model-based research is the publishing of guidelines for the development of research studies (Fawcett, 1995, table 32-1). These rules are applicable to any health-care discipline and have been refined over the years. The latest rendition is given in Neuman and Fawcett (2011, p. 162, table 10-1). These rules can apply to both quantitative and qualitative studies. An excellent example of a CTE structure for a quantitative study of multiple role stress in mothers attending college (Gigliotti, 1997, 1999) is displayed in Neuman and Fawcett (2002, p. 290, Figure 21-1). Note that the midrange theory concepts are specific attributes of the NSM concepts but do not include all model concepts. An excellent example of a CTE for a qualitative study is found in Neuman and Fawcett (2002, p. 179, Figure 10-3). Note that this diagram moves from the Neuman model concepts (Level 1) to empirical research methods (Level 3), from which Level 2 midrange theory concepts have been derived from patient interviews. If the guidelines for conducting model-based research are followed, resulting studies will be logically consistent and will advance nursing knowledge by helping to explain the effects of using the NSM (Louis, Gigliotti, Neuman, & Fawcett, 2011; Gigliotti). The ultimate goal of all research is to develop conceptual model-based middle-range theories (Fawcett & Garrity, 2009; Gigliotti, 2012).

The fourth step of the research guidelines is research methodology. Appropriate research instruments for data collection must be selected. This means that the items in each instrument are either derived from the NSM or are compatible with concepts within the NSM. For example, Loescher, Clark, Atwood, Leigh, and Lamb (1990) created the Cancer Survivors Questionnaire, which collects data on the client's perception of physiological, psychological, and sociocultural stressors. Each item in each of these categories is a descriptor of something physical, psychological, and sociocultural. A second example is the "Client System Perception Guides" for structured interviews. The items listed in the guide were developed from the NSM for measuring spirituality (Clark, Cross, Deane, & Lowry, 1991), dialysis treatment (Breckenridge, 1997), and elder abuse (Kottwitz & Bowling, 2003). To date, 25 instruments have been directly derived from the NSM and can measure stressors, client systems perceptions, client system needs, the five system variables, coping strategies, the lines of defense and resistance, and client system responses.

Four reviews of NSM-based studies from the 1980s and 1990s focused on how the studies reflected the research rules. Gigliotti (2001) presented an integrative review of 10 studies to determine the extent of support for Neuman propositions that link various concepts of the model. Gigliotti reported her difficulty interpreting the results due to investigators' failures to link the research concepts to the NSM in their designs. Fawcett and Giangrande (2002) presented a full integrative-review project that linked all the available NSM-based research. The authors found that about one-half of published research journal articles and book chapters included conceptual linkages between NSM propositions and the study variables. Master's theses and doctoral dissertations (about two-thirds) did not make the conceptual linkages. Researchers are reminded to pay more attention to conceptual aspects of their studies and make explicit references to these so that nursing theoretical knowledge is advanced. Throughout this chapter, one can find the network of researchers who have conducted model-based studies.

Fawcett and Giangrande (2002) presented a literature review of 212 studies and identified the instruments used for data collection that are compatible with the NSM concepts and propositions as well as the middle-range theory measured by each instrument. Compatible with the NSM concepts are 75 instruments, such as the State-Trait Anxiety Inventory, used to measure anxiety; the Beck Depression Inventory, used to measure depression; and the Norbeck Social Support Questionnaire, used to measure client's perception of social support in their lives. When using an instrument not deducted directly from the model, researchers must describe the linkages between the concepts in the instruments and those from the NSM to demonstrate logical congruence between the NSM and the instrument. The evidence of validity and reliability of the instruments selected must be provided in the study. The ultimate goal is to accumulate a group of instruments that measure the complete spectrum of NSM concepts, such as the five variables; the central core; the four environments; client system stability; reconstitution; variances from wellness; primary, secondary, and tertiary prevention interventions; and client perceptions. Finally, Gigliotti and Manister (2012) presented an article to guide novice researchers through the writing of the conceptual model-based theoretical rationale. This is a must-read for every beginning researcher.

Focus of Current Research

Neuman concepts *of stressors,* and the three *preventions as intervention* have been the foci most frequently studied by descriptive methodology. Gigliotti (1999, 2004, 2007) has a program of research on the subject of women's maternal-student role stress in which she tests the NSM flexible line of defense. *Spirituality* is the variable that has been researched most recently. Neuman (1989) claimed that spirituality is the unifying variable of all personal systems. She states that the "spirit controls the mind, and the mind controls the body" (pp. 29–30). A spiritual encounter occurs between clients and caregivers, thus, nurses must assess spirituality as part of their data collection. These beliefs have influenced the development of spirituality studies. Some of the studies focus on the development of spirituality in students, and others aim to understand the concept of spirituality. Because student nurses must learn to assess the spiritual variable, it is imperative that they develop spiritually. A team of faculty from Indiana Purdue–Ft. Wayne are studying the evolution of student nurses' awareness of the concept of spirituality (Beckman, Boxley-Harges, Bruick-Sorge, & Salmon, 2007; Beckman, Boxley-Harges, &

Kaskel, 2012; Bruick-Sorge, Beckman, Boxley-Harges, & Salmon, 2010). If the NSM is to be used for assessment of the spiritual variable, then caregivers must be confident that the Neuman definition is congruent with client beliefs (Lowry, 2012). Several studies have addressed the importance of spirituality to quality care (Clark, Cross, Deane & Lowry, 1991), to aging persons (Lowry, 2002, 2012), and to adults living with HIV (Cobb, 2012). Finally, Burkhart, Schmidt, and Hogan (2012) published a new spiritual care inventory instrument within the context of the NSM to measure spiritual interventions that facilitate health and wellness.

The Neuman Systems Model Research Institute

At the 2003 Biennial International Neuman Systems Model Symposium in Philadelphia, PA, the NSM Trustees formally approved the formation of a Research Institute to test and generate midrange theories derived from the NSM (Gigliotti & Fawcett, 2011). Activities of this institute include the funding of two distinct types of fellowships for novice researchers: the John Crawford Awards (up to 10 per biennium) and the Patricia Chadwick Research Grant (one per biennium). For more information, see http://www.neumansystemsmodel.org/NSMdocs/research_institute.htm.

Each biennium, the Neuman Systems Model Trustees Group conducts an international symposium where the recipients of the fellowships can join other scholars and present their findings. All researchers, educators, and nurses who practice from the NSM perspective are welcome to attend these events to share new insights and to advance understanding of various model concepts. The networking among these scholars helps to integrate the growing body of knowledge about the use of the model in education, research, practice, and administration of nursing services.

Value of the Neuman Systems Model for the Future

Theory development is the hallmark of any profession. The NSM continues to be researched and validated through studies; thus, it becomes more valuable as the basis for quality patient care and for the advancement of the nursing profession. The addition of the spiritual variable to the client system in 1989 accentuated the importance of this dimension. The plethora of research on spirituality and the recognition of the importance of the concept are increasingly being recognized by the health-care community. The development of middle-range theories from the NSM is imperative because it is the integration of theories from other disciplines that are compatible with Neuman concepts. The concepts of holism, wellness, and prevention interventions used to attain, retain, and maintain client system stability are as viable today in our complex health-care system as they were in 1970. Our global colleagues find that these philosophical beliefs are congruent with beliefs in their own health-care systems. More than 12 countries have been introduced to the model over two decades, with Belgium being the most recent in 2012. Holland has adopted the model most widely due to its translation into Dutch and hosts the annual International Neuman Systems Model Association symposium (Merks, Verberk, de Kuiper, & Lowry, 2012).

Networking to Enhance Applications of the Model

There are opportunities to network with others using the model in a variety of applications and settings. One way is to attend the Neuman Systems Model International Symposium, which is held every 2 years, in the odd year. International scholars gather to share ideas, insights, innovations, practice, and research from the model. The Neuman Systems Model website provides the latest information: www .neumansystemsmodel.org.

The Neuman Archives were established to preserve and protect the work of Betty Neuman and others working with the model. The archives, previously located at Newmann University in Aston, PA, are now housed in the Barbara Bates Center for the Study of the History of Nursing at the University of Pennsylvania (http://www.nursing.upenn .edu/history/Pages/default.aspx). Contact Gail Farr, MA, CA, for information and an appointment to access the collection (gfarr@nursing.upenn.edu).

Practice Exemplar

A nurse guided by the Neuman systems model met Gloria Washington while providing care for her mother in Gloria's home. Gloria's 74-year-old mother has Alzheimer's disease, and Gloria has been her caregiver for 4 years. The nurse was aware that, according to Neuman, the family client system includes Gloria and her mother. This nurse uses practice-based research to guide her work (best practice). She recently read Jones-Cannon and Davis's (2005) research study that examined the coping strategies of African American daughters who have functioned as caregivers. In their study, African American caregivers of a family member with dementia or a stroke believed that attending support groups and knowing that their parent needed them influenced their caregiving experience positively. Most caregivers identified that religion gave them a

strong tolerance for the caregiving situation and served to mediate strain. Caregivers who voiced a lack of support from family, especially siblings, had much anger and resentment.

The nurse used this new knowledge to enhance the nursing process with Gloria. By using the Neuman systems model Assessment and Intervention Tool, she learned that Gloria is a 52-year-old divorced African American woman who is employed full-time by a company for which she enjoys working. She also has a teenage daughter who lives with her and a grown son who lives away from home. Gloria attends the Baptist church in her neighborhood 2 or 3 times a week and attributes this experience to her ability to care for her mother.

The nurse assessed for stressors as they were perceived by Gloria and by herself. The nurse assessed for discrepancies between their

Continued

perceptions and found none. She identified the intrapersonal, interpersonal, and extrapersonal factors that made up Gloria's environment. To ensure the assessment was holistic and comprehensive, she identified the physiological, psychological, sociocultural, developmental, and spiritual variables for each of these factors. Gloria identified caring for her mother with Alzheimer's disease as her major stressor.

Assessment

The nurse's assessment of Gloria's environmental factors is identified below. Examples of assessment data for each variable are included.

Intrapersonal factors

Physiological: Gloria experiences occasional signs and symptoms of increased anxiety such as rapid heart rate and increased blood pressure.

Psychological: Gloria occasionally worries about the future, but she tries to focus on the present and prides herself on her sense of humor.

Sociocultural: Gloria values her belief that African American families take care of their elderly.

Developmental: Gloria is in Erickson's (1959) developmental stage of middle adulthood with its crisis of generativity versus stagnation. She strives to look outside of herself to care for others.

Spiritual: Gloria reports that religion, faith, and prayer help her cope with caregiving demands.

Interpersonal factors

Physiological: Gloria occasionally has interrupted sleep when her mother awakens and wanders during the night.

Psychological: Gloria reminds herself when physically caring for her mother that this is an expected part of her mother's aging.

Sociocultural: Gloria is the full-time caregiver of her mother, who has Alzheimer's disease. She works full-time with supportive people but does not attend an Alzheimer's support group because she didn't know anything about them.

Developmental: Gloria has significant relationships with her co-workers.

Spiritual: Gloria is supported by her pastor and friends at church.

Extrapersonal factors

Physiological: From a co-worker, Gloria received the gift of a comfortable bed mattress that promotes her sleep.

Psychological: Gloria shared that reading her Bible helps her think positive thoughts.

Sociocultural: Gloria earns $35,000 per year.

Developmental: Gloria can feel "in charge of the situation" with a comfortable house for her mom.

Spiritual: Gloria attends church services in her neighborhood 2 or 3 times a week.

The nurse applied the NSM nursing process format (Neuman & Fawcett, 2011, p. 338) focusing on the following: (1) nursing diagnosis (based on valid database), (2) nursing goals negotiated with the client including appropriate levels of prevention as interventions, and (3) nursing outcomes.

The nurse prepared a comprehensive list of nursing diagnoses based on her holistic and comprehensive assessment and then prioritized the list. She validated her findings with Gloria to ensure that their perceptions were in agreement.

The nurse and Gloria identified Gloria's full-time role as a caregiver for her mother with Alzheimer's disease as a significant stressor. The nurse considered the research study by Jones-Cannon and Davis (2005), which reported that caregivers of a family member with dementia believed attendance at a support group influenced their caregiving in a positive way. One of the nursing diagnoses they determined was "*risk for* caregiver role strain." Although this was identified as a risk, they both agreed there was not a supporting sign or symptom to validate the existence of caregiver role strain at this time. However, it was important to prevent this strain in the future.

The nurse recognized that their observations provided a glimpse of Gloria's normal line of defense; then they identified an

Practice Exemplar cont.

immediate goal to strengthen her flexible line of defense.

The goal is that Gloria will report that she has participated in a monthly Alzheimer support group session by (date). They could have identified intermediate and future goals at that time. Together they planned nursing actions for primary prevention as intervention.

The nurse also used the tool and nursing process to provide holistic comprehensive care for Gloria's mother, and the family client system was strengthened. By strengthening Gloria's lines of defense, the nurse helped strengthen Gloria's mother's lines of defense. The model is dynamic as the individual and family client systems are assessed continuously, leading to new diagnoses, goals, and interventions that promote optimal holistic comprehensive nursing care. The desired outcome goal for Gloria in the case example was optimal health retention.

If this had been an actual problem of caregiver role strain, they would have identified secondary prevention as interventions and tertiary prevention as interventions that would activate resource factors (lines of resistance) to protect Gloria's basic structure (organ

strength or ability to cope). An example of each follows.

Secondary prevention as intervention: Assist Gloria to schedule respite care for a determined period of time.

Tertiary prevention as intervention: Provide ongoing education at each visit about practical resources that will provide caregiver support.

The nurse would have continued to use the nursing process by implementing and evaluating their plan; reassessing, as part of evaluation, for a reduction or elimination of caregiver role strain; and maintenance of system stability. Neuman refers to this as *reconstitution.*

Reconstitution represents the return and maintenance of system stability after treatment of a stressor reaction, which may result in a higher or lower level of wellness than previously. It represents successful mobilization of energy resources (Neuman, 2002c, p. 324).

The desired outcome goals are for optimal health retention, restoration, and maintenance. In Neuman's model, high importance is placed on validating nurse and client perceptions and validating data.

Summary

"The Neuman Systems Model is well positioned as a contemporary and future guide for health care practice, research, education and administration far into the 21st century. The concepts and processes of the model are so universal and timeless that they are easily understood by all members of the health care teams worldwide" (Neuman and Fawcett, 2011, p. 317).

The NSM has been used for more than three decades, first as a teaching tool and later

as a conceptual model to observe and interpret the phenomena of nursing and health care globally. The model is well accepted by the nursing profession and is guided by the Neuman Systems Model Trustees, Inc. The Trustees are dedicated to the improvement of health for people worldwide through development and use of the NSM to guide practice, education, research, and administration (www .neumansystemsmodel.org/trustees).

References

Amaya, M. A. (2002). The Neuman systems model and clinical practice: An integrative review 1974–2000. In B. Neuman & J. Fawcett (Eds.), *The Neuman systems model* (4th ed., pp. 216–243). Upper Saddle River, NJ: Prentice-Hall. Archives of the Neuman Systems

Beckman, S. J., Boxley-Harges, S., Bruik-Sorge, C., & Echenauer, J. (1998). Evaluation modalities for assessing student and program outcomes. In L. Lowry (Ed.), *Neuman systems model and nursing education: Teaching strategies and outcomes* (pp. 149–160). Indianapolis, IN: Sigma Theta Tau International Center Nursing Press.

Beckman, S. J., Boxley-Harges, S., Bruick-Sorge, C., & Salmon, B. (2007). Five strategies that heighten nurses' awareness of spirituality to impact client care. *Holistic Nursing Practice, 21*(3),135–139.

Beckman, S. J., Boxley-Harges, S., & Kaskel, B.L. (2012) Experience informs: Spanning three decades with the Neuman systems model. *Nursing Science Quarterly, 25*(4), 341–346.

Beddome, G. (1995). Community-as-client assessment. A Neuman-based guide for education and practice. In B. Neuman, *The Neuman systems model* (3rd ed., pp. 567–579). Norwalk, CT: Appleton & Lange.

Beynon, C. E. (1995). Neuman-based experiences of the Middlesex-London Health Unit. In B. Neuman (Ed.), *The Neuman systems model* (3rd ed., pp. 537–547). Norwalk, CT: Appleton & Lange.

Boxer, B. (2009). *The Neuman systems model as a professional model of care for a magnet hospital health care system.* Unpublished manuscript.

Breckenridge, D. M. (1995). Nephrology practice and directions for nursing research. In B. Neuman (Ed.), *The Neuman systems model* (3rd ed., pp. 499–507). Norwalk, CT: Appleton & Lange.

Breckenridge, D. M. (1997). Patients' perceptions of why, how and by whom dialysis treatment modality was chosen. *American Nephrology Nurses Association Journal, 24*, 313–319.

Breckenridge, D. M. (2011). The Neuman systems model and evidence-based practice. In B. Neuman & J. Fawcett, (Eds.) *The Neuman systems model* (5th ed. pp. 245–252). Upper Saddle River, NJ: Pearson.

Bruick-Sorge, C., Beckman, S. J., Boxley-Harges, S., & Salmon, B. (2010). The evolution of student nurses concepts of spirituality. *Holistic Nursing Practice, 24*(2), 73–78.

Bueno, M. M., & Sengin, K. K. (1995). The Neuman systems model for critical care nursing. A framework for practice. In B. Neuman (Ed.), *The Neuman systems model* (3rd ed., pp. 275–291. Norwalk, CT: Appleton & Lange.

Burkhart, L., Schmidt, L., & Hogan, N. (2011). Development and psychometric testing of the spiritual care inventory instrument. *Journal of Advanced Nursing, 67*, 2463–2472.

Burnett, H. M., & Johnson-Crisanti, K. J. (2011). Nursing services at Allegiance Health. In B. Neuman & J. Fawcett (Eds.), *The Neuman systems model* (5th ed., pp. 267–275). Upper Saddle River, NJ: Pearson.

Chiverton, P., & Flannery J. C. (1995). Cognitive impairment. Use of the Neuman systems model. In: B. Neuman, *The Neuman systems model* (3rd ed., pp. 249–259). Norwalk, CT: Appleton & Lange.

Clark, C. C., Cross, J. R. Deane, D. M., & Lowry, L. W. (1991). Spirituality: Integral to quality care. *Holistic Nursing Practice, 5*(3), 67–76.

Cobb, R. K. (2012). How well does spirituality predict health status in adults living with HIV-disease: A Neuman systems model study. *Nursing Science Quarterly, 25*(4), 347–355.

Craig, D. M. (1995). Community/public health nursing in Canada. Use of the Neuman systems model in a new paradigm. In B. Neuman (Ed.), *The Neuman systems model* (3rd ed., pp. 529–535). Norwalk, CT: Appleton & Lange.

Damant, M. (1995). Community nursing in the United Kingdom. A case for reconciliation using the Neuman Systems Model. In B. Neuman (Ed.), *The Neuman systems model* (3rd ed., pp. 607–620). Norwalk, CT: Appleton & Lange.

Davies, P., & Proctor, H. (1995). In Wales: Using the model in community mental health. In B. Neuman (Ed.), *The Neuman systems model* (3rd ed., pp. 621–627). Norwalk, CT: Appleton & Lange.

de Kuiper, M. (2011). The created environment. In B. Neuman & J. Fawcett. (Eds.), The Neuman systems model (5th ed., pp. 100–104). Upper Saddle Creek, NJ: Pearson.

Engberg, I. B., Bjalming, E., & Bertilson, B. (1995). A structure for documenting primary health care in Sweden using the Neuman systems model. In B. Neuman (Ed.), *The Neuman systems model* (3rd ed., pp. 637–651). Norwalk, CT: Appleton & Lange.

Erikson, E. H. (1959). *Identity and the life cycle.* New York: International Universities Press.

Fawcett, J. (1989). Analysis and evaluation of Nueman's systems model. In B. Neuman (Ed.), *The Neuman systems model. Application to nursing education and practice* (2nd ed., pp. 65–92). Norwalk, CT: Appleton and Lange.

Fawcett, J. (1995). Constructing conceptual-theoretical-empirical structures for research. Future implications for use of the Neuman systems model. In B. Neuman (Ed.), *The Neuman systems model* (3rd ed., pp. 459–471). Norwalk, CT: Appleton & Lange.

Fawcett, J. (2011). Neuman systems model bibliography and web site information. In B. Neuman & J. Fawcett (Eds.), *The Neuman systems model* (5th ed., pp. 375–422). Upper Saddle Creek, NJ: Pearson. Available at: http://www.neumansystemsmodel.org/Bibliography.

CHAPTER 11 • *Betty Neuman's Systems Model* **183**

Fawcett, J. & Garrity, J. (2009). *Evaluating research for evidence-based nursing practice.* Philadelphia, PA: F.A. Davis.

Fawcett, J., & Giangrande, S. K. (2002). The Neuman systems model and research: An integrative review. In B. Neuman & J. Fawcett (Eds.), *The Neuman systems model* (4th ed., pp. 120–149). Upper Saddle River, NJ: Prentice-Hall.

Felix, M., Hinds, C., Wolfe, C., & Martin, A. (1995). The Neuman systems model in a chronic care facility: A Canadian experience. In B. Neuman (Ed.), *The Neuman systems model* (3rd ed., pp. 549–566). Norwalk, CT: Appleton & Lange.

Fulton, R. A. (1995). The spiritual variable. In B. Neuman (Ed.), *The Neuman systems model* (3rd ed., pp. 77–91). Norwalk, CT: Appleton & Lange.

Gigliotti, E. (1997). Use of Neuman's lines of defense and resistance in nursing research: Conceptual and empirical considerations. *Nursing Science Quarterly, 10,* 136–143.

Gigliotti, E. (1999). Women's multiple role stress: Testing Neuman's flexible line of defense. *Nursing Science Quarterly, 12,* 36–44.

Gigliotti, E. (2001). Empirical tests of the Neuman systems model: Relational statements analysis. *Nursing Science Quarterly, 14,* 149–157.

Gigliotti, E., (2004). Etiology of maternal-student role stress. *Nursing Science Quarterly, 17,* 156–164.

Gigliotti, E. (2007). Improving external and internal validity of a model of midlife Women's maternal-student role stress. *Nursing Science Quarterly, 20,* 161–170.

Gigliotti, E. (2012). Deriving middle-range theories from the Neuman systems model. In B. Neuman & J. Fawcett (Eds.), The Neuman systems model (5th ed., pp. 283–298). Upper Saddle Creek, NJ: Pearson.

Gigliotti, E. & Fawcett, J. (2011) The Neuman systems model research institute. In B. Neuman & J. Fawcett (Eds.) *The Neuman systems model* (5th ed., pp. 351–354). Upper Saddle Creek, NJ: Pearson. http://neumansystemsmodel.org/NSMdocs/research_institute.htm.

Gigliotti, E., & Manister, N. N. (2011). A beginner's guide to writing the nursing conceptual model-based theoretical rationale. *Nursing Science Quarterly,25*(4), 301–306.

Groesbeck, M. J. (2011). Reflections on Neuman systems model-based advanced psychiatric nursing practice. In B. Neuman & Fawcett (Eds.) *The Neuman systems model* (5th ed., pp. 237-244). Upper Saddle River, NJ: Prentice-Hall.

Jones-Cannon, S., & Davis, B. (2005, November-December). Coping among African-American daughters caring for aging parents. *The ABNF Journal,* 118–123.

Kinder, L., Napier, D., Rubertino, M., Surace, A., & Burkholder, J. (2011). Utilizing the Neuman systems model to maintain and enhance the health of a nursing service: Riverside Methodist Hospital. In

B. Neuman & J. Fawcett (Eds.), *The Neuman systems model* (5th ed., pp. 276–280). Upper Saddle Creek, NJ: Pearson.

Kottwitz , D., & Bowling, S. (2003). A pilot study of the elder abuse questionnaire. *Kansas Nurse, 78*(7), 4–6.

Loescher, L. J., Clark, L., Atwood, J.R., Leigh, S., & Lamb, S. (1990). The impact of the cancer experience on long-term survivors. *Oncology Nursing Forum, 17, 223–*229.

Louis, M., Gigliotti, E., Neuman, B., & Fawcett, J. (2011). Neuman model-based research: Guidelines and instruments. In B. Neuman & J. Fawcett (Eds.), *The Neuman systems model* (5th ed., pp. 160–174.) Upper Saddle Creek, NJ: Pearson.

Lowry, L., (1998). Efficacy of the Neuman systems model as a curricular framework: A longitudinal study. In L. Lowry (Ed.), *The Neuman systems model and nursing education: Teaching strategies and outcomes* (pp. 139–147). Indianapolis, IN: Sigma Theta Tau International Center Nursing Press.

Lowry, L. (2002). The Neuman systems model and education. An integrative review. In B. Neuman & J. Fawcett (Eds.), *The Neuman systems model* (4th ed., pp. 216–237). Upper Saddle River, NJ: Prentice-Hall.

Lowry, L.W. (2012). A qualitative descriptive study of spirituality guided by the Neuman systems model. *Nursing Science Quarterly, 25*(4), 356–361.

Lowry, L. W., & Conco, D. (2002). Exploring the meaning of spirituality with aging adults in Appalachia. *Journal of Holistic Health, 20,* 388–402.

McGee, M. (1995). Implications for use of the Neuman systems model in occupational health nursing. In B. Neuman (Ed.), *The Neuman systems model* (3rd ed., pp. 657–667). Norwalk, CT: Appleton & Lange.

McClure, M. (2005). Magnet hospitals insights and issues. *Nursing Administration Quarterly, 29*(3), 158–161.

Merks, A., van Tilburg, C., & Lowry, L. (2011). Excellence in practice. In B. Neuman & J. Fawcett (Eds.), *The Neuman systems model* (5th ed. pp. 253–264). Upper Saddle Creek, NJ: Pearson.

Merks, A., Verberk, F., de Kuiper, M., & Lowry, L. W. (2012). Neuman systems model in Holland: An update. *Nursing Science Quarterly, 25*(4), 364–368.

Neuman, B. (1982). *The Neuman systems model: Application to nursing education and practice.* Norwalk, CT: Appleton-Century-Crofts.

Neuman, B. (1989). *The Neuman systems model* (2nd ed.). Norwalk, CT: Appleton & Lange.

Neuman, B. (1995). *The Neuman systems model* (3rd ed.). Norwalk, CT: Appleton & Lange.

Neuman, B. (2002a). Assessment and intervention based on the Neuman systems model. In B. Neuman & J. Fawcett (Eds.), *The Neuman systems model* (4th ed., pp. 347–359). Upper Saddle River, NJ: Prentice-Hall. Available at: http://neumansystemsmodel.org/index.html

Neuman, B. (2002b). Betty Neuman's autobiography and chronology of the development and utilization of the Neuman systems model. In: B. Neuman & J. Fawcett, *The Neuman systems model* (4th ed., pp. 325–346). Upper Saddle River, NJ: Prentice-Hall.www.neumansystemsmodel.org/Autobiography

Neuman, B. (2002c). The Neuman systems model. In B. Neuman & J. Fawcett (Eds.), *The Neuman systems model* (4th ed., pp. 3–33). Upper Saddle River, NJ: Prentice-Hall.

Neuman, B. (2011a). The Neuman systems model. In B. Neuman & J. Fawcett (Eds.), *The Neuman systems model* (5th ed., pp. 1–33). Upper Saddle River, NJ: Prentice-Hall.

Neuman, B. (2011b). Assessment and intervention based on the Neuman systems model. In B. Neuman & J. Fawcett (Eds.). *The Neuman systems model* (5th ed., pp. 343–350). Upper Saddle River, NJ: Prentice-Hall.

Neuman, B., & Fawcett, J. (Eds.). (2002). *The Neuman systems model* (4th ed.). Upper Saddle River, NJ: Prentice-Hall.

Neuman, B., & Fawcett, J. (2011). *The Neuman systems model* (5th ed.). Upper Saddle Creek, NJ: Pearson.

Neuman, B., & Lowry, L. (2011). The Neuman systems model and the future. In B. Neuman & J. Fawcett (Eds.), *The Neuman systems model* (5th ed., pp. 317–326). Upper Saddle Creek, NJ: Pearson.

Newman, D. M. L., Gehring, K. R., Lowry, L., Taylor, R., Neuman, B. & Fawcett, J. (2011). Neuman systems model-based education for the health professions: Guidelines and educational tools. In B. Neuman & J. Fawcett (Eds.), *The Neuman systems model* (5th ed., pp. 117–135). Upper Saddle River, NJ: Prentice-Hall.

Peirce, A. G., & Fulmer, T. T. (1995). Application of the Neuman systems model to gerontological nursing. In B. Neuman (Ed.), *The Neuman systems model* (3rd ed., pp. 293–308). Norwalk, CT: Appleton & Lange.

Pew Health Professions Commission. (1995). *Critical challenges: Revitalizing the health professions for the twenty-first century*. San Francisco: UCSF Center for the Health Professions.

Russell, J., Hileman, J. W., & Grant, J. S. (1995). Assessing and meeting the needs of home caregivers using the Neuman systems model. In B. Neuman (Ed.), *The Neuman systems model* (3rd ed., pp. 331–341). Norwalk, CT: Appleton & Lange.

Sanders, N. F., & Kelley, J. A. (2002). The Neuman systems model and administrative nursing services: An integrative review. In B. Neuman & J. Fawcett (Ed.), *The Neuman systems model* (4th ed., pp. 271–287). Upper Saddle River, NJ: Prentice-Hall.

Stuart, G. W., & Wright, L. K. (1995). Applying the Neuman systems model to psychiatric nursing practice. In B. Neuman (Eds.), *The Neuman systems model* (3rd ed., pp. 263–273). Norwalk, CT: Appleton & Lange.

Tarko, M. A., & Helewka, A. M. (2011). Psychiatric nursing education at Douglas College. In B. Neuman & J. Fawcett (Eds.), *The Neuman systems model* (5th ed., pp. 216–220). Upper Saddle River, NJ: Pearson.

Trepanier, M., Dunn, S. I., & Sprague, A. E. (1995). Application of the Neuman systems model to perinatal nursing. In B. Neuman (Eds.), *The Neuman systems model* (3rd ed., pp. 309–320). Norwalk, CT: Appleton & Lange.

Ume-Nwagbo, P. N., DeWan, S. A., & Lowry, L. (2006). Using the Neuman systems model for best practices. *Nursing Science Quarterly, 19*(1), 31–35.

Vaughan, B., & Gough, P. (1995). Use of the Neuman systems model in England. In B. Neuman (Ed.), *The Neuman systems model* (3rd ed., pp. 599–605). Norwalk, CT: Appleton & Lange.

Verberk, F. (1995). In Holland: Application of the Neuman model in psychiatric nursing. In B. Neuman (Ed.), *The Neuman systems model* (3rd ed., pp. 629–636). Norwalk, CT: Appleton & Lange.

Ware, L. A., & Shannahan, M. K. (1995). Using Neuman for a stable parent support group in neonatal intensive care. In B. Neuman, *The Neuman systems model* (3rd ed., pp. 321–330). Norwalk, CT: Appleton & Lange.

Chapter 12

Helen Erickson, Evelyn Tomlin, and Mary Ann Swain's Theory of Modeling and Role Modeling

HELEN L. ERICKSON

Introducing the Theorist
Overview of Modeling and Role-Modeling Theory
Practice Applications
Practice Exemplar
Summary
References

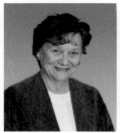

Helen L. Erickson

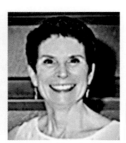

Mary Ann Swain

Introducing the Theorist

My life journey, filled with challenges and opportunities, helped me discover the essence of my Self, understand my Reason for Being, and uncover my Life Purpose (H. Erickson, 2006a). My Self is reflected in my values and beliefs; my Reason for Being is to learn that unconditional love is the key to human relationships; and my Life Purpose is to facilitate growth in others. The following snippets of my journey offer an occasional glimpse into my Self and the underlying philosophy of modeling and role-modeling (MRM).

Born and raised in north-central Michigan with one older brother and two younger sisters, I learned that our early experiences affect who we become. My father worked for the highway department; our mother cared for the family and worked part-time as a retail clerk. I learned that family connections, caring about others, positive attitudes, respect for the environment, and hard work are essential.

I was 5 years old when World War II was declared. Although too young to understand the implications of the war, I learned that it was important to stand up for our beliefs and life principles.

I learned that anything is possible if we are persistent, our goals have integrity, and we are honest with others and ourselves. I started working when I was about 10 years old. My jobs included babysitting, keeping house for a family in need, waitressing, and clerking. Each was an opportunity to learn about myself, and each was a step toward nursing school.

I enrolled in a diploma program for nurses, and in my junior year, I met my future husband and his family. His father, Milton Erickson,

185

well known for his work with mind–body healing, taught me that people know more about themselves than health-care providers do, that their *inner-knowing* is essential to healing, and that we can help them by attending to their worldview. I committed to married life, moved to Texas, and accepted the position of head nurse in the emergency room of the Midland Memorial Hospital.

Between 1959 and 1967, I worked in a variety of settings in Texas, Michigan, and Puerto Rico and welcomed four children into our family. I learned valuable lessons about blind prejudice, discrimination, and staying true to self; about how personal stories provide insight into client needs; and about the uniqueness of people and how limiting labels did not capture their wholeness. I had opportunities to develop a professional practice model.

In 1974, I completed my RN-BSN program at the University of Michigan and was recruited as a faculty member and consultant at the University Hospital.

I enrolled in the master's program in medical–surgical and psychiatric nursing and graduated in 1976. During this time, Evelyn Tomlin and I talked freely about the nursing model I had derived from practice. I labeled and developed the adaptive potential assessment model and worked with Mary Ann Swain to test some of my hypotheses (H. Erickson & Swain, 1982). I continued in my faculty position and advanced to chairman of the undergraduate program and assistant dean.

Over the next 10 years, my model of nursing acquired a life of its own. By the early 1980s, I had speaking invitations but little had been written (H. Erickson, 1976; H. Erickson & Swain, 1982). Together Evelyn, Mary Ann, and I further elaborated some of the concepts. The term modeling and role-modeling (MRM), first coined by Milton Erickson, was selected as the best descriptor of this work. The original edition was printed in November 1982 (H. Erickson, Tomlin, & Swain, 2009), has had eight reprints, and is now considered a classic by the Society for the Advancement of Modeling and Role-Modeling (SAMRM). I completed my PhD in 1984, left Michigan in 1986, spent 2 years at the University of South Carolina School of Nursing

as associate dean of academic affairs and then moved to the University of Texas, where I assumed the role of professor and chair of adult health nursing. When I retired in 1997, the Helen L. Erickson Endowed Lectureship on Holistic Nursing was established at the University of Texas in Austin.

I have authored or coauthored chapters on MRM and/or holistic nursing (Clayton, Erickson, & Rogers, 2006; H. Erickson, 1996, 2002, 2006b, 2006c, 2006d, 2006e, 2007, 2008; M. Erickson, Erickson, & Jensen, 2006; Walker & Erickson, 2006), some of which are included in the second book on MRM, and more recently, a book on the relationship between the philosophy and discipline of holistic nursing. I know now that advancing holistic health care is my mission, my life work; MRM is a vehicle for that purpose.[1]

Overview of Modeling and Role-Modeling Theory

MRM is based in several nursing principles that guide the assessment, intervention, and evaluation aspects of practice. These principles, reflected in the data collection categories (H. Erickson et al., 2009, pp. 148–168), are linked to *intervention aims* and *goals* (H. Erickson et al., 2009, pp. 168–201). Although both intervention aims and goals involve nursing actions, they differ in their purpose. Nursing interventions *should have intent;* nurses should *aim to make something happen that facilitates health and healing when they interact with clients.* There should also be markers that help us evaluate the efficacy of our activities— *intervention goals.* Table 12-1 shows the relations among MRM principles of nursing, data needed to practice this model, the aims of nursing actions, and specific goals.

Modeling

The *modeling* process involves assessment of a client's situation. It starts when we initiate an interaction with an individual and concludes with

---

[1]For additional information, please see the bonus chapter content available at http://davisplus.fadavis.com.

Table 12 • 1 **Relations Among Principles, Data Categories, Intervention Goals, and Aims**

Principles	Categories of Data	Goals	Aims
The nursing process requires that a trusting and functional relationship exist between nurse and client.	Description of the situation	Develop a trusting and functional relationship between self and your client.	Build trust.
Affiliated-individuation is contingent on the individual's perceiving that he or she is an acceptable, respectable, and worthwhile human being.	Expectation	Facilitate a self-projection that is futuristic and positive.	Promote client's positive orientation.
Human development is dependent on the individual's perceiving that he or she has some control over life while concurrently sensing a state of affiliation.	(External) Resource potential	Promote affiliated-individuation with the minimum degree of ambivalence possible.	Promote client's control.
There is an innate drive toward holistic health that is facilitated by consistent and systematic nurturance.	(Internal) Resource potential	Promote a dynamic, adaptive, and holistic state of health.	Affirm and promote client's strengths.
Human growth is dependent on satisfaction of basic needs and is facilitated by growth-need satisfaction.	(Internal) Resource potential	Promote (and nurture) coping mechanisms that satisfy basic needs and permit growth-need satisfaction.	Set mutual goals that are health directed.
	Goal and life tasks	Facilitate congruent actual and chronological development stages.	

Adapted with permission from Erickson, H., Tomlin, E., & Swain, M. A. (Eds.). (2009). *Modeling and role-modeling: A theory and paradigm for nursing* (p. 171). Cedar Park, TX: EST.

an understanding of that person's perspective of their circumstances. We aim to learn how that individual describes the situation, what he or she expects will happen, and his or her perceived resources and life goals. As we listen and observe, we interpret the information using the constructs embedded in the theory. Stated simplistically, *modeling is the process we use to build a mirror image of an individual's worldview. This worldview helps us understand what that person perceives to be important, what has caused his or her problems, what will help, and how he or she wants to relate to others.*

Table 12-2 shows the categories of data and the type of information needed in the modeling process.

Table 12-3 shows the priority given to the information we collect. Primary data are acquired from the client; secondary data include the nurse's observations and information from the family. Tertiary data include information from medical records and other sources. Primary and secondary data are essential for professional practice, whereas tertiary data are added as needed.

Role-Modeling

The *role-modeling* process requires both objective and artistic actions. First, we analyze the data using theoretical *propositions* in the MRM model (Table 12-4; H. Erickson et al., 2009,

Table 12 • 2	Categories of Data and Purpose for Obtaining Data
Categories of Data Collection	**Purpose of Data Is to Obtain**
Description of the Situation	1. An overview of client's perception of the problem 2. The etiology of the problem including stressors and distressors 3. Client's perceived therapeutic needs
Expectations	1. Immediate expectations 2. Long-term expectations
Resource Potential	1. External: Social network, support system, and health-care system 2. Internal: Self-strengths, adaptive potential, feeling states, physiological states
Goal and Life Tasks	1. Current goals 2. Plans for future

Adapted with permission from Erickson, H., Tomlin, E., & Swain, M. A. (Eds.). (2009). *Modeling and role-modeling: A theory and paradigm for nursing* (p. 119). Cedar Park, TX: EST.

Table 12 • 3	Sources of Information
Primary Source	**Client's self-care knowledge**
Secondary Source	Information from family and nurses' observations
Tertiary Source	Medical records and other information related to client's case

Table 12 • 4	Selected Theoretical Propositions in MRM Theory

1. Developmental task resolution is related to basic need status.
2. Growth depends on basic need status and is facilitated by growth need satisfaction.
3. Basic need satisfaction leads to object attachment.
4. Object loss leads to basic need deficits.
5. Affiliated-individuation is dependent on one's perception of acceptance and worth.
6. Feelings of worth result in a sense of futurity.
7. Development of self-care resources is related to basic need satisfaction.
8. Ability to mobilize coping resources is related to need satisfaction.
9. Responses to stressors are mediated by internal and external resources.
10. Ability to mobilize appropriate and adequate resources determines resultant health status.

pp. 148–167). We interpret the meaning of what has been provided and search for linkages among the data that will help us understand the client's worldview. As we analyze the data, implications for nursing actions emerge (H. Erickson et al., 2009, pp. 168–220). Nursing actions are then artistically designed with *intent* (i.e., the aims of interventions) and specific *outcomes* (i.e., intervention goals). Our overall objectives are to help people grow and heal and to find meaning in their experiences. The following

sections elaborate each of these objectives. The first section addresses the philosophical assumptions that underlie this model; theoretical underpinnings follow with implications for practice. Finally, the global applications of MRM are presented.

Philosophical Assumptions

Nursing has a metaparadigm that includes four extant constructs: person, environment, health, and nursing; sometimes social justice is added as a fifth construct (Schim, Benkert, Bell, Walker, & Danford, 2007). The operational definitions of these constructs provide the context necessary to clarify how an individual's actions are unique to nursing as opposed to the actions of another profession. Although all nursing theories are developed and articulated within this context, our personal philosophy affects how we define and operationalize the constructs of nursing and therefore how we articulate our models (H. Erickson, 2010). For this reason, it is important to be clear about our own philosophical beliefs and how they affect our conceptual definitions and our theoretical models. Nurses can use clear philosophical statements to determine whether the underpinnings of a theoretical model are consistent with their own belief systems (H. Erickson, 2010). When they are not, discrepancies among nursing's philosophical beliefs, the nurse's personal belief system, and the theoretical propositions often create dissonance that impedes the nurses' ability to use the model (H. Erickson et al., 2009). The philosophical assumptions underlying the MRM theory and paradigm are described in the text that follows. The first section presents MRM's orientation toward two of nursing's metaparadigm constructs: person and environment. Health, nursing, and social justice are described in the following sections.

Person and Environment

Humans are inherently holistic. This means that all aspects of the human are interconnected and dynamically interactive; what affects one part affects another. This is different from the wholistic person, wherein the parts are associated but not necessarily interconnected or interactive (Fig. 12-1). When we approach people from a wholistic perspective, we can break them down into systems, organs, and other parts. When we view them as holistic, we understand that all the dimensions of the human being are interconnected; what affects one part has the potential to affect other parts. Our holistic nature is manifested through our innate instincts and drives: instincts and drives necessary for *humans* to maneuver through the pathways of their life

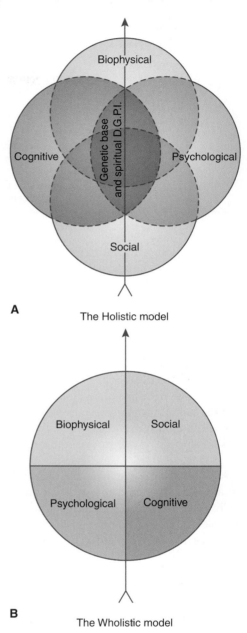

A   The Holistic model

B   The Wholistic model

Fig 12 • 1 Holism versus wholism.

journey. Table 12-5 provides examples of each of these. Although some might argue that all animals have an *innate instinct* to cope and some have an innate ability to receive and interpret stimuli, most would agree that not all animals have an *innate drive* to receive stimuli in a cognitive form, to acquire skills necessary to perceive and understand stimuli, to give and receive feedback, the freedom to speak, or the

Table 12 · 5   Selected List of Human Instincts and Drives

Instincts Inherent in Human Nature	To receive and interpret stimuli
	To cope and adapt to stressors
	To experience mind–body–spirit intraconnectedness, or holistic well-being
Drives That Motivate Our Behavior	To cognitively interpret stimuli
	To acquire skills necessary to perceive and interpret stimuli
	To give and receive feedback
	To communicate freely
	To choose and act freely
	To experience balanced affiliated-individuation
	To be self-actualized

freedom to choose. These latter characteristics are unique to the human species, are innate, and often motivate our behavior (Maslow, 1968, 1982). I have added one instinct—an inherent instinct for holistic well-being—and two human drives: the drive for healthy affiliated-individuation and the drive for self-actualization. These instincts and drives affect how we function as *holistic beings.* The holistic person is one in whom the whole is greater than the sum of the parts, whereas a wholistic person is one in whom the whole is equal to the sum of the parts (H. Erickson et al., 2009, pp. 45–46).

As holistic beings, our mind, body, and spirit are inextricably interrelated with continuous feedback loops. Cells in each dimension can produce stimuli affecting responses in cells of other dimensions. Cellular responses have the potential to become new stimuli, moving the chain reaction around and among the dimensions of the human being. These interactions are dynamic and ongoing. Because we have an internal environment (i.e., within the confines of our physical being) and an external environment (i.e., outside the confines of the biopsychosocial being), external stimuli have the potential to create multiple internal responses, and vice versa. To agree that we are holistic is to believe that we are human beings, living in a context that includes all that is within us and within our external environment—holistic beings, constantly in process both internally and externally. These dynamically interactive dimensions cannot be separated without a loss of information about the person, a loss that

diminishes our ability to fully understand the person's situation.

Humans are inherently intuitive. We know (at some level) what we need. We know what has made us sick and what will help us get well, grow, develop, and heal. We have *instinctual* information about our own personhood and our mind–body–spirit linkages. This information is called *self-care knowledge.* Our perceptions of what we have available to help us are called *self-care resources.* Self-care resources are both internal and external. We have resources within ourselves as well as resources within our external environment. Our actions, thoughts, biophysical responses, and behavior that help us get our needs met are our *self-care* actions. We are *inherently* social beings with an innate drive to grow and develop, to become the most that we can be, find meaning in our lives, fulfill our potential, and self-actualize. However, we are vulnerable. Our ability to grow and develop is dependent on *repeated satisfaction* of our needs. We want and *need* to be connected or *affiliated* to others in some way. Simultaneously, we also need to perceive ourselves as unique and *individuated* from these same people. We call this affiliated-individuation (Acton, 1992; H. Erickson et al., 2009, p. 47; M. Erickson et al., 2006, pp. 182–207). Our drive to be both affiliated and individuated at the same time mandates a balance between being connected while perceiving a sense of one's self as a unique human being, separate from others. We achieve our drive for a balanced affiliated-individuation through our interactions with others. How well we achieve this balance at any point in our life will determine how we relate to others in the following years.

Although we are social beings with a drive for affiliated-individuation with others, we are also spiritual beings with an inherent drive to be connected with our soul (H. Erickson et al., 2009, 2006). More specifically, our drive for individuation is to fulfill our psychosocial needs while doing soul-work unique to our life journey.

Health

Health is a matter of perception. It is a state of well-being in the whole person, not just a part of the person. It is not the presence, absence, or control of disease; one's ability to adapt; or one's ability to perform social roles. Instead, it is a *eudemonistic health* that incorporates all of these and more. It is a *sense of well-being* in the holistic, social being. It includes one's perceptions of her life quality, her ability to find meaning in her existence, and a capacity to enjoy a positive orientation toward the future. As a result, personal perceptions of health may differ from those of others. It is possible for persons with no obvious physical problem to perceive a low level of health, while at the same time others, taking their last mortal breath, may perceive themselves as very healthy. The perception of health status is always related to perceived balance of affiliated-individuation.

Nursing

Nursing is the unconditional acceptance of the inherent worth of another human being. When we have unconditional acceptance for another person, we recognize that all humans have an innate need to be loved, to belong, to be respected, and to feel worthy. Unconditional acceptance of a person as a worthwhile being is not the same as accepting all behaviors without conditions. It does mean, however, that we recognize that behaviors are motivated by unmet needs. Our work, then, is to help people find ways to get their needs met without harming themselves or others.

We do this through nurturance and facilitation of the holistic person. Our goal is to help people grow, develop, and, when necessary, to heal. We use all of our skills acquired through formal education as well as our own innate ability to connect with others to help them recover from illnesses and to live meaningful lives. We do this from the beginning of physical life to the end, even as people are taking their last breath. Within this context, our *intent*, or what we aim to facilitate when we interact with another human being, is important.

Social Justice

As professional nurses, we are committed to live by the ethics of our profession, serve as advocates for our clients, and serve the public as defined by our professional standards. For nurses who use the MRM theory, this means that we are committed to recognize the individual's worldview as valid information, to act on that information with the intent of nurturing and facilitating growth and well-being in our clients, and to practice within the context of the Standards of Holistic Nursing as defined by the American Holistic Nurses Association (AHNA, 2013) and recognized by the American Nurses Association (ANA, 2008).

Theoretical Constructs

People have an innate instinct to *cope* and *adapt* to stressors and related stress responses that confront us constantly. We adapt as much as we are able to, given our life situation. We need oxygen, glucose, and protein to maintain our physical systems; we also need to feel safe and to be loved. When these needs are perceived to be unmet, they create stressors; stressors produce the stress response. Stress responses can become new stressors mandating still more responses, and so on (Benson, 2006, pp. 240–266; H. Erickson, 1976; H. Erickson et al., 2009). Many of our stress responses are instinctual, a part of our human makeup; however, some have to be learned and developed. As our needs are met, the stressors decrease; and we are able to work through the stress response.

Adaptive Potential

Our ability to mobilize resources at any moment in time can be identified as our *Adaptive*

Potential. The adaptive potential assessment model (APAM; Fig. 12-2), first labeled in 1976 (H. Erickson, 1976; H. Erickson & Swain, 1982; H. Erickson et al., 2009), was derived by synthesizing Selye's (1974, 1976, 1980, 1985) work with that of George Engel (1964). Our adaptive potential has three states: equilibrium, arousal, and impoverishment. Equilibrium, a state of nonstress or eustress, represents maximum ability to mobilize resources. The individual in equilibrium is in a healthy balance between need demands and need resources.

Arousal and impoverishment are both stress states; needs are unmet, creating stressors and the related stress responses. However, people in arousal are temporarily able to mobilize their resources, whereas those in impoverishment are not. Persons in the first group (arousal) need help solving their problem, finding alternatives. They tend to be tense and anxious but do not demonstrate depleted resources through the expression of fatigue and sadness. On the other hand, impoverished people show the wear and tear of prolonged stress. They have diminished physical resources and are fatigued and sad. People in arousal are at risk for becoming impoverished, and impoverished people are at risk for depleting their resources, getting sick, developing complications, and even dying (Barnfather, 1987; Barnfather & Ronis, 2000; Benson, 2006, pp. 242–254; H. Erickson, 1976; H. Erickson et al., 2009, pp. 75–83; H. Erickson & Swain, 1982). As indicated, a person's ability to cope is related to how well his or her needs are met at any given point in time.

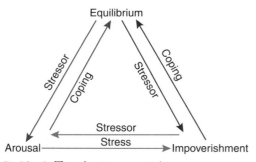

Fig 12 • 2 The adaptive potential assessment model.

Human Needs

Human needs, classified as basic, social, and growth needs, *drive* our behavior. They provide motivation for our self-care actions and emerge in a quasi-hierarchical order. Physiological needs must be met to some degree before social needs emerge. Growth or higher-level needs emerge after the basic and social needs have been met to some degree (for a more detailed taxonomy of human needs, see H. Erickson, 2006a, pp. 484–485). Basic needs are related to survival of the species. When they are unmet, tension rises, motivating behavioral response(s) necessary to decrease the tension. When self-care actions decrease the tension, the need dissipates. When the need is completely satisfied, the tension disappears. When needs are met repeatedly, need assets are built. Conversely, when the need is not met, the tension rises, and need deficits emerge. When the tension continues, need deprivation exists. Need status can be classified on a 0 to 5 scale ranging from deprivation to asset status (Fig. 12-3). Growth needs are different. Because people have an innate drive for self-actualization, growth needs emerge when basic needs are met (to some degree). Unmet growth needs do not create tension unless they are related to a basic need. Instead, *satisfaction* of growth needs creates tension. The need increases in intensity. Until one feels satiated, the need to continue to behave in ways that will meet growth needs continues.

Need Satisfaction and the Object Attachment Process

Objects that repeatedly meet humans needs become *attachment objects*. These objects take on significance unique to the individual, are both human and nonhuman, have a physical form (so they stimulate one of the five senses) or are abstract (such as an idea), and are necessary throughout life. When a person perceives that the object is or will be lost, a grieving response occurs. Loss is a subjective

Deprivation	Deficit	Unmet	Met	Satisfied	Assets
0	1	2	3	4	5

Fig 12 • 3 The needs status scale, 0 to 5.

experience known by the individual; it can be real, threatened, or perceived. Any loss produces a grieving process. One's difficulty in resolving the loss depends on the significance of the lost object. The grieving response is normal, occurs in a predetermined sequence, and is self-limited. Normal grieving processes take about 1 year (Fig. 12-4). Grief resolution occurs as the individual finds new ways to view the lost object or finds alternative objects that meet their needs. Commonly accepted processes of grief include sequential phases of shock/disbelief, anger, bargaining, sadness, and acceptance (Kübler-Ross, 1969). Other models (Engel, 1964; Bowlby, 1973) indicate slightly different phases (M. Erickson, 2006, p. 229). Table 12-6 compares three of these models. I believe that their differences are based in the nature of the lost object, its meaning to the individual, and the resources accrued

before the experienced loss. Resources are based on one's ability to work through the normal developmental tasks encountered during the human journey. This issue is discussed further in the text that follows.

Attachment to new objects is necessary for continued growth and grief resolution. The new object can be the *same* object, perceived in a new way, or a completely new object. Sometimes *transitional objects* are used to facilitate this process. Transitional objects are those that symbolize the lost object and are never human, but are almost always concrete. For example, mothers attached to their children as preschoolers often experience a loss when their children start school and become increasingly independent. It is common to see these mothers attach to their child's baby shoes, pictures, or some other symbol of who they were in their previous life stage.

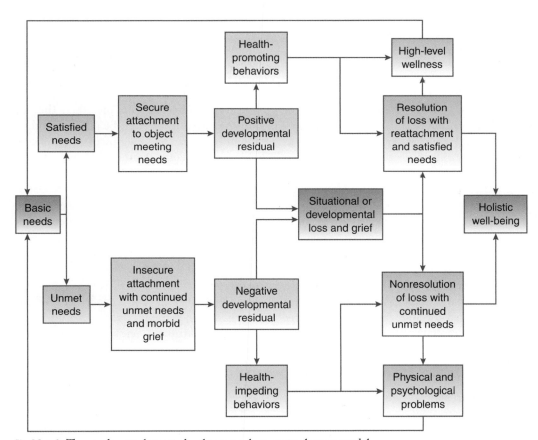

Fig 12 • 4 The needs–attachment–development–loss–reattachment model.

Table 12·6	**Stages of Grief According to Contributing Authors**	
Engel	**Kübler-Ross**	**Bowlby**
Shock/disbelief	Denial/shock	
Awareness	Anger/hostility	Protest
Resolution	Bargaining	
Loss resolution	Depression	*Despair*
Idealization	Acceptance	*Detachment*

Italicized stages indicate unresolved loss with movement toward morbid grief.
Reprinted with permission from Erickson, H. (Ed.). (2006). *Modeling and role-modeling: A view from the client's world* (p. 229). Cedar Park, TX: Unicorns Unlimited.

Morbid grief emerges when the individual is unable to find alternative objects that will repeatedly meet their needs. Because we are holistic beings, morbid grief has the potential to result in physical symptoms, illness, and over the long period, disease. What happens in one part of the holistic person has the potential of creating disease in another part, disease that becomes distressful, mandates mobilization of resources often not available, and therefore producing alternative biophysical responses, depleting psychoneuroimmunological resources (Walker & Erickson, 2006

Behaviors that indicate emergence of morbid grief include an inability to move on and let go of the lost object, combined with vacillation between *anger* and *sadness* (M. Erickson, 2006, pp. 209–239; Lindeman, 1944, pp. 141–148). Initially individuals are able to focus their anger and sadness, but with time, anger grows into hostility and sadness into depression. When this happens, people are less able to articulate the focus of their feelings or recognize the loss that produced the grieving response in the beginning. They often use language that describes giving up rather than letting go, and sometimes express nostalgia for the lost object. In contrast, those who have let go of the lost object, worked through the normal grief response, and reattached to a new object can usually describe the importance of *moving on.*

Need Satisfaction and Life Orientation

The degree to which a person's needs are met repeatedly determines how he or she relates to others; it affects his or her life orientation. When needs are met repeatedly, people are able to grow and develop, to integrate mind–body–spirit, to perceive themselves as worthy human beings, and to experience a healthy balance of affiliated-individuation. When this happens, they are interested in others as individuals who are unique and worthwhile. They enjoy both a sense of connectedness and a sense of individuation. Their life orientation is called a *being orientation* because they are interested in becoming all they can be and in participating in the same way with others.

However, when needs are repeatedly unmet, growth is limited, and people have difficulty with their developmental processes. Their relationships with others exist within a context of what can be obtained from the other. They are not interested in the well-being of the other, might be threatened by growth in significant others, and are intolerant of the uniqueness of others. More interested in what they can get from someone than what they can give, these people often view others as a source of getting their basic needs met. As a result, often unable to meet the needs of significant others, they are perceived as "needy people." Their life orientation is called a *deficit orientation.* Being and deficit orientations exist on a scale; most people have some of both. The balance between the two is what determines one's overriding traits or personal attributes, one's values and virtues, and one's ways of interacting with others.

Developmental Processes

People have an inherent drive for self-actualization. This requires that they pass through predetermined chronological developmental stages—stages with *task*s that mandate attention as they emerge. Our ability to work on these *developmental tasks* depends on our ability to mobilize resources. Resources are derived by getting our needs met at any given time as well as our past experiences. Because our experiences are always contextual, how we resolve our developmental tasks will determine the resources we have to work on current tasks. As we work through a stage-related task, a *developmental residual* is produced. This residual includes positive *and* negative attributes, strengths, and virtues. In our original work, we followed Erik Erikson's (1994) work to define eight stages, their tasks, and the associated residual. Our more recent work has expanded the stages to include one prebirth and another at the time of death because the work of the soul affects the developmental processes during one's physical life (M. Erickson, 2006, pp. 121–181; Table 12-7).

Sequential Development

Development occurs as a series of predetermined stages with specific tasks in each stage. It is also chronological: unique, sequential

stages, and their related tasks emerge during a specific time frame in our lives. During that time, the task becomes predominate in our life journey, drawing resources, focusing attention, and motivating behaviors.

Epigenesis

Development is also epigenetic. Although we have specific tasks that focus our attention at specific times in life, we also rework earlier life tasks and set the framework for later tasks at the same time. This later work is done within the context of the appointed life task. Simply stated, we repeatedly work on all of the developmental tasks at every stage of life, although we have a key task that dominates at any given time. Our ability to manage multiple tasks is dependent on the residual we have produced throughout the process and our current ability to have our needs met.

Linkages

Three key theoretical linkages exist in the MRM model. Relations exist between or among (1) adaptive potential and need status;

Table 12 · 7 Developmental Stages, Residual, Virtues, and Strengths

Stages/Age	Residual	Virtue	Strength(s)
Integration of Spirit (pre–post birth)	Unity vs. duality	Groundedness	Awareness
Building Trust (birth–15 months)	Trust vs. mistrust	Hope	Drive toward future
Acquiring Autonomy (12–36 months)	Autonomy vs. introspection	Willpower	Self-control
Taking Initiative (2–7 years)	Initiative vs. responsibility	Purpose	Drive
Developing Industry (5–13 years)	Competency vs. inferiority	Competence	Methodological problem-solving
Developing Identity (11–30 years)	Self-identity vs. role confusion	Fidelity	Devotion
Building Intimacy (20–50 years)	Intimacy vs. isolation	Love	Affiliation with individuation
Developing Generativity (midlife to 60s)	Generativity vs. stagnation	Caring	Production
Ego Integrity (60s to transformation)	Ego integrity vs. despair	Wisdom	Renunciation
Transformation (end of physical life)	Reconnecting vs. disconnecting	Oneness	Peace, cosmic understanding, compassion

Adapted with permission from Erickson, H. (Ed.). (2006). *Modeling and role-modeling: A view from the client's world* (Table 5.1, pp. 128–129). Cedar Park TX: Unicorns Unlimited.

(2) need status, object attachment, loss, and new attachment status; and (3) developmental task resolution and need satisfaction. Selected theoretical propositions, derived from these linkages, are shown in Table 12-4. Others exist, limited only by an understanding of MRM.

MRM Practice Strategies

Initiating the Relationship

Three sequential strategies are important for those using the MRM model: (1) establishing a mindset, (2) creating a nurturing space, and (3) facilitating the story (H. Erickson, 2006b, pp. 309–317; Table 12-8). Each can be done in seconds once the essence of the strategy is understood. However, before you can start, it is necessary to reflect on your own beliefs about human nature and nursing and to consider how these affect your practice. This helps you clarify *how to get your needs met*—a prerequisite to meeting the needs of others. Unless we know how to initiate our own self-care, we have difficulty mobilizing the energy necessary to focus on the needs of our clients. Finally, we have to open ourselves to the worth of each individual, to unconditionally accept that each human has an inherent need to be valued, to be treated with respect, and to live with dignity.

Establishing a Mindset

Establishing a mindset involves three strategies: centering, focusing, and opening. *Centering* helps to organize our resources so that we can connect energetically with our client. It requires that we temporarily put aside other thoughts, worries, or concerns and believe that at some level we can discover what we need to know to help our clients; it requires us to focus on the other with the intent of nurturing their growth and facilitating their healing. When we focus on our client's needs, we initiate an energetic connection, necessary for a caring–healing environment.

Creating a Nurturing Space

Creating a nurturing space follows naturally when we have established a mind-set. Our goal is to create a caring–healing environment. Although one cannot force growth in others, we can create environments that nurture growth. We do this by decreasing adverse stimuli while increasing positive ones. It is important to remember that you are entering the client's space and to respect it. Even though you may think it is important to close the door, turn on the radio, or fluff pillows, you will want to assess whether your actions serve to comfort the client. Each of these processes helps you connect with your client in such a

Table 12 · 8 Three Strategies That Facilitate a Trusting–Functional Relationship

Establish a Mindset	Self-care preliminaries Moving forward	Enhance sense-of-self. Center self. Focus intent. Open self to the essence of other.
Create a Nurturing Space	Reduce distracting stimuli. Respect client's space. Connect spirit to spirit.	Attend to sounds, lights, smells, and other stimuli that are distracting and discomforting. Recognize and respect client's physical/ energetic space. Use eye contact, soft tones, and gentle touch to connect with client.
Facilitate the Client's Story	Tap self-care knowledge.	Address stimuli, encourage focus on nurse–client linkage. Relate to beliefs about client's self-care knowledge as primary. Encourage client's perceptions of the situation.

Adapted with permission from Erickson, H. (Ed.). (2006). *Modeling and role-modeling: A view from the client's world* (pp. 307–317). Cedar Park, TX: Unicorns Unlimited.

way that you will initiate a trusting relationship and create a caring–healing environment. Any stimuli that affects the five senses has the possibility of being comforting, uncomfortable, or discomforting. We can influence these by our actions in the milieu and by our interactions with our client. For example, a noisy hallway or bright lights shining in our eyes are stimuli that seem to drain energy from us, and no doubt our clients experience the same thing. Or consider a beautiful picture, the glimpse of a fully leafed tree swaying in a gentle breeze, soft music of our choice, clean sheets against our skin, or the gentle touch of a loving person. In thinking about how you respond to these stimuli, you will understand that these have the possibility of comforting another human being. You will also understand that how you touch, look, or speak to someone conveys a message about your intent to comfort or not to comfort. Of course, it is extremely important that we consider the individual's cultural perspectives and values as we consider how to create a nurturing space; what works for one person does not for another. The only way we can know is to ask our clients or, when they are unable to speak for themselves, to ask their significant others.

Facilitating the Story

Facilitating the story is the third strategy that MRM nurses use. Disclosure of our clients' self-care knowledge provides basic information needed before we can decide what nursing actions are required—information that provides insight into their worldview. We learn about their perceptions and beliefs, what they believe about their current situation, what they expect will happen, what resources they believe they have, and what they would like to do to alter the situation. It also allows them to "contextualize life experiences and present them in a way that softens associated feelings" (H. Erickson, 2006b, p. 315).

Our clients' self-care knowledge is best obtained by allowing them to tell their story in their own way. We use active listening to facilitate our clients to tell their stories. This can be done very quickly by initiating the discussion with statements such as, "Tell me about your situation" followed by "Why do you think

this has happened?" or "What do you think has caused it?" and "How do you feel about that?" and so forth (H. Erickson et al., 2009, pp. 153–167). The data are then organized into four distinct but interrelated categories: description of the situation, expectations, resource potential, and goals (see Table 12-2). Information provided by our clients has to be interpreted, aggregated, and analyzed before we can use it to plan interventions (H. Erickson et al., 2009, pp. 153–168).

Phases of Understanding the Data

There are three phases in understanding the information gained in MRM practice model. In data interpretation, we use the philosophical and theoretical underpinnings discussed earlier as we attend to words, affects, and nonverbal cues, searching for evidence of coping potential (i.e., adaptive potential), needs status, and developmental residual. Sometimes it is necessary to clarify what we observe to avoid superimposing our own interpretations on these data. For example, clients might have a spouse or significant other but not perceive this individual as supportive. When this happens, they often describe them as "draining" rather than invigorating. We cannot always make these distinctions without asking the client how they perceive their relationship with their significant other (H. Erickson et al., 2009, pp. 160–163). A person's story usually includes information about interactions among the dimensions of the holistic person, but nurses often have trouble understanding the significance of what they have heard. For example, when people say they are sick because they are too stressed, our first response might be to think about the cause and effect of disease—for example, bacteria (not stress) cause infections. However, the MRM model supports a holistic perspective; we know that mind and body are inextricably interactive. Therefore, we recognize that psychosocial stress stimulates the hypothalamic–pituitary–adrenal axis interactions, compromising the immune system. When this happens, we have more difficulty fighting bacterial invasions. As a result, we know that psychosocial stress has the potential of causing signs and symptoms of physical illness and/or disease.

The second phase, data aggregation, sometimes occurs as we interpret data derived from the primary source (i.e., the client), but not always. To aggregate data accurately, we need to consider data derived from the secondary and tertiary sources as well as the data derived from the client. Although data can be aggregated with only the client's story and the nurse's clinical knowledge, it is also helpful to hear the family's perspective. Sometimes it is important to include the information collected from tertiary sources as well.

When aggregating data, we consider all the information and look for consistencies as well as inconsistencies across the sources of information. Additional information may be necessary to clarify perspectives. Usually, this phase helps determine what needs to be done when moving into the intervention phase of the nursing process.

Data analysis is the next phase. Again, you may be doing all three—interpreting, aggregating, and analyzing—simultaneously. During the analysis phase, you look for theoretical linkages among the data and make diagnoses.

Proactive Nursing Care

Often the process of assessing our clients' worldview serves as a therapeutic intervention. People in arousal commonly state that they feel much better after talking. Some will ask for minimal help, but some require more sophisticated help. In any case, based on our diagnoses, nursing care is planned within the context of the MRM principles of care, aimed at facilitating well-being in our clients, and designed specifically to meet intervention goals. We do this as we manage technical care such as wound management, intravenous insertion, and so forth. We use nonjudgmental language, caring tones, and direct statements that relay information needed to feel safe and cared about. We also use Ericksonian hypnotherapeutic techniques to promote growth and facilitate healing (H. Erickson et al., 2009, pp. 84–85, 145–147; H. Erickson, 2006b, pp. 315–317; 372–374; Zeig, 1982).

We can also do this without ever touching the person because we use ourselves as conduits of healing energy. Sometimes knowing that someone cares about us will help us grow and heal. We project these messages through our actions when we unconditionally accept the worth of another human being and set intent to facilitate health and healing. Watzlawick (1967) stated that "we cannot not communicate." Our attitudes, nonverbal behaviors, and touch are often more important than what we say when we convey our intent to help others heal and grow; words are not always necessary. Our demeanor, the way we look at the person, what we focus on first, and how we touch our clients relays our intent. When we enter a relationship with the intent to comfort and nurture the other person, our energy field connects with his; we convey presence and initiate a caring–healing environment (H. Erickson, 2006b, pp. 300–324).

Practice Applications

MRM, recognized by AHNA as one of the extant holistic nursing theories, is used in a variety of settings including educational institutions as a framework for entire programs or specific courses, hospitals to guide practice, and for independent practice (Table 12-9).

The Society for the Advancement of Modeling and Role-Modeling (SAMRM; www.mrmnursingtheory.org), established in 1985, meets biennially with retreats in alternate years. Selected publications (Table 12-10) demonstrate how MRM has been applied across populations and settings from pediatrics to the elderly, chronically ill to the well, and intensive care to home care. Others (such as publications by Baas, Barnfather, Duke, Frisch, Hertz, Kelly, and Perese; see Table 12-10) describe MRM with those who have heart failure, undereducated adult learners, and/or employed mothers with preschool children. For example, Baas (2004) has tested relations between self-care resources and activities and quality of life and developed protocol for nursing practice. Baas, Past President of the American Association of Heart Failure (AAFH) Nurses and Director of Nursing Research at the University of Cincinnati Medical Center (2009–2012), continues to be actively involved in setting practice protocol for nurses working

Table 12 · 9 Agencies Using or Teaching Modeling and Role-Modeling

Harding University, School of Nursing, Searcy, Arkansas	Theoretical foundation for pediatric clinical course
Metro State University, School of Nursing, St. Paul, Minnesota	Theoretical foundation, and student advising
The College of St. Catherine's, School of Nursing, St. Paul, Minnesota	Theoretical foundation, ADN Program
The University of Texas at Austin, School of Nursing	Theoretical foundation, the Alternate Entry Program
Contemporary Health Care, Austin, Texas	Independent Nurse Practice Agency

with people experiencing congestive heart failure. Duke, Professor of Nursing and Associate Dean for Research, University of Texas at Tyler, previously interested in the experiences of single mothers (published in Weber, 1999), is currently studying attitudes about and preferences for end-of-life care in persons of Jewish, Hindu, Muslim, Buddhist, and Bhai'I faiths and living in Texas. Both Frisch & Frisch (2010) and Perese (2012) have published textbooks for mental health practitioners; Frisch & Frisch's book is used as a foundational book, whereas Perese's was written specifically for advanced practice nurses. Hertz has developed and tested a midrange

theory derived from MRM that measures *perceived enactment of autonomy in the elderly*. Hertz, Professor and Director of Graduate Studies, Northern Illinois University, is currently involved with mentoring graduate students interested in advancing holistic care for the elderly. Case studies are reported by practitioners in each of the SAMRM newsletters; these and additional publications (Hertz, 2013; Hertz, Irving, & Bowman, 2010; Hertz, Koren, Rossetti, & Robertson, 2008; Jablonski & Duke, 2012; Mitty, Resnick, Allen, Bakerjian, Hertz, Gardner et al., 2010) can be found on the SAMRM website (www.mrmnursingtheory.org).

Table 12 · 10 Practice/Intervention Studies Related to Modeling and Role-Modeling (MRM) Theory and Paradigm

Author	Tested	Source
Erickson, H. (1976)	Identification of states of coping	Unpublished master's thesis, University of Michigan, Ann Arbor
Erickson, H., & Swain, M. (1982)	MRM and well-being	*Research in Nursing & Health, 5,* 93–101
Erickson, H. (1984)	Exploration of self-care knowledge	*Dissertation Abstracts International, 45,* 171. University Microfilms No. AAD84–12136
Darling-Fisher, C., & Kline-Leidy, N. (1988)	Measuring Eriksonian developmental residual in the adult	*Psychological Reports, 62,* 747–754
Walsh, K., Vanden Bosch, T., & Boehm, S. (1989)	MRM applied to two clinical cases	*Journal of Advanced Nursing, 14*(9), 755–761
Barnfather, J., Swain, M. A. P., & Erickson, H. (1989).	Construct validity the APAM	*Issues in Mental Health Nursing, 10,* 23–40
Erickson, H., & Swain, M. (1990)	MRM and hypertension reduction	*Issues in Mental Health Nursing, 11*(3), 217–235

Continued

Table 12 · 10   **Practice/Intervention Studies Related to Modeling and Role-Modeling (MRM) Theory and Paradigm—cont'd**

Author	Tested	Source
Finch, D. (1990)	MRM nursing assessment model	*Modeling and Role-Modeling: Theory, Practice and Research, 1*(1), 203–213
Kline-Leidy, N. (1990)	Relations among stress, resources, and symptoms of chronic illness	*Nursing Research, 39,* 230–236
Erickson, H. (1990)	MRM with mind–body problems	In J.K. Zeig & Gilligan, S. (Eds.) Brief Therapy: Myths, Methods, and Metaphors. New York: Brunner/Mazel, 473–491.
Acton, G., Irvin, B., & Hopkins, B. (1991)	Theory testing research: Building the science	*Advances in Nursing Science, 14*(1), 52–61.
Barnfather, J. (1993)	Testing a theoretical proposition of MRM	*Issues in Mental Health Nursing, 14,* 1–18.
Holl, R. (1993)	MRM vs. restricted visiting	*Critical Care Nursing Quarterly, 16*(2), 70–82
Baas, L., Deges-Curl, E., Hertz, J., & Robinson, K. (1994)	Innovative approaches to theory based measurement: MRM research	*Advances in Nursing Science Series: Advances in Methods of Inquiry, 5,* 147–159.
Webster, D., Vaughn, K., Webb, M., & Player, A. (1995)	MRM and brief solution-focused therapy	*Issues in Mental Health Nursing, 16*(6), 505–518
Kline-Leidy, N., & Travis, G. (1995)	Relations between psychophysiological factors and physical functioning	*Research in Nursing & Health, 18,* 535–546
Hertz, J. (1996)	Perceived enactment of autonomy (PEA)	*Issues in Mental Health Nursing, 17,* 261–273
Baldwin, C. (1996)	Perceptions of hope	*The Journal of Multicultural Nursing & Health, 2*(3), 41–45
Erickson, M. (1996)	EMBAT and maternal well-being	*Issues in Mental Health Nursing, 17,* 185–200
Sappington, J., & Kelly, J. (1996)	A case study	*Journal of Holistic Nursing, 14*(2), 130–141
Baas, L., Fontana, J., & Bhat, G. (1997)	Self-care resources and the quality of life	*Progress in Cardiovascular Nursing, 12*(1), 25–38
Raudonis, B., & Acton, G. (1997)	Theory-based nursing practice	*Journal of Advanced Nursing, 26*(1), 138–145
Acton, G., Mayhew, P., Hopkins, B., & Yauk, S. (1999)	Communicating with persons with dementia	*Journal of Gerontological Nursing, 25*(2), 6–13
Acton, G. (1997)	The mediating effect of affiliated-individuation	*Journal of Holistic Nursing, 15*(4), 336–357
Irvin, B., & Acton, G. (1997)	Stress, hope and well-being	*Holistic Nursing Practice, 11*(2), 69–79
Jensen, B. (1997)	Caring for the caregiver	*Home Care Provider, 2*(6), 34–36
Baas, L., Berry, T., Fontana, J., & Wagoner, L. (1999)	Developmental growth in adults with heart failure	*Journal of Holistic Nursing, 17*(2), 117–138
Jensen, B. (1999)	Caregiver responses to MRM	*Dissertation Abstracts International, B 56/06, 3127*
Scheela, R. (1999)	Remodeling sex offenders	*Journal of Psychosocial Nursing and Mental Health Services, 37*(9), 25–31
Weber, G. (1999)	The meaning of well-being (self-care knowledge)	*Western Journal of Nursing Research, 21*(6), 785–795

Table 12 • 10	Practice/Intervention Studies Related to Modeling and Role-Modeling (MRM) Theory and Paradigm—cont'd	
Author	**Tested**	**Source**
Barnfather, J., & Ronis, D. (2000)	Psychosocial resources, stress, and health	*Research in nursing & health, 23,* 55–66.
Timmerman, G., & Acton, G. (2001)	Relations between needs and emotional eating	*Issues in Mental Health Nursing,* 22(7), 691–701
Mayhew, P., Acton, G., Yauk, S., & Hopkins, B. (2001)	Communication, dementia, and well-being	*Gerontological Nursing, 22,* 106–110
Berry, T., Baas, L., Fowler, C., & Allen, G. (2002)	Spirituality in persons with heart failure	Journal of Holistic Nursing, 20(1), pp. 5–30
Perese, E. (2002)	Integrating psychiatric nursing into educational models	*Journal of American Association of Psychiatric Nurses,* 8(5), 152–158
Hertz, J., Anschutz, C. (2002)	Relationships among PEA, self-care, and holistic health	*Journal of Holistic Nursing, 20,* 166–186
Baas, L. (2004)	Self-care resources, activities as predictors of quality of life	*Dimensions of Critical Care Nursing, 23*(3), 131–138
Baas, L., Berry, T., Allen, G., Wizer, M., &Wagoner, L. (2004)	Awareness in persons with heart failure or transplant	*Journal of Cardiovascular Nursing,* 19(1), 32–40
Lombardo, S. L., & Roof, M. (2005)	Application MRM to person with morbid obesity	*Home Healthcare Nurse, 23*(7), 425–428.
Berry, T., Baas, L., & Henthorn, C. (2007)	Self-reported adjustment to implanted cardiac devices	*Journal of Cardiovascular Nursing,* 22(6), 516–524

We cannot cure people, but we can help them heal and grow, even as they are taking their first or last breath. When people heal, they become more fully connected with the multiple dimensions of their mind, body, and spirit, and as a result, they become more fully actualized. A caring–healing environment, created by the nurses' intent, fosters growth and well-being in their clients. Because people have inherent instincts and drives to grow, develop, and heal, all nursing actions focus on facilitation and nurturance of these innate abilities. We use ourselves to connect with our clients in such a way that we can create trusting functional relationships with them, relationships that have a purpose or are aimed at some outcome. In the MRM model, these relationships aim to affirm clients' worth; to help them mobilize and build resources needed to cope with their stressors/stress; foster hope for the future; and promote a sense of affiliated-individuation. When people have these experiences, a sense of well-being follows. Although we use every professional skill we have

acquired, these are secondary to using ourselves as healing agents. As nurses, we nurture and facilitate people to become the most that they can be. We help them actualize their life roles and find meaning in their existence. When this happens, it affects not only our clients but also those who are significant in their lives.

As nurses, every interaction with our clients and their loved ones provides us with opportunities to affect the future; I call this the "long-arm affect" (H. Erickson, 2006b, p. 390). How we perceive our roles as nurses will determine our intent. This in turn affects what we do, how we interact, the focus of our work, and the outcomes of our relationships. We cannot always change what will happen in our lives or those of others, but we can set the intent to help people grow, heal, and move on. J. M.'s letter (see Practice Exemplar 1) suggests that I not only helped his family deal with a life tragedy but also helped them discover ways to find meaning in the experience. I helped them grow, heal, and move on.

Practice Exemplar 1

A man who was the strong, dominant member of his family was lying in bed, incontinent, riddled with cancer, and feeling hopeless. When I learned that he no longer allowed his family to visit, I gently took his hand and told him I was happy to be his nurse that evening. He "looked at me with very sad eyes . . . [and said] that he didn't want his family to see him in this condition. . . . [H]e had always taken care of his family, and now . . . he couldn't take care of himself" (H. Erickson, 2006a, p. 325). I rephrased his words and then told him that although he had been the breadwinner in the past and his family members had enjoyed and appreciated that, all they wanted now was to be with him, to share his life, to show him that he was important because he loved them and they loved him. He agreed, and for the next few days his family members took turns just being with him. On the third day when he quietly passed, he and his family were able to grieve with dignity and peace.

Eight years later, I received a letter from his son (only 16 at the time of his father's death), notifying me that his mother had died. He knew I would want to know that because of what they had learned from me, she was able to pass at home with her family at her side, singing her favorite songs and strumming on the guitar. He went on to state:

In the year my Dad was with you people in Ann Arbor, you were of incalculable aid and comfort to both my parents—you gave them confidence in you and your staff, and the dignity and respect which makes life worth living; no one else could, or did, more genuinely have their gratitude and respect. When I would come down and all seemed to be lost, the one bright spot was that Mrs. Erickson would be coming on, and we could breathe a little more easily as Dad's anxiety visibly receded. Your kindness and humanity made the world a better place at that time and without you the experience would have been more difficult than you probably believe. Thank you, J. M.

Practice Exemplar 2

Most data are easy to understand although there are some that are symbolic of earlier losses. A middle-aged man I worked with a number of years ago had just been admitted to the hospital for a "workup." Mr. S. had complained of chronic fatigue for the past 6 months. An hour or so before I saw him, he had learned that he had acute leukemia. When I asked him to tell me about his situation, he told me about his leukemia and then launched into a story about his childhood. He described a time when he was about 16 years old, had been told to watch his younger sister and had let her ride a horse without supervision. She fell off and was killed. He remembered his father telling him that he had not been responsible and that he needed to grow-up and be a man.

Mr. S. looked surprised and said he didn't know what had made him think of that event and hadn't thought about it for years. When I asked him what he expected to happen to him, he said he guessed that he was going to die. He went on to say that he thought he had developed leukemia because he hadn't been responsible, and when he wasn't responsible; people died. As we explored his resources, he explained that he had been promoted about 9 months earlier and that his new job required skills he didn't think he had. His conclusions were that he was sick because he had "worried himself to death." He also stated that he didn't want his wife to come see him, that he needed to decide what he wanted to do first, and how he could take care of her now that he was sick? When I asked if she or someone else could

Practice Exemplar 2 cont.

help him consider options, he said no, that it was his responsibility to take care of himself. To understand these data, I needed to recognize the following:

• People who link new stressful experiences to past experiences are usually dealing with a loss related to the past experience. In his case, it was not only the loss of his sister but also the meaning of the loss. As a 16-year-old boy, he was learning about his ability to make sound decisions, to be independent, to determine who he was as a unique human being in society. He had learned that "when he wasn't responsible, people died."

• Although he identified his wife as his significant other, he was overindividuated. He needed to decide how to "tell" his wife about his problem—his problem of not being responsible, not being a "man." He did not perceive that it was appropriate to seek comfort from her or others.

• Mr. S. is in arousal with unmet safety and belonging needs, unresolved loss with morbid grief, and both positive and negative residual from adolescence on. Strong positive residual from early childhood provides some resources that could be mobilized with assistance.

• Although Mr. S. is chronologically in the stage of Intimacy versus Isolation, his stressors are related to residuals from the stage of Competency versus Limitations.

• Mr. S's healthy affiliated–individuation has been threatened due to overindividuation.

• Mr. S. wished to be "responsible" to "take care of his wife."

Specific interventions used in this case are as follows:

• I centered myself and set intent to be energetically connected, using myself as a conduit of healing energy from the universe. Setting an intent to connect and serve as a healing instrument is a prerequisite to facilitating a client's storytelling. It is also an important strategy for helping people mobilize resources needed to help themselves heal. Centering, setting intent to connect, and to

serve as an energetic conduit were strategies used throughout our time together, purposefully initiated with each visit.

• When I asked him to tell me about his situation, I also stated that he could talk about anything that popped into his mind, even if it didn't seem to be related to his current situation. This strategy is used because people have state-dependent memory, their current experiences are often related to losses incurred in the past. Although they are unaware of these relations, it may be important to help them "uncover" these experiences in their own time and their own way so that they can begin to heal—a prerequisite for mobilizing resources needed to contend with the current situation.

• I used active listening skills as he told his story, using nonverbal communications to encourage him to open up, staying energetically connected, and remaining quiet when he paused, allowing him an opportunity to express his self-care knowledge.

• My question: *What do you expect will happen?* was used to assess self-care resources and to allow him to identify associated factors and express his worse fears. His response indicated that he was depleted of resources (i.e., impoverished), his definition of being responsible no longer worked for him, and he needed help reframing his behaviors and identifying new resources. I further explored his resources with the follow-up questions.

• Considering that the loss had occurred during the age of adolescence and the task of developing Identity and that healthy resolution of *Identify* is important for the development of healthy intimacy in the next stage of life, follow-up interventions included exploring alternative ways to think about "being responsible"—the role he had chosen for himself. Using open-ended questions, I helped him consider his relationship with his family by thinking about *how he was like* the 16-year-old boy and how he was different; *how he wanted to be*

Continued

Practice Exemplar 2 cont.

like that boy and how he wanted to be different; and *how he wanted* to relate to his wife in the future and how he might start. Rhetorical questions, stated as curiosities rather than a demand for a response, were used to stimulate growth. Examples include statements such as *I wonder how you are like that 16-year-old boy now, and how you are different? It might even be interesting to think about how you want to be like that boy—or different.*

• Biophysical care was also offered and provided with consideration for his developmental resources. Adolescents with healthy developmental resources often vacillate in their need to be independent in their activities of daily life and their needs to have care consistent with earlier stages provided. The only way to know is to offer care and follow the client's responses. Thus, when asked to help with foot care, it was provided; when told that he could manage making his own outpatient appointments, he was given the information needed to make his appointments and asked if he needed any other information after the appointments were confirmed.

• As he prepared for discharge to the outpatient clinic for chemotherapy, I explored his perceptions of the effects of chemotherapy. He stated that chemotherapy was a poison and would make him sick, that he didn't look forward to that. I agreed that chemotherapy was a poison, but that there were several things he could do to help himself. Aiming to reframe the perception of chemotherapy outcomes, I suggested that chemotherapy was designed to fight with the bad cells, but he didn't need to have the chemotherapy fight with his good cells, that he could protect them if he wanted. When he expressed curiosity about protecting his good cells, I helped him learn how to use guided imagery so that the chemotherapy would seek out bad cells and attach them, but leave the others alone. We then talked about ensuring that the chemotherapy had a good chance of doing its work by proactively getting sufficient sleep, drinking fluids, seeking nurturing relations, participating in activities that help him laugh, and other activities that made him feel loved, happy, and at peace.

• Upon discharge, I offered him a business card as a transitional object. I explained that it contained my name and contact information in the event that he wanted to talk with me at any time. I also stated that many people find they are able remember our time together—what they felt, heard, smelled, and saw—by holding the card and/or even just by thinking about it.

I followed this gentleman for several weeks, visiting him occasionally in the outpatient clinic. He always had my business card with him and often commented that it was magic and that it helped him get through the bad days. Two years later I received a letter thanking me for helping him and stating that he was in remission. He and his wife were planning a trip to celebrate their anniversary.

■ Summary

Nurses who use modeling and role-modeling believe the human is holistic with ongoing, dynamic mind–body–spirit interactions; clients are the primary source of information; and nurses are instruments of healing. Modeling is the process used to gain an understanding of their clients' perceptions and understandings of their conditions, health needs, and possible therapeutic interventions. During the modeling process, nurses gain an understanding of their clients perceptions of what has caused their health problem, what impedes their healing, and what will facilitate healing and growth. Modeling the client's worldview also helps nurses to understand their clients' relationships and related roles, identify those that impede health and wellness and those that are meaningful and facilitate healing and growth.

Role-modeling is helping clients find alternative ways to fulfill their desired roles in life. This requires interventions including biophysical care as well as psychosocial strategies designed to help people articulate their self-care knowledge, mobilize resources, and participate

in healthy self-care actions. Strategies are designed within the context of developmental residual and with consideration for losses and related attachment objects. Verbal and nonverbal communication and basic biophysical nursing skills are considered essential prerequisites in the use of MRM.

References

Acton, G. (1992). *The relationships among stressors, stress, affiliated-individuation, burden, and well-being in caregivers of adults with dementia: A test of the theory and paradigm for nursing, modeling and role-modeling.* Doctoral dissertation, University of Texas at Austin. *Dissertation Abstracts International,* AAT 9323314.

American Holistic Nurses Association (AHNA). (2007). *Holistic nursing: Scope and standards of practice.* Silver Spring, MD: American Holistic Nurses Association, American Nurses Association.

American Nurses Association (ANA). Retrieved June 3, 2008, from www.ahna.org/AboutUs/ANASpecialtyRecognition/tabid/1167/Default.aspx

Baas, L. (2004). Self-care resources, activities as predictors of quality of life. *Dimensions of Critical Care Nursing, 23*(3), 131–138.

Barnfather, J. (1987). *Mobilizing coping resources related to basic need status in healthy, young adults.* Doctoral dissertation, University of Texas at Austin. *Dissertation Abstracts International,* 49-02B (AAF8801275).

Barnfather, J., & Ronis, D. (2000). Test of a model of psychosocial resources, stress, and health among undereducated adults. *Research in Nursing & Health, 23*(1), 55–66.

Benson, D. (2006). Adaptation: Coping with stress. In: H. Erickson (Ed.), *Modeling and role-modeling: A view from the client's world* (pp. 240–274). Cedar Park, TX: Unicorns Unlimited.

Bowlby, J. (1973). *Separation.* New York: Basic Books.

Clayton, D., Erickson, H., & Rogers, S. (2006). Finding meaning in our life journey. In: H. Erickson (Ed.), *Modeling and role-modeling: A view from the client's world* (pp. 391–410). Cedar Park, TX: Unicorns Unlimited.

Engel, G. (1964). Grief and grieving. *American Journal of Nursing, 64,* 93.

Erikson, E. (1994). *Identity and the life cycle.* New York, NY: Norton & Company.

Erickson, H. C. (1976). *Identification of states of coping utilization physiological and psychological data.* Unpublished master's thesis, University of Michigan, Ann Arbor, MI.

Erickson, H. (Guest ed.). (1996). Holistic healing: Intra/inter relations of person and environment. *Issues of Mental Health Nursing, 17*(3), vii–viii.

Erickson, H. (2002). Facilitating generativity and ego integrity: Applying Ericksonian methods to the aging population. In B. B. Geary & J. K. Zeig (Eds.), *The handbook of Ericksonian psychotherapy.* Phoenix, AZ: Zeig Tucker.

Erickson, H. (Ed.). (2006a). *Modeling and role-modeling: A view from the client's world.* Cedar Park, TX: Unicorns Unlimited.

Erickson, H. (2006b). Connecting. In H. Erickson (Ed.), *Modeling and role-modeling: A view from the client's world* (pp. 300–322). Cedar Park, TX: Unicorns Unlimited.

Erickson, H. (2006c). Facilitating development. In: H. Erickson (Ed.), *Modeling and role-modeling: A view from the client's world* (pp. 346–390). Cedar Park, TX: Unicorns Unlimited.

Erickson, H. (2006d). Nurturing growth. In H. Erickson (Ed.), *Modeling and role-modeling: A view from the client's world* (pp. 324–345). Cedar Park, TX: Unicorns Unlimited.

Erickson, H. (2006e). The healing process. In H. Erickson (Ed.), *Modeling and role-modeling: A view from the client's world* (pp. 411–434). Cedar Park, TX: Unicorns Unlimited.

Erickson, H. (2007). Philosophy and theory of holism. *Nursing Clinics of North America, 42,* 140.

Erickson, H. (2008). Nursing of the body, mind & spirit? *Advance for Nurses, 6*(20), 31–32.

Erickson, H. (2010). Paradigm choices: Implications for nursing knowledge. In H. Erickson (Ed.), *Exploring the context and essence of holistic nursing: Modeling and role-modeling for nurse educators.* Cedar Park, TX: Unicorns Unlimited. In press.

Erickson, H., Tomlin, E., & Swain, M. A. (2009). *Modeling and role-modeling: A theory and paradigm for nursing.* Cedar Park, TX: EST.

Erickson, H. C., & Swain, M. A. (1982). A model for assessing potential adaptation to stress. *Research in Nursing and Health, 5,* 93–101.

Erickson, M. (2006). Attachment, loss and reattachment. In H. Erickson (Ed.), *Modeling and role-modeling: A view from the client's world* (pp. 208–237). Cedar Park, TX: Unicorns Unlimited.

Erickson, M., Erickson, H., & Jensen, B. (2006). Affiliated-individuation and self-actualization: Need satisfaction as prerequisite. In H. Erickson (Ed.), *Modeling and role-modeling: A view from the client's world* (pp. 182–207). Cedar Park, TX: Unicorns Unlimited.

Frisch, N. C., & Frisch, L. E. (2010). *Psychiatric mental health nursing.* (2nd ed.). Albany, NY: Delmar.

Jablonski, K. & Duke, G. (2012). Pain management in persons who are terminally ill in rural acute care: Barriers and facilitators. *Journal of Hospice and Palliative Nursing. 14*(8), 533–540.

Hertz, J. E. (2013). Self-care. In I. M. Lubkin & P. D. Larsen (Eds.), *Chronic illness: Impact and intervention* (8th ed., chap. 14). Sudbury, MA: Jones and Bartlett.

Hertz, J. E., Irving, B. L., & Bowman, S. S. (2010). Issues for a culturally-diverse society. In H. L. Erickson (Ed.), *Exploring the interface between the philosophy and discipline of holistic nursing: Modeling and role-modeling at work* (pp. 228-261). Cedar Park, TX: Unicorns Unlimited.

Hertz, J. E., Koren, M. E., Rossetti, J., & Robertson, J. F. (2008). Early identification of relocation risk in older adult with critical illness. *Critical Care Nursing Quarterly, 31*(1), 59–64.

Kübler-Ross, E. (1969). *On death and dying.* London: Tavistock.

Lach, H. W., Hertz, J. E., Pomeroy, S. H., Resnick, B., & Buckwalter, K. C. (2013). The challenges and benefits of distance mentoring. *Journal of Professional Nursing, 29*(1), 39–48.

Lindeman, E. (1944). Symptomatology and management of acute grief. *American Journal of Psychiatry, 101*, 141–148.

Maslow, A. (1968). *Toward a psychology of being* (2nd ed.). New York: D. Van Nostrand.

Maslow, A. (1982). *The farthest reaches of human nature.* New York: D. Van Nostrand.

Mitty, E., Resnick, B., Allen, J., Bakerjian, D., Hertz, J., Gardner, W. et al. (2010). Nursing delegation and medication administration in assisted living. *Nursing Administration Quarterly, 34*(2), 162–171.

Perese, E. (2012). *Psychiatric advanced practice nursing: A biopsychosocial foundation for practice.* Philadelphia: F. A. Davis.

Schim, S., Benkert, R., Bell, S., Walker, D., & Danford, C. (2007). Social justice: Added metaparadigm concept for urban health nursing. *Public Health Nursing, 24*(1), 73–80.

Selye, H. (1974). *Stress without distress.* Philadelphia: J. B. Lippincott.

Selye, H. (1976). *The stress of life* (rev. ed.). New York: McGraw-Hill.

Selye, H. (1980). *Selye's guide to stress research* (vol. 1). New York: Van Nostrand Reinhold.

Selye, H. (1985). History and present status of the stress concept. In A. Monat & R. S. Lazarus (Eds.), *Stress and coping: An anthology* (pp. 17–29). New York: Columbia University Press.

Walker, M., & Erickson, H. (2006). Mind, body and spirit relations. In: H. Erickson (Ed.), *Modeling and role-modeling: A view from the client's world* (pp. 67–91). Cedar Park, TX: Unicorns Unlimited.

Wazlawick, P. (1967). *Pragmatics of human communication: A study of interactional patterns, pathologies, and paradoxes.* New York: W. W. Norton.

Weber, G.J. (1999). The experiential meaning of well-being for employed mothers. *Western Journal of Nursing Research, 21*(6), 785–795.

Zeig, J. (Ed.) (1982). *Ericksonian approaches to hypnosis and psychotherapy.* New York: Brunner/Mazel.

Barbara Dossey's Theory of Integral Nursing

Barbara Montgomery Dossey

Introducing the Theorist
Overview of the Theory
Applications to Practice
Practice Exemplar
Summary
References

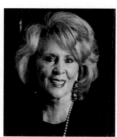

Barbara Montgomery Dossey

Introducing the Theorist

Barbara Montgomery Dossey, PhD, RN, AHN-BC, FAAN, HWNC-BC, is internationally recognized as a pioneer in the holistic nursing movement and the integrative nurse coach movement as well as a Florence Nightingale scholar. She is Co-Director, International Nurse Coach Association (INCA), and Core Faculty, Integrative Nurse Coach Certificate Program (INCCP); International Co-Director, Nightingale Initiative for Global Health (NIGH); and Director, Holistic Nursing Consultants. She is the author or coauthor of 25 books. Her most recent books include *Nurse Coaching: Integrative Approaches for Health and Wellbeing (2015), Holistic Nursing: A Handbook for Practice* (6th ed., 2013), *The Art and Science of Nurse Coaching: The Provider's Guide to Coaching Scope and Competencies* (2013), *Florence Nightingale: Mystic, Visionary, Healer (Commemorative Edition, 2010), and Florence Nightingale Today: Healing, Leadership, Global Action* (2005).

B. M. Dossey's *theory of integral nursing* (2008, 2013) is considered a grand theory that presents the science and art of nursing. Her collaborative global nursing project, the Nightingale Initiative for Global Health (NIGH) and its initiative the Nightingale Declaration Campaign (NDC), recognizes the contributions of nurses worldwide as they engage in the promotion of global health, including the United Nations Millennium Development Goals and the Post-2015 Sustainable Development Goals. Dossey has received many awards and recognitions. She is a Fellow of the American Academy of Nursing, Board Certified by the American Holistic Nurses credentialing corporation as an advanced holistic nurse (AHN-BC), and a health and wellness nurse coach (HWNC-BC). She is a ten-time recipient of the prestigious *American Journal of Nursing* Book of the Year Award. Dossey received the 2014 Lifetime Achievement Award and was named the 1985 Holistic Nurse of the Year by the American Holistic Nurse's Association. With her husband, Larry, she received the 2003 Archon Award from Sigma Theta Tau International, the International Honor Society of Nursing, honoring the contribution that they have made to promote global health. In 2004, Barbara and Larry also received the Pioneer of Integrative Medicine Award from the Aspen Center for Integrative Medicine, Aspen, Colorado.

Overview of the Theory

As you begin to explore the theory of integral nursing, I invite you to reflect on the following questions: Why am I here? Are my personal and professional actions sourced from my soul's purpose and wisdom? What is my calling, mission, and vision for my work in the world? How can I strengthen my passion in nursing and in my life? What am I currently doing to become more aware of my personal health and the health of my home and workplace? What am I doing locally that can affect the health and well-being of humanity and our Earth? How am I connected to my nursing colleagues and concerned citizens in my community, in other cities, and nations? What is my calling?

The theory of integral nursing is a grand theory that guides the science and art of integral nursing practice, education, research, and health-care policy. It incorporates physical, mental, emotional, social, spiritual, cultural, and environmental dimensions and an expansive worldview. It invites nurses to think widely and deeply about personal health and client, patient, and family health, as well as that of the local community and the global village. This theory recognizes the philosophical foundation and legacy of Florence Nightingale (1820–1910; Dossey, 2010; Dossey, Selanders, Beck, & Attewell, 2005) healing and healing research, the metaparadigm of

nursing (nurse, person[s], health, and environment [society]), six patterns of knowing (personal, empirics, aesthetics, ethics, not knowing, sociopolitical), integral theory, and theories outside of the discipline of nursing. It builds on the existing integral, integrative, and holistic ultidimensional theoretical nursing foundations and has been informed by the work of other nurse theorists; it is not a free-standing theory. It incorporates concepts from various philosophies and fields that include holistic, multidimensionality, integral, chaos, spiral dynamics, complexity, systems, and many other paradigms. [*Note: Concepts specific to the theory of integral nursing are in italics throughout this chapter. Please consider these words as a frame of reference and a way to explain and explore what you have observed or experienced with yourself and others.*]

Integral nursing is a comprehensive integral worldview and process that includes integrative and holistic theories and other paradigms; holistic nursing is included (embraced) and transcended (goes beyond); this integral process and integral worldview enlarges our holistic nursing knowledge and understanding of body–mind–spirit connections and our knowing, doing, and being to more comprehensive and deeper levels. To delete the word "integral" or to substitute the word "holistic" diminishes the impact of the expansiveness of the integral process and integral worldview and its implications.

The theory of integral nursing includes an integral process, integral worldview, and integral dialogues that compose *praxis*—theory in action (B. M. Dossey, 2008; 2013). An *integral process* is defined as a comprehensive way to organize multiple phenomena of human experience and reality from four perspectives: (1) the individual interior (personal/intentional), (2) individual exterior (physiology/behavioral), (3) collective interior (shared/cultural), and (4) collective exterior (systems/structures). An *integral worldview* examines values, beliefs, assumptions, meaning, purpose, and judgments related to how individuals perceive reality and relationships from the four perspectives. *Integral dialogues* are transformative and visionary explorations of ideas and possibilities across disciplines, where these four perspectives are considered as equally important to all exchanges, endeavors, and outcomes. With an increased integral awareness and an integral worldview, we are more likely to raise our collective nursing voice and power to engage in social action in our role and work of service for society—local to global.

As you read this chapter, 35 million nurses and midwives are engaged in nursing and health care around the world (World Health Organization [WHO], 2009). Together, we are collectively addressing human health—of individuals, of communities, of environments (interior and exterior) and the world as our first priority. We are educated and prepared—physically, emotionally, socially, mentally, and spiritually—to accomplish the required activities effectively—on the ground—to create a healthy world. Nurses are key in mobilizing new approaches in health education and health-care delivery in all areas of the profession and society as a whole. Theories, solutions, and evidence-based practice protocols can be shared and implemented around the world through dialogues, the Internet, and publications.

We are challenged to "act locally and think globally" and to address ways to create healthy environments (B. M. Dossey, 2013; B. M. Dossey et al., 2005). For example, we can address global warming in our personal habits at home as well as in our workplace (using green products, turning off lights when not in the room, using water efficiently) and simultaneously address our personal health and the health of the communities where we live (National Prevention Council, 2011). In 2000, the United Nations Millennium Goals were recommended to articulate clearly how to achieve health and decrease health disparities (United Nations, 2000). As we expand our awareness of individual and collective states of healing consciousness and integral dialogues, we are able to explore integral ways of knowing, doing, and being. We can unite 35 million nurses and midwives and concerned citizens through the Internet to create a healthy world through many endeavors such as the Nightingale Declaration (B. M. Dossey et al., 2013; NIGH,

2013; WHO, 2009). You are invited to sign the Nightingale Declaration at www.nightingaledeclaration.net. Our Nightingale nursing legacy, as discussed in the next section, is foundational to the theory of integral nursing and to understanding our important roles as 21st-century nurses.

Philosophical Foundation: Florence Nightingale's Legacy

Florence Nightingale, the philosophical founder of modern secular nursing and the first recognized nurse theorist, was an *integralist.* Her worldview focused on the individual and the collective, the inner and outer, and human and nonhuman concerns. She identified environmental determinants (clean air, water, food, houses, etc.) and social determinants (poverty, education, family relationships, employment)—local to global. She also experienced and recorded her personal understanding of the connection with the Divine—that is, awareness that something greater than she, the Divine, was present in all aspects of her life.

Nightingale's work was *social action* that clearly articulated the science and art of an integral worldview for nursing, health care, and humankind. Her social action was also *sacred activism* (Harvey, 2007), the fusion of the deepest spiritual knowledge with radical action in the world. Nightingale was ahead of her time; her dedicated and focused 50 years of work and service still inform and affect the nursing profession and our global mission of health and healing. In the 1880s, Nightingale began to write in letters that it would take 100 to 150 years before sufficiently educated and experienced nurses would arrive to change the health-care system. We are that generation of 21st-century Nightingales who can transform health care and carry forth her vision to create a healthy world (B. M. Dossey, 2013; B. M. Dossey, Luck, & Schaub, 2015; Beck, Dossey, & Rushton, 2011; McDonald, 2001–2012; Mittelman et al., 2010).

Personal Journey Developing the Theory of Integral Nursing

As a young nurse attending my first nursing theory conference in the late 1960s, I was captivated by nursing theory and the eloquent visionary words of these theorists as they spoke about the science and art of nursing. This opened my heart and mind to exploration and to the necessity to understand and use nursing theory. Thus, I began my professional commitment to address theory in all endeavors as well as to increase my knowledge of other disciplines that could inform a deeper understanding about the human experience. I realized that nursing was not either "science" or "art," but both. From the beginning of my critical care and cardiovascular nursing focus, I learned how to combine science and technology with the art of nursing. For example, for patients with severe pain after an acute myocardial infarction, I gave pain medication while simultaneously guiding them in a relaxation or imagery practice to enhance relaxation and release anxiety. I also experienced a difference in myself when I used this approach to combine the science and art of nursing.

In the late 1960s, I began to study and attend workshops on holistic and mind–body-related ideas and to read in other disciplines, such as systems theory, quantum physics, integral theory, Eastern and Western philosophy, and mysticism. I was reading theorists from nursing and other disciplines that informed my knowing, doing, and being in caring, healing, and holism. My husband, a physician of internal medicine who was caring for critically ill patients and their families, was with me at the beginning of this journey of discovery. As we cared for patients and families— some of our greatest teachers—we reflected on how to blend the art of caring–healing modalities with the science of technology and traditional modalities. I discussed these ideas with a critical care and cardiovascular nursing soulmate, Cathie Guzzetta. We began writing teaching protocols and presenting in critical care courses as well as writing textbooks and articles with other contributors.

My husband and I both had health challenges—mine was postcorneal transplant rejection, and my husband's challenge was blinding migraine headaches. We both began to take courses related to body–mind–spirit

therapies (biofeedback, relaxation, imagery, music, meditation, and other reflective practices and touch therapies) and began to incorporate them into our daily lives. As we strengthened our capacities with self-care and self-regulation modalities, our personal and professional philosophies and clinical practices changed. As we integrated these modalities into our own lives, we began to introduce them into the traditional health-care setting that today is called integrative and integral health care.

As a founding member in 1980 of the American Holistic Nurses Association (AHNA) and with my AHNA colleagues, our collective holistic nursing endeavors were recognized as the specialty of holistic nursing by the American Nurses Association (ANA) in November 2006 (AHNA & ANA, 2007, 2013). Holistic nursing can now be expanded by using an integral lens. An integral perspective can also further our endeavors in national health-care reform and the implementation of Healthy People 2020 as a national strategy. The emerging movement for professional nurse coaching (Dossey, Luck, & Schaub, 2015; Hess et al., 2013) and strategies to increase patient engagement (Weil, 2013) can be strengthened when considered from an integral perspective.

Beginning in 1992 in London, my Florence Nightingale primary, historical research of studying and synthesizing her original letters, army and public health documents, manuscripts, and books, deepened my understanding of her relevance for nursing. My professional mission now is to articulate and use the integral process and integral worldview in my nursing, integrative nurse coaching, and interprofessional endeavors, and to explore rituals of healing with many. My sustained nursing career focus with nursing colleagues on wholeness, unity, and healing and my Florence Nightingale scholarship have resulted in numerous protocols and standards for practice, education, research, and health-care policy. My integral focus since 2000 and my many conversations with Ken Wilber and the integral team and other interdisciplinary integral colleagues has led to my development of the theory of integral nursing.

Theory of Integral Nursing Developmental Process and Intentions

The theory of integral nursing advances the evolutionary growth processes, stages, and levels of human development and consciousness toward a comprehensive integral philosophy and understanding. It can assist nurses to map human capacities that begin with healing and evolve to the transpersonal self in connection with the Divine, however defined or identified, in their endeavors to create a healthy world.

The theory of integral nursing has three intentions: (1) to embrace the unitary whole person and the complexity of the nursing profession and health care; (2) to explore the direct application of an integral process and integral worldview that includes four perspectives of realities—the individual interior and exterior and the collective interior and exterior; and (3) to expand nurses' capacities as 21st-century Nightingales, health diplomats, and integral nurse coaches for integral health—local to global.

Integral Foundation and the Integral Model

The theory of integral nursing adapts the work of Ken Wilber, one of the most significant American new-paradigm philosophers, to strengthen the central concept of healing. His elegant, four-quadrant model was developed over 35 years. In the eight-volume *The Collected Works of Ken Wilber* (Wilber, 1999, 2000a), Wilber synthesizes the best known and most influential thinkers to show that no individual or discipline can determine reality or lay claim to all the answers. Many concepts within the integral nursing theory have been researched or are in formative stages of development within integral medicine, integral health-care administration, integral business, integral health-care education, and integral psychotherapy (Wilber, 2000a, 2000b, 2005a, 2005b, 2006). Within the nursing profession, other nurses are exploring integral and related theories and ideas. When nurses use an integral lens, they are more likely to expand nurses' roles in transdisciplinary dialogues and to explore commonalities and differences across

disciplines (J. Baye, personal communication, 2007; Clark, 2006; Fiandt et al., 2003; Frisch, 2013; Jarrin, 2007; Quinn, Smith, Rittenbaugh, Swanson, & Watson, 2003; Watson, 2005; Zahourek, 2013).

Content, Context, and Process

To present the theory of integral nursing, Barbara Barnum's (2005) framework to critique a nursing theory—content, context, and process—provides an organizing structure that is most useful. The philosophical assumptions of the theory of integral nursing are as follows:

1. An integral understanding recognizes the individual as an energy field connected to the energy fields of others and the wholeness of humanity; the world is open, dynamic, interdependent, fluid, and continuously interacting with changing variables that can lead to greater complexity and order.
2. An integral worldview is a comprehensive way to organize multiple phenomena of human experience from four perspectives of reality: (a) individual interior (subjective, personal); (b) individual exterior (objective, behavioral); (c) collective interior (interobjective, cultural); and (d) collective exterior (interobjective, systems/structures).
3. Healing is a process inherent in all living things; it may occur with curing of symptoms, but it is not synonymous with curing.
4. Integral health is experienced by a person as wholeness with development toward personal growth and expanding states of consciousness to deeper levels of personal and collective understanding of one's physical, mental, emotional, social, spiritual, cultural, environmental dimensions.
5. Integral nursing is founded on an integral worldview using integral language and knowledge that integrates integral life practices and skills each day.
6. Integral nursing is broadly defined to include knowledge development and all ways of knowing that also recognizes the emergent patterns of not knowing.

7. An integral nurse is an instrument in the healing process and facilitates healing through her or his knowing, doing, and being.

8. Integral nursing is applicable in practice, education, research, and health-care policy.

Content Components

Content of a nursing theory includes the subject matter and building blocks that give a theory its form. It comprises the stable elements that are acted on or that do the acting. In the theory of integral nursing, the subject matter and building blocks are (1) healing, (2) the meta-paradigm of nursing, (3) patterns of knowing, (4) the four quadrants that are adapted from Wilber's (2000a) integral theory (individual interior [subjective, personal/intentional], individual exterior [objective, behavioral], collective interior [intersubjective, cultural], and collective exterior [interobjective, systems/structures]), and (5) Wilber's "all quadrants, all levels, all lines" (Wilber, 2000a, 2006).

Content Component 1: Healing. The first content component in a theory of integral nursing is *healing*, illustrated as a diamond shape in Figure 13-1A. The theory of integral nursing enfolds from the central core concept of healing. Healing includes knowing, doing, and being, and is a lifelong journey and process of bringing together aspects of oneself at deeper levels of harmony and inner knowing leading toward integration. This healing process places us in a space to face our fears, to seek and express self in its fullness where we can learn to trust life, creativity, passion, and love. Each aspect of healing has equal importance and value that leads to more complex levels of understanding and meaning.

Healing capacities are inherent in all living things. No one can take healing away from life; however, we often get "stuck" in our healing or forget that we possess it due to life's continuing challenges and perceived barriers to wholeness. Healing can take place at all levels of human experience, but it may not occur simultaneously in every realm. In truth, healing will most likely not occur simultaneously or even in all realms, and yet the person may still

Fig 13 • 1   *A,* Healing.   *Source: Copyright © Barbara Dossey, 2007.*

have a perception of healing having occurred (B. M. Dossey, 2013; Gaydos, 2004, 2005).

Healing embraces the individual as an energy field that is connected with the energy fields of all humanity and the world. Healing is transformed when we consider four perspectives of reality in any moment: (1) the individual interior (personal/intentional), (2) individual exterior (physiology/behavioral), (3) collective interior (shared/cultural), and (4) collective exterior (systems/structures). Using our reflective integral lens of these four perspectives of reality assists us to more likely experience a unitary grasp within the complexity that emerges in healing.

Healing is not predictable; it may occur with curing of symptoms, but it is not synonymous with curing. Curing may not always occur, but the potential for healing is always present even until one's last breath. Intention and intentionality are key factors in healing (Barnum, 2004; Engebretson, 1998; Zahourek, 2004; 2013). Intention is the conscious determination to do a specific thing or to act in a specific manner; it is the mental state of being committed to, planning to, or trying to perform an action. Intentionality is the quality of an intentionally performed action.

Content Component 2: Metaparadigm of Nursing. The second content component in the theory of integral nursing is the recognition of the *metaparadigm* in a nurse theory: nurse, person/s, health, and environment (society; Fig. 13-1B) (Fawcett, Watson, Neuman, Walker, & Fitzpatrick, 2001). Starting with healing at the center, a Venn diagram surrounds healing and implies the interrelation, interdependence, and effect of these domains as each informs and influences the others; a change in one will create a degree(s) of change in the other(s), thus affecting healing at many

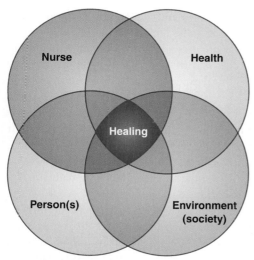

Fig 13 • 1 *B,* Healing and Meta-Paradigm of Nursing. *Source: Copyright © Barbara Dossey, 2007.*

levels. These concepts are important to the theory of integral nursing because they are encompassed within the quadrants of human experience as seen in Content Component 4.

An *integral nurse* is defined as a 21st-century Nightingale. Using terms coined by Patricia Hinton Walker, PhD, RN, FAAN (personal communication, May 15, 2007), nurses' endeavors of social action and sacred activism engage "nurses as health diplomats" and "integral nurse coaches" that are "coaching for integral health." As nurses strive to be integrally informed, they are more likely to move to a deeper experience of a connection with the Divine or Infinite, however defined or identified. *Integral nursing* provides a comprehensive way to organize multiple phenomena of human experience in the four perspectives of reality as previously described. The nurse is an instrument in the healing process, bringing her or his whole self into relationship to the whole self of another or a group of significant others and thus reinforcing the meaning and experience of oneness and unity.

A *person(s)* is defined as an individual (patient/client, family members, significant others) who is engaged with a nurse who is respectful of this person's subjective experiences about health, health beliefs, values, sexual orientation, and personal preferences. It also includes an individual nurse who interacts with a nursing colleague, other interprofessional health-care team members, or a group of community members or other groups.

Integral health is the process through which we reshape basic assumptions and worldviews about well-being and see death as a natural process of the cycle of life. Integral health may be symbolically seen as a jewel with many facets that is reflected as a "bright gem" or a "rough stone" depending on one's situation and personal growth that influence states of health, health beliefs, and values (Gaydos, 2004). The jewel may also be seen as a spiral or as a symbol of transformation to higher states of consciousness to more fully understand the essential nature of our beingness as energy fields and expressions of wholeness (Newman, 2003). This includes evolving one's state of consciousness to higher levels of personal and collective understanding of one's physical, mental, emotional, social, and spiritual dimensions. It acknowledges the individual's interior and exterior experiences and the shared collective interior and exterior experiences with others, where authentic power is recognized within each person. Disease and illness at the physical level may manifest for many reasons and variables. It is important *not* to equate physical health, mental health, and spiritual health, as they are not the same thing. They are facets of the whole jewel of integral health.

An *integral environment(s)* has both interior and exterior aspects (Samueli Institute, 2013). The *interior* environment includes the individual's mental, emotional, and spiritual dimensions, including feelings and meanings as well as the brain and its components that constitute the internal aspect of the exterior self. It includes patterns that may not be understood or may manifest related to various situations or relationships. These patterns may be related to living and nonliving people and things—for example, a deceased relative, a pet, lost precious object(s) that surface through flashes of memories stimulated by a current situation (e.g., a touch may bring forth past memories of abuse, suffering). Insights gained through dreams and other reflective practices that reveal symbols, images, and other connections also influence one's internal environment. The *exterior* environment includes objects that can be seen and measured that are related to the physical and social in some form in any of the gross, subtle, and causal levels that are expanded later in Content Component 4.

Content Component 3: Patterns of Knowing. The third content component in a theory of integral nursing is the recognition of the patterns of knowing in nursing (Fig. 13-1C). These six patterns of knowing are personal, empirics, aesthetics, ethics, not knowing, and sociopolitical. As a way to organize nursing knowledge, Carper (1978) in her now-classic 1978 article identified the four fundamental patterns of knowing (personal, empirics, ethics, aesthetics) followed by the introduction of the pattern of not knowing by Munhall (1993) and the pattern of sociopolitical knowing by White (1995). All of these patterns continue to be refined and reframed with new applications and interpretations (Averill & Clements, 2007; Barnum, 2003; Burkhardt & Najai-Jacobson, 2013; Chinn & Kramer, 2010; Cowling, 2004; Fawcett et al., 2001; Halifax, Dossey, & Rushton, 2007; Koerner, 2011; McElligott, 2013; McKivergin, 2008; Meleis,

2012; Newman, 2003). These patterns of knowing assist nurses in bringing themselves into a full presence in the moment, integrating aesthetics with science, and developing the flow of ethical experience with thinking and acting.

Personal knowing is the nurse's dynamic process of being whole that focuses on the synthesis of perceptions and being with self. It may be developed through art, meditation, dance, music, stories, and other expressions of the authentic and genuine self in daily life and nursing practice.

Empirical knowing is the science of nursing that focuses on formal expression, replication, and validation of scientific competence in nursing education and practice. It is expressed in models and theories and can be integrated into evidence-based practice. Empirical indicators are accessed through the known senses that are subject to direct observation, measurement, and verification.

Aesthetic knowing is the art of nursing that focuses on how to explore experiences and meaning in life with self or another that includes authentic presence, the nurse as a facilitator of healing, and the artfulness of a healing environment. It calls forth resources and inner strengths from the nurse to be a facilitator in the healing process. It is the integration and

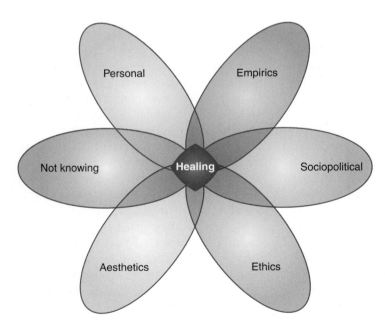

Fig 13 • 1 *C,* Healing and patterns of knowing in nursing. *Source: Adapted from B. Carper (1978). Copyright © Barbara Dossey, 2007.*

expression of all the other patterns of knowing in nursing praxis. By combining knowledge, experience, instinct, and intuition, the nurse connects with a patient/client to explore the meaning of a situation about the human experiences of life, health, illness, and death.

Ethical knowing is the moral knowledge in nursing that focuses on behaviors, expressions, and dimensions of both morality and ethics. It includes valuing and clarifying situations to create formal moral and ethical behaviors intersecting with legally prescribed duties. It emphasizes respect for the person, the family, and the community that encourages connectedness and relationships that enhance attentiveness, responsiveness, communication, and moral action.

Not knowing is the capacity to use healing presence, to be open spontaneously to the moment with no preconceived answers or goals to be obtained. It engages authenticity, mindfulness, openness, receptivity, surprise, mystery, and discovery with self and others in the subjective space and the intersubjective space that allows for new solutions, possibilities, and insights to emerge.

Sociopolitical knowing addresses the important contextual variables of social, economic, geographic, cultural, political, historical, and other key factors in theoretical, evidence-based practice and research. This pattern includes informed critique and social justice for the voices of the underserved in all areas of society along with protocols to reduce health disparities. [*Note: Because all patterns of knowing in the theory of integral nursing are superimposed on Wilber's four quadrants, these patterns will be primarily positioned as seen; however, they may also appear in one, several, or all quadrants and inform all other quadrants.*]

Content Component 4: Quadrants. The fourth content component in the theory of integral nursing examines four perspectives for all known aspects of reality; expressed another way, it is how we look at and/or describe anything (Fig. 13-1D). Healing, the core concept in the theory of integral nursing, is transformed by adapting Ken Wilber's (2000b) integral model. Starting with healing at the

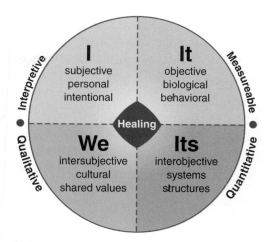

Fig 13 • 1   *D,* Healing and the four quadrants (I, We, It, Its).   *Source: Adapted with permission from Ken Wilber. http://www.kenwilber.com. Copyright © Barbara Dossey, 2007.*

center to represent our integral nursing philosophy, human capacities, and global mission, dotted horizontal and vertical lines illustrate that each quadrant can be understood as permeable and porous, with each quadrant's experience(s) integrally informing and empowering all other quadrant experiences. Within each quadrant, we see "I," "We," "It," and "Its" to represent four perspectives of realities that are already part of our everyday language and awareness.

Virtually all human languages use first-person, second-person, and third-person pronouns to indicate three basic dimensions of reality (Wilber, 2000b). First-person is "the person who is speaking," which includes pronouns like *I, me, mine* in the singular, and *we, us, ours* in the plural (Wilber, 2000b, 2005a). Second-person means "the person who is spoken to," which includes pronouns like *you* and *yours.* Third-person is "the person or thing being spoken about," such as *she, her, he, him,* or *they, it,* and *its.* For example, if I am speaking about my new car, "I" am first-person, and "you" are second-person, and the new car is third-person. If you and I are communicating, the word "we" is used to indicate that we understand each other. "We" is technically first person plural, but if you and I are communicating, then you are second person and my first person is part of this extraordinary "we." So we represent first-, second- and third-person as: "I," "We," "It" and "Its."

These four quadrants show the four primary dimensions or perspectives of how we experience the world; these are represented graphically as the upper-left (UL), upper-right (UR), lower-left (LL), and lower-right (LR) quadrants. It is simply the inside and the outside of an individual and the inside and outside of the collective. It includes expanded states of consciousness where one feels a connection with the Divine and the vastness of the universe, the infinite that is beyond words. Integral nursing considers all of these areas in our personal development and any area of practice, education, research, and healthcare policy—local to global. Each quadrant, which is intricately linked and bound to each

other, carries its own truths and language (Wilber, 2000b). The specifics of the quadrants are provided in Table 13-1.

• **Upper-left (UL).** In this "I" space (subjective), the world of the individual's interior experiences can be found. These are the thoughts, emotions, memories, perceptions, immediate sensations, and states of mind (imagination, fears, feelings, beliefs, values, esteem, cognitive capacity, emotional maturity, moral development, and spiritual maturity). Integral nursing starts with "I."
(*Note: When working with various cultures, it is important to remember that within many cultures, the "I" comes last or is never verbalized or recognized as the focus is on the "We" and relationships. However, this development of the "I" and an awareness of one's personal value, beliefs, and ethics is critical.*)

Table 13 • 1   Integral Model and Quadrants

Upper left	Upper right
Individual interior (intentional/personal)	Individual exterior (behavioral/biological)
"I" space includes self and consciousness (self-care, fears, feelings, beliefs, values, esteem, cognitive capacity, emotional maturity, moral development, spiritual maturity, personal communication skills, etc.)	"It" space that includes brain and organisms (physiology, pathophysiology [cells, molecules, limbic system, neurotransmitters, physical sensations], biochemistry, chemistry, physics, behaviors [skill development in health, nutrition, exercise, etc.])
• **Subjective** • **Interpretive** • **Qualitative** **I** **It**	• **Objective** • **Observable** • **Quantitative**
We **Its**	
Collective interior (cultural/shared)	Collective exterior (systems/structures)
"We" space includes the relationship to each other and the culture and worldview (shared understanding, shared vision, shared meaning, shared leadership and other values, integral dialogues and communication/morale, etc.)	"Its" space includes the relation to social systems and environment, organizational structures and systems [in healthcare—financial and billing systems], educational systems, infomation technology, mechanical structures and transportation, regulatory structures [environmental and governmental policies, etc.]
Lower left	**Lower right**

Source: Ken Wilber, Integral Psychology: Consciousness, Spirit, Psychology, Therapy (Boston: Shambhala, 2000). Table adapted with permission from Ken Wilber. http://www.kenwilber.com. Copyright © by Barbara M. Dossey, 2007.

- **Upper-right (UR).** In this "It" (objective) space, the world of the individual's exterior can be found. This includes the material body (physiology [cells, molecules, neuro-transmitters, limbic system], biochemistry, chemistry, physics), integral patient care plans, skill development (health, fitness, exercise, nutrition, etc.), behaviors, leadership skills, and integral life practices and anything that we can touch or observe scientifically in time and space. Integral nursing with our nursing colleagues and health-care team members includes the "It" of new behaviors, integral assessment and care plans, leadership, and skills development.
- **Lower-left (LL).** In this "We" (intersubjective) space resides the interior collective of how we can come together to share our cultural background, stories, values, meanings, vision, language, relationships, and to form partnerships to achieve a healing mission. This can decrease our fragmentation and enhance collaborative practice and deep dialogue around things that really matter. Integral nursing is built on "We."
- **Lower-right (LR).** In this "Its" space (interobjective) the world of the collective, exterior things can be found. This includes social systems/structures, networks, organizational structures, and systems (including financial and billing systems in health care), information technology, regulatory structures (environmental and governmental policies, etc.), any aspect of the technological environment, and the natural world. Integral nursing identifies the "Its" in the structure that can be enhanced to create more integral awareness and integral partnerships to achieve health and healing—local to global.

We see that the left-hand quadrants (UL, LL) describe aspects of reality as interpretive and qualitative (see Fig. 13-1D). In contrast, the right-hand quadrants (UR, LR) describe aspects of reality as measurable and quantitative. When we fail to consider these subjective, intersubjective, objective, and interobjective aspects of reality, our endeavors and initiatives

become fragmented and narrow, inhibiting our ability to reach meaningful outcomes and goals. The four quadrants are a result of the differences and similarities in Wilber's investigation of the many aspects of identified reality. The model describes the territory of our own awareness that is already present within us and an awareness of things outside of us. These quadrants help us connect the dots of the actual process to more deeply understand who we are, and how we are related to others and all things.

Content Component 5: AQAL (All Quadrants, All Levels). The fifth content component in the theory of integral nursing is the exploration of Wilber's "all quadrants, all levels, all lines, all states, all types" or A-Q-A-L (pronounced *ah-qwul*), as seen in Figure 13-1E. These levels, lines, states, and types are important elements of any comprehensive map of reality. The integral model simply assists us in further articulating and connecting all areas, awareness, and depth in these four quadrants.

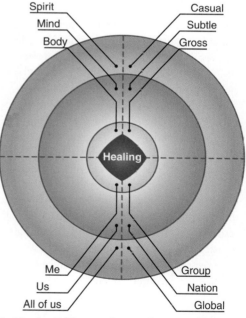

Fig 13 • 1 *E*, Theory of integral nursing (healing, metaparadigm, patterns of knowing in nursing, four quadrants, and AQAL). *Source: Adapted with permission from Ken Wilber. http://www.kenwilber.com. Copyright © Barbara Dossey, 2007.*

Briefly stated, these levels, lines, states, and types are as follows:

• **Levels:** Levels of development that become permanent with growth and maturity (e.g., cognitive, relational, psychosocial, physical, mental, emotional, spiritual) that represent a level of increased organization or level of complexity. These levels are also referred to as waves and stages of development. Each individual possesses both the masculine and the feminine voice or energy. One is not superior to the other; they are two equivalent types at each level of consciousness and development.

• **Lines:** Developmental areas that are known as multiple intelligences (e.g., cognitive line [awareness of what is]; interpersonal line [how I relate socially to others]; emotional/affective line [the full spectrum of emotions]; moral line [awareness of what should be]; needs line [Maslow's hierarchy of needs]; aesthetics line [self-expression of art, beauty, and full meaning]; self-identity line [who am I?]; spiritual line [where "spirit" is viewed as its own line of unfolding, and not just as ground and highest state], and values line [what a person considers most important; studied by Clare Graves and brought forward by Don Beck, 2007, in his spiral dynamics integral, which is beyond the scope of this chapter]).

• **States:** Temporary changing forms of awareness (e.g., waking, dreaming, deep sleep, altered meditative states [such as occurs in meditation, yoga, contemplative prayer, etc.]; altered states [due to mood swings, physiology and pathophysiology shifts with disease/illness, seizures, cardiac arrest, low or high oxygen saturation, drug-induced]; peak experiences [triggered by intense listening to music, walks in nature, lovemaking, mystical experiences such as hearing the voice of God or of a deceased person, etc.].

• **Types:** Differences in personality and masculine and feminine expressions and development (e.g., cultural creative types, personality types, enneagram).

This part of the theory of integral nursing (see Fig. 13-1E) starts with healing at the center surrounded by three increasing concentric circles with dotted lines of the four quadrants. This part of the integral theory moves to higher orders of complexity through personal growth, development, expanded stages of consciousness (permanent and actual milestones of growth and development), and evolution. These levels or stages of development can also be expressed as being self-absorbed (such as a child or infant) to ethnocentric (centers on group, community, tribe, nation) to world-centric (care and concern for all peoples regardless of race or national origin, color, sex, gender, sexual orientation, creed, and to the global level).

In the UL, the "I" space, the emphasis is on the unfolding "awareness" from body to mind to spirit. Each increasing circle includes the lower as it moves to the higher level.

In the UR, the "It" space, is the external of the individual. Every state of consciousness has a felt energetic component that is expressed from the wisdom traditions as three recognized bodies: gross, subtle, and causal (Wilber, 2000b, 2005). We can think of these three bodies as the increasing capacities of a person toward higher levels of consciousness. Each level is a specific vehicle that provides the actual support for any state of awareness. The *gross* body is the individual physical, material, sensorimotor body that we experience in our daily activities. The *subtle* body occurs when we are not aware of the gross body of dense matter, but of a shifting to a light, energy, emotional feelings, and fluid and flowing images. Examples might be in our shift during a dream, during different types of bodywork, walks in nature, or other experiences that move us to a profound state of bliss. The causal body is the body of the infinite that is beyond space and time. Causal also includes *nonlocality* in which minds of individuals are not separate in space and time (L. Dossey, 1989; 2013). When this is applied to consciousness, separate minds behave as if they are linked, regardless of how far apart in space and time they may be. Nonlocal consciousness may underlie phenomena such as remote healing, intercessory prayer, telepathy, premonitions, as well as so-called miracles. Nonlocality also implies that the soul does not die with the death of the physical body—hence, immortality forms some dimension of consciousness. Nonlocality can also be both upper and lower quadrant phenomena.

The LL, the "We" space, is the interior collective dimension of individuals that come together. The concentric circles from the center outward represent increasing levels of complexity of our relational aspect of shared cultural values, as this is where teamwork and the interdisciplinary and transpersonal disciplinary development occur. The inner circle represents the individual labeled as *me;* the second circle represents a larger group labeled *us;* the third circle is labeled as *all of us* to represent the largest group consciousness that expands to all people. These last two circles may include people but also animals, nature, and nonliving things that are important to individuals.

The LR, the "Its" space, the exterior social system and structures of the collective, is represented with concentric circles. An example within the inner circle might be a *group* of health-care professionals in a hospital clinic or department or the complex hospital system and structure. The middle circle expands in increased complexity to include a *nation;* the third concentric circle represents even greater increased complexity to the *global* level where the health of all humanity and the world are considered. It is also helpful to emphasize that these groupings are the physical dynamics such as the working structure of a group of health care professionals versus the relational aspect that is a LL aspect, and the physical and technical structural of a hospital or a clinic.

Integral nurses strive to integrate concepts and practices related to body, mind, and spirit (the all-levels) in self, culture, and nature ("all quadrants" part). The individual interior and exterior—"I" and "It"—as well as the collective interior and exterior—"We" and "Its"—must be developed, valued, and integrated into all aspects of culture and society. The AQAL integral approach suggests that we consciously touch all of these areas and do so in relation to self, to others, and the natural world. Yet to be integrally informed does *not* mean that we have to master all of these areas; we just need

to be aware of them and choose to integrate integral awareness and integral practices. Because these areas are already part of our being-in-the-world and cannot be imposed from the outside (they are part of our makeup from the inside), our challenge is to identify specific areas for development and find new ways to deepen our daily integral life practices.

Structure

The structure of the theory of integral nursing is shown in Figure 13-1F. All content components are represented together as an overlay that creates a mandala to symbolize wholeness. Healing is placed at the center, then the metaparadigm of nursing, the patterns of knowing, the four quadrants, and all quadrants and all levels of growth, development, and evolution. [*Note: Although the patterns of knowing are superimposed as they are in the various quadrants, they can also fit into other quadrants.*]

Using the language of Ken Wilber (2000b) and Don Beck (2007) and his spiral dynamics integral, individuals move through primitive, infantile consciousness to an integrated language that is considered *first-tier* thinking. As they move up the spiral of growth, development, and evolution and expand their integral worldview and integral consciousness, they move into what is *second-tier* thinking and participation. This is a *radical leap* into holistic, systemic, and integral modes of consciousness. Wilber also expands to a *third-tier* of stages of consciousness that addresses an even deeper level of transpersonal understanding that is beyond the scope of this chapter (Wilber, 2006).

Context

Context in a nursing theory is the environment in which nursing acts occur and the nature of the world of nursing. In an integral nursing environment, the nurse strives to be an *integralist,* which means that she or he strives to be integrally informed and is challenged to further develop an integral worldview, integral life practices, and integral capacities, behaviors, and skills. The term *nurse healer* is used to describe that a nurse is an instrument in the healing process and a major part of the external

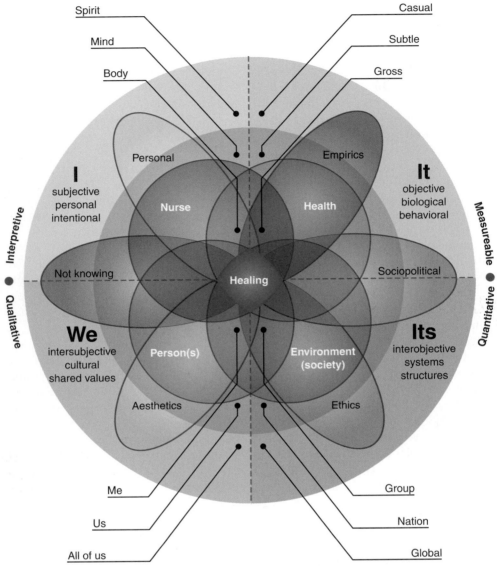

Fig 13 • 1 *F,* Healing and AQAL (all quadrants, all levels). *Source: Adapted with permission from Ken Wilber. http://www.kenwilber.com. Copyright © Barbara Dossey, 2007.*

healing environment of a patient or family. An integral nurse values, articulates, and models the integral process and integral worldview and integral life practices and self-care. Nurses assist and facilitate the individual person/s (client/patient, family, and coworkers) to access their own healing process and potentials; they do not do the actual healing. An integral nurse recognizes herself or himself as a healing environment interacting with a person, family, or colleague in a *being with* rather than always

doing to or *doing for* another person, and enters into a shared experience (or field of consciousness) that promotes healing potentials and an experience of well-being.

Relationship-centered care is valued and integrated as a model of caregiving that is based in a vision of community where three types of relationships are identified: (1) patient–practitioner relationship, (2) community–practitioner relationship, and (3) practitioner–practitioner relationship (Tresoli, 1994). *Relationship–based care* is also valued as it provides the map and highlights the most direct routes to achieve the highest levels of care and serve to patients and families (Koloroutis, 2004).

Process

Process in a nursing theory is the method by which the theory works. An *integral healing process* contains both nurse processes and patient/family and health-care worker processes (individual interior and individual exterior), and collective healing processes of individuals and of systems/structures (interior and exterior). This is the understanding of the unitary whole person interacting in mutual process with the environment.

Applications to Practice

The theory of integral nursing can guide nursing practice and strengthen our 21st-century nursing endeavors. It considers equally important data, meanings, and experiences from the personal interior, the collective interior, the individual exterior, and the collective exterior. Nursing and health care are fragmented. Collaborative practice has not been realized because only portions of reality are seen as being valid within health care and society.

The nursing profession asks nurses to wrap around "all of life" on so many levels with self and others that we can often feel overwhelmed. So how do we get a handle on "all of life?" The following questions always arise: How can overworked nurses and student nurses use an integral approach or apply the theory of integral nursing? How do we connect the complexity of so much information that arises in clinical practice? The answer is to start right now. Remember that healing, the core concept in this theory, is the innate natural phenomenon that comes from within a person and reflects the indivisible wholeness, the interconnectedness of all people, all things. The practice situation that follows addresses these questions.

Imagine that you are caring for a very ill patient who needs to be transported to the radiology department for a procedure. The current transportation protocol between the unit and the radiology department lacks continuity. In this moment, shift your feelings and your interior awareness (and believe it!) to "I am doing the best I can in this moment" and "I have all the time needed to take a deep breath and relax my tight chest and shoulder muscles." This helps you connect these four perspectives as follows: (1) the interior self (caring for yourself in this moment), (2) the exterior self (using a research-based relaxation and imagery integral practice to change your physiology), (3) the self in relationship to others (shifting your awareness creates another way of being with your patient and the radiology team member), and (4) the relationship to the exterior collective of systems/structures (considering how to work with the radiology team and department to improve a transportation procedure in the hospital).

Professional burnout is high, with many nurses disheartened. Self-care is a low priority; time is not given or valued within practice settings to address basic self-care such as short breaks for personal needs and meals. This is worsened by short staffing and overtime. Also, we do not consistently listen to the pain and suffering that nurses experience within the profession, nor do we consistently listen to the pain and suffering of the patient and family members or our colleagues (Dossey, Luck, & Schaub, 2015; McEligott, 2013). Often there is a lack of respect for each other, with verbal abuse occurring on many levels in the workplace.

Nurse retention and a global nursing shortage are at a crisis level throughout the world (International Council of Nurses, 2004). As nurses deepen their understanding related to an integral process and integral worldview and use daily integral life practices, we will more consistently be healthy and model health and understand the complexities within healing and society. This enhances nurses' capacities for empowerment, leadership, and acting as change agents for a healthy world.

An integral worldview and approach can help each nurse and student nurse increase her or his self-awareness, as well as the awareness of how self affects others—that is the patient, family, colleagues, and the workplace and community. As the nurse discovers her or his own innate healing from within, she or he is able to model self-care and how to release stress, anxiety, and fear that manifest each day in this human journey. All nursing curricula can be mapped in the integral quadrants so that students learn to think integrally about how these four perspectives create the whole (Clark 2006; Hess, 2013).

Meaning of the Theory of Integral Nursing for Practice

A key concept in the theory of integral nursing is *meaning*, which addresses that which is indicated, referred to, or signified (L. Dossey, 2003). *Philosophical meaning* is related to one's view of reality and the symbolic connections that can be grasped by reason. *Psychological meaning* is related to one's consciousness, intuition, and insight. *Spiritual meaning* is related to how one deepens personal experience of a connection with the Divine, to feel a sense of oneness, belonging and feeling of connection in life. In the next section, four integral nursing principles are discussed that provide further insight into how the theory of integral nursing guides nursing practice and meaning in practice. See Figure 13-1F for specifics for each principle.

Integral Nursing Principle 1: Nursing Starts With "I"

Integral Nursing Principle 1 recognizes the interior individual "I" (subjective) space. Each of us must value the importance of exploring one's health and well-being starting with our own personal work on many levels. In this "I" space, *integral self-care* is valued, which means that integral reflective practices become part of and can be transformative in our developmental process. This includes how each of us continually addresses our own stress, burnout, suffering, and soul pain. It can assist us to understand the necessity of personal healing and self-care related to nursing as art where we develop qualities of nursing presence and inner reflection.

Nurse presence is also used and is a way of approaching a person in a way that respects and honors the person's essence; it is relating in a way that reflects a quality of "being with" and "in collaboration with." Our own inner work also helps us to hold deeply a conscious awareness of our own roles in creating a healthy world. We recognize the importance of addressing one's own shadow as described by Jung (1981). This is a composite of personal characteristics and potentials that have been denied expression in life and of which a person is unaware; the ego denies the characteristics because they are in conflict and incompatible with a person's chosen conscious attitude.

Mindfulness is the practice of giving attention to what is happening in the present moment such as our thoughts, feelings, emotions, and sensations. To cultivate the capacity of mindfulness practice, one may include mindfulness meditation practice, centering prayer, and other reflective practices such as journaling, dream interpretation, art, music, or poetry that leads to an experience of nonseparateness and love; it involves developing the qualities of stillness and being present for one's own suffering that will also allow for full presence when with another.

In our personal process, we recognize *conscious dying* where time and thought is given to contemplate one's own death. Through a reflective practice, one rehearses and imagines one's final breath to practice preparing for one's own death. The experience prepares us to not be so attached to material things nor to spend so much time thinking about the future but to live in the moment as often as we can and to live fully until death comes. We are more likely to participate with deeper compassion in the death process and to become more fully engaged in the death process. *Death* is seen as the mirror in which the entire meaning and mystery of life is reflected—the moment of liberation. Within an integral perspective, the state of *transparency*, the understanding that there is no separation between our practice and our everyday life is recognized. This is a mature practice that is wise and empty of a separate self.

Integral Nursing Principle 2: Nursing Is Built on "We"

Integral Nursing Principle 2 recognizes the importance of the "We" (intersubjective) space. In this "We" space, nurses come together and are conscious of sharing their worldviews, beliefs, priorities, and values related to working together in ways to enhance integral self-care and integral health care. *Deep listening*, being present and focused with intention to understand what another person is expressing or not expressing, is used. *Bearing witness* to others, the state achieved through reflective and mindfulness practices, is also valued (Beck et al., 2011; B. M. Dossey, 2013; B. M. Dossey, Beck, & Rushton, 2013; Halifax et al., 2007). Through mindfulness one is able to achieve states of *equanimity*—that is, the stability of mind that allows us to be present with a good and impartial heart no matter how beneficial or difficult the conditions; it is being present for the sufferer and suffering just as it is while maintaining a spacious mindfulness in the midst of life's changing conditions. *Compassion* is where bearing witness and lovingkindness manifest in the face of suffering, and it is part of our integral practice. The realization of the self and another as *not* being separate is experienced; it is the ability to open one's heart and be present for all levels of suffering so that suffering may be transformed for others, as well as for the self. A useful phrase to consider is "I'm doing the best I can." Compassionate care assists us in living as well as when being with the dying person, the family, and others. We can touch the roots of pain and become aware of new meaning in the midst of pain, chaos, loss, grief, and also in the dying process.

An integral nurse considers *transpersonal* dimensions. This means that interactions with others move from conversations to a deeper dialogue that goes beyond the individual ego; it includes the acknowledgment and appreciation for something greater that may be referred to as spirit, nonlocality, unity, or oneness. Transpersonal dialogues contain an integral worldview and recognize the role of *spirituality* that is the search for the sacred or holy that involves feelings, thoughts, experiences, rituals, meaning, value, direction, and purpose as valid aspects of the universe. It is a unifying force of a person with all that is—the essence of beingness and relatedness that permeates all of life and is manifested in one's knowing, doing, and being; it is usually, although not universally, considered the interconnectedness with self, others, nature, and God/Life Force/Absolute/Transcendent.

Within nursing, health care, and society, there is much suffering (physical, mental, emotional, social, spiritual), moral suffering, moral distress, and soul pain. We are often called on to "be with" these difficult human experiences and to use our nursing presence. Our sense of "We" supports us to recognize the phases of suffering—"mute" suffering, "expressive" suffering, and "new identity" in suffering (Halifax et al., 2007). When we feel alone, as nurses, we experience mute suffering; this is an inability to articulate and communicate with others one's own suffering. Our challenge in nursing is to more skillfully enter into the phase of "expressive" suffering, where sufferers seek language to express their frustrations and experiences such as in sharing stories in a group process (Levin & Reich, 2013). Outcomes of this experience often move toward new identity in suffering through new meaning-making in which one makes new sense of the past, interprets new meaning in suffering, and can envision a new future. A shift in one's consciousness allows for a shift in one's capacity to be able to transform her or his suffering from causing distress to finding some new truth and meaning of it. As we create times for sharing and giving voice to our concerns, new levels of healing may happen.

From an integral perspective, *spiritual care* is an interfaith perspective that takes into account dying as a developmental and natural human process that emphasizes meaningfulness and human and spiritual values. *Religion* is recognized as the codified and ritualized beliefs, behaviors, and rituals that take place in a community of like-minded individuals involved in spirituality. Our challenge is to enter into deep dialogue to more fully understand religions different than our own so that we may be tolerant where there are differences.

Integral action is the actual practice and process that creates the condition of trust wherein a plan of care is cocreated with the patient and care can be given and received. Full attention and intention to the whole person, not merely the current presenting symptoms, illness, crisis, or tasks to be accomplished, reinforce the person's meaning and experience of community and unity. Engagement between an integral nurse and a patient and the family or with colleagues is done in a respectful manner; each patient's subjective experience about health, health beliefs, and values are explored. We deeply care for others and recognize our own mortality and that of others.

The integral nurse uses *intention*, the conscious awareness of being in the present moment with self or another person, to help facilitate the healing process; it is a volitional act of love. An awareness of the role of *intuition* is also recognized, which is the perceived knowing of events, insights, and things without a conscious use of logical, analytical processes; it may be informed by the senses to receive information. Integral nurses recognize *love* as the unconditional unity of self with others. This love then generates *lovingkindness* and the open, gentle, and caring state of mindfulness that assist one's with nursing presence.

Integral communication is a free flow of verbal and nonverbal interchange between and among people and pets and significant beings such as God/Life Force/Absolute/Transcendent. This type of sharing leads to explorations of meaning and ideas of mutual understanding and growth and loving kindness. *Intuition* is a sudden insight into a feeling, a solution, or problem in which time and actions and perceptions fit together in a unified experience such as understanding about pain and suffering, or a moment in time with another. This is an aspect that may lead to recognizing and being with the pattern of not knowing.

Integral Nursing Principle 3: "It" Is About Behavior and Skill Development

Integral Nursing Principle 3 recognizes the importance of the individual exterior "It" (objective) space. In this "It" space of the individual exterior, each person develops and integrates her or his integral self-care plan. This includes skills, behaviors, and action steps to achieve a fit body and to consider body strength training and stretching and conscious eating of healthy foods. It also includes modeling integral life skills. For the integral nurse and patient, it is also the space where the "doing to" and "doing for" occurs. However, if the patient has moved into the active dying process, the integral nurse combines her or his nursing presence with nursing acts to assist the patient to access personal strengths, to release fear and anxiety, and to provide comfort and safety. Most often the patient has an awareness of conscious dying and a time of sacredness and reverence in this dying transition.

Integral nurses, with nursing colleagues and health-care team members, compile the data around physiological and pathophysiological assessment, nursing diagnosis, outcomes, plans of care (including medications, technical procedures, monitoring, treatments, traditional and integrative practice protocols), implementation, and evaluation. This is also the space that includes patient education and evaluation. Integral nurses cocreate plans of care with patients, when possible combining *caring–healing interventions/modalities* and integral life practices that can interface and enhance the success of traditional medical and surgical technology and treatment. Some common interventions are relaxation, music, imagery, massage, touch therapies, stories, poetry, healing environment, fresh air, sunlight, flowers, soothing and calming pictures, pet therapy, and more.

Integral Nursing Principle 4: "Its" Is Systems and Structures

Integral Nursing Principle 4 recognizes the importance of the exterior collective "Its" (interobjective) space. In this "Its" space, integral nurses and the health-care team come together to examine their work, their priorities, use of technologies and any aspect of the technological environment, and create exterior healing environments that incorporate nature and the natural world when possible such as with outdoor healing gardens, green materials inside with soothing colors, and sounds of music and nature. Integral nurses identify how they might work together as an interdisciplinary team to deliver more effective patient care and to coordinate care while creating external healing environments.

Application of the Theory of Integral Nursing in Practice, Education, Research, Health-Care Policy, Global Nursing

The world is currently anchored in one of the most dramatic social shifts in health-care history, and the theory of integral nursing can inform and shape nursing practice, education, research, and policy—local to global—to achieve a healthy world. The theory of integral nursing engages us to think deeply and purposefully about our role as nurses as we face a changing picture of health due to globalization that knows no natural or political boundaries.

Practice

The theory of integral nursing was published in this author's coauthored text in 2008 and 2013 (Dossey, Beck, & Rushton, 2008; 2013) and is currently being used in many clinical settings. The textbook clearly develops the integral, integrative, and holistic processes and clinical application in traditional settings. It includes guidance about the use of complementary and integrative interventions.

Education

The theory of integral nursing can assist educators to be aware of all quadrants while organizing and designing curriculum, continuing education courses, health education presentations, teaching guides, and protocols. In most nursing curricula, there is minimal focus on the individual subjective "I" and the collective intersubjective "We"; the emphasis is on teaching concepts such as physiology and pathophysiology and passing an examination or learning a new skill or procedure. Thus, the learner retains only small portions of what is taught. Before teaching any technical skills, the instructor might guide a student or patient in an integral practice such as relaxation and imagery rehearsal of the event to encourage the student to be in the present moment.

The following are examples of how the theory of integral nursing is being used. At Quinnipiac University, Hamden, Connecticut, Cynthia Barrere, PhD, RN, CNS, AHN-BC, and Mary Helming, PhD, APRN, FNP-BC, AHN-BC, introduced the theory of integral nursing to their nurse educator colleagues, who use the theory in their holistic undergraduate and graduate curricula as they prepare holistic nurses for the future (Barrere, 2013). Darlene Hess, PhD, NP, AHN-BC, HWNC-BC, (Hess, 2013) used the theory of integral nursing in her Brown Mountain Visions consulting practice to design an RN-to-BSN program at Northern New Mexico State (NNMC), in Espanola, New Mexico. This RN-to-BSN program prepares registered nurses to assume leadership roles as integral nurses at the bedside, within organizations, in the community, and other areas of professional practice. Hess also uses the integral process in her private nurse coaching practice. In the Integrative Nurse Coach Certificate Program (2013), the integral perspectives and change are major components (Dossey, Luck, & Schaub, 2015). Juliann S. Perdue, DNP, RN, FNP, has adapted the theory of integral nursing into her integrative rehabilitation model (Perdue, 2011). Diane Pisanos, RNC, MS, NNP (personal communication, June 15, 2012) integrates integral theory and process to organize her life and health coaching practice.

Research

A theory of integral nursing can assist nurses to consider the importance of qualitative and quantitative research (B. M. Dossey, 2008, 2013; Esbjorn-Hargens, 2006; Frisch, 2013; Quinn, 2003; Zahourek, 2013). Our challenges in integral nursing are to consider the findings from both qualitative and quantitative data and always consider triangulation of data when appropriate. We must always value introspective, cultural, and interpretive experiences and expand our personal and collective capacities of consciousness as evolutionary progression toward achieving our goals. In other words, knowledge emerges from all four quadrants.

Health-Care Policy

A theory of integral nursing can guide us to consider many areas related to health-care policy. Compelling evidence in all of the health-care professions shows that the origins of health and illness cannot be understood by focusing only on the physical body. Only by expanding the equations of health, exemplified by an integral approach or an AQAL approach to include our entire physical, mental, emotional, social, and spiritual dimensions and interrelationships can we account for a host of health events. Some of these include, for example, the correlations among poverty, poor health, and shortened life span; job dissatisfaction and acute myocardial infarction; social shame and severe illness; immune suppression and increased death rates during bereavement; and improved health and longevity as spirituality and spiritual awareness is increased.

Global Health Nursing

The theory of integral nursing can assist us as we engage in global health partnerships and projects. Global health is the exploration of the value base and new relationships and agendas that emerge when health becomes an essential component and expression of global citizenship (Beck et al., 2011; B. M. Dossey, Beck, & Rushton, 2013; Gostin, 2007; Karpf , Swift, Ferguson, & Lazarus, 2008; Karph, Ferguson, & Swift, 2010); J. Kreisberg, personal communication, August 25, 2011; WHO, 2007). It is an increased awareness that health is a basic human right and a global good that needs to be promoted and protected by the global community. Severe health needs exist in almost every community and nation throughout the world as previously described in the UN Millennium Goals. Thus, all nurses must raise their voices and speak about global nursing as their health and healing endeavors assist individuals to become healthier. As Nightingale (1892) said, "We must create a public opinion, which must drive the government instead of the government having to drive us . . . an enlightened public opinion, wise in principle, wise in detail."

Practice Exemplar

A nurse can use the theory of integral nursing in any clinical situation; it assists us in integrating the art and science of nursing simultaneously with all actions/interactions. As discussed previously, healing, the core concept, can occur on many levels (physical, mental, emotional, social, spiritual). Having an integral awareness and creating a space for the possibility that healing can occur allows for a unique field of experience. As nurses engage in their own healing, reflective integral practices, personal development and self-care, they literally embody a special way of being with others. That is, they "walk their talk" of caring–healing. There is a mutual respect for self and others in each encounter as the nurse is always part of the patient's external environment. Even while giving medications and performing various acute care technical skills, a nurse's healing presence in each encounter can reflect a "being with" and "in collaboration with." Nurses must engage in their own development and also personally experience the various reflective practices (relaxation, imagery, reframing) before engaging the patient in these practices.

Background

J. D. is a lean, extroverted, competitive, 6'4," 200-pound, 64-year-old global energy corporate executive who travels internationally. J. D., an avid jogger, had a recent executive physical with normal stress test and blood work and was declared "a picture of good health." His father and paternal grandfather both died of heart attacks in their 60s. He eats a Mediterranean diet when possible and drinks several glasses of wine with meals. He uses a treadmill or runs daily. J. D. has been a widower for 2 years after a tragic head-on automobile accident in which his wife was killed by an intoxicated driver. He has four grown children who live in the same city and who quarrel over loopholes in their inheritance left by their mother and maternal grandmother. Two children are executives and have problems with alcohol abuse; two others are happily married, and each has two preschool children.

Practice Exemplar cont.

One Sunday, J. D. placed second in a city marathon and was disappointed he didn't win. On finishing a morning shower on Monday morning after a restful night's sleep before a scheduled international trip, J. D. had severe back pain. He tried stretching exercises, and the pain went away, so he related it to a back strain from the marathon. He then drove to his office and collapsed onto the steering wheel after he parked his car. A friend saw this and immediately called 911. He was taken to a nearby emergency room, where he was immediately assessed and sent for cardiac catheterization where he received a stent to open the complete occlusion of his right coronary artery. Later that night his cardiologist confirmed from his electrocardiogram that he had had a severe inferior myocardial infarction with cardiac irritability; a few days later, he developed pericarditis secondary to the infarction and was placed on pain medication.

His cardiac situation was even more complicated. His cardiologist informed him that he also had an 80% blockage at the bifurcation in his left anterior descending coronary artery and circumflex that was in a difficult place for a stent. Because he had excellent collateral circulation, he was placed on cardiac medications and told that he would be monitored over the next few months to determine whether he needed further invasive procedures or possibly open heart surgery. He was started on gradual CCU cardiac rehabilitation.

J. D. was very quiet when the nurse entered the room after the cardiologist left. The nurse had a hunch that J. D. might want to talk about what he was experiencing. After a brief exchange, the nurse followed with further exploration of the meaning and negative images that he conveyed. She asked him if he wanted to pursue some new ideas that might help him relax and to engage in a guided imagery to access his inner healing resources and strengths. He said that he would. This encounter took 10 minutes. After the guided imagery, the following dialogue unfolded.

Nurse: *In your recovery now with your heart healing, how do you experience your healing?*

J. D.: *There is this sac around my heart; every time I take a deep breath, my breath is cut off by the pain [pericarditis]. My heart is like a broken vase. I don't think it is healing. The pain medication is helping.*

Nurse: *I can understand some of your frustration and concern. However, some important things that are present right now show me that you are better than when you first came to the CCU. Your persistent chest pain is gone, and your heartbeats are now regular, which shows that the stent is very effective. If you focus on what is going right, you can help your heart and lift your spirits. Let me share some ideas so that you might be able to shift to some positive thoughts.*

J. D.: *I don't know if I can.*

Nurse: *I would like to show you how to breathe more comfortably. Place your right hand on your upper chest and your left hand on your belly and begin to breathe with your belly. With your next breath in, through your nose, let the breath fill your belly with air. And as you exhale through your mouth, let your stomach fall back to your spine. As you focus on this way of breathing, notice how still your upper chest feels.*

J. D.: *(After three complete breaths) This is the easiest breathing I've done today.*

Nurse: *As you focused on breathing with your belly, you let go of fearing the discomfort with your breathing. Can you tell me more about the image you have of your heart as a broken vase?*

J. D.: *I saw this crack down the front of my heart right after the doctor told me about my big arteries that have the 80% blockage. This is very scary.*

Nurse: *(Taking a small plastic bag full of crayons out of her pocket and picking up a piece of paper) Is it possible for you to choose a few crayons and draw your heart as you just described it?*

J. D.: *I can't draw.*

Nurse: *This has nothing to do with drawing, but something usually happens when you place a few marks to create an image of your words.*

J. D.: *If you mean the image of a broken vase, I can draw that.*

Continued

Practice Exemplar cont.

He began to place an image on the paper. When halfway through with the drawing, he said, "I know this sounds crazy, but my father had a heart attack when he was 63. I was visiting my parents. Dad hadn't been feeling well, even complained of his stomach hurting that morning. He was in the living room, and as he fell, he knocked over a large Chinese porcelain vase that broke in two pieces. I can remember so clearly running to his side. I can see that vase now, cracked in a jagged edge down the front. He made it to the hospital, but died 2 days later. You know, I think that might be where that image of a broken heart came from."

Nurse: *Your story contains a lot of meaning. Remembering this image and event can be very helpful to you in your healing. What are some of the things that you are most worried about just now?*
J. D.: *Dying young.*

(Tears fill his eyes) I have this funny feeling in my stomach just now. I don't want to die. I'm too young. I have so much to contribute to life. I've been driving myself to excess at work. I need to learn to relax and manage my stress and change my life.

Nurse: *J., each day you are getting stronger. This time over the next few weeks can be a time to reflect on what are the most important things in your life. Whenever you feel discouraged, let images come to you of a beautiful vase that has a healed crack in it. This is exactly what your heart is doing right now. Even as we are talking, the area that has been damaged is healing. As it heals, there will be a solid scar that will be very strong, just in the same way that a vase can be mended and become strong again. New blood supplies also come into the surrounding area of your heart to help it heal. Positive images can help you heal because you send a different message from your mind to your body when you are relaxed and thinking about becoming strong and well. You help your body, mind, and spirit function at their highest level. Is it possible for you to once again draw an image*

of your heart as a healed vase and notice any difference in your feelings?
J. D.: *Thanks for this talk.*

With a smile, he picked up several crayons and began to draw a healing image to encourage hope and healing.

When J. D. entered the outpatient cardiac rehabilitation program, he was motivated to learn stress management skills and express his emotions. Two weeks into the program, J. D. did not appear to be his usual extroverted self. The cardiac rehabilitation nurse engaged him in conversation, and before long, he had tears in his eyes. He stated that he was very discouraged about having heart disease. He said, "It just has a grip on me." The nurse took him into her office, and they continued the dialogue. After listening to his story, she asked J. D. if he would like to explore his feelings further. He nodded yes. This next session took 15 minutes.

To facilitate the healing process, she thought it might be helpful to have J. D. get in touch with his images and their locations in his body. She began by saying, "If it seems right to you, close your eyes and begin to focus on your breathing just now." She guided him in a general exercise of head-to-toe relaxation, accompanied by an audiocassette music selection of sounds in nature. As his breathing patterns became more relaxed and deeper, indicating relaxation, she began to guide him in exploring "the grip" in his imagination.

Nurse: *Focus on where you experience the grip. Give it a size, ... a shape, ... a sound, ... a texture, ... a width, ... and a depth.*
J. D.: *It's in my chest, but not like chest pain. It's dull, deep, and blocks my knowing what I need to think or feel about living. I can't believe that I'm using these words. Well, it's bigger than I thought. It's very rough, like heavy jute rope tied in a knot across my chest. It has a sound like a rope that keeps a sailboat tied to a boat dock. I'm now rocking back and forth. I don't know why this is happening.*
Nurse: *Stay with the feeling, and let it fill you as much as it can. If you need to change the*

Practice Exemplar cont.

experience, all you have to do is take several deep breaths.

J. D.: *It's filling me up. Where are these sounds, feelings, and sensations coming from?*

Nurse: *They are coming from your wise, inner self, your inner healing resources. Just let yourself stay with the experience. Continue to use as many of your senses as you can to describe and feel these experiences.*

J. D.: *Nothing is happening. I've gone blank.*

Nurse: *Focus again on your breath in ... and feel the breath as you let it go. ... Can you allow an image of your heart to come to you under that tight grip?*

J. D.: *It is so small I can hardly see it. It's all wrapped up.*

Nurse: *In your imagination, can you introduce yourself to your heart as if you were introducing yourself to a person for the first time? Ask your heart if it has a name.*

J. D.: *It said hello, but it was with a gesture of hello, no words.*

Nurse: *That's fine. Just say, "Nice to meet you," and see what the response might be.*

J. D.: *My heart seems like an old soul, very wise. This feels very comfortable.*

Nurse: *Ask your heart a question for which you would like an answer. Stay with this and listen for what comes.*

After long pause:

J. D.: *The answer is practice patience, that I am on the right track, that my heart disease has a message, don't know what it is.*

Nurse: *Just stay with your calmness and inner quiet. Notice how the grip has changed for you. There are many more answers to come for you. This is your wise self that has much to offer you. Whenever you want, you can get back to this special kind of knowing. All you have to do is take the time. When you set aside time to be quiet with your rich images, you will get more information. You might also find special music to assist you in this process. ... Your skills with this way of knowing will increase each time you use this process ... now that whatever is right for you in this moment is unfolding, just as it should.*

In a few moments, I will invite you back into a wakeful state. On five, be ready to come back into the room and feel wide-awake and relaxed. One ... two ... three ... four ... eyelids lighter, taking a deep breath ... and five, back into the room, awake and alert, ready to go about your day.

J. D.: *Where did all that come from? I've never done that before.*

Nurse: *All of these experiences are your inner healing resources that are always with you to help you recognize quality and purpose in living each day. All you have to do is take the time to remember to use them and direct your self-talk and images toward a desired outcome. If you want, I can teach and share more of these skills.*

J. D.: *Ever since my wife died, I have had a sense of "What is the meaning of my life? what is my purpose?" Some days I feel like I have lost my soul. I go through my days doing and doing, and yes I do accomplish a lot. But deep down I am not happy. I have been asking myself the question, "What am I doing ... or NOT doing ... that is feeding the problems I don't want and believing that I can find happiness out there?" Today with you in this experience, a light switch got turned on in me. My happiness is buried inside me. I have to gain access to it again somehow. I try to fix my kids by giving them more money. I actually don't really sit down with them. Sometimes I feel like I don't really know anything about them. I have grandkids that I rarely see. I get frustrated with my corporation as I feel we are contributing to environmental pollution. We [the corporation] can do more about changing this. You helped me identify my needs and how I can contribute differently. I feel a new kind of ownership about my life.*

Evaluation and Outcomes

Together the patient and the nurse evaluate the encounter and determine whether the relaxation and imagery experiences were useful and discuss future outcomes. Such sessions frequently open up profound information and possibilities. To evaluate the session further,

Continued

Practice Exemplar cont.

the nurse may again explore the subjective effects of the experience with the patient. Relaxation and imagery are integral life practices for connecting with our unlimited capabilities and capacities. The patient can experience more self-awareness, self-acceptance, self-love, and self-worth. These integral life practices can be transferred to daily life as resources for self-care. The best way to develop confidence and skill in using relaxation and imagery in a clinical setting is for the nurse to embody these practices in her or his own life as a part of personal self-care and enrichment.

Learning how to be authentic and fresh in interactions and in each moment can be enhanced as we learn to bear witness by deep listening and "simply noticing" what is going on. It is so easy to get locked into our analytical logic that we block ourselves from reaching into our hearts and moving into our intuitions or emotions. With time and practice, we give space to what might appear. Both good and negative thoughts always contain some wisdom. After such a patient encounter, it is a time to really reflect on what happened: How did you stay focused for the patient and stay in the moment? In this kind of encounter, we can never predict what will happen. As we engage in our work, our challenge is to be aware of learning to bear witness, not trying to fix anything, and just exploring the moment with self and other(s). It seems that when we least expect it, we might experience or access a deeper place on inner wisdom. Reflection is often how the contrast of the light and shadow, the "dark nights of the soul" are resolved.

■ Summary

The theory of integral nursing addresses how we can increase our integral awareness, our wholeness and healing, and strengthen our personal and professional capacities to more fully open to the mysteries of life's journey and the wondrous stages of self-discovery with self and others. There are many opportunities to increase our integral awareness, application, and understanding each day. Reflect on all that you do each day in your work and life—analyzing, communicating, listening, exchanging, surveying, involving, synthesizing, investigating, interviewing, mentoring, developing, creating, researching, teaching, and creating new schemes for what is possible. Before long, you will realize how all the quadrants and realities fit together. You might find you are completely missing a quadrant, thus an important part of reality. As we address and value the individual interior and exterior, the "I" and "It," as well as the collective interior and exterior, the "We" and "Its," a new level of integral understanding emerges, and we may also experience more balance and harmony each day.

Our time demands a new paradigm and a new language in which we take the best of what we know in the science and art of nursing that includes holistic and human caring theories and modalities. With an integral approach and worldview, we are in a better position to share with others the depth of nurses' knowledge, expertise, and critical-thinking capacities and skills for assisting others in creating health and healing. Only an attention to the heart of nursing, for "sacred" and "heart" reflect a common meaning, can we generate the vision, courage, and hope required to unite nursing in healing. This assists us as we engage in health-care reform to address the challenges in these troubled times—local to global. It is not an abstract matter of philosophy, but of survival.[1]

---

[1] For additional information please go to bonus chapter content available at http://davisplus.fadavis.com
See Barbara Dossey's website at www.dosseydossey.com to download the theory of integral nursing PowerPoint and one-page handout.

References

American Holistic Nurses Association and the American Nurses Association. (2007). *Holistic nursing: Scope and standards of practice*. Silver Spring, MD: American Nurses Association.

American Holistic Nurses Association and the American Nurses Association. (2013). *Holistic nursing: Scope and standards of practice* (2nd ed.). Silver Spring, MD: American Nurses Association.

Averill, J. B., & Clements, P. T. (2007). Patterns of knowing as a foundation for action-sensitive pedagogy. *Qual Health Research, 17*(3), 386–399.

Barnum, B. (2004). *Spirituality in nursing: From traditional to new age* (2nd ed.). New York: Springer.

Barnum, B. S. (2005). *Nursing theory: Analysis, application, evaluation* (6th ed.). Philadelphia: Lippincott Williams & Wilkins.

Barrere, C. C. (2013). Teaching our future holistic nurses: Integration of holistic and Quality Safety Education for Nurses (QSEN) concepts. In B. M. Dossey & L. Keegan (Eds.), *Holistic nursing: A handbook for practice* (6th ed., pp. 815–823). Burlington, MA: Jones and Bartlett Learning.

Beck, D. E. (2007). *Spiral dynamics integral*. Retrieved July 20, 2007, from http://www.spiraldynamics.net

Beck, D. M., Dossey, B. M., & Rushton, C. H. (2011). Integral nursing and the Nightingale Initiative for Global Health. *Journal of Integral Theory and Practice 6*(4), 71–92.

Burkhardt, M. A., & Najai-Jacobson, M. G. (2013). Spirituality and healing. In B. M. Dossey & L. Keegan (Eds.), *Holistic nursing: A handbook for practice* (6th ed., 721–740). Sudbury, MA: Jones and Bartlett Learning.

Carper, B. A. (1978). Fundamental patterns of knowing in nursing. *Advances in Nursing Science, 1*(1), 13–23.

Chinn, P. L., & Kramer, M. K. (2010). *Theory and nursing: Integrated knowledge development* (8th ed.). St. Louis, MO: Elsevier/Mosby.

Clark, C. S. (2006). An integral nursing education: Exploration of the Wilber quadrant model. *International Journal of Human Caring, 10*(3), 22–29.

Cowling, W. R. (2004). Pattern, participation, praxis, and power in unitary appreciative inquiry. *Advances in Nursing Science, 27*(3), 202–214.

Cowling, W. R., & Repede, E. (2010). Unitary appreciative inquiry: Evolution and refinement *Advances in Nursing Science* 33(1), 64–77.

Dossey, B. M. (2008). Theory of integral nursing. *Advances in Nursing Science, 31*(1), E52–73.

Dossey, B. M. (2010). *Florence Nightingale: Mystic, visionary, healer* (commemorative ed.). Philadelphia: F. A. Davis.

Dossey, B. M. (2013). Nursing: Integral, integrative, holistic—Local to global. In: B. M. Dossey & L. Keegan (Eds.), *Holistic nursing: A handbook for practice* (6th ed., pp. 3–57). Burlington, MA: Jones and Bartlett Learning.

Dossey, B. M., Beck, D. M., & Rushton, C. H. (2008). Nightingale's vision for collaboration. In: S. Weinstein & A. M. Brooks (Eds.), *Nursing without borders: Values, wisdom and success markers*. Indianapolis, IN: Sigma Theta Tau.

Dossey, B. M., Beck, D. M., & Rushton, C. H. (2013). Global activism, advocacy and transformation: Florence Nightingale's legacy for the 21st century. In M. J. Kreitzer & M. Koithan (Eds.), *Integrative nursing*. New York: Oxford Press.

Dossey, B. M., Luck, S., & Schaub, B. G. (2015). *Nurse Coaching: Integrative approaches for health and wellbeing*. North Miami, FL: International Nurse Coach Association.

Dossey, B. M., Selanders, L. C., Beck, D. M., & Attewell, A. (2005). *Florence Nightingale today: Healing, leadership, global action*. Washington, DC: American Nurses Association.

Dossey, L. (1989). *Recovering the soul: A scientific and spiritual search*. New York: Bantam.

Dossey, L. (2003). Samueli conference on definitions and standards in healing research: Working definitions and terms. *Alternative Therapies in Health and Medicine, 9*(3), A11.

Dossey, L. (2013). *One mind: How our individual mind is part of a greater mind, and why it matters*. Carlsbad, CA: Hay House International.

Engebretson, E. (1998). A heterodox model of healing. *Alternative Therapy in Health and Medicine, 4*(2), 37–43.

Esbjorn-Hargens, S. (2006). Integral research: A multimethod approach to investigating phenomena. *Constructivism in the Human Sciences, 11*(1), 79–107.

Fawcett, J., Watson, J., Neuman, B., Walker, P. H., & Fitzpatirck, J. J. (2001). On nursing theories and evidence. *Journal of Nursing Scholarship, 33*(2), 115–119. ff102–105.

Fiandt, K., Forman, J., Megel, M. E., Pakieser, R. A., & Burge, S. (2003). Integral nursing: An emerging framework for engaging the evolution of the profession. *Nursing Outlook, 51*(3), 130–137.

Frisch, N. C. (2013). Nursing theory in holistic nursing practice. In: B. Dossey & L. Keegan (Eds.), *Holistic nursing: A handbook for practice* (6th ed., p. 126). Burlington, MA: Jones and Bartlett Learning.

Gaydos, H. L. (2004). The co-creative aesthetic process: A new model for aesthetics in nursing. *International Journal of Human Caring, 7*, 40–43.

Gaydos, H. L. (2005). The experience of immobility due to trauma. *Holistic Nursing Practice, 19*(1), 40–43.

Gostin, L. O. (2007). Meeting the survival needs of the world's least healthy people. *JAMA, 298*(2), 225–227.

Halifax, J., Dossey, B. M., & Rushton, C. H. (2007). *Being with dying: Compassionate end-of-life care*. Santa Fe, NM: Prajna Mountain Press.

Harvey, A. (2007). Sacred activism. Retrieved July 18, 2007, from http://www.andrewharvey.net/sacred_activism.html

Hess, D. R. (2013). *Curriculum for an RN-to-BSN program using the theory of integral nursing.* In B. M. Dossey & L. Keegan (Eds.), *Holistic nursing: A handbook for practice* (6th ed., pp. 45–51). Burlington, MA: Jones and Bartlett Learning.

Hess, D. R., Dossey, B. M., Southard, M. E., Luck, S., Schaub, B. G., & Bark, L. (2013). *The art and science of nurse coaching: The provider's guide to coaching scope and competencies.* Silver Spring, MD: American Nurses Association.

Integrative Nurse Coach Certificate Program. Retrieved February 1, 2013, from http://www.inursecoach .com.

International Council of Nurses. (2004). *The global shortage of registered nurses: An overview of issues and action.* Geneva: International Council of Nurses. Retrieved April 1, 2007, from http://www.icn.ch/global/shortage.pdf

Jarrín, O. F. (2007). An integral philosophy and definition of nursing. *AQAL: Journal of Integral Theory and Practice, 2*(4), 79–101.

Jung, C. G. (1981). *The archetypes and the collective unconscious* (2nd ed., vol. 9, part I). Princeton, NJ: Bollingen.

Karph, J. T., Ferguson, R., & Swift R. (2010). Light still shines in the darkness: Decent care for all. *Journal of Holistic Nursing 28*(4), 266–274.

Karpf, T., Swift, R., Ferguson, T., & Lazarus, J. (2008). *Restoring hope: Decent care in the midst of HIV/AIDS.* London: Palgrave MacMillan Press and World Health Organization.

Koerner, J. G. (2011). *Nursing presence: The essence of nursing* (2nd ed.). New York: Springer.

Koloroutis, M. (Ed.). (2004). *Relationship-based care: A model for transforming practice.* Minneapolis, MN: Creative Health Care Management.

Levin, J. D., & Reich, J. L. (2013). Self-reflection. In B. M. Dossey & L. Keegan (Eds.), *Holistic nursing: A handbook for practice* (6th ed., 247–259). Burlington, MA: Jones and Bartlett Learning.

McDonald, L. (2001-2012*). The collected works of Florence Nightingale* (volumes 1–16) Waterloo, Canada: Wilfred Laurier University Press.

McElligott, D. (2008). Self-care. In B. M. Dossey & L. Keegan (Eds.), *Holistic nursing: A handbook for practice* (6th ed., pp. 827–842). Burlington, MA: Jones & Bartlett Learning.

McKivergin, M. (2008). Nurse as an instrument of healing. In B. M. Dossey & L. Keegan (Eds.), *Holistic nursing: A handbook for practice* (5th ed.). Burlington, MA: Jones and Bartlett Learning.

Meleis, A. L. (2012). *Theoretical nursing: Development and progress* (5th. ed.). Philadelphia: Lippincott Williams & Wilkins.

Mittelman, M., S. Y. Alperson, S. Y, Arcari, P. M., Donnelly, G. F., Ford, L. C., Koithan, M., & Kreitzer, M. J. (2010). Nursing and integrative health care. *Alternative Therapies in Health and Medicine 16*(5), 84–94.

Munhall, P. L. (1993). Unknowing: Toward another pattern of knowing in nursing. *Nursing Outlook, 41*(3), 125–128.

National Prevention Council. (2011, June 16). *National prevention strategy: American's plan for better health and wellness.* Retrieved from www.surgeongeneral. gov/initiatives/prevention/strategy/report.pdf

Newman, M. A. (2003). A world of no boundaries. *Advances in Nursing Science, 26*(4), 240–245.

Nightingale, F. Letter to Sir Frederick Verney. 23 November 1892, Add. Mss. 68887.

Nightingale Initiative for Global Health. (2013). *Nightingale declaration.* Retrieved January 1, 2013, from www.nightingaledeclaration.net

Perdue, J. S. (2011). *Integration of complementary and alternative therapies in an acute rehabilitation hospital, a readiness assessment.* Unpublished doctoral dissertation, Western University of Health Sciences, Pomona, CA.

Quinn, J. F., Smith, M., Rittenbaugh, C., Swanson, K., & Watson, J. (2003). Research guidelines for assessing the impact of the healing relationship in clinical nursing. *Alternative Therapies in Health and Medicine, 9*(3), A65–A79.

Samueli Institute. (2013). *Optimal healing environments:Your healing journey.* Alexandria, VA: Samueli Institute. Retrieved from http://www.samueliinstitute.org/File%20Library/Health%20Policy/YourHealingJourney.pdf

Tresoli, C. (1994). *Pew-Fetzer Task Force on Advancing Psychosocial Health Education: Health professions education and relationship-centered care.* San Francisco: Commission at the Center for the Health Professions, University of California.

United Nations. (2000). *United Nations Millennium Development Goals.* Retrieved July 20, 2007, from www.un.org/millenniumgoals

Watson, J. (2005). *Caring science as sacred science.* Philadelphia: F. A. Davis.

Weil, A. R. (Ed.). (2013, February). A new era of patient engagement. *Health Affairs, 32*(2).

White, J. (1995). Patterns of knowing: Review, critique, and update. *Advances in Nursing Science 17*(4), 73–86.

Wilber, K. (1999). *The collected works of Ken Wilber* (vols. 1–4). Boston: Shambhala.

Wilber, K. (2000a). *The collected works of Ken Wilber* (vols. 5–8). Boston: Shambhala.

Wilber, K. (2000b). *Integral psychology.* Boston: Shambhala.

Wilber, K. (2005a). *Integral operating system.* Louisville, CO: Sounds True.

Wilber, K. (2005b). *Integral life practice.* Denver, CO: Integral Institute.

Wilber, K. (2006). *Integral spirituality.* Boston: Shambhala.

World Health Organization. World Health Organization Statistics Report 2009. Global Standards for the Initial Education of Professional Nurses and Midwives. http://www.who.int/hrh/nursing_midwifery/hrh_global_standards_education.pdf. (Accessed December 18, 2014).

World Health Organization (WHO). *Primary care.* Retrieved from http://www.paho.org/English/DD/PIN/ptoday12_nov05.htm (Accessed July 20, 2007).

Zahourek, R. (2004). Intentionality forms the matrix of healing: A theory. *Alternative Therapies in Health and Medicine, 10*(6), 40–49.

Zahourek, R. (2013). Holistic nursing research: Challenges and opportunities. In B. M. Dossey & L. Keegan (Eds.), *Holistic nursing: A handbook for practice* (6th ed., pp. 775–794). Burlington, MA: Jones and Bartlett.

IV

Conceptual Models and Grand Theories in the Unitary–Transformative Paradigm

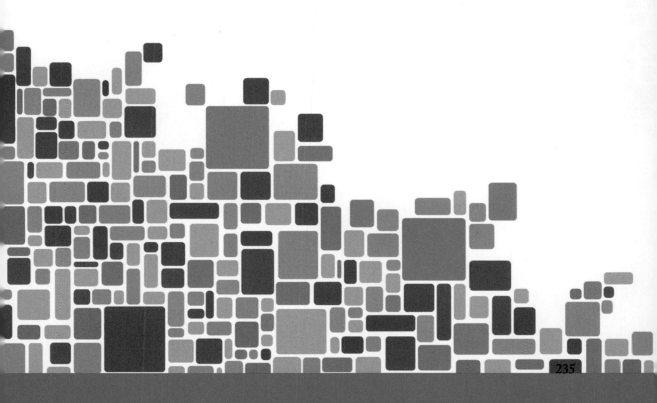

Conceptual Models and Grand Theories in the Unitary–Transformative Paradigm

There are three grand theories clustered in the Unitary–Transformative Paradigm. In this paradigm, the human being and environment are conceptualized as irreducible fields, open with the environment. The person and environment are continuously changing and evolving through mutual patterning.

In Chapter 14, Rogers' science of unitary human beings (SUHB) is explicated by Howard Butcher and Violet Malinski. The SUHB is based on the premise that humans and environments are patterned, pandimensional energy fields in continuous mutual process with each other. Persons participate in their well-being, which is relative and personally defined. Several theories, research traditions, and practice traditions have evolved from this conceptual system. While Parse has recently called humanbecoming a paradigm rather than a school of thought, the editors continue to situate humanbecoming within the Unitary-Transformative Paradigm. Humanbecoming is featured in Chapter 15, written by the theorist herself. Humanbecoming is defined as a basic human science that has cocreated human experiences as its central focus. Humanbecoming portends a view that unitary human beings are expert in their own health and lives. For Parse, human beings choose meanings that reflect value priorities cocreated in transcending with the possibles. Humanbecoming has well-developed research and practice methods that guide the inquiry and practice of nurses embracing it.

Newman's theory of health as expanding consciousness (HEC) is explicated in Chapter 17 by Margaret Dexheimer Pharris. According to HEC, health is an evolving unitary pattern of the whole, including patterns of disease. Consciousness, or the informational capacity of the whole, is revealed in the evolving pattern. Pattern identifies the human–environmental process and is characterized by meaning. Concepts important to nursing practice include expanding consciousness, time, presence, resonating with the whole, pattern, meaning, insights as choice points, and the mutuality of the nurse–patient relationship. These concepts are reflected in the praxis method developed to guide practice-research.

Martha E. Rogers' Science of Unitary Human Beings

Chapter 14

Howard Karl Butcher and
Violet M. Malinski

Introducing the Theorist
Overview of Rogers' Science of Unitary
Human Beings
Applications of the Conceptual System
Practice Exemplar
Summary
References

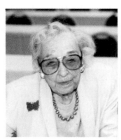

Martha E. Rogers

Introducing the Theorist

Martha E. Rogers, one of nursing's foremost scientists, was a staunch advocate for nursing as a basic science from which the art of practice would emerge. A common refrain throughout her career was the need to differentiate skills, techniques, and ways of using knowledge from the actual body of knowledge needed to guide practice to promote well-being for humankind. Rogers identified the human–environmental mutual process as nursing's central focus, not health and illness. She repeatedly emphasized the need for nursing science to encompass human beings in space and on Earth. Who was this visionary who introduced a new worldview to nursing?

Martha Elizabeth Rogers was born in Dallas, Texas, on May 12, 1914, a birthday she shared with Florence Nightingale. Her parents soon returned home to Knoxville, Tennessee, where Martha and her three siblings grew up. Rogers spent 2 years at the University of Tennessee in Knoxville before entering the nursing program at Knoxville General Hospital. She then attended George Peabody College in Nashville, Tennessee, where she earned her bachelor of science degree in public health nursing, choosing that field as her professional focus. Rogers spent the next 13 years in rural public health nursing in Michigan, Connecticut, and Arizona, where she established the first visiting nurse service in Phoenix, serving as its executive director (Hektor, 1989/1994). In 1945, recognizing the need for advanced education, she earned a master's degree in nursing from Teachers College, Columbia University, in the program developed by another nurse theorist, Hildegard Peplau. In

1951, she left public health nursing in Phoenix to return to academia, this time earning both a master's of public health and a doctor of science degree from Johns Hopkins University in Baltimore, Maryland.

In 1954, after her graduation from Johns Hopkins, Rogers was appointed head of the Division of Nursing at New York University (NYU), beginning the second phase of her career overseeing baccalaureate, master's, and doctoral programs in nursing and developing the nursing science she knew was integral to the knowledge base nurses needed. During the 1960s, she successfully shifted the focus of doctoral research from nurses and their functions to humans in mutual process with the environment. She wrote three books that explicated her ideas: *Educational Revolution in Nursing* (1961), *Reveille in Nursing* (1964), and the landmark *An Introduction to the Theoretical Basis of Nursing* (1970). From 1963 to 1965, she edited *Nursing Science,* a journal that was far ahead of its time; it offered content on theory development and the emerging science of nursing, as well as research and issues in education and practice.

Rogers died in 1994, leaving a rich legacy in her writings on nursing science, the space age, research, education, and professional and political issues in nursing.

Overview of Rogers' Science of Unitary Human Beings

The historical evolution of the Science of Unitary Human Beings has been described by Malinski and Barrett (1994). This chapter presents the science in its current form and identifies work in progress to expand it further.

Rogers' Worldview

Rogers (1992) articulated a new worldview in nursing, one that was commensurate with new knowledge emerging across disciplines, which rooted nursing science in "a pandimensional view of people and their world" (p. 28). Rogers (1992) described the evolution from older to newer worldviews in such shifting perspectives as cell theory to field theory, entropic to negentropic universe, three-dimensional to pandimensional, person–environment as dichotomous to person–environment as integral, causation and adaptation to mutual process, dynamic equilibrium to innovative growing diversity, homeostasis to homeodynamics, waking as a basic state to waking as an evolutionary emergent, and closed to open systems. She pointed out that in a universe of open systems, energy fields are continuously open, infinite, and integral with one another. A view of change as predictable, or even probabilistic, yields to change as diverse, creative, innovative, and unpredictable.

Rogers (1994a) identified the unique focus of nursing as "the irreducible human being and its environment, both defined as energy fields" (p. 33). "Human" encompasses both *Homo sapiens* and *Homo spatialis,* the evolutionary transcendence of humankind as we voyage into space; environment encompasses outer space, the cosmos itself.

Rogers was aware that the world looks very different from the vantage point of this newer view as contrasted with the older, traditional worldview. She pointed out that we are already living in a new reality, one that is "a synthesis of rapidly evolving, accelerating ways of using knowledge" (Rogers, 1994a, p. 33), even if people are not always fully aware that these shifts have occurred or are in process. She urged that nurses be visionary, looking forward and not backward and not allowing themselves to become "stuck" in the present, in the details of how things are now, but envision how they might be in a universe where continuous change is the only given. Rogers (1994b) cautioned that although traditional modalities of practice and methods of research serve a purpose, they are inadequate for the newer worldview, which urges nurses to use the knowledge base of Rogerian nursing science creatively to develop innovative new modalities and research approaches that would promote the betterment of humankind.

Postulates of Rogerian Nursing Science

Rogers (1992) identified four fundamental postulates that form the basis of the new reality:

• Energy fields
• Openness

- Pattern
- Pandimensionality (formerly called both four-dimensionality and multidimensionality)

Rogers (1990) defined the energy field as "the fundamental unit of the living and the non-living," noting that it is dynamic, infinite, and continuously moving (p. 7). Although Rogers did not define energy per se, Todaro-Franceschi's (1999) wide-ranging philosophical study of the enigma of energy sheds light on a Rogerian conceptualization of energy. She highlighted the communal, transformative nature of energy, noting that energy is everywhere and is always changing and actualizing potentials. Energy transformation is the basis of all that is, both in living and dying.

Rogers identified two energy fields of concern to nurses, which are distinct but not separate: the human field and the environmental field. The human field can be conceptualized as person, group, family, or community. The human and environmental fields are irreducible; they cannot be broken down into component parts or subsystems. For example, the unitary human is neither understood nor described as a bio–psycho–sociocultural or body–mind–spirit entity. Instead, she maintained that each field, human and environmental, is identified by pattern, defined as "the distinguishing characteristic of an energy field perceived as a single wave" (Rogers, 1990, p. 7). Pattern manifestations and characteristics are specific to the whole, the unitary human–environment in mutual process. Change occurs simultaneously for human and environment.

The fields are pandimensional, defined as "a non-linear domain without spatial or temporal attributes" (Rogers, 1992, p. 29). Pandimensional reality transcends traditional notions of space and time, which can be understood as perceived boundaries only. Examples of pandimensionality include phenomena commonly labeled "paranormal" that are, in Rogerian nursing science, manifestations of the changing diversity of field patterning and examples of pandimensional awareness.

The postulate of openness resonates throughout the preceding discussion. In an open universe, there are no boundaries other than perceptual ones. Therefore, human and environment are not separated by boundaries. The energy of each flows continuously through the other in an unbroken wave. Rogers repeatedly emphasized that person and environment are themselves energy fields; they do not have energy fields, such as auras, surrounding them. In an open universe, there are multiple potentials and possibilities. People experience their world in multiple ways, evidenced by the diverse manifestations of field patterning that continuously emerge.

Rogers (1992, 1994a) described pattern as changing continuously while giving identity to each unique human–environmental field process. Although pattern is an abstraction, not something that can be observed directly, "it reveals itself through its manifestations" (Rogers, 1992, p. 29). Individual characteristics of a particular person are not characteristics of field patterning. Pattern manifestations reflect the human–environmental field mutual process as a unitary, irreducible whole. They reveal innovative diversity flowing in lower and higher frequency rhythms within the human–environmental mutual field process. Rogers identified some of these manifestations as lesser and greater diversity; longer, shorter, and seemingly continuous rhythms; slower, faster, and seemingly continuous motion; time experienced as slower, faster, and timeless; pragmatic, imaginative, and visionary; and longer sleeping, longer waking, and beyond waking. Beyond waking refers to emergent experiences and perceptions such as hyperawareness, unitive experiences attained in meditation, precognition, déjà vu, intuition, tacit knowing, mystical experiences, clairvoyance, and telepathy. She explained "seems continuous" as "a wave frequency so rapid that the observer perceives it as a single, unbroken event" (Rogers, 1990, p. 10). This view of the ongoing process of change is captured in Rogers' principles of homeodynamics.

Principles of Homeodynamics

Homeodynamics conveys the dynamic, ever-changing nature of life and the world. Her three principles of homeodynamics—resonancy, helicy, and integrality—describe the nature and process of change in the human–environmental field process.

Resonancy is "the continuous change from lower to higher frequency wave patterns in human and environmental fields" (Rogers, 1992, p. 31). Although she verbalized the need to delete the "from–to" language, which seems to imply linearity and directionality, Rogers never actually deleted it in print. However, it is important to remember that this process is nonlinear and nondirectional because in a pandimensional universe there is no space and no time (Phillips, 2010a). Resonancy specifies the nonlinear, continuous flow of lower and higher frequency wave patterning in the human–environmental field process, the way change occurs.

Both lower and higher frequency awareness and experiencing are essential to the wholeness of rhythmical patterning. As Phillips (1994, p. 15) described it, "[W]e may find that growing diversity of pattern is related to a dialectic of low frequency–high frequency, similar to that of order–disorder in chaos theory. When the rhythmicities of lower-higher frequencies work together, they yield innovative, diverse patterns."

Helicy is "the continuous, innovative, unpredictable, increasing diversity of human and environmental field patterns (Rogers, 1992, p. 31). It describes the creative and diverse nature of ongoing change in field patterning, a "diversity of pattern that is innovative, creative, and unpredictable" (Phillips, 2010a, p. 57).

Integrality is "continuous mutual human field and environmental field process" (Rogers, 1992, p. 31). It specifies the process of change within the integral human–environmental field process where person and environment are unitary, thus inseparable.

Together the principles suggest that the mutual patterning process of human and environmental fields changes continuously, innovatively, and unpredictably, flowing in lower and higher frequencies. Rogers (1990, p. 9) believed that they serve as guides both to the practice of nursing and to research in the science of nursing.

Theories Derived From the Science of Unitary Human Beings

Rogers clearly stated her belief that multiple theories can be derived from the science of unitary human beings. They are specific to nursing and reflect not what nurses do but an understanding of people and our world (Rogers, 1992). Nursing education is identified by transmission of this theoretical knowledge, and nursing practice is the creative use of this knowledge. "Research is done in relation to the theories" (Rogers, 1994a, p. 34) to illuminate the nature of the human–environmental field change process and its many unpredictable potentials.

Theory of Accelerating Change

Rogers derived the theory of accelerating change, formerly known as the theory of accelerating evolution, to illustrate that the only "norm" is accelerating change. Higher frequency field patterns that manifest growing diversity open the door to wider ranges of experiences and behaviors, calling into question the very idea of "norms" as guidelines. Human and environmental field rhythms are accelerating. We experience faster environmental motion now than ever before. It is common for people to experience time as rapidly speeding by. People are living longer. Rather than viewing aging as a process of decline or as "running down," as in an entropic worldview, this theory views aging as a creative process in which field patterns show increasing diversity in such manifestations as sleeping, waking, and dreaming. "[I]n fact, as evolutionary diversity continues to accelerate, the range and variety of differences between individuals also increase; the more diverse field patterns evolve more rapidly than the less diverse ones" (Rogers, 1992, p. 30).

The theory of accelerating change provides the basis for reconceptualizing the aging process. Rogers (1970, 1980) used the principle of helicy and the theory of accelerating change to put forward the notion that aging is a continuously creative process of growing diversity of field patterning. Therefore, aging is not a process of decline or running down. Rather, field patterns become increasingly diverse as we age as older adults need less sleep; are more satisfied with personal relationships; are better able to handle their emotions; are better able to cope with stress; and have increasing crystallized intelligence, wisdom, and improved problem-solving abilities (Whitbourne & Whitbourne, 2011). Butcher (2003) expanded on Rogers "negentropic" view of aging in outlining key elements for a "unitary model of aging as emerging brilliance" that includes replacing ageist stereotypes with new positive images of aging and developing policies, lifestyles, and technologies that enhance successful aging and longevity. Within a unitary view of aging, later life becomes a potential for growth, "a life imbued with splendor, meaning, accomplishment, active involvement, growth, adventure, wisdom, experience, compassion, glory, and brilliance" (Butcher, 2003, p. 64).

Theory of Emergence of Paranormal Phenomena

Another theory derived by Rogers is the emergence of paranormal phenomena, in which she suggests that experiences commonly labeled "paranormal" are actually manifestations of changing diversity and innovation of field patterning. They are pandimensional forms of awareness, examples of pandimensional reality that manifest visionary, beyond waking potentials. Meditation, for example, transcends traditionally perceived limitations of time and space, opening the door to new and creative potentials. Therapeutic Touch provides another example of such pandimensional awareness. Both participants often share similar experiences during Therapeutic Touch, such as a visualization of common features that evolves spontaneously for both, a shared experience arising within the mutual process both are experiencing, with neither able to lay claim to it as a personal, private experience.

The idea of a pandimensional or nonlinear domain provides a framework for understanding paranormal phenomena. A nonlinear domain unconstrained by space and time provides an explanation of seemingly inexplicable events and processes. Rogers (1992) asserted

that within the science of unitary human beings, psychic phenomena become "normal" rather than "paranormal." Dean Radin, director of the Conscious Research Laboratory at the University of Nevada in Las Vegas, suggests that an understanding of nonlocal connections along with the relationship between awareness and quantum effects provides a framework for understanding paranormal phenomena (Radin, 1997). "Deep interconnectedness" demonstrated by Bell's Theorem embraces the interconnectedness of everything unbounded by space and time. In addition, the work of L. Dossey (1993, 1999), Nadeau and Kafatos (1999), Sheldrake (1988), and Talbot (1991) explicate the role of nonlocality in evolution, physics, cosmology, consciousness, paranormal phenomena, healing, and prayer. Tart (2009), in his excellent text *The End of Materialism: How Evidence of the Paranormal Is Bringing Science and Spirit Together*, reviews the research supporting common paranormal experiences with separate chapters on telepathy, clairvoyance/remote viewing, precognition, psychokinesis, psychic healing, out-of-body experiences, near-death experiences, postmortem survival, and mystical experiences. Murphy (1992) in his highly referenced and researched text presents the evidence supporting what he refers to as emergent extraordinary human abilities such as placebo effects, paranormal experiences, spiritual healing, meditative, mystical, and contemplative practices on health and healing. The relevance of these experiences and practices to nursing is in the number that occur in health-related contexts, and Rogers's nursing science provides a theoretical and scientific understanding that accounts for the occurrence of paranormal experiences.

Within a nonlinear–nonlocal context, paranormal events are our experience of the deep nonlocal interconnections that bind the universe together. Existence and knowing are locally and nonlocally linked through deep connections of awareness, intentionality, and interpretation. Pandimensionality embraces the infinite nature of the universe in all its dimensions and includes processes of being more aware of naturally occurring changing energy patterns. Pandimensionality also includes intentionally participating in mutual process with a nonlinear–nonlocal potential of creating new energy patterns. Distance healing, the healing power of prayer, Therapeutic Touch, out-of-body experiences, phantom pain, precognition, déjà vu, intuition, tacit knowing, mystical experiences, clairvoyance, and telepathic experiences are a few of the energy field manifestations patients and nurses experience that can be better understood as natural events in a pandimensional universe characterized by nonlinear–nonlocal human–environmental field integrality propagated by increased awareness and intentionality.

Manifestations of Field Patterning

Rogers' third theory, rhythmical correlates of change, was changed to manifestations of field patterning in unitary human beings, discussed earlier. Here Rogers suggested that evolution is an irreducible, nonlinear process characterized by increasing diversity of field patterning. She offered some manifestations of this relative diversity, including the rhythms of motion, time experience, and sleeping–waking, encouraging others to suggest further examples. In addition to the theories that Rogers derived, a number of others have been developed by Rogerian scholars that are useful in informing Rogerian pattern–based practice and research. The first such theory to be developed was Barrett's (1989, 2010) theory of power as knowing participation in change, described in Chapter 29.

Butcher's (1993) theory of kaleidoscoping in life's turbulence is an example of a theory derived from Rogers' science of unitary human beings, chaos theory (Briggs & Peat, 1989; Peat, 1991), and Csikszentmihalyi's (1990) theory of flow. It focuses on facilitating well-being and harmony amid turbulent life events. Turbulence is a dissonant commotion in the human–environmental field characterized by chaotic and unpredictable change. Any crisis may be viewed as a turbulent event in the life process. Nurses often work closely with clients who are in a "crisis." Turbulent life events are often chaotic in nature, unpredictable, and always transformative. The theory of kaleidoscoping in life's

turbulence is described in more detail in the Bonus content for the chapter.[1]

Other theories derived from Rogers's nursing science include Reed's (1991, 2003; see Chapter 23 in this volume) theory of self-transcendence, the theory of enfolding health-as-wholeness-and-harmony (Carboni, 1995a), Bultemeier's (1997) theory of perceived dissonance, the theory of enlightenment (Hills & Hanchett, 2001), Alligood and McGuire's theory of aging (2000), Butcher's theory of aging as emerging brilliance (2003), and Zahourek's (2004, 2005) theory of intentionality in healing.

Applications of the Conceptual System

New worldviews require new ways of thinking, sciencing, languaging, and practicing. Rogers's nursing science postulates a pandimensional universe of human–environmental energy fields manifesting as continuously innovative, increasingly diverse, creative, and unpredictable unitary field patterns. The principles of homeodynamics provide a way to understand the process of human–environmental change, paving the way for Rogerian theory–based practice. Rogers often reminded us that unitary means whole. Therefore, people are always whole, regardless of what they are experiencing in the moment, and therefore do not need nurses to facilitate their wholeness. Rogers identified noninvasive modalities as the basis for nursing practice now and in the future. She stated that nurses must use "nursing knowledge in non-invasive ways in a direct effort to promote well-being" (Rogers, 1994a, p. 34). This focus gives nurses a central role in health care rather than medical care. She also noted that health services should be community based, not hospital based. Hospitals are properly used to provide satellite services in specific instances of illness and trauma; they do not provide health services. Rogers urged nurses to develop autonomous, community-based nursing centers. See Boxes 14-1 and 14-2.

---

[1] For additional information please go to bonus chapter content available at FA Davis http://davisplus.fadavis.com

The relevance of Rogerian nursing science to both human well-being and nursing is precisely the transformative vision of people and the world that it offers. Recognizing this, the nursing department at Bronx Lebanon Hospital Center, Bronx, New York, has made the decision to use Rogerian nursing science as the framework for practice throughout the hospital. People are complex, society is changing, and nursing's image is changing and so is our practice, which is driven by the science of nursing, according to Dr. Jeanine M. Frumenti, Vice President, Patient Care Services/Chief Nursing Officer. Rogerian nursing science was chosen because it is inclusive and reflective of people's ever-changing relationship to their environment, whereas many other nursing theories are reflective of the art of nursing. According to Frumenti, nurses need to be open to unfolding pattern and pandimensional experiences; everything is integrated and changing. The Rogerian nursing science assists Bronx Lebanon nurses in actualizing transformative practice for themselves and their clients.

In 2008, Howard Butcher launched a wiki site on Rogerian science with the purpose of providing a website to gather Rogerian scholars so they can mutually cocreate a comprehensive and easily accessible and in-depth explication of the science of unitary human beings. The wiki can be viewed by anyone and is organized like a textbook with chapters on the following: Rogers' life, the aim of nursing science, Rogerian cosmology and philosophy, Rogers' postulates, Rogerian science, Rogerian theories, practice methods, and research methods. There are links of all the issues of *Visions: The Journal of Rogerian Nursing Science* as well as photos. The wiki is not complete; it is ever evolving. However, it is a valuable resource to all interested in learning more about the science of unitary human beings.

Rogers (1986) identified the living–dying process as one characterized by rhythmical patterning, opening the door to new ways of studying and working with the dying process.

For example, Todaro-Franceschi (2006) identified the existence of synchronicity experiences, meaningful coincidences, in many who were grieving the loss of a spouse, a pioneering effort in delineating a unitary view of death and dying. From the results of her qualitative study, she described how such experiences help the bereaved to relate to their deceased loved ones in a new, meaningful way, one that is potentially healing, rather than in the traditional view of learning to let go and move on. Malinski (2012) conceptualized the unitary rhythm of dying–grieving, highlighting the shared nature of this process, for the one grieving is also dying a little just as the one dying is simultaneously grieving. She synthesized this unitary rhythm as "a process of kaleidoscopic patterning flowing now swiftly now gently, spiraling creatively through shifting rhythms of now-elsewhen-elsewhere, becoming in solitude and silence alone-all one, timeless-boundaryless" (p. 242). Pandimensional awareness and experience of this rhythm means recognition that there is no space or time, no boundary or separation. The reality is one of unity amid changing configurations of patterning, with endless potentials.

Unfortunately, a number of ideas relevant to nursing practice that Rogers discussed verbally never made it into print, for example, healing, intentionality, and expanded views on Therapeutic Touch. In three audiotaped and transcribed dialogues among Rogers, Malinski, and Meehan on January 26, 1988, for example, she described healing as a process, everything that happens as persons actualize potentials they identify as enhancing health and wellness for themselves. Todaro-Franceschi (1999) described healing in a similar way, with nurses knowingly participating in the healing process by helping people actualize "their unique potentials—whatever those potentials may be" (p. 104). Cowling (2001) described healing as appreciating wholeness, offering unitary pattern appreciation as the praxis for exploring wholeness within the unitary human–environmental mutual process.

Rogers also reminded us that change is a neutral process, neither good nor bad, one that we cannot direct but in which we participate. In this vein, in the transcribed dialogue among

Rogers, Malinski, and Meehan on Therapeutic Touch, Rogers described this modality as a neutral process, one that facilitates the patterning most commensurate with well-being for the person, whatever that is. There is no exchange of energy, no identification of desired outcomes in Therapeutic Touch. Rather than intentionality, Rogers suggested knowing participation as most congruent with her thinking, seeing intentionality as too closely tied to will and intent. However, she did suggest that a unitary view of intentionality was worthy of study.

Rogers also questioned the concept of spirituality, which she saw as too often confused with religiosity. Smith (1994) and Malinski (1991, 1994) have both explored a Rogerian view of spirituality. Barrett (2010) suggested that the interrelationships of pandimensionality, consciousness, and spirituality will become clearer and increasingly important. She defined consciousness "as the *Spirit* in all that is, was, and will be" and spirituality "as *experiencing the Spirit* in all that is, was, and will be" (italics in the original; p. 53).

Phillips (2010b) created the terms *energyspirit* and *Homo pandimensionalis* to highlight expanding "pandimensional relative present awareness" (p. 8). In a discussion about the big bang, he suggested that if energy is indeed unitary, discussions of physical energy are not only incomplete but inaccurate. Phillips speculated, "What if the big bang was a cataclysm of spirit integral with energy that was not separated into physical and spirit, but made their presence as a unitary whole. Then, we have a new phenomenon known as energyspirit, one word. This energyspirit was the origin of the universe and human beings and all their changes" (p. 9). Energyspirit thus replaces any discussion of mindbodyspirit. Already of no relevance to Rogerian nursing science, perhaps mindbodyspirit can be replaced now with energyspirit throughout the unitary perspective. As pandimensional relative present awareness is continuously changing, it is possible that we will see the emergence of new, unanticipated pattern manifestations characterizing the human–environmental mutual field process. Phillips suggests that this emerging life form is *Homo pandimensionalis*.

Evolution of Rogerian Practice Methods

A hallmark of a maturing scientific practice discipline is the development of specific practice and research methods evolving from the discipline's extant conceptual systems. Rogers (1992) asserted that practice and research methods must be consistent with the science of unitary human beings to study irreducible human beings in mutual process with a pandimensional universe. Therefore, Rogerian practice and research methods must be congruent with Rogers' postulates and principles if they are to be consistent with Rogerian science.

The goal of nursing practice is the promotion of well-being and human betterment. Nursing is a service to people wherever they may reside. Nursing practice—the art of nursing—is the creative application of substantive scientific knowledge developed through logical analysis, synthesis, and research. Since the 1960s, the nursing process has been the dominant nursing practice method. The nursing process is an appropriate practice methodology for many nursing theories. However, there has been some confusion in the nursing literature concerning the use of the traditional nursing process within Rogers's nursing science.

In early writings, Rogers (1970) did make reference to nursing process and nursing diagnosis. But in later years she asserted that nursing diagnoses were not consistent with her scientific system. Rogers (quoted in Smith, 1988, p. 83) stated:

Nursing diagnosis is a static term that is quite inappropriate for a dynamic system. . . . it [nursing diagnosis] is an outdated part of an old worldview, and I think by the turn of the century, there are going to be new ways of organizing knowledge.

Furthermore, nursing diagnoses are particularistic and reductionist labels describing cause and effect (i.e., "related to") relationships inconsistent with a "nonlinear domain without spatial or temporal attributes" (Rogers, 1992, p. 29).

The nursing process is a stepwise sequential process inconsistent with a nonlinear or pandimensional view of reality. In addition, the term *intervention* is not consistent with Rogerian science. Intervention means to "come, appear, or lie between two things" (*American Heritage Dictionary*, 2000, p. 916). The principle of integrality describes the human and environmental field as integral and in mutual process. Energy fields are open, infinite, dynamic, and constantly changing. The human and environmental fields are inseparable, so one cannot "come between." The nurse and the client are already inseparable and interconnected. Outcomes are also inconsistent with Rogers' principle of helicy: expected outcomes infer predictability. The principle of helicy describes the nature of change as being unpredictable. Within an energy-field perspective, nurses in mutual process assist clients in actualizing their field potentials by enhancing their ability to participate knowingly in change. Given the inconsistency of the traditional nursing process with Rogers' postulates and principles, the science of unitary human beings requires the development of new and innovative practice methods derived from and consistent with the conceptual system. A number of practice methods have been derived from Rogers's postulates and principles.

Barrett's Rogerian Practice Method

Barrett's Rogerian practice methodology for health patterning was the first accepted alternative to the nursing process for Rogerian practice (see Chapter 29). It was followed by Cowling's conceptualization.

Cowling's Rogerian Practice

Cowling (1990) proposed a template comprising 10 constituents for the development of Rogerian practice models. Cowling (1993b, 1997) refined the template and proposed that "pattern appreciation" was a method for unitary knowing in both Rogerian nursing research and practice. Cowling preferred the term *appreciation* rather than *assessment* or *appraisal* because appraisal is associated with evaluation. Appreciation has broader meaning, which includes "being fully aware or sensitive to or realizing; being thankful or grateful for; and enjoying or understanding critically or emotionally" (Cowling, 1997, p. 130). Pattern

appreciation has a potential for deeper understanding. For a description of the constituents, see Bonus content for the chapter.[2]

Unitary Pattern-Based Praxis Method

Butcher (1997a, 1999a, 2001) synthesized Cowling's Rogerian practice constituents with Barrett's practice method to develop a more inclusive and comprehensive practice model. In 2006, Butcher expanded the "praxis" model by illustrating how the Rogerian cosmology, ontology, epistemology, esthetics, ethics, postulates, principles, and theories all form an "interconnected nexus" informing both Rogerian-based practice and research models (Butcher, 2006a, p. 9). The unitary pattern–based practice (Fig. 14-1) consists of two nonlinear and simultaneous processes: pattern manifestation appreciation and knowing, and voluntary mutual patterning. The focus of nursing care guided by Rogers's nursing science is on pattern transformation by facilitating pattern recognition during pattern manifestation knowing and appreciation and by facilitating the client's ability to participate knowingly in change, harmonizing person–environment integrality, and promoting healing potentialities and well-being through voluntary mutual patterning

Pattern Manifestation Knowing and Appreciation

Pattern manifestation knowing and appreciation is the process of identifying manifestations of patterning emerging from the human–environmental field mutual process and involves focusing on the client's experiences, perceptions, and expressions. "Knowing" refers to apprehending pattern manifestations (Barrett, 1988), whereas "appreciation" seeks a perception of the "full force of pattern" (Cowling, 1997). Pattern is the distinguishing feature of the human–environmental field. Everything experienced, perceived, and expressed is a manifestation of patterning. During the process of pattern manifestation knowing and appreciation, the nurse and client are coequal

Unitary pattern-based praxis

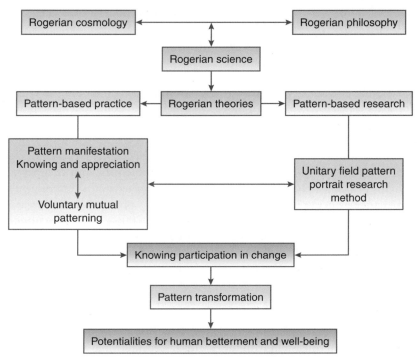

Fig 14 • 1 The unitary pattern-based praxis model. *(Model from Butcher, H. K. [2006a]. Unitary pattern-based praxis: A nexus of Rogerian cosmology, philosophy, and science.* Visions: The Journal of Rogerian Nursing Science, 14*[2], 8–33.)*

participants. In Rogerian practice, nursing situations are approached and guided by a set of Rogerian-ethical values, a scientific base for practice, and a commitment to enhance the client's desired potentialities for well-being.

Unitary pattern–based practice begins by creating an atmosphere of openness and freedom so that clients can freely participate in the process of knowing participation in change. Approaching the nursing situation with an appreciation of the uniqueness of each person and with unconditional love, compassion, and empathy can help create an atmosphere of openness and healing patterning (Butcher, 2002; Malinski, 2004). Rogers (1966/1994) defined nursing as a humanistic science dedicated to compassionate concern for humans. Compassion includes energetic acts of unconditional love and means (1) recognizing the interconnectedness of the nurse and client by being able to fully understand and know the

suffering of another, (2) creating actions designed to transform injustices, and (3) not only grieving in another's sorrow and pain but also rejoicing in another's joy (Butcher, 2002).

Pattern manifestation knowing and appreciation involves focusing on the experiences, perceptions, and expressions of a health situation, revealed through a rhythmic flow of communion and dialogue. In most situations, the nurse can initially ask the client to describe his or her health situation and concern. The dialogue is guided toward focusing on uncovering the client's experiences, perceptions, and expressions related to the health situation as a means to reaching a deeper understanding of unitary field pattern. Humans are constantly all-at-once experiencing, perceiving, and expressing (Cowling, 1993a). Experience involves the rawness of living through sensing and being aware as a source of knowledge and includes any item or ingredient the client senses (Cowling, 1997). The client's own observations and description of his or her health situation includes his or her experiences. "Perceiving is the apprehending of experience or the ability to reflect while experiencing" (Cowling, 1993a, p. 202). Perception is making sense of the experience through awareness, apprehension, observation, and interpreting. Asking clients about their concerns, fears, and observations is a way of apprehending their perceptions. Expressions are manifestations of experiences and perceptions that reflect human field patterning. In addition, expressions are any form of information that comes forward in the encounter with the client. All expressions are energetic manifestations of field patterns. Body language, communication patterns, gait, behaviors, laboratory values, and vital signs are examples of energetic manifestations of human–environmental field patterning.

Because all information about the client–environment–health situation is relevant, various health assessment tools, such as the comprehensive holistic assessment tool developed by B. M. Dossey, Keegan, and Guzzetta (2004), may also be useful in pattern knowing and appreciation. However, all information must be interpreted within a unitary context. A unitary context refers to conceptualizing all information as energetic/dynamic manifestations of pattern emerging from a pandimensional human–environmental mutual process. All information is interconnected, is inseparable from environmental context, unfolds rhythmically and acausally, and reflects the whole. Data are not divided or understood by dividing information into physical, psychological, social, spiritual, or cultural categories. Rather, a focus on experiences, perceptions, and expressions is a synthesis more than and different from the sum of parts. From a unitary perspective, what may be labeled as abnormal processes, nursing diagnoses, or illness or disease are conceptualized as episodes of discordant rhythms or nonharmonic resonancy (Bultemeier, 2002).

A unitary perspective in nursing practice leads to an appreciation of new kinds of information that may not be considered within other conceptual approaches to nursing practice. The nurse is open to using multiple forms of knowing, including pandimensional modes of awareness (intuition, meditative insights, tacit knowing) throughout the pattern manifestation knowing and appreciation process. Intuition and tacit knowing are artful ways to enable seeing the whole, revealing subtle patterns, and deepening understanding. Pattern information concerning time perception, sense of rhythm or movement, sense of connectedness with the environment, ideas of one's own personal myth, and sense of integrity are relevant indicators of human–environment–health potentialities (Madrid & Winstead-Fry, 1986). A person's hopes and dreams, communication patterns, sleep–rest rhythms, comfort–discomfort, waking–beyond waking experiences, and degree of knowing participation in change provide important information regarding each client's thoughts and feelings concerning a health situation.

The nurse can also use a number of pattern appraisal scales derived from Rogers's postulates and principles to enhance the collecting and understanding of relevant information specific to Rogerian science. For example, nurses can use Barrett's (1989) power as knowing participation in change tool as a way of knowing clients' energy field patterns in relation to their capacity to knowingly participate in the continuous patterning of human and environmental fields as manifest in frequencies of awareness, choice making ability, sense of freedom to act intentionally, and degree of involvement in creating change. Watson's (1993) assessment of dream experience scale can be used to know and appreciate the clients' dream experiences, and Ference's (1979, 1986) human field motion tool is an indicator of the wave frequency pattern of the energy field.

Hastings-Tolsma's (1992) diversity of human field pattern scale may be used as a means for knowing and appreciating a clients' perception of the diversity of their energy field pattern, Johnston's (1994) human image metaphor scale can be used as a way of knowing and appreciating the clients' perception of the wholeness of their energy field, and the well-being picture scale for adults (Gueldner et al., 2005; Johnson, Guadron, Verchot, & Gueldner, 2011) and for children (Terwillinger, Gueldner, & Bronstein, 2012) afford a way to measure a person's sense of unitary well-being. Paletta (1990) developed a tool consistent with Rogerian science that measures the subjective awareness of temporal experience.

The pattern manifestation knowing and appreciation is enhanced through the nurse's ability to grasp meaning, create a meaningful connection, and participate knowingly in the client's change process (Butcher, 1999a). "Grasping meaning entails using sensitivity, active listening, conveying unconditional acceptance, while remaining fully open to the rhythm, movement, intensity, and configuration of pattern manifestations" (Butcher, 1999a, p. 51). Through integrality, nurse and client are always connected in mutual process. However, a meaningful connection with the client is facilitated by creating a rhythm and flow through the intentional expression of unconditional love, compassion, and empathy. Together, in mutual process, the nurse and client explore the meanings, images, symbols, metaphors, thoughts, insights, intuitions, memories, hopes, apprehensions, feelings, and dreams associated with the health situation.

Rogerian ethics are integral to all unitary pattern–based practice situations. Rogerian ethics are pattern manifestations emerging from the human–environmental field mutual process that reflect those ideals concordant with Rogers' most cherished values and are indicators of the quality of knowing participation in change (Butcher, 1999b). Thus, unitary pattern–based practice includes making the Rogerian values of reverence, human betterment, generosity, commitment, diversity, responsibility, compassion, wisdom, justice-creating, openness, courage, optimism, humor, unity, transformation, and celebration intentional in the human–environmental field mutual process (Butcher, 1999b, 2000).

When initial pattern manifestation knowing and appreciation is complete, the nurse synthesizes all the pattern information into a meaningful pattern profile. The pattern profile is an expression of the person–environment–health situation's essence. The nurse weaves together the expressions, perceptions, and experiences in a way that tells the client's story. The pattern profile reveals the hidden meaning embedded in the client's human–environmental mutual field process. Usually the pattern profile is in a narrative form that describes the essence of the properties, features, and qualities of the human–environment–health situation. In addition to a narrative form, the pattern profile may also include diagrams, poems, listings, phrases, metaphors, or a combination of these. Interpretations of any measurement tools may also be incorporated into the pattern profile.

Voluntary Mutual Patterning

Voluntary mutual patterning is a process of transforming human–environmental field patterning. The goal of voluntary mutual patterning is to facilitate each client's ability to participate knowingly in change, harmonize person–environment integrality, and promote healing potentialities, lifestyle changes, and well-being in the client's desired direction of change without attachment to predetermined outcomes. The process is mutual in that both the nurse and the client are changed with each encounter, each patterning one another and coevolving together. "Voluntary" signifies freedom of choice or action without external compulsion (Barrett, 1998). The nurse has no investment in changing the client in a particular way.

Whereas patterning is continuous, voluntary mutual patterning may begin by sharing the pattern profile with the client. Sharing the pattern profile with the client is a means of validating the interpretation of pattern information and may spark further dialogue, revealing new and more in-depth information. Sharing the pattern profile with the client facilitates pattern recognition and also may enhance the client's knowing participation in his or her own change process. An increased awareness of one's own pattern may offer new insight and increase one's desire to participate in the change process. In addition, the nurse and client can continue to explore goals, options, choices, and voluntary mutual patterning strategies as a means to facilitate the client's actualization of his or her human–environmental field potentials.

A wide variety of mutual patterning strategies may be used in Rogerian practice, including many "interventions" identified in the Nursing Intervention Classification (Bulechek, Butcher, & Dochterman, 2013). However, "interventions," within a unitary context, are not linked to nursing diagnoses and are reconceptualized as voluntary mutual patterning strategies, and the activities are reconceptualizied as patterning activities. Rather than linking voluntary mutual patterning strategies to nursing diagnoses, the strategies emerge in dialogue whenever possible out of the patterns and themes described in the pattern profile. Furthermore, Rogers (1988, 1992, 1994a) placed great emphasis on modalities that are traditionally viewed as holistic and noninvasive. In particular, the use of sound, dialogue, affirmations, humor, massage, journaling, exercise, nutrition, reminiscence, aroma, light, color, artwork, meditation, storytelling, literature, poetry, movement, and dance are just a few of the voluntary mutually patterning strategies consistent with a unitary perspective. In addition, patterning modalities have been developed that are conceptualized within the science of unitary human beings such as Butcher's metaphoric unitary landscape narratives (2006b) and written emotional expression (2004a), Therapeutic Touch (Malinski, 1993), guided imagery (Butcher & Parker, 1988; Levin, 2006), magnet therapy (Kim, 2001), and music (Horvath, 1994; Johnston, 2001). Sharing of knowledge through health education and providing health education literature and teaching also have the potential to enhance knowing participation in change. These and other noninvasive modalities are well described and documented in both the Rogerian (Barrett, 1990; Madrid, 1997; Madrid & Barrett, 1994) and the holistic nursing practice literature (B. M. Dossey, 1997; B. M. Dossey, Keegan, & Guzzetta, 2004).

The nurse continuously apprehends changes in patterning emerging from the human–environmental field mutual process throughout the simultaneous pattern manifestation knowing and appreciation and voluntary mutual patterning processes. Although the concept of "outcomes" is incompatible with Rogers' notions of unpredictability, outcomes in the

Nursing Outcomes Classification (Moorhead, Johnson, Maas, & Swanson, 2013) can be reconceptualized as potentialities of change or "client potentials" (Butcher, 1997a, p. 29), and the indicators can be used as a means to evaluate the client's desired direction of pattern change. At various points in the client's care, the nurse can also use the scales derived from Rogers's science (previously discussed) to co-examine changes in pattern. Regardless of which combination of voluntary patterning strategies and evaluation methods is used, the intention is for clients to actualize their potentials related to their desire for well-being and betterment.

The unitary pattern–based practice method identifies the aspect that is unique to nursing and expands nursing practice beyond the traditional biomedical model dominating much of nursing. Rogerian nursing practice does not necessarily need to replace hospital-based and medically driven nursing interventions and actions for which nurses hold responsibility. Rather, unitary pattern–based practice complements medical practices and places treatments and procedures within an acausal, pandimensional, rhythmical, irreducible, and unitary context. Unitary pattern–based practice provides a new way of thinking and being in nursing that distinguishes nurses from other health care professionals and offers new and innovative ways for clients to reach their desired health potentials.

Applications of Theory and Research
Research is the bedrock of nursing practice. The science of unitary human beings has a long history of theory-testing research. As new practice theories and health patterning modalities evolve from the science of unitary human beings, there remains a need to test the viability and usefulness of Rogerian theories and voluntary health patterning strategies. The mass of Rogerian research has been reviewed in a number of publications (Butcher, 2008; Caroselli & Barrett, 1998; Dykeman & Loukissa, 1993; Fawcett, 2013; Fawcett & Alligood, 2003; Kim, 2008; Malinski, 1986a; Phillips, 1989; Watson, Barrett, Hastings-Tolsma, Johnston, & Gueldner, 1997). Rather

than repeat the reviews of Rogerian research, the following section describes current methodological trends within the science of unitary human beings to assist researchers interested in Rogerian science in making methodological decisions.

Rogers (1994b) maintained that both quantitative and qualitative methods may be useful for advancing Rogerian science. Similarly, Barrett (1996), Barrett and Caroselli (1998), Barrett, Cowling, Carboni, and Butcher (1997), Cowling (1986), Rawnsley (1994), and Smith and Reeder (1996) have all advocated for the appropriateness of multiple methods in Rogerian research. Conversely, Butcher (cited in Barrett et al., 1997), Butcher (1994), and Carboni (1995b) have argued that the ontological and epistemological assumptions of causality, reductionism, particularism, control, prediction, and linearity of quantitative methodologies are inconsistent with Rogers's unitary ontology and participatory epistemology. Later, Fawcett (1996) also questioned the congruency between the ontology and epistemology of Rogerian science and the assumptions embedded in quantitative research designs; like Carboni (1995b) and Butcher (1994), she concluded that interpretive/qualitative methods may be more congruent with Rogers's ontology and epistemology. This chapter presents an inclusive view of methodologies.

Approaches to Rogerian Research

Cowling (1986) was among the first to suggest a number of research designs that may be appropriate for Rogerian research, including philosophical, historical, and phenomenological ones. There is strong support for the appropriateness of phenomenological methods in Rogerian science. Reeder (1986) provided a convincing argument demonstrating the congruence between Husserlian phenomenology and the Rogerian science of unitary human beings. Experimental and quasi-experimental designs are problematic because of assumptions concerning causality; however, these designs may be appropriate for testing propositions concerning differences in the change process in relation to "introduced environmental change" (Cowling, 1986, p. 73). The researcher must be careful to interpret the findings in a way that is consistent with Rogers's notions of unpredictability, integrality, and nonlinearity. Emerging interpretive evaluation methods, such as Guba and Lincoln's (1989) Fourth Generation Evaluation, offer an alternative means for testing for differences in the change process within or between groups (or both) more consistent with the science of unitary human beings.

Cowling (1986) contended that in the early stages of theory development, designs that generate descriptive and explanatory knowledge are relevant to the science of unitary human beings. For example, correlational designs may provide evidence of patterned changes among indices of the human field. Advanced and complex designs with multiple indicators of change that may be tested using linear structural relations (LISREL) statistical analysis may also be a means to uncover knowledge about the pattern of change (Phillips, 1990). Barrett (1996) suggested that canonical correlation may be useful in examining relationships and patterns across domains and may also be useful for testing theories pertaining to the nature and direction of change. Another potentially promising area yet to be explored is participatory action and cooperative inquiry (Reason, 1994), because of their congruence with Rogers's notions of knowing participation in change, continuous mutual process, and integrality. Cowling (1998) proposed that a case-oriented approach is useful in Rogerian research because case inquiry allows the researcher to attend to the whole and strives to comprehend his or her essence.

Selecting a Focus of Rogerian Inquiry

In selecting a focus of inquiry, concepts that are congruent with the science of unitary human beings are most relevant. The focus of inquiry flows from the postulates, principles, and concepts relevant to the conceptual system. Noninvasive voluntary patterning modalities, such as guided imagery, Therapeutic Touch, humor, sound, dialogue, affirmations, music, massage, journaling, written emotional expression, exercise, nutrition, reminiscence, aroma, light, color, artwork, meditation, storytelling, literature, poetry, movement, and dance, provide a rich source for Rogerian science-based research. Creativity, mystical experiences, transcendence, sleeping-beyond-waking experiences, time experience, and paranormal experiences as they relate to human health and well-being are also of interest in this science. Feelings and experiences are a manifestation of human–environmental field patterning and are a manifestation of the whole (Rogers, 1970); thus, feelings and experiences relevant to health and well-being are an unlimited source for potential Rogerian research. Discrete particularistic biophysical phenomena are usually not an appropriate focus for inquiry because Rogerian science focuses on irreducible wholes. An exception could be the use of such phenomena, for example blood pressure, as part of diverse data collected to obtain different views of pattern manifestations and pattern change.

For example, see Madrid, Barrett, and Winstead-Fry's (2010) study of Therapeutic Touch and blood pressure, pulse, and respirations in the operative setting with patients undergoing cerebral angiography, and Malinski and Todaro-Franceschi's (2011) study of comeditation and anxiety and relaxation in a nursing school setting.

Rogers clearly identified that everything is a manifestation of the whole, of field patterning. However, one cannot use just the numerical data, mere "facts," so interpretation would differ accordingly (Rogers, 1989). Researchers need to ensure that concepts and measurement tools used in the inquiry are defined and conceptualized within a unitary perspective and congruent with Rogers's principles and postulates. Diseases or medical diagnoses are not the focus of Rogerian inquiry. Disease conditions are conceptualized as labels and as manifestations of patterning emerging acausally from the human–environmental mutual process.

Measurement of Rogerian Concepts

The Human Field Motion Test (HFMT) is an indicator of the continuously moving position and flow of the human energy field. Two major concepts—"my motor is running" and "my field expansion"—are rated using a semantic differential technique (Ference, 1979, 1986). Examples of indicators of higher human field motion include feeling imaginative, visionary, transcendent, strong, sharp, bright, and active. Indicators of relative low human field motion include feeling dull, weak, dragging, dark, pragmatic, and passive. The tool has been widely used in numerous Rogerian studies.

The Power as Knowing Participation in Change Tool (PKPCT) has been used in more than 26 major research studies (Caroselli & Barrett, 1998) and is a measure of one's capacity to participate knowingly in change as manifested by awareness, choices, freedom to act intentionally, and involvement in creating changes using semantic differential scales. Statistically significant correlations have been found between power as measured by the PKPCT and the following: human field motion, life satisfaction, spirituality, purpose in life, empathy, transformational leadership style, feminism, imagination, and socioeconomic status. Inverse relations with power have been found with anxiety, chronic pain, personal distress, and hopelessness (Caroselli & Barrett, 1998).

Diversity is inherent in the evolution of the human–environmental mutual field process. The evolution of the human energy field is characterized by the creation of more diverse patterns reflecting the nature of change. The Diversity of Human Field Pattern Scale measures the process of diversifying human field pattern and may also be a useful tool to test theoretical propositions derived from the postulates and principles of Rogerian science to examine the extent of selected patterning modalities designed to foster harmony and well-being (Hastings-Tolsma, 1992; Watson et al., 1997). Other measurement tools developed within a unitary science perspective may be used in a wide variety of research studies and in combination with other Rogerian measurements. For example, there are the Assessment of Dream Experience Scale, which measures the diversity of dream experience as a beyond-waking manifestation using a 20-item Likert scale (Watson, 1993; Watson et al., 1997);

Temporal Experience Scale, which measures the subjective experience of temporal awareness (Paletta, 1990); and Mutual Exploration of the Healing Human Field–Environmental Field Relationship Creative Measurement Instrument developed by Carboni (1992), which is a creative qualitative measure designed to capture the changing configurations of energy field pattern of the healing human–environmental field relationship.

A number of new tools have been developed that are rich sources of measures of concepts congruent with unitary science. The Human Field Image Metaphor Scale used 25 metaphors that capture feelings of potentiality and integrality rated on a Likert-type scale. For example, the metaphor "I feel at one with the universe" reflects a high degree of awareness of integrality; "I feel like a worn-out shoe" reflects a more restricted perception of one's potential (Johnston, 1994; Watson et al., 1997). Future research may focus on developing an understanding of how human field image changes in a variety of health-related situations or how human field image changes in mutual process with selected patterning strategies.

Research Methods Specific to Science of Unitary Human Beings

The criteria for developing Rogerian research methods are presented in the supplementary material (for a description of the constituents see Bonus content for the chapter.)[3] They are a synthesis and modification of the Criteria of Rogerian Inquiry developed by Butcher (1994) and the Characteristics of Operational Rogerian Inquiry developed by Carboni (1995b). The criteria are a useful guide in designing research methods that are consistent with Rogers's principles and postulates. Two Rogerian research methods were developed using the criteria and the Unitary Field Pattern Portrait research method and Rogerian Process Inquiry. A third method developed by Cowling (2001), Unitary Appreciative Inquiry is also described in the bonus content for the chapter.[3]

---

[3] For additional information please go to bonus chapter content available at FA Davis http://davisplus.fadavis.com

Rogerian Process of Inquiry

Carboni (1995b) developed the Rogerian process of inquiry from her characteristics of Rogerian inquiry. The method's purpose is to investigate the dynamic enfolding-unfolding of the human field–environmental field energy patterns and the evolutionary change of configurations in field patterning of the nurse and participant. Rogerian process of inquiry transcends both matter-centered methodologies espoused by empiricists and thought-bound methodologies espoused by phenomenologists and critical theorists (Carboni, 1995b). Rather, this process of inquiry is evolution-centered and focuses on changing configurations of human and environmental field patterning.

The flow of the inquiry starts with a summation of the researcher's purpose, aims, and visionary insights. Visionary insights emerge from the study's purpose and researcher's understanding of Rogerian science. Next, the researcher focuses on becoming familiar with the participants and the setting of the inquiry. Shared descriptions of energy field perspectives are identified through observations and discussions with participants and processed through mutual exploration and discovery. The researcher uses the Mutual Exploration of the Healing Human Field–Environmental Field Relationship Creative Measurement Instrument (Carboni, 1992) as a way to identify, understand, and creatively measure human and environmental energy field patterns. Together, the researcher and the participants develop a shared understanding and awareness of the human–environmental field patterns manifested in diverse multiple configurations of patterning. All the data are synthesized using inductive and deductive data synthesis. Through the mutual sharing and synthesis of data, unitary constructs are identified. The constructs are interpreted within the perspective of unitary science, and a new unitary theory may emerge from the synthesis of unitary constructs. Carboni (1995b) also developed special criteria of trustworthiness to ensure the scientific rigor of the findings conveyed in the form of a Pandimensional Unitary Process

Report. Carboni's research method affords a way of creatively measuring manifestations of field patterning emerging during coparticipation of the researcher and participant's process of change.

The Unitary Field Pattern Portrait Research Method

The unitary field pattern portrait (UFPP) research method (Butcher, 1994, 1996, 1998, 2005) was developed at the same time Carboni was developing the unitary process of inquiry and was derived directly from the criteria of Rogerian inquiry. The purpose of the UFPP research method is to create a unitary understanding of the dynamic kaleidoscopic and symphonic pattern manifestations emerging from the pandimensional human–environmental field mutual process as a means to enhance the understanding of a significant phenomenon associated with human betterment and well-being. The UFPP research method is part of the unitary pattern–based praxis model (see Fig. 14-1) illustrating the inherent unity of Rogerian philosophy, science, theory, practice, and research (Butcher, 2006a). There are eight essential aspects and three essential processes in the method. The aspects include initial engagement, a priori nursing science, immersion, manifestation knowing and appreciation, the unitary field pattern profile, mutually constructed unitary field pattern profile, the unitary field pattern portrait, and theoretical unitary field pattern portrait. The UFPP (see Fig. 14-2) and the three essential processes are creative pattern synthesis, immersion and crystallization, and evolutionary interpretation.

1. Initial Engagement: Inquiry within the UFPP begins with initial engagement, which is a passionate search for a research question of central interest to understanding unitary phenomena associated with human betterment and well-being. For example, experiences, perceptions, and expressions related to noninvasive voluntary patterning modalities such as guided imagery, Therapeutic Touch, humor, sound, dialogue, affirmations, music, massage,

journaling, written emotional expression, exercise, nutrition, reminiscence, aroma, light, color, artwork, meditation, storytelling, literature, poetry, movement, and dance provide a rich source for UFPP research. Creativity, mystical experiences, transcendence, sleeping-beyond-waking experiences, time experience, and paranormal experiences as they relate to human health and well-being are also experiences that can be researched using the UFPP. The UFPP research method can also be used to create a unitary conceptualization and understanding of an unlimited number of human experiences relevant to understanding health and well-being within a unitary perspective. New concepts that describe unitary phenomena may also be developed through research using this method.

2. A priori nursing science identifies the science of unitary human beings as the researcher's perspective. As in all research, the perspective of the researcher guides all aspects and processes of the research method, including the interpretation of findings.

3. Immersion involves becoming steeped in the research topic. The researcher may immerse in poetry, art, literature, music, dialogue with self and/or others, research literature, or any activity that enhances the integrality of the researcher and the research topic.

4. Pattern manifestation knowing and appreciation includes participant selection, in-depth dialoguing, and recording pattern manifestations. Participant selection is made using intensive purposive sampling. Patterning manifestation knowing and appreciation occurs in a natural setting and involves using pandimensional modes of awareness during in-depth dialoguing. The activities described earlier in the pattern manifestation knowing and appreciation process in the practice method are used in this research method. However, in the UFPP research method the focus of pattern appreciation and knowing is on experiences, perceptions, and expressions

Unitary Field Pattern Portrait Research Method

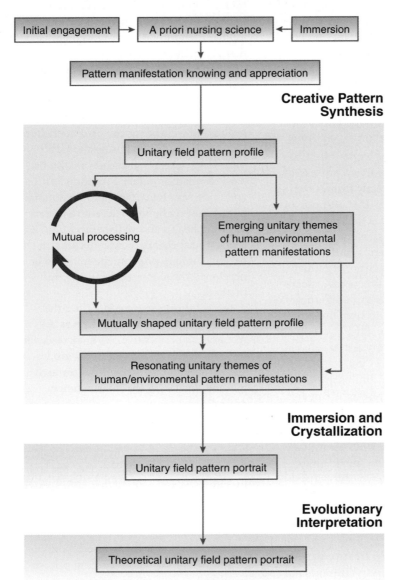

Fig 14 • 2 The unitary field pattern portrait research method. *(Model from Butcher, H. K. (2005). The unitary field pattern portrait research method: Facets, processes and findings.* Nursing Science Quarterly, 18, *293–297.)*

associated with the phenomenon of concern. The researcher also maintains an informal conversational style while focusing on revealing the rhythm, flow, and configurations of the pattern manifestations emerging from the human–environmental mutual field process associated with the research topic. The dialogue is taped and transcribed. The researcher maintains observational, methodological, and theoretical field notes, and a reflexive journal. Any artifacts the participant wishes to share that illuminate the meaning of the phenomenon may also be included. Artifacts may include pictures, drawings, poetry, music, logs, diaries, letters, notes, and journals.

5. Unitary field pattern profile is a rich description of each participant's experiences, perception, and expressions created through a process of creative pattern synthesis. All the information collected for each participant is synthesized into a narrative statement (profile) revealing the essence of the participant's description of the phenomenon of concern. The field pattern profile is in the language of the participant and is then shared with the participant for revision and validation.

6. Mutual processing involves constructing the mutual unitary field pattern profile by mutually sharing an emerging joint or shared profile with each successive participant at the end of each participant's pattern manifestation knowing and appreciation process. For example, at the end of the interview of the fourth participant, a joint construction of the phenomenon is shared with the participant for comment. The joint construction (mutual unitary field pattern profile) at this phase would consist of a synthesis of the profiles of the first three participants. After verification of the fourth participant's pattern profile, the profile is folded into the emerging mutual unitary field pattern profile. Pattern manifestation knowing and appreciation continues until there are no new pattern manifestations to add to the mutual unitary field pattern profile. If it is not possible to either share the pattern profile with each participant or create a mutually constructed unitary field pattern profile, the research may choose to bypass the mutual processing phase.

7. The UFPP is created by identifying emerging unitary themes from each participant's field pattern profile, sorting the unitary themes into common categories, creating the resonating unitary themes of human–environmental pattern manifestations through immersion and crystallization, which involves synthesizing the resonating themes into a descriptive portrait of the phenomenon. The UFPP is expressed in the form of a vivid, rich, thick, and accurate aesthetic rendition of the universal patterns, qualities, features, and themes exemplifying the essence of the dynamic kaleidoscopic and symphonic nature of the phenomenon of concern.

8. The UFPP is interpreted from the perspective of the science of unitary human beings using the process of evolutionary interpretation to create a theoretical UFPP of the phenomenon. The purpose of theoretical UFPP is to explicate the theoretical structure of the phenomenon from the perspective of nursing science using the Rogers's postulates and principles. The theoretical UFPP is expressed in the language of Rogerian science, thereby lifting the UFPP from the level of description to the level of unitary science. Scientific rigor is maintained throughout processes by using the criteria of trustworthiness and authenticity (Butcher, 1998, 2005).

Butcher's (1997b) study on the experience of dispiritedness in later life was the first published study using the UFPP. Ring (2009) used the method to investigate and describe changes in pattern manifestations in individuals receiving Reiki, and Fuller (2011) used the UFPP method to create a vivid portrait of adult substance users and family pattern in rehabilitation.

Practice Exemplar

The focus of nursing care guided by Rogers's nursing science is on pattern transformation by facilitating pattern recognition during pattern manifestation knowing and appreciation and by facilitating the client's ability to participate knowingly in change, harmonizing person–environment integrality, and promoting healing potentialities and well-being through voluntary mutual patterning. The unitary pattern–based practice model consists of two nonlinear and simultaneous processes: pattern manifestation appreciation and knowing, and voluntary mutual patterning. To illustrate practice guided by Rogerian science, consider

Continued

Practice Exemplar cont.

Amanda, who is a 20-year-old college student at a local university. She entered a nurse owned and managed wellness center with her mother. Pattern manifestation appreciation and knowing as well as voluntary mutual patterning begin simultaneously upon meeting as the nurse practitioner apprehends that Amanda's eyes are downcast, she manifests low energy, and she did not say a word when first greeted. Amanda's initial visit was 2 years ago during her freshman year when she was experiencing depressive symptoms. Amanda had major life changes at the time: she broke up with her boyfriend, her parents were going through a divorce, and her grades were falling; she was spending less time with her friends and more time in her room; and she had obviously lost weight. Today was similar as Amanda and her mother entered the center to see the nurse. After spending a few moments in silence, the nurse ask Amanda to describe her current situation, paying close attention to her body language, words, and meanings as she described her fears of failing school. Engaged in dialogue, Amanda revealed that for the past 3 months, she has been increasingly missing classes, having difficulty concentrating and falling asleep, eating less, and spending more time in her apartment. Her mother explained that Amanda had not come home for the weekend in several weeks and doesn't call anymore.

Once her mother stepped out of the room, Amanda began crying. She stated that she was very stressed with school and misses her friends. "Really, I just find myself staying in bed and I don't want to get out from under the covers. I can't seem to shut my brain off anymore either. I don't sleep. Yeah, that's it if I could just get some sleep, I know I would be better." Amanda was asked how she felt her mood was. "I know I am depressed. I can feel it." Amanda continued to cry as she speaks with her eyes down cast. When asked about sleep, she stated that she was in bed a lot but couldn't seem to shut off her mind. "I can't even concentrate on one topic, and my brain is off on another. I don't even get hungry

anymore. The reason I haven't come in is because I didn't want you to see me like this again. I was trying to get better." Amanda was having a difficult time focusing on one topic and stated, "that big cloud is back again." She denied napping but does admit to feeling tired "all the time." The nurse invited Amanda to participate in a brief deep-breathing and focusing exercise to help her become more relaxed and to enable her to reflect and describe more deeply what she was experiencing in her life situation. She revealed that her real fear was failure and disappointing her mother. The nurse then asked if Amanda would complete a standard depression scale and the PKPCT (Power as Knowing Participation in Change Tool), and both were scored immediately. Within Rogerian science, all information is relevant, and even though the depression scale was not specific to Rogerian science, the tool can be interpreted within a unitary context. Her score on the depression scale indicated that Amanda was moderately depressed, which is an indication her human–environmental field mutual process. Rather than labeling or diagnosing Amanda having "minor depression," the nurse understood Amanda's field pattering as lower frequency energy pattering and discordant with her environmental field. Amanda's scores on the 48-item PKPCT are helpful in revealing her ability to participate in change in a knowingly matter. In all four dimensions of the tool (awareness, choices, freedom to act intentionally, and involvement in creating changes), Amanda's scores were low, indicating she manifested low power in her change process. As the nurse shared and dialogues with her about the scores on the scales, she confirmed that she was feeling helpless and unable to develop a plan to help change her situation.

The nurse and Amanda worked together in mutual process to develop a plan that would help her experience her power to deal more effectively with her feelings and her academic work. The nurse documented the encounter by writing a health pattern profile that included descriptions of Amanda's experiences,

Practice Exemplar cont.

expressions, and perceptions of her health situation using her words as much as possible, and they mutually agreed on a plan that was designed to enhance her energy, help her better manage her school work and diet, and facilitate rest at night. During voluntary mutual patterning, the nurse first asked Amanda's mother to come back into the room. Together they explored her mother's feelings about the importance of Amanda's academic performance. Her mother revealed that she was more concerned about her daughter's health than her grades, which actually helped relieve much of the pressure she was feeling about her academic performance. A plan was developed that included Amanda meeting with the faculty instructors in two of the courses in which she was performing poorly to see what she can do to make up for any missed assignments. In one other course, both she and her mother agreed it might be best to withdraw from the course and retake it the following semester. The nurse developed a "Power Prescription Plan" that included Amanda developing a daily activity schedule so that her time would be more structured with a balance of study time, exercise at the recreational center, increased nutrition, and rest. Amanda enjoyed swimming, so the schedule included her swimming 4 of 7 days for 1 hour each time initially. Amanda also was interested in but had never tried yoga, which she admitted was popular with a number of her friends. She agreed to reengage with several of her close friends and join one of the local yoga clubs on campus. Together the nurse and Amanda developed an imagery exercise that was meaningful to her, and Amanda agreed to practice it daily. Amanda also agreed to weekly sessions with the nurse practitioner so that they can together monitor Amanda's progress and her involvement in her change process. In the weekly sessions, the nurse and Amanda would also continue to explore the deeper meanings of "depressed" feelings, mutually explore the choices she was making, and identify new options that would allow her to achieve her hopes and dreams. The session concluded with Therapeutic Touch with both Amanda and her mother.

■ Summary

If nursing's content and contribution to the betterment of the health and well-being of a society is not distinguishable from other disciplines and has nothing unique or valuable to offer, then nursing's continued existence may be questioned. Thus, nursing's survival rests on its ability to make a difference in promoting the health and well-being of people. The science of unitary human beings offers nursing a new way of conceptualizing health events concerning human well-being that is congruent with the most contemporary scientific theories. As with all major theories embedded in a new worldview, new terminology is needed to create clarity and precision of understanding and meaning. There is an ever-growing body of literature demonstrating the application of Rogerian science to practice and research. Rogers's nursing science is applicable in all nursing situations. Rather than focusing on disease and cellular biological processes, the science of unitary human beings focuses on human beings as irreducible wholes inseparable from their environment.

For 30 years, Rogers advocated that nurses should become the experts and providers of noninvasive modalities that promote health. Now, the growth of "complementary/integrative," noninvasive practices is outpacing the growth of allopathic medicine. If nursing continues to be dominated by biomedical frameworks that are indistinguishable from medical care, nursing will lose an opportunity to become expert in unitary health-care modalities.

References

Alligood, M. R., & McGuire, S. L. (2000). Perception of time, sleep patterns, and activity in senior citizens: A test of a Rogerian theory of aging. *Visions: The Journal of Rogerian Nursing Science, 8,* 6–14.

American Heritage Dictionary. (2000). (4th ed.). New York: Houghton Mifflin.

Barrett, E. A. M. (1988). Using Rogers' science of unitary human beings in nursing practice. *Nursing Science Quarterly, 1,* 50–51.

Barrett, E. A. M. (1989). A nursing theory of power for nursing practice: Derivation from Rogers' paradigm. In J. Riehl-Sisca (Ed.), *Conceptual models for nursing practice* (3rd ed., pp. 207–217). Norwalk, CT: Appleton & Lange.

Barrett, E. A. M. (1990). Health patterning with clients in a private practice environment. In E. A. M. Barrett (Ed.), *Visions of Rogers' science-based practice* (pp. 105–115). New York: National League for Nursing.

Barrett, E. A. M. (1996). Canonical correlation analysis and its use in Rogerian research. *Nursing Science Quarterly, 9,* 50–52.

Barrett, E. A. M. (1998). A Rogerian practice methodology for health patterning. *Nursing Science Quarterly, 11,* 136–138.

Barrett, E. A. M. (2010). Power as knowing participation in change: What's new and what's next. *Nursing Science Quarterly, 23,* 47–54.

Barrett, E. A. M., & Caroselli, C. (1998). Methodological ponderings related to the power as knowing participation in change tool. *Nursing Science Quarterly, 11,* 17–22.

Barrett, E. A. M., Cowling, W. R., Carboni, J. T., & Butcher, H. K. (1997). Unitary perspectives on methodological practices. In M. Madrid (Ed.), *Patterns of Rogerian knowing* (pp. 47–62). New York: National League for Nursing.

Briggs, J., & Peat, F. D. (1989). *Turbulent mirror: An illustrated guide to chaos theory and the science of wholeness.* New York: Harper & Row.

Bulechek, G. M., Butcher, H. K., & Dochteman, J. M. (2013). *Nursing interventions classification (NIC)* (6th ed.). St. Louis, MO: Elsevier.

Bultemeier, K. (1997). Photo-disclosure: A research methodology for investigating unitary human beings. In M. Madrid (Ed.), *Patterns of Rogerian knowing* (pp. 63–74). New York: National League for Nursing.

Bultemeier, K. (2002). Rogers' science of unitary human beings in nursing practice. In M. R. Alligood & A. Marriner-Tomey (Eds.), *Nursing theory: Utilization and application* (pp. 267–288). St. Louis, MO: Mosby.

Butcher, H. K. (1993). Kaleidoscoping in life's turbulence: From Seurat's art to Rogers' nursing science. In M. E. Parker (Ed.), *Patterns of nursing theories in practice* (pp. 183–198). New York: National League for Nursing.

Butcher, H. K. (1994). The unitary field pattern portrait method: Development of research method within Rogers' science of unitary human beings. In M. Madrid & E. A. M. Barrett (Eds.), *Rogers' scientific art of nursing practice* (pp. 397–425). New York: National League for Nursing.

Butcher, H. K. (1996). A unitary field pattern portrait of dispiritedness in later life. *Visions: The Journal of Rogerian Nursing Science, 4,* 41–58.

Butcher, H. K. (1997a). Energy field disturbance. In G. K. McFarland & E. A. McFarlane, (Eds.), *Nursing diagnosis and intervention* (3rd ed., pp. 22–33). St. Louis, MO: Mosby.

Butcher, H. K. (1997b). A unitary field pattern portrait of dispiritedness in later life. *Visions: The Journal of Rogerian Nursing Science, 4,* 41–58.

Butcher, H. K. (1998). Crystallizing the processes of the unitary field pattern portrait research method. *Visions: The Journal of Rogerian Nursing Science, 6,* 13–26.

Butcher, H. K. (1999a). The artistry of Rogerian practice. *Visions: The Journal of Rogerian Nursing Science, 7,* 49–54.

Butcher, H. K. (1999b). Rogerian-ethics: An ethical inquiry into Rogers' life and science. *Nursing Science Quarterly, 12,* 111–117.

Butcher, H. K. (2000). Critical theory and Rogerian science: Incommensurable or reconcilable. *Visions: The Journal of Rogerian Nursing Science, 8,* 50–57.

Butcher, H. K. (2001). Nursing science in the new millennium: Practice and research within Rogers' science of unitary human beings. In: M. Parker (Ed.), *Nursing theories and nursing practice* (pp. 205–226). Philadelphia: F. A. Davis.

Butcher, H. K. (2002). Living in the heart of helicy: An inquiry into the meaning of compassion and unpredictability in Rogers' nursing science. *Visions: The Journal of Rogerian Nursing Science, 10,* 6–22.

Butcher, H. K. (2003). Aging as emerging brilliance: Advancing Rogers' unitary theory of aging. *Visions: The Journal of Rogerian Nursing Science, 11,* 55–66.

Butcher, H. K. (2004). Written expression and the potential to enhance knowing participation in change. *Visions: The Journal of Rogerian Nursing Science, 12,* 37–50.

Butcher, H. K. (2005). The unitary field pattern portrait research method: Facets, processes and findings. *Nursing Science Quarterly, 18,* 293–297.

Butcher, H. K. (2006a). Unitary pattern-based praxis: A nexus of Rogerian cosmology, philosophy, and science. *Visions: The Journal of Rogerian Nursing Science, 14*(2), 8–33.

Butcher, H. K. (2006b). Using metaphoric unitary landscape narratives to facilitate pattern transformation: Fires in the tallgrass prairie as a wellspring of possibilities. *Visions: The Journal of Rogerian Nursing Science, 13,* 41–58.

Butcher, H. K. (2008). Progress in the explanatory power of the science of unitary human beings: Frubes in a lull or surfing in the barrel of the wave. *Visions: The Journal of Rogerian Nursing Science, 15*(2), 23–26.

Butcher, H. K., & Parker, N. (1988). Guided imagery within Martha Rogers' science of unitary human beings: An experimental study. *Nursing Science Quarterly, 1,* 103–110.

Carboni, J. T. (1992). Instrument development and the measurement of unitary constructs. *Nursing Science Quarterly, 5,* 134–142.

Carboni, J. T. (1995a). Enfolding health-as-wholeness-and-harmony: A theory of Rogerian nursing practice. *Nursing Science Quarterly, 8,* 71–78.

Carboni, J. T. (1995b). A Rogerian process of inquiry. *Nursing Science Quarterly, 8,* 22–37.

Caroselli, C., & Barrett, E. A. M. (1998). A review of the power as knowing participation in change literature. *Nursing Science Quarterly, 11,* 9–16.

Cowling, W. R. (1986). The science of unitary human beings: Theoretical issues, methodological challenges, and research realities. In V. M. Malinski (Ed.), *Explorations on Martha Rogers' science of unitary human beings* (pp. 65–78). Norwalk, CT: Appleton-Century-Crofts.

Cowling, W. R. (1990). A template for unitary pattern-based nursing practice. In E. A. Barrett (Ed.), *Visions of Rogers' science-based nursing* (pp. 45–65). New York: National League for Nursing.

Cowling, W. R. (1993a). Unitary knowing in nursing practice. *Nursing Science Quarterly, 6,* 201–207.

Cowling, W. R. (1993b). Unitary practice: Revisionary assumptions. In M. E. Parker (Ed.), *Patterns of nursing theories in practice* (pp. 199–212). New York: National League for Nursing.

Cowling, W. R. (1997). Pattern appreciation: The unitary science/practice of reaching essence. In M. Madrid (Ed.), *Patterns of Rogerian knowing* (pp. 129–142). New York: National League for Nursing.

Cowling, W. R. (1998). Unitary case inquiry. *Nursing Science Quarterly, 11,* 139–141.

Cowling, W. R. (2001). Unitary appreciative inquiry. *Advances in Nursing Science, 23*(4), 32–48.

Cowling, W. R. (2001). Unitary appreciative inquiry. *Advances in Nursing Science, 23*(4), 32–48.

Csikszentmihalyi, M. (1990). *Flow: The psychology of optimal experience.* New York: Harper & Row.

Deutsch, D. (1997). *The fabric of reality: The science of parallel universes—and its implications.* New York: Allen Lane.

Deutsch, D. (2011). *The beginnings of infinity: Explanations that transform the world.* New York: Viking.

Dossey, B. M. (1997). *Core curriculum for holistic nursing.* Gaithersburg, MD: Aspen.

Dossey, B. M., Keegan, L., & Guzzetta, C. (2004). *Holistic nursing: A handbook for practice* (4th ed.). Boston: Jones & Bartlett.

Dossey, L. (1993). *Healing words: The power of prayer and the practice of medicine.* New York: HarperCollins

Dossey, L. (1999). *Reinventing medicine: Beyond mind-body to a new era of healing.* New York: HarperCollins.

Dykeman, M. C., & Loukissa, D. (1993). The science of unitary human beings: An integrative review. *Nursing Science Quarterly, 6,* 179–188.

Fawcett, J. (1996). Issues of (in) compatibility between the worldview and research views of the science of unitary human beings: An invitation to dialogue. *Visions: The Journal of Rogerian Nursing Science, 4,* 5–11.

Fawcett, J. (2013). *Contemporary nursing knowledge: Analysis and evaluation of nursing models and theories* (3rd ed.). Philadelphia: F. A. Davis.

Fawcett, J., & Alligood, M. R. (2003). The science of unitary human beings: Analysis of qualitative research approaches. *Visions: The Journal of Rogerian Nursing Science, 11,* 7–20.

Ference, H. (1979). *The relationship of time experience, creativity traits, differentiation, and human field motion.* Unpublished doctoral dissertation, New York University, New York.

Ference, H. M. (1986). The relationship of time experience, creativity traits, differentiation, and human field motion. In V. M. Malinski (Ed.), *Explorations on Rogers' science of unitary human beings* (pp. 95–105). Norwalk, CT: Appleton-Century-Crofts.

Fuller, J. M. (2011). *A family unitary field pattern portrait of power as knowing participation in change among adult substance users in rehabilitation.* Unpublished doctoral dissertation, Hampton University, Hampton, Virginia.

Guba, E. G., & Lincoln, Y. S. (1989). *Fourth generation evaluation.* Newbury Park, CA: Sage.

Gueldner, S. H., Michel, Y., Bramlett, M. H., Liu, C-F., Johnston, L. W., Endo, E., et al. (2005). The Well-Being Picture Scale: A revision of the Index of Field Energy. *Nursing Science Quarterly, 18,* 42–50.

Hastings-Tolsma, M. T. (1992). *The relationship among diversity and human field pattern, risk taking, and time experience: An investigation of Rogers' principles of homeodynamics.* Unpublished doctoral dissertation, New York University, New York.

Hektor, L. M. (1989/1994). Martha E. Rogers: A life history. In V. M. Malinski & E. A. M. Barrett (Eds.). *Martha E. Rogers: Her life and her work* (pp. 10-27). Philadelphia: F. A. Davis. (Reprinted from *Nursing Science Quarterly, 2,* 63–73).

Hills, R. G. S., & Hanchett, E. (2001). Human change and individuation in pivotal life situation: Development and testing of the theory of enlightenment. *Visions: The Journal of Rogerian Nursing Science, 9,* 6–19.

Horvath, B. (1994). The science of unitary human beings as a foundation for nursing practice with persons experiencing life patterning difficulties: Transforming theory into motion. In M. Madrid & E. A. M. Barrett (Eds.), *Rogers' scientific art of nursing practice* (pp. 163–176). New York: National League for Nursing.

Johnson, N., Guadron, M., Verchot, C., & Gueldner, S. (2011). Validation of the Well-being Picture Scale (WPS). *Vision: The Journal of Rogerian Nursing Science, 18*(1), 8–21.

Johnston, L. W. (1994). Psychometric analysis of Johnson's Human Field Metaphor Scale. *Visions: The Journal of Rogerian Nursing Science, 2,* 7–11.

Johnston, L. W. (2001). An exploration of individual preferences for audio enhancement of the dying experience. *Visions: The Journal of Rogerian Nursing Science, 9,* 20–26.

Kim, T. S. (2001). The relation of magnetic field therapy to pain and power over time in persons with chronic primary headache: A pilot study. *Visions: The Journal of Rogerian Nursing Science, 9,* 27–42.

Kim, T. S. (2008). Science of unitary human beings: An update on research. *Nursing Science Quarterly, 21,* 294–299.

Levin, J. D. (2006). Unitary transformative nursing: using metaphor and imagery for self-reflection and theory informed practice. *Visions: The Journal of Rogerian Nursing Science, 14,* 27–35.

Lorenz, E. N. (1994). *The essence of chaos.* Seattle: University of Washington Press.

Madrid, M. (Ed.). (1997). *Patterns of Rogerian knowing.* New York: National League for Nursing.

Madrid, M. (Ed.). (1997). *Patterns of Rogerian knowing.* New York: National League for Nursing.

Madrid, M., & Barrett, E. A. M. (Eds.). (1994). *Rogers' scientific art of nursing practice.* New York: National League for Nursing.

Madrid, M., Barrett, E. A. M., & Winstead-Fry, P. (2010). A study of the feasibility of introducing therapeutic touch into the operative environment with patients undergoing cerebral angiography. *Journal of Holistic Nursing, 28,* 168–174.

Madrid, M., & Winstead-Fry, P. (1986). Rogers' conceptual model. In P. Winstead-Fry (Ed.), *Case studies in nursing theory* (pp. 73–102). New York: National League for Nursing.

Malinski, V. M. (Ed.). (1986a). *Explorations on Martha Rogers' science of unitary human beings.* Norwalk, CT: Appleton-Century-Crofts.

Malinski, V. M. (1986b). Further ideas from Martha Rogers. In V. M. Malinski (Ed.), *Explorations on Martha Rogers' science of unitary human beings* (pp. 9–14). Norwalk, CT: Appleton-Century-Crofts.

Malinski, V. M. (1991). Spirituality as integrality: A Rogerian perspective on the path of healing. *Journal of Holistic Nursing, 9,* 54–64.

Malinski, V. (1993). Therapeutic touch: The view from Rogerian nursing science. *Visions: The Journal of Rogerian Nursing Science, 1,* 45–54.

Malinski, V. M. (1994). Spirituality: A pattern manifestation of the human/environmental mutual process. *Visions: The Journal of Rogerian Nursing Science, 2,* 12–18.

Malinski, V. M. (2004). Compassion and loving-kindness: Heartsongs for healing spirit. *Spirituality and Health International, 5,* 89–98.

Malinski, V. M. (2012). Meditations on the unitary rhythm of dying-grieving. *Nursing Science Quarterly, 25,* 239–244.

Malinski, V. M., & Barrett, E. A. M. (Eds.). (1994). *Martha E. Rogers: Her life and her work.* Philadelphia: F. A. Davis.

Malinski, V. M., & Todaro-Franceschi, V. (2011). Exploring co-meditation as a means of reducing anxiety and facilitating relaxation in a nursing school setting. *Journal of Holistic Nursing, 29,* 242–248.

Moorhead, S., Johnson, M., Maas, M., & Swanson, E. (2013). *Nursing outcomes classification (NOC)* (5th ed.). St. Louis, MO: Elsevier.

Murphy, M. (1992). *The future of the body: Explorations into the further evolution of human nature.* Los Angeles, CA: Tarcher.

Nadeau, R., & Kafatos, M. (1999). *The non-local universe: The new physics and matters of the mind.* Oxford: Oxford University Press.

Paletta, J. L. (1990). The relationship of temporal experience to human time. In: E. A. M. Barrett (Ed.), *Visions of Rogers' science-based nursing* (pp. 239–253). New York: National League for Nursing.

Peat, F. D. (1991). *The philosopher's stone: Chaos, synchronicity, and the hidden world of order.* New York: Bantam.

Phillips, J. (1989). Science of unitary human beings: Changing research perspectives. *Nursing Science Quarterly, 2,* 57–60.

Phillips, J. R. (1990). Research and the riddle of change. *Nursing Science Quarterly, 3,* 55–56.

Phillips, J. R. (1994). The open-ended nature of the science of unitary human beings. In M. Madrid & E. A. M. Barrett (Eds.), *Rogers' scientific art of nursing practice* (pp. 11–25). New York: National League for Nursing.

Phillips, J. R. (2010a). The universality of Rogers' science of unitary human beings. *Nursing Science Quarterly, 23,* 55–59.

Phillips, J. R. (2010b). Perspectives of Rogers' relative present. *Visions: The Journal of Rogerian Nursing Science, 17,* 8–18.

Radin, D. (1997). *The conscious universe: The scientific truth of psychic phenomena.* San Francisco: Harper.

Rawnsley, M. M. (1994). Multiple field methods in unitary human field science. In M. Madrid & E. A. M. Barrett (Eds.), *Rogerian scientific art of nursing practice* (pp. 381–395). New York: National League for Nursing.

Reason, P. (1994). Three approaches to participative inquiry. In N. K. Denzin & Y. S. Lincoln (Eds.), *Handbook of qualitative research* (pp. 324–339). Thousand Oaks, CA: Sage.

Reed, P. G. (1991). Self-transcendence and mental health in the oldest-old adults. *Nursing Research, 40*(1), 5–11.

Reed, P. G. (2003). The theory of self-transcendence. In M. J. Smith & P. R. Liehr (Eds.). *Middle range theory for nursing* (pp. 145–166). New York: Springer.

Reeder, F. (1986). Basic theoretical research in the conceptual system of unitary human beings. In V. M. Malinski (Ed.), *Explorations on Martha E. Rogers' science of unitary human beings* (pp. 45–64). Norwalk, CT: Appleton-Century-Crofts.

Ring, M. E. (2009). Reiki and changes in pattern manifestations. *Nursing Science Quarterly, 22,* 250–258.

Rogers, M. F. (1961). *Educational revolution in nursing.* New York: Macmillan.

Rogers, M. F. (1964). *Reveille in nursing.* Philadelphia: F. A. Davis.

Rogers, M. E. (1966/1994). Epilogue. In V. M. Malinski & E. A. M. Barrett (Eds.), *Martha E. Rogers and her work* (pp. 337–338). Philadelphia: F. A. Davis. (Reprinted from the *Education Violet,* the New York University newspaper, 1966.)

Rogers, M. E. (1970). *An introduction to the theoretical basis of nursing.* Philadelphia: F. A. Davis.

Rogers, M. E. (1980). Nursing: A science of unitary man. In J. P. Riehl & C. Roy (Eds.), *Conceptual models for nursing practice* (2nd ed., pp. 329–337). New York: Appleton-Century-Crofts.

Rogers, M. E. (1986). Science of unitary human beings. In V. M. Malinski (Ed.), *Explorations on Martha Rogers' science of unitary human beings* (pp. 3–8). Norwalk, CT: Appleton-Century-Crofts.

Rogers, M. E. (1988). Nursing science and art: A prospective. *Nursing Science Quarterly, 1,* 99–102.

Rogers, M. E. (1989). Response to questions for Dr. Martha E. Rogers. *Rogerian Nursing Science News, 1*(3), 6.

Rogers, M. E. (1990). Nursing: Science of unitary, irreducible human beings: Update 1990. In E. A. M. Barrett (Ed.), *Visions of Rogers' science-based nursing* (pp. 5–11). New York: National League for Nursing.

Rogers, M. E. (1992). Nursing and the space age. *Nursing Science Quarterly, 5,* 27–34.

Rogers, M. E. (1994a). The science of unitary human beings: Current perspectives. *Nursing Science Quarterly, 7,* 33–35.

Rogers, M. E. (1994b). Nursing science evolves. In: M. Madrid & E. A. M. Barrett (Eds.), *Rogers' scientific art of nursing practice* (pp. 3–9). New York: National League for Nursing.

Sheldrake, R. (1988). *The presence of the past: Morphic resonance and the habits of nature.* New York: Times Books.

Smith, D. W. (1994). Toward developing a theory of spirituality. *Visions: The Journal of Rogerian Nursing Science, 2,* 35–43.

Smith, M. C., & Reeder, F. (1996). Clinical outcomes research and Rogerian science: Strange or emergent bedfellows. *Visions: The Journal of Rogerian Nursing Science, 6,* 27–38.

Smith, M. J. (1988). Perspectives on nursing science. *Nursing Science Quarterly, 1,* 80–85.

Tart, C. T. (2009). *The end of materialism: How evidence of the paranormal is bringing science and spirit together.* Oakland, CA: New Harbinger.

Talbot, M. (1991). *The holographic universe.* New York: HarperCollins.

Terwilliger, S. H., Gueldner, S. H., & Bronstein, L. (2012). A preliminary evaluation of the well-being picture scale-children's version (WPS-CV) in a sample of fourth and fifth graders. *Nursing Science Quarterly, 25,* 155–159.

Todaro-Franceschi, V. (1999). *The enigma of energy: Where science and religion converge.* New York: Crossroad.

Todaro-Franceschi, V. (2006). Synchronicity related to dead loved ones: A natural healing modality. *Spirituality and Health International, 7,* 151–161.

Watson, J. (1993). *The relationships of sleep-wake rhythm, dream experience, human field motion, and time experience in older women.* Unpublished doctoral dissertation, New York University, New York.

Watson, J., Barrett, E. A. M., Hastings-Tolsma, M., Johnston, L., & Gueldner, S. (1997). Measurement in Rogerian Science: A review of selected instruments. In M. Madrid (Ed.), *Patterns of Rogerian knowing* (pp. 87–99). New York: National League for Nursing.

Whitbourne, S. K., & Whitbourne, S.B. (2011). *Adult development and aging* (4th ed.). New York: Wiley

Zahourek, R. P. (2004). Intentionality forms the matrix of healing: A theory. *Alternative Therapies in Health and Medicine, 10*(6), 40–49.

Zahourek, R. P. (2005). Intentionality: Evolutionary development in healing: A grounded theory study for holistic nursing. *Journal of Holistic Nursing, 23,* 89–109.

Rosemarie Rizzo Parse's Humanbecoming Paradigm

ROSEMARIE RIZZO PARSE

Introducing the Theorist
Overview of Parse's Humanbecoming
Paradigm
Application of Theory
Summary
References

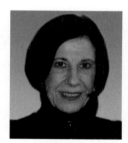

Rosemarie Rizzo Parse

Introducing the Theorist

Rosemarie Rizzo Parse is a Distinguished Professor Emerita at Loyola University Chicago as well as a Fellow in the American Academy of Nursing, where she initiated and is immediate past chair of the Nursing Theory–Guided Practice Expert Panel. She is founder and editor of *Nursing Science Quarterly;* president of Discovery International, which sponsors international nursing theory conferences; and founder of the Institute of Humanbecoming, where each summer in Pittsburgh she teaches new material on the ontological, epistemological, and methodological aspects of the humanbecoming paradigm. There are also sessions on the Humanbecoming Community Change Model (Parse, 2003a, 2012a, 2013a, 2014), the Humanbecoming Teaching–Learning Model (Parse, 2004, 2014), the Humanbecoming Mentoring Model (Parse, 2008c, 2014), the Humanbecoming Leading–Following Model (Parse, 2008b, 2011a, 2014), and the Humanbecoming Family Model (Parse, 2008a, 2009a, 2014). The goal of all sessions is the understanding of the meaning of humanuniverse from a humanbecoming perspective.

Dr. Parse has published more than 300 articles and 10 books. Her books include *Nursing Fundamentals* (Parse, 1974); *Man-Living-Health: A Theory of Nursing* (Parse, 1981); *Nursing Research: Qualitative Methods* (Parse, Coyne, & Smith, 1985); *Nursing Science: Major Paradigms, Theories, and Critiques* (Parse, 1987); *Illuminations: The Human Becoming Theory in Practice and Research* (Parse, 1995); *The Human Becoming School of Thought* (Parse, 1998a); *Hope: An International Human Becoming Perspective* (Parse, 1999a); *Qualitative Inquiry: The Path of Sciencing* (Parse, 2001); *Community: A Human Becoming Perspective* (Parse, 2003a); and *The Humanbecoming Paradigm: A Transformational Worldview* (Parse, 2014). Her books and other publications have been translated into many languages, as her theory is a guide for practice in health-care settings, and her research methodologies are used by nurse scholars in Australia, Canada, Denmark, Finland, Greece, Italy, Japan, South Korea, Sweden, Switzerland, Taiwan, the United Kingdom, the United States, and many other countries on five continents.

Dr. Parse has received two lifetime achievement awards, one from the Midwest Nursing Research Society and one from the Asian Nurses' Association. The Rosemarie Rizzo Parse Scholarship was endowed in her name at the Henderson State University School of Nursing. She is a sought-after speaker and consultant for local, national, and international venues. She also received the Medal of Honor from the University of Lisbon.

Dr. Parse is a graduate of Duquesne University in Pittsburgh and received her master's and doctorate from the University of Pittsburgh. She was a member of the faculty of the University of Pittsburgh, dean of the School of Nursing at Duquesne University, professor and coordinator of the Center for Nursing Research at Hunter College of the City University of New York (1983–1993), and professor and Niehoff Chair in Nursing Research at Loyola University Chicago (1993–2006). Since January 2007, she has been a consultant, visiting scholar, and adjunct professor at the New York University College of Nursing.

Overview of Parse's Humanbecoming Paradigm

Prologue: Reflections on the Discipline and Profession of Nursing

At present, nurse leaders in research, administration, education, and practice are focusing attention on expanding the knowledge base of nursing through enhancement of the discipline's frameworks and theories. Nursing is both a discipline and a profession (Parse, 1999b). The goal of the *discipline* is to expand knowledge about human experiences through creative conceptualization and research (Parse, 2005, 2009c). The knowledge base of the discipline is the scientific guide to living the art of nursing. The discipline-specific knowledge is born and fostered in academic settings where research and education advance knowledge to new realms of understanding (Parse, 2008d, 2009b). The goal of the *profession* is to provide service to humankind through living the art of the science. Members of the nursing profession are responsible for regulating the standards of practice and education based on disciplinary knowledge that reflects safe health service to society in all settings (Parse, 1999b, 2012b, 2013b).

The Profession of Nursing

The profession of nursing consists of people educated according to nationally regulated, defined, and monitored standards that are intended to preserve the integrity of health care for members of society. The standards are specified predominantly in medical terms, according to a tradition largely related to nursing's early subservience to medicine. Recently, nurse leaders in health-care systems and in regulating organizations have been developing standards (Mitchell, 1998) and regulations (Damgaard, 2012; Damgaard & Bunkers, 1998, 2012) consistent with discipline-specific knowledge as articulated in the theories and frameworks of nursing. This is a significant development that has fortified the identity of nursing as a discipline with its own body of knowledge—one that specifies the service that society can expect from members of the profession (Parse, 2011c). With the rapidly changing health policies and the general dissatisfaction of consumers with health-care delivery, clearly stated expectations for services from each of nursing's paradigms are a welcome change (Parse, 1999b, 2013a).

The Discipline of Nursing

The discipline of nursing encompasses at least three paradigmatic perspectives about humanuniverse (Parse, 2012a, 2013a). The totality paradigm posits the human as body–mind–spirit whose health is considered a state of biological, psychological, social, and spiritual well-being. The body–mind–spirit perspective is particulate—focusing on the bio–psycho–social–spiritual parts of the whole human as the human interacts with and adapts to the environment. The ontology leads to research and practice on phenomena related to preventing disease and maintaining and promoting health according to societal norms. The totality paradigm frameworks and theories are more closely aligned with the medical model tradition. Nurses practicing according to this paradigm are concerned with participation of persons in health-care decisions but have specific regimens and goals to bring about change for the people they serve (Parse, 1999b).

In contrast, the simultaneity paradigm views the human as unitary—indivisible, unpredictable, and everchanging (Parse, 1987, 1998a, 2007b), wherein health is considered a value and a process. The ontology leads research and practice scholars to focus on, for example, energy and environmental field patterns (Rogers, 1992). Nurses focus

on power in knowing participation (Barrett, 2010; Rogers, 1992).

In 2012, Parse identified a third paradigm, the humanbecoming paradigm (Parse, 2012a, 2013a). (Fig. 15-1) This was created inasmuch as the ontology, epistemology, and methodologies of the humanbecoming school of thought have moved on from the traditional metaparadigm conceptualization and beyond the totality and simultaneity paradigms (Parse, 2013a, 2014). With the humanbecoming paradigm in the ontology, humanuniverse is an indivisible, unpredictable everchanging cocreation, and living quality is the becoming visible-invisible becoming of the emerging now. The ethos of humanbecoming is also described and this is unlike any other paradigm. With the epistemology, the focus of study is on universal *living* experiences. With the methodologies, sciencing (the research process) is qualitative (Parse research method and the humanbecoming hermeneutic method), and living the art of humanbecoming is in true presence with illuminating meaning, shifting rhythms, and inspiring transcending (Parse, 1981, 1992, 1997a, 1998a,

Paradigms of the Discipline of Nursing

Totality Paradigm	Simultaneity Paradigm	Humanbecoming Paradigm
Ontology	**Ontology**	**Ontology**
Human Biopsychosocialspiritual being	*Human* Unitary pattern	*Humanuniverse* Indivisible, unpredictable, everchanging cocreation
Universe Internal and external environment	*Universe* Unitary pattern in mutual process with the human	*Ethos of Humanbecoming-Dignity* Presence, existence, trust, worth
Health A state and process of well-being	*Health* A value and a process	*Living quality* Becoming visible-invisible Becoming of the emerging now
Epistemology Human attributes	*Epistemology* Human patterns	*Epistemology* Universal living experiences
Methodologies (research and practice) Quantitative, qualitative, mixed Steps of the nursing process	*Methodologies* (research and practice) Quantitative, qualitative, praxis Pattern recognition	*Methodologies* (sciencing and living the art) Qualitative True presence illuminating meaning, shifting rhythms, inspiring transcending

Copyright, Rosemarie Rizzo Parse, 2014

Fig 15 • 1 Paradigms of the discipline of nursing. *(Copyright ©2014, Rosemarie Rizzo Parse.)*

2010, 2014). Nurses living the humanbecoming paradigm beliefs hold that their primary concern is people's perspectives of living quality with human dignity (Parse, 1981, 1992, 1997a, 1998a; 2010, 2012a, 2013a, 2014). The new conceptualization *living quality* is described in detail in Parse (2013a). (See Parse, 2012a and 2013a, for details about the humanbecoming paradigm.)

Because the ontologies of these three paradigmatic perspectives are different, they lead to different research and practice modalities, different ethical considerations, and different professional services to humankind. (See Parse, 2010, for the humanbecoming ethical tenets of human dignity, which are reverence, awe, betrayal, and shame.) Humanbecoming is a basic *human science* that has cocreated universal humanuniverse living experiences as a central focus. It is called a paradigm and a school of thought because it encompasses a unique ontology, epistemology, and methodologies (Parse, 1997b, 2010, 2012a, 2013a, 2014).

Parse's (1981) original work was titled *Man-Living-Health: A Theory of Nursing.* When the term *mankind* was replaced with *male gender* in the dictionary definition of *man,* the name of the theory was changed to *human becoming* (Parse, 1992). No aspect of the principles changed at that time. With the publication of *The Human Becoming School of Thought* (1998a), Parse expanded the original work to include descriptions of three research methodologies and additional specifics related to the practice methodology (Parse, 1987), thus classifying the science of humanbecoming as a school of thought (Parse, 1997b). The fundamental idea of humanbecoming—that humans are indivisible, unpredictable, everchanging, as specified in the ontology—precludes any use of terms such as *physiological, biological, psychological,* or *spiritual* to describe the human. These terms are particulate, thus inconsistent with the ontology. Other terms inconsistent with humanbecoming include words often used to describe people, such as *noncompliant, dysfunctional,* and *manipulative.*

In 2007, Parse set forth a clarification of the ontology of the school of thought. She specified *humanbecoming* as one word and *humanuniverse* as one word (Parse, 2007b). Joining the words creates one concept and further confirms the idea of indivisibility. She also described postulates to clarify the ontology further (Parse, 2007b). The ontology—that is, the assumptions, postulates, and principles—sets forth beliefs that are clearly different from other nursing frameworks and theories. Discipline-specific knowledge is articulated in unique language specifying a position on the phenomenon of concern for each discipline. The humanbecoming language is unique to nursing. For example, the three humanbecoming principles contain nine concepts written in verbal form with *-ing* endings to make clear the importance of the ongoing process of change as basic to humanuniverse emergence. In addition, each concept is explicated with paradoxes, not opposites, but rhythms, further specifying the uniqueness of the humanbecoming language.

The humanbecoming encompasses the ontology, the epistemology, and the research and practice methodologies as described here. In 2012, the school of thought was expanded and new conceptualizations created the humanbecoming paradigm (Parse 2012a, 2013a, 2014).

The Ontology

The assumptions, postulates, and principles of the humanbecoming paradigm comprise the ontology (Parse, 2007b, 2012a, 2013a; Fig. 15-2).

Philosophical Assumptions

The assumptions of the humanbecoming paradigm are written at the philosophical level of discourse (Parse, 1998a, 2010, 2012a, 2013a, 2014). There are nine fundamental assumptions about humanuniverse, ethos of humanbecoming, and living quality (Parse, 2013a, 2014). The assumptions arose beginning with the first book in 1981, from a synthesis of ideas from the science of unitary human beings (Rogers, 1992) and from existential phenomenological thought, particularly Heidegger, Merleau-Ponty, and Sartre; see Parse, 1981, 1992, 1994a, 1995, 1997a, 1998a,

The Humanbecoming Ontology

Assumptions	Postulates	Principles	Concepts and Paradoxes
Humanuniverse is indivisible, unpredictable, everchanging. Humanuniverse is cocreating reality as a seamless symphony of becoming. Humanuniverse is an illimitable mystery with contextually construed pattern preferences. Ethos of humanbecoming is dignity. Ethos of humanbecoming is august presence, a noble bearing of immanent distinctness. Ethos of humanbecoming is abiding truths of presence, existence, trust, and worth. Living quality is the becoming visible-invisible becoming of the emerging now. Living quality is the everchanging whatness of becoming. Living quality is the personal expression of uniqueness.	Illimitability is the indivisible unbounded knowing extended to infinity, the all-at-once remembering-prospecting with the emerging now. Paradox is an intricate rhythm expressed as a pattern preference. Freedom is contextually construed liberation. Mystery is the unexplainable, that which cannot be completely known unequivocally.	Structuring meaning is the imaging and valuing of languaging. Configuring rhythmical patterns is the revealing-concealing and enabling-limiting of connecting-separating. Cotranscending with possibles is the powering and originating of transforming.	**Imaging:** explicit-tacit; reflective-prereflective **Valuing:** confirming–not confirming **Languaging:** speaking–being silent; moving–being still **Revealing-concealing:** disclosing–not disclosing **Enabling-limiting:** potentiating-restricting **Connecting-separating:** attending-distancing **Powering:** pushing-resisting; affirming–not affirming; being-nonbeing **Originating:** certainty-uncertainty; conforming–not conforming **Transforming:** familiar-unfamiliar

Copyright, Rosemarie Rizzo Parse, 2014

Fig 15 • 2 The humanbecoming ontology. *(Copyright ©2014, Rosemarie Rizzo Parse.)*

2013a, 2014). In the assumptions, Parse posits humanuniverse as indivisible, unpredictable, and everchanging, cocreating unique becoming. She also posits additional descriptions of humanuniverse, ethos of humanbecoming, and *living quality. Living quality* is the chosen way of being in the becoming visible-invisible becoming of the emerging now (2012a, 2013a, 2014). Humans live an all-at-onceness, which *is* the becoming visible-invisible of the emerging now, in freely choosing meanings that arise with the illimitable (2007b, 2012a, 2013a, 2014). The chosen meanings are the value priorities cocreated in transcending with the possibles (Parse, 1998a).

Postulates and Principles

In 2007, Parse elaborated certain truths embedded in the conceptualizations of the ontology (2007b). In so doing she expanded the idea of cocreating reality as a seamless symphony of becoming (Parse, 1996), a central thought foundational to the ontology, as foregrounded with four postulates of illimitability, paradox, freedom, and mystery [See Parse (2007b) for detailed descriptions of the postulates]. The meanings of the postulates permeate all three of the principles; the words of the postulates are not used in the statements of the principles. Thus, the wording has been clarified to provide semantic consistency without changing the original meaning of the principles. The principles of humanbecoming, often referred to as the theory, describe the central phenomenon of nursing (humanuniverse), and arise from the three major themes of the assumptions: meaning, rhythmicity, and transcendence. Each principle describes a theme with three concepts. Each of the concepts explicates fundamental paradoxes of humanbecoming (Parse, 1998a, 2007b). The paradoxes are rhythms lived all-at-once as pattern preferences (Parse, 2007b). Paradoxes are not opposites or problems to be solved but rather are ways humans live their chosen meanings. This way of viewing paradox is unique to the humanbecoming school of thought (Mitchell, 1993a; Parse, 1981, 1994b, 2007b).

Statements of Principles

The statements of principles are presented in detail in Parse (2007b, 2010, 2012a, 2013a, 2014). With the *first* principle (see Parse 1981, 1998a, 2007b, 2013a, 2014), Parse explicates the idea that humans construct personal realities with unique choosings arising with illimitable humanuniverse options. Reality, the meaning given to a situation, is the individual human's everchanging seamless symphony of becoming (Parse, 1996). The seamless symphony is the unique story of the human as mystery emerging with the explicit-tacit knowings of *imaging*. The human lives the confirming–not confirming of *valuing* as cherished beliefs, while *languaging* with speaking–being silent and moving–being still in the becoming visible-invisible of the emerging now (for details, see Parse 2007b, 2012a, 2013a, 2014).

The *second* principle (Parse, 1981, 1998a, 2007b, 2010) describes rhythmical humanuniverse patterns. The paradoxical rhythm "*revealing–concealing* is disclosing–not disclosing all-at-once" (Parse, 1998a, p. 43). Not all is explicitly known or can be told in the unfolding mystery of humanbecoming. "*Enabling–limiting* is living the opportunities–restrictions present in all choosings all-at-once" (Parse, 1998a, p. 44). There are opportunities and restrictions whatever the choice; all choosings are potentiating–restricting (see Parse, 2007b and 2014 for details). "*Connecting–separating* is being with and apart from others, ideas, objects and situations all-at-once" (Parse, 1998a, p. 45). It is a coming together and moving apart; there is closeness in the separation and distance in the closeness—a rhythmical attending–distancing (for details, see Parse 2007b, 2012a, 2013a).

With the *third* principle, Parse (1981, 1998a, 2007b, 2010, 2012a, 2013a) explicated the idea that humans are everchanging, that is, moving on with the possibilities of their intended hopes and dreams. A changing diversity unfolds as humans affirm and do not affirm in the pushing–resisting of *powering*, as creating new ways of living the conformity–nonconformity and certainty–uncertainty of *originating* sheds new light on the familiar–unfamiliar of *transforming*. *Powering* is the pushing–resisting of affirming–not affirming being in light of nonbeing (Parse, 1998a, 2007b, 2012a, 2013a, 2014). The being–nonbeing rhythm is all-at-once living the everchanging becoming visible-invisible becoming of the emerging now. Humans, in *originating*, seek to conform–not conform, that is, to be like others and unique all-at-once, while living the ambiguity of the certainty–uncertainty embedded in all change. The changing diversity arises with *transforming* the familiar–unfamiliar, as illimitable possibles are viewed in a different light.

The three principles, together with the postulates and assumptions, comprise the ontology of the humanbecoming school of thought. The principles are referred to as the humanbecoming theory. The concepts, with the paradoxes, describe humanuniverse. This ontological base gives rise to the epistemology and methodologies of humanbecoming. Epistemology refers to the focus of inquiry. Consistent with the humanbecoming school of thought, the focus of inquiry is universal living experiences (Parse, 2005, 2012a, 2013a).

Applications of Theory
Humanbecoming Research Methodologies

Sciencing humanbecoming is coming to know; it is an ongoing inquiry to discover and understand the meaning of living experiences.

The humanbecoming research tradition has two basic research methods (Parse, 1998a, 2005, 2011b). These two methods flow from the ontology of the school of thought. The basic research methods are the *Parse method* (Parse, 1987, 1990, 1992, 1995, 1997a, 1998a, 2001, 2005, 2011b, 2012a, 2013a, 2014) and the *humanbecoming hermeneutic method* (Cody, 1995; Parse, 1995, 1998a, 2001, 2005, 2011b, 2012a, 2013a, 2014). The humanbecoming hermeneutic method was created in congruence with the assumptions and principles of Parse's theory, drawing from works by Bernstein (1983), Gadamer (1976, 1960/1998), Heidegger (1962), Langer (1976), and Ricoeur (1976, 1981).

The purpose of these two basic research methods is to advance the science of humanbecoming by studying universal living experiences from participants' descriptions (Parse method) and from written texts and art forms (humanbecoming hermeneutic method). The phenomena for study with the Parse method are universal living experiences such as joy, sorrow, hope, grieving, and courage, among others. Written texts from any literary source or art form may be the subject of sciencing with the humanbecoming hermeneutic method. The processes of both methods call for a unique dialogue, researcher with participant, or researcher with text or art form. The researcher in the Parse Method is in true presence as the participant moves with an unstructured dialogue about the living experience under study. The researcher in the humanbecoming hermeneutic method is in true presence with the emerging possibilities in the horizon of meaning arising in dialogue with texts or art forms. True presence is an intense attentiveness to unfolding essences and emergent meanings. The researcher's intent with these research methods is to discover structures (Parse method) and emergent meanings (humanbecoming hermeneutic method; see Parse, 2001, 2005, 2011b, 2012a, 2013a, 2014). The contributions of the findings from studies using these two methods include "new knowledge and understanding of humanly lived experiences" (Parse, 1998a, p. 62).

Many nurse scholars worldwide have conducted studies using the Parse method, many of which have been published (for example, Baumann, 2000, 2003, 2009, 2013; Bunkers, 2010, 2012; Condon, 2010; Doucet, 2012a, 2012b; Doucet & Bournes, 2007; MacDonald & Jonas-Simpson, 2009; Maillard-Struby, 2012; Morrow, 2010; Naef & Bournes, 2009; S. M. Smith, 2012, and many others). Parse (1999a) was the principal investigator for a nine-country research study on the living experience of hope using the Parse method, with participants from Australia, Canada, Finland, Italy, Japan, Sweden, Taiwan, the United Kingdom, and the United States. The findings from these studies and the stories of the participants are published in *Hope: An International Human Becoming Perspective* (Parse, 1999a). Collaborative research projects using the Parse research method have also been published on feeling very tired (Baumann, 2003; Huch & Bournes, 2003; Parse, 2003b). Six studies have been published in which authors used the humanbecoming hermeneutic method (Baumann, 2008; Baumann, Carroll, Damgaard, Millar, & Welch, 2001; Cody, 1995, 2001; Ortiz, 2003; Parse, 2007a)

Living-the-art projects are initiated when a researcher wishes to describe the changes, satisfactions, and effectiveness when humanbecoming guides practice (Parse, 1998a, 2001, 2006). The major purpose of the project is to understand what happens when humanbecoming is living nurse with person, family, and community. A number of researchers have conducted such living-the-art projects, all of which demonstrated enhanced satisfaction among persons, families, and communities (Bournes & Ferguson-Paré, 2007, 2008; Bournes et al., 2007; Jonas, 1995a; Legault & Ferguson-Paré, 1999; Maillard-Strüby, 2007; Mitchell, 1995; Northrup & Cody, 1998; Santopinto & Smith, 1995), and a synthesis of the findings of these and other such studies was written and published (Bournes, 2002; Doucet & Bournes, 2007).

Humanbecoming: Living the Art

The goal of the nurse living the humanbecoming beliefs is true presence in bearing witness and being with others in their changing patterns of living quality. True presence is lived nurse with person, family, and community in illuminating meaning, synchronizing rhythms, and mobilizing transcendence (Parse, 1987, 1992, 1994a, 1995, 1997a, 1998a, 2010, 2012a, 2013a, 2014). The nurse with individuals or groups is in true presence with the unfolding meanings as persons explicate, dwell with, and move on with changing patterns of diversity.

Living true presence is unique to the art of humanbecoming. True presence is not to be confused with terms now prevalent in the literature such as *authentic presence, transforming presence, presencing*, and others. It is sometimes misinterpreted as simply asking persons what they want. Often nurses say it is what they always do (Mitchell, 1993b); this is not true presence. "True presence is an intentional reflective love, an interpersonal art grounded in a strong knowledge base" (Parse, 1998a, p. 71). The knowledge base underpinning true presence is specified in the assumptions, postulates, and principles of humanbecoming (Parse, 1981, 1992, 1995, 1997a, 1998a, 2007b, 2010, 2012a, 2013a, 2014). True presence is a free-flowing attentiveness in the emerging now that arises from the belief that the humanuniverse is indivisible, unpredictable, everchanging. Humans freely choose with situations, structure personal meaning, live paradoxical rhythms, and move beyond with changing diversity (Parse, 1998a, 2007b, 2012a, 2013a, 2014). Parse (1987, 1998b) states that to know, understand, and live the beliefs of humanbecoming requires concentrated study of the ontology, epistemology, and methodologies and a commitment to a different way of being with people. The different way that arises from the humanbecoming beliefs is true presence.

True presence is a powerful humanuniverse connection. It is lived in face-to-face discussions, silent immersions, and lingering presence (Parse, 1987, 1998a). Nurses may be with persons, families, and communities in discussions, imaginings, or remembrances through stories, films, drawings, photographs, movies, metaphors, poetry, rhythmical movements, and other expressions (Parse, 1998a).

Many publications explicate the art of true presence with a variety of persons and groups. (See, for example, Arndt, 1995; Banonis, 1995; Bournes, 2000, 2003, 2006; Bournes, Bunkers, & Welch, 2004; Bournes & Flint, 2003; Bournes & Naef, 2006; Butler, 1988; Butler & Snodgrass, 1991; Chapman, Mitchell, & Forchuk, 1994; Cody, Mitchell, Jonas-Simpson, & Maillard-Strüby, 2004; Hansen-Ketchum, 2004; Hutchings, 2002; Jonas, 1994, 1995b; Jonas-Simpson & McMahon, 2005; Karnick, 2005, 2007; Lee & Pilkington, 1999; Mattice & Mitchell, 1990; Mitchell, 1988, 1990; Mitchell & Bournes, 2000; Mitchell, Bournes, & Hollett, 2006; Mitchell & Bunkers, 2003; Mitchell & Cody, 1999; Mitchell & Copplestone, 1990; Mitchell & Pilkington, 1990; Naef, 2006; Norris, 2002; Paille & Pilkington, 2002; Quiquero, Knights, & Meo, 1991; Rasmusson, 1995; Rasmusson, Jonas, & Mitchell, 1991; M. K. Smith, 2002; Stanley & Meghani, 2001; and others).

Living the Art of Humanbecoming With Persons and Groups

It is important here to clarify some terminology. *Nursing practice* is a generic term that refers to the genre of activities of the profession in general. The term *practice* is not appropriate to use when referring to humanbecoming, because according to various dictionary definitions it means a habit, or to drill, exercise, try repeatedly, or do over and over again. The word *practice* is antithetical to the ontology, as a major focus of humanbecoming is reverence, awe, human freedom, and dignity (Parse, 2010). Humanbecoming nurses live the art of the science of humanbecoming. The art of humanbecoming refers to living true presence, which arises directly from a sound understanding of the ontology of the school of thought. True presence flows only from nurses and health professionals who have studied, understand, believe in, and live the humanbecoming assumptions, postulates, and principles. *Living* is the proper term to describe what nurses experience when with recipients of health care. Nurses and others who live humanbecoming believe that persons, families, and communities are the experts on their own health-care situations, and all are treated with dignity (Parse, 2010).

In nurse-with-person health-care situations, nurses in true presence come to persons with an availability to be with and bear witness, as persons illuminate the meaning of the situations, shift rhythms, and inspire transcending in focusing on the becoming visible-invisible becoming of the emerging now (Parse, 1981, 1987, 1998a, 2007b, 2010, 2012a, 2013a, 2014). Illuminating meaning, shifting rhythms, and inspiring transforming occur in the true presence of the humanbecoming nurse, as persons explicate their situations, dwell with the becoming visible-invisible becoming of the emerging now. In explicating, dwelling with, and moving on, persons experience new insights and even surprises, as situations are seen in the new light that arises with the true presence of nurses who bear witness and do not label. Labeling or diagnosing is objectifying, ignoring the importance of persons' dignity and freedom (Parse, 2010). Humanbecoming nurses believe that persons know their way and live quality according to their unique value priorities (Parse, 2012a, 2013a). Humanbecoming nurses do not have a preset agenda or teaching plan about what persons should or ought do but rather listen carefully to the intents and desires stated by persons because these intents are value priorities that are the living choices of persons. With recipients of health care, humanbecoming nurses ask what is most important for the moment and explore meanings, wishes, intents, and desires related to what is emerging now from the perspective of the recipients and these guide nurses' participation (Parse, 2008e, 2012a, 2013a, 2014). What may seem important to the nurse may not be what is important to the person. For example, when a nurse (not living humanbecoming) thought that fear about the new diagnosis of lung cancer was the most important issue for a person, she began to design a teaching plan to inform the person about the disease; however, when a humanbecoming nurse asked the person, "What is the most important issue for you right now?" the gentleman answered, "Telling my family and continuing to work to care for them." The humanbecoming nurse continued to discuss these concerns with the gentleman with no agenda except the one set by the gentleman. Humanbecoming nurses are with persons in ways that honor their wishes and desires. Persons are seamless symphonies of becoming, and nurses are only one note in the symphony (Parse, 1996).

Living the Art of Humanbecoming With Community

The humanbecoming school of thought is a guide for research, practice, education, and administration in settings throughout the world. Scholars from five continents have embraced the belief system and live humanbecoming in a variety of venues, including health-care centers and university nursing programs. The Humanbecoming Community Model (Parse, 2003a, 2014), the Humanbecoming Teaching–Learning Model (Parse, 2004, 2014), The Humanbecoming Mentoring Model (Parse, 2008c, 2014), the Humanbecoming Leading–Following Model (Parse, 2008b, 2011a, 2014) , and the Humanbecoming family model (Parse 2008a, 2009a, 2014) are disseminated and used in practice settings worldwide. Many health centers throughout the world have humanbecoming as a guide to health care (Bournes et al., 2004; Cody et al., 2014). In several university-affiliated practice settings in Canada, humanbecoming practice has been evaluated, and the theory has provided underpinnings for standards of care (Bournes, 2002; Legault & Ferguson-Paré, 1999; Mitchell, 1998; Mitchell, Closson, Coulis, Flint, & Gray, 2000; Northrup & Cody, 1998) and nursing best practice guidelines (Nelligan et al., 2002). For example, in Toronto, Sunnybrook Health Science Centre and University Health Network had created multidisciplinary standards of care that arise from the beliefs and values of the humanbecoming school of thought.

In settings worldwide where humanbecoming has guided nursing practice on a large scale, researchers examined the effects on the nurses and persons who were involved (Bournes & Ferguson-Paré, 2007, 2008; Bournes et al., 2007; Jonas, 1995a; Legault & Ferguson-Paré, 1999; Maillard-Strüby, 2007; Mitchell, 1995; Northrup & Cody, 1998; Santopinto & Smith, 1995). The findings of the studies describe what happened when humanbecoming was used as a guide for nursing practice on an orthopedic surgery and rheumatology unit (Bournes & Ferguson-Paré, 2007), on a cardiac surgery unit (Bournes et al., 2007), on a medical oncology unit and a general surgery unit (Bournes & Ferguson-Paré, 2008), in a family practice unit affiliated with a large teaching hospital (Jonas, 1995a), on a 41-bed vascular and general surgery unit (Legault & Ferguson-Paré, 1999), on an acute care medical unit (Mitchell, 1995), on three acute care psychiatry units (Northrup & Cody, 1998), on three units in a 400-bed community teaching hospital (Santopinto & Smith, 1995), and on a medical oncology unit (Maillard-Strüby, 2007). The findings from five of the studies are summarized in Bournes (2002) and are consistent with those of more recent evaluations (Bournes & Ferguson-Paré, 2007, 2008; Bournes et al., 2007; Maillard-Strüby, 2007).

Bournes and Ferguson-Paré (2007, 2008) and Bournes, Plummer, Hollett, and Ferguson-Paré (2008) examined the impact of an innovative academic employment model (the humanbecoming 80/20 model—in which nurses spent 80 percent of their paid work time in direct patient care guided by humanbecoming and 20 percent of their paid work time learning about humanbecoming and engaging in related professional development activities). The humanbecoming 80/20 model has been implemented on four units—three in Toronto, Ontario (Bournes & Ferguson-Paré, 2007, 2008) and one in Regina, Saskatchewan (Bournes et al., 2007). The Regina project was implemented in collaboration with Regina Qu'Appelle Health Region and the Saskatchewan Union of Nurses.

Findings from the research (Bournes & Ferguson-Paré, 2007, 2008; Bournes et al., 2007) to evaluate implementation of the humanbecoming 80/20 model have been extremely positive. For example, interviews with nurses, patients, families, and other health professionals in the Bournes and Ferguson-Paré (2007) study "supported the humanbecoming theory as an effective basis for learning and implementing patient-entered care that benefits both nurses and patients" (p. 251). Patients and families in that study "reported that they appreciated the reverent consideration given to them by nurses who had learned about humanbecoming-guided patient-centered care"

(p. 251). They also described "being confident engaging in discussions with nurses who understood and attentive experts interested in who they were and what was important to them" (p. 251). Similarly, the nurse participants in Bournes and Ferguson-Paré's (2007) and Bournes and colleagues' (2008) studies reported that after learning about humanbecoming-guided nursing practice, they were more concerned with listening to patients and families, being with them, getting to know what is important to them, and respecting them as the experts about their quality of life. They also reported being more satisfied with their work—a theme noted by nurse leaders and allied health participants who shared that nurses listened more and focused on patients' perspectives. (Bournes & Ferguson-Paré, 2007, p. 251)

Participants in both studies described the benefits of the program—not only in relation to how it changed their relationships with patients but also in relation to how it changed their view of how to be with their colleagues in more meaningful ways (see Bournes & Ferguson-Paré, 2007; Bournes et al., 2007). In addition, study findings show that the cost of providing education about humanbecoming-guided practice and staffing the 80/20 aspect of the model is offset by higher nurse and patient satisfaction scores and a reduction in sick time and overtime (Bournes & Ferguson-Paré, 2007; Bournes et al., 2007). At a large academic teaching hospital, the humanbecoming 80/20 model has been tested as the basis for a mentoring program among experienced critical care nurses and new nurses who want to work in critical care (Bournes et al., 2008). The mentoring program is based on the Humanbecoming Mentoring Model (Parse, 2008c).

In South Dakota, a parish nursing model was built on the Eight Beatitudes and the principles of humanbecoming to guide nursing practice in the health model at the First Presbyterian Church in Sioux Falls (Bunkers, 1998a, 1998b; Bunkers, Michaels, & Ethridge, 1997; Bunkers & Putnam, 1995). Bunkers and Putnam (1995) stated, "The nurse, in practicing from the human becoming perspective and emphasizing the teachings of the Beatitudes, believes in the endless possibilities present for persons when there is openness, caring, and honoring of justice and human freedom" (p. 210). Also, the Board of Nursing of South Dakota has adopted a decisioning model based on the humanbecoming school of thought (Damgaard & Bunkers, 1998, 2012). Augustana College (in Sioux Falls) has humanbecoming as one theoretical focus of the curricula for the baccalaureate and master's programs. The humanbecoming theory was the basis of Augustana's Health Action Model for Partnership in Community (Bunkers, Nelson, Leuning, Crane, & Josephson, 1999). "The purpose of the model is to respond in a new way to nursing's social mandate to care for the health of society by gaining an understanding of what is wanted from those living these health experiences" (Bunkers et al., 1999, p. 94). The creation of the model was "for persons homeless and low income who are challenged with the lack of economic, social and interpersonal resources" (Bunkers et al., 1999, p. 92).

The humanbecoming school of thought is the theoretical foundation of the baccalaureate and master's curricula at the California Baptist University College of Nursing in Riverside, California. Faculty and students learn and live the art of humanbecoming in the various venues where they practice. The Nursing Center for Health Promotion with the Charlotte Rainbow PRISM Model was established in Charlotte, North Carolina, as a venue for nurses to offer health-care delivery to homeless women and children with diverse backgrounds. The PRISM Model, based on humanbecoming, was the guide to practice (Cody, 2003). At the Espace Mediane community nursing center in Geneva, Switzerland (for persons who have concerns about cancer and palliative care), practice and teaching–learning are guided by humanbecoming, meaning that nurses in the center live true presence with visitors. They also link with academic partners to provide an academic service for postgraduate nursing students

specializing in oncology and palliative care (Cody et al., 2004). The purpose of another project was to evaluate what happens when the art of humanbecoming was initiated in a palliative care inpatient setting in Fribourg, Switzerland (F. Maillard-Strüby, personal communication, August, 7, 2008).

Shifting practice from the traditional medical model mode to living the art of humanbecoming is a challenge for health-care institutions and requires high-level administrative commitment for resources, including educational opportunities for nurses. The commitment to humanbecoming practice requires a change in value priorities systemwide (Bournes, 2002; Bournes & DasGupta, 1997; Linscott, Spee, Flint, & Fisher, 1999; Mitchell et al., 2000).

Approximately 300 participants worldwide who are interested in living the art of humanbecoming subscribe to Parse-L, an e-mail listserv where Parse scholars share ideas. There is a Parse home page on the Internet that is updated regularly (see www.humanbecoming.org). Every other year, most of the 100 or more members of the International Consortium of Parse Scholars meet in Canada or the United States for a weekend immersion in humanbecoming theory, research, and practice. The DVD *The Human Becoming School of Thought: Living the Art of Human Becoming* (International Consortium of Parse Scholars, 2007; available from the Consortium at www.humanbecoming.org) shows Parse nurses in true presence with persons in different settings and features Rosemarie Rizzo Parse talking about humanbecoming in practice. Parse is also featured on the video in the Portraits of Excellence Series called *Rosemarie Rizzo Parse: Human Becoming* (Fitne, 1997), available from Fitne (www.fitne.net). Another video showing nurse with persons is *The Grief of Miscarriage* (Gerretsen & Pilkington, 1990). There is also a video called *I'm Still Here*, which is a humanbecoming research-based drama on living with dementia (Ivonoffski, Mitchell, Krakauer, & Jonas-Simpson, 2006). It is available from the Murray Alzheimer Research and Education Program at the University of Waterloo.

■ Summary

Through the efforts of Parse scholars, the humanbecoming paradigm continues to emerge as a major force in the 21st-century evolution of nursing knowledge. Knowledge gained from basic research studies continue to be synthesized to explicate further the meaning of living experiences. The findings from living the art research projects related to fostering understanding of humanbecoming with persons, families, and communities also continue to be synthesized. These syntheses guide decisions for continually creating the vision for sciencing and living the art of the humanbecoming paradigm for the betterment of humankind.

References[1]

Arndt, M. J. (1995). Parse's theory of human becoming in practice with hospitalized adolescents. *Nursing Science Quarterly, 8,* 86–90.

Banonis, B. C. (1995). Metaphors in the practice of the human becoming theory. In R. R. Parse (Ed.), *Illuminations: The human becoming theory in practice and research* (pp. 87–95). New York: National League for Nursing Press.

Barrett, E. A. M. (2010). Power as knowing participation in change: What's new and what's next. *Nursing Science Quarterly, 23,* 47–55.

Baumann, S. L. (2000). The lived experience of feeling loved: A study of mothers in a parolee program. *Nursing Science Quarterly 13,* 332–338.

Baumann, S. L. (2003). The lived experience of feeling very tired: A study of adolescent girls. *Nursing Science Quarterly, 16,* 326–333.

Baumann, S. (2008). Wisdom, compassion & courage in the Wizard of Oz: A humanbecoming hermeneutic study. *Nursing Science Quarterly, 21,* 322-329.

Baumann, S. L. (2009). Feeling fear: A humanbecoming study with older adults. *Nursing Science Quarterly, 22,* 346–354.

Baumann, S. L. (2013). Feeling bored: A Parse research method study. *Nursing Science Quarterly, 26,* 42-52.

Baumann, S., Carroll, K. A., Damgaard, G. A., Millar, B., Welch, A. J. (2001). An International Human Becoming Hermeneutic Study of Tom Hegg's *A Cup of Christmas Tea. Nursing Science Quarterly. 14,* 316-322.

Benedict, L. L., Bunkers, S. S., Damgaard, G. A., Duffy, C. E., Hohman, M. L., & Vander Woude, D. L. (2000). The South Dakota board of nursing theory–based regulatory decisioning model. *Nursing Science Quarterly, 13,* 167–171.

Bernstein, R. J. (1983). *Beyond objectivism and relativism: Science, hermeneutics, and praxis.* Philadelphia: University of Pennsylvania Press.

Bournes, D. A. (2000). A commitment to honoring people's choices. *Nursing Science Quarterly, 13,* 18–23.

Bournes, D. A. (2002). Research evaluating human becoming in practice. *Nursing Science Quarterly, 15,* 190–195.

Bournes, D. A. (2003). Stories of courage and confidence: Interpretation with the human becoming community change concepts. In R. R. Parse, *Community: A human becoming perspective* (pp. 131–145). Sudbury, MA: Jones and Bartlett.

Bournes, D. A. (2006). Human becoming–guided practice. *Nursing Science Quarterly, 19,* 329–330.

Bournes, D. A., Bunker, S. S., & Welch, A. J. (2004). The theory of human becoming in action: Scope and challenges. *Nursing Science Quarterly, 17*(3), 227–232.

Bournes, D. A., & DasGupta, D. (1997). Professional practice leader: A transformational role that addresses human diversity. *Nursing Administration Quarterly, 21*(4), 61–68.

Bournes, D. A., & Ferguson-Paré, M. (2007). Human becoming and 80/20: An innovative professional development model for nurses. *Nursing Science Quarterly, 20,* 237–253.

Bournes, D. A., & Ferguson-Paré, M. (2008). *The humanbecoming 80/20 study: Second study in Toronto.* Unpublished manuscript.

Bournes, D. A., Ferguson-Paré, M., Plummer, C., Kyle, C., Larrivee, D., & LeMoal, L. (2007, November). *Innovations in nurse retention and patient centered care: The 80/20 study in Regina.* Poster panel presentation at Celebrating New Knowledge and Innovation, University Health Network Nursing Research Day, Old Mill Inn and Spa, Toronto, ON.

Bournes, D. A., & Flint, F. (2003). Mis-Takes: Mistakes in the nurse-person process. *Nursing Science Quarterly, 16,* 127–130.

Bournes, D. A., & Naef, R. (2006). Human becoming practice around the globe: Exploring the art of living true presence. *Nursing Science Quarterly, 19,* 109–115.

Bournes, D. A., Plummer, C., Hollett, J., & Ferguson-Paré, M. (2008). *Critical care mentoring study: Testing a humanbecoming mentoring program to enhance retention and recruitment of nurses.* Unpublished manuscript.

Bunkers, S. S. (1998a). A nursing theory–guided model of health ministry: Human becoming in parish nursing. *Nursing Science Quarterly, 11,* 7–8.

[1] For additional information please go to bonus chapter content available at FA Davis http://davisplus.fadavis.com

Bunkers, S. S. (1998b). Translating nursing conceptual frameworks and theory for nursing practice in the parish community. In A. Solari-Twadell & M. McDermott (Eds.), *Parish nursing* (pp. 205–214). Thousand Oaks, CA: Sage.

Bunkers, S. S. (2010). The lived experience of feeling sad. *Nursing Science Quarterly, 23*, 231-239.

Bunkers, S. S. (2012). The lived experience of feeling disappointed: A Parse research method study. *Nursing Science Quarterly, 25*, 53-61.

Bunkers, S. S., Michaels, C., & Ethridge, P. (1997). Advanced practice nursing in community: Nursing's opportunity. *Advanced Practice Nursing Quarterly, 2*(4), 79–84.

Bunkers, S. S., Nelson, M. L., Leuning, C. J., Crane, J. K., & Josephson, D. K. (1999). The health action model: Academia's partnership with the community. In E. L. Cohen & V. DeBack (Eds.), *The outcomes mandate: Case management in health care today* (pp. 92–100). St. Louis, MO: C. V. Mosby.

Bunkers, S. S., & Putnam, V. (1995). A nursing theory–based model of health ministry: Living Parse's theory of human becoming in the parish community. In *Ninth Annual Westberg Parish Nurse Symposium: Parish nursing: Ministering through the arts.* Northbrook, IL: International Parish Nursing Resource Center–Advocate Health Care.

Butler, M. J. (1988). Family transformation: Parse's theory in practice. *Nursing Science Quarterly, 1*, 68–74.

Butler, M. J., & Snodgrass, F. G. (1991). Beyond abuse: Parse's theory in practice. *Nursing Science Quarterly, 4*, 76–82.

Chapman, J. S., Mitchell, G. J., & Forchuk, C. (1994). A glimpse of nursing theory–based practice in Canada. *Nursing Science Quarterly, 7*, 104–112.

Cody, W. K. (1995). Of life immense in passion, pulse, and power: Dialoguing with Whitman and Parse, a hermeneutic study. In R. R. Parse (Ed.), *Illuminations: The human becoming theory in practice and research* (pp. 269–307). New York: National League for Nursing Press.

Cody, W. K. (2001). "Mendacity" as the refusal to bear witness: A human becoming hermeneutic study of a theme from Tennessee Williams' "Cat on a Hot Tin Roof." In R. R. Parse (Ed.), *Qualitative inquiry: The path of sciencing* (pp. 205–220). Sudbury, MA: Jones and Bartlett.

Cody, W. K. (2003). Human becoming community change concepts in an academic nursing practice setting. In R. R. Parse (Ed.), *Community: A human becoming perspective* (pp. 49–71). Sudbury, MA: Jones and Bartlett.

Cody, W. K., Mitchell, G. J., Jonas-Simpson, C., & Maillard-Strüby, F. V. (2004). Human becoming: Scope and challenges continued. *Nursing Science Quarterly, 17*, 324–329.

Condon, B. B. (2010). The lived experience of feeling misunderstood. *Nursing Science Quarterly, 23*(2), 138-147.

Damgaard, G. (2012). High altitude leadership and the humanbecoming leading-following model: An executive director's perspective. *Nursing Science Quarterly, 25*, 370-374.

Damgaard, G., & Bunkers, S. S. (1998). Nursing science–guided practice and education: A state board of nursing perspective. *Nursing Science Quarterly, 11*, 142–144.

Damgaard, G., & Bunkers, S. S. (2012). Revisited: The South Dakota Board of Nursing theory-based regulatory decisioning model. *Nursing Science Quarterly, 25*, 211–216.

Doucet, T. J. (2012a). Feeling strong: A Parse research method study. *Nursing Science Quarterly, 25*, 62–71.

Doucet, T. J. (2012b). A humanbecoming program of research: Having faith. *Nursing Science Quarterly, 25*, 20–24.

Doucet, T., & Bournes, D. A. (2007). Review of research related to Parse's theory of human becoming. *Nursing Science Quarterly, 20*, 16–32.

Fitne. (1997). Portraits of excellence: Rosemarie Rizzo Parse: Human becoming [CD-ROM]. Athens, OH: Author. (Available from www.fitne.net)

Gadamer, H. -G. (1976). *Philosophical hermeneutics* (D. E. Linge, trans.). Berkeley, CA: University of California.

Gadamer, H.-G. (1998). *Truth and method* (2nd rev. ed.; J. Weinsheimer & D. G. Marshall, Trans.). New York: Continuum. (Original work published 1960)

Gerretsen, P. (Producer), & Pilkington, F. B. (Consultant). (1990). *The grief of miscarriage* [video]. Toronto, Canada: St. Michael's Hospital.

Hansen-Ketchum, P. (2004). Parse's theory in practice. *Journal of Holistic Nursing, 22*, 57–72.

Heidegger, M. (1962). *Being and time* (J. Macquarrie & E. Robinson, trans.). New York: Harper & Row.

Huch, M. H., & Bournes, D. A. (2003). Community dwellers' perspectives on the experience of feeling very tired. *Nursing Science Quarterly, 16*, 334–339.

Hutchings, D. (2002). Parallels in practice: Palliative nursing practice and Parse's theory of human becoming. *American Journal of Hospice and Palliative Care, 19*, 408–414.

International Consortium of Parse Scholars. (2007). *The human becoming school of thought: Living the art of human becoming* [DVD]. Toronto, Canada: Author.

Ivonoffski, V., Mitchell, G. J., Krakauer, R., Jonas-Simpson, C. (Writers), & Dennis, G. (Producer). (2006). *I'm still here* [DVD]. Waterloo, Canada: Murray Alzheimer Research and Education Program.

Jonas, C. M. (1994). True presence through music. *Nursing Science Quarterly, 7*, 102–103.

Jonas, C. M. (1995a). Evaluation of the human becoming theory in family practice. In R. R. Parse (Ed.), *Illuminations: The human becoming theory in practice and research* (pp. 347–366). New York: National League for Nursing Press.

Jonas, C. M. (1995b). True presence through music for persons living their dying. In R. R. Parse (Ed.), *Illuminations: The human becoming theory in practice and research* (pp. 97–104). New York: National League for Nursing Press.

Jonas-Simpson, C., & McMahon, E. (2005). The language of loss when a baby dies prior to birth: Cocreating human experience. *Nursing Science Quarterly, 18*, 124–130.

Karnick, P. M. (2005). Human becoming theory with children. *Nursing Science Quarterly, 18*, 221–226.

Karnick, P. M. (2007). Nursing practice: Imaging the possibles. *Nursing Science Quarterly, 20*, 44–47.

Langer, S. (1976). *Philosophy in a new key.* Cambridge, MA: Harvard University Press.

Lee, O. J., & Pilkington, F. B. (1999). Practice with persons living their dying: A human becoming perspective. *Nursing Science Quarterly, 12*, 324–328.

Legault, F., & Ferguson-Paré, M. (1999). Advancing nursing practice: An evaluation study of Parse's theory of human becoming. *Canadian Journal of Nursing Leadership, 12*(1), 30–35.

Linscott, J., Spee, R., Flint, F., & Fisher, A. (1999). Creating a culture of patient-focused care through a learner-centred philosophy. *Canadian Journal of Nursing Leadership, 12*(4), 5–10.

MacDonald, C. A., & Jonas-Simpson, C. M. (2009). Living with changing expectations for women living with high risk pregnancies: A Parse method study. *Nursing Science Quarterly, 22*(1), 74–82.

Maillard-Strüby, F. (2007, March). *Evaluation of the humanbecoming theory in practice.* Paper presented at the 2nd International Congress of the University of Applied Studies. Freiburg, Switzerland.

Maillard-Struby, F. (2012). Feeling unsure: A lived experience of humanbecoming. *Nursing Science Quarterly, 25*, 72–81.

Mattice, M., & Mitchell, G. J. (1990). Caring for confused elders. *The Canadian Nurse, 86*(11), 16–18.

Mitchell, G. J. (1988). Man-living-health: The theory in practice. *Nursing Science Quarterly, 1*, 120–127.

Mitchell, G. J. (1990). Struggling in change: From the traditional approach to Parse's theory-based practice. *Nursing Science Quarterly, 3*, 170–176.

Mitchell, G. J. (1993a). Living paradox in Parse's theory. *Nursing Science Quarterly, 6*, 44–51.

Mitchell, G. J. (1993b). The same-thing-yet-different phenomenon: A way of coming to know—or not? *Nursing Science Quarterly, 6*, 61–62.

Mitchell, G. J. (1995). The lived experience of restriction-freedom in later life. In R. R. Parse (Ed.), *Illumina-tions: The human becoming theory in practice and research* (pp. 159–195). New York: National League for Nursing Press.

Mitchell, G. J. (1998). Standards of nursing and the winds of change. *Nursing Science Quarterly, 11*, 97–98.

Mitchell, G. J., & Bournes, D. A. (2000). Nurse as patient advocate? In search of straight thinking. *Nursing Science Quarterly, 13*, 204–209.

Mitchell, G. J., Bournes, D. A., & Hollett, J. (2006). Human becoming–guided patient-centered care: A new model transforms nursing practice. *Nursing Science Quarterly, 19*, 218–224.

Mitchell, G. J., & Bunkers, S. S. (2003). Engaging the abyss: A mis-take of opportunity? *Nursing Science Quarterly, 16*, 121–125.

Mitchell, G. J., Closson, T., Coulis, N., Flint, F., & Gray, B. (2000). Patient-focused care and human becoming thought: Connecting the right stuff. *Nursing Science Quarterly, 13*, 216–224.

Mitchell, G. J., & Cody, W. K. (1999). Human becoming theory: A complement to medical science. *Nursing Science Quarterly, 12*, 304–310.

Mitchell, G. J., & Copplestone, C. (1990). Applying Parse's theory to perioperative nursing: A nontraditional approach. *AORN Journal, 51*, 787–798.

Mitchell, G. J., & Pilkington, B. (1990). Theoretical approaches in nursing practice: A comparison of Roy and Parse. *Nursing Science Quarterly, 3*, 81–87.

Morrow, M. R. (2010). Feeling unsure: A universal lived experience. *Nursing Science Quarterly, 23*(4), 315–325.

Naef, R. (2006). Bearing witness: A moral way of engaging in the nurse-person relationship. *Nursing Philosophy, 3*, 146–156.

Naef, R., & Bournes, D. A. (2009). The lived experience of waiting: A Parse method study. *Nursing Science Quarterly, 22*(2), 141-53.

Nelligan, P., Balfour, J., Connolly, L., Grinspun, D., Jonas-Simpson, C., Lefebre, N., et al. (2002). *Nursing best practice guideline: Client centred care.* Toronto, Canada: Registered Nurses Association of Ontario.

Norris, J. R. (2002). One-to-one teleapprenticeship as a means for nurses teaching and learning Parse's theory of human becoming. *Nursing Science Quarterly, 15*, 113–116.

Northrup, D., & Cody, W. K. (1998). Evaluation of the human becoming theory in practice in an acute care psychiatric setting. *Nursing Science Quarterly, 11*, 23–30.

Ortiz, M. R. (2003). Lingering presence: A study using the human becoming hermeneutic method. *Nursing Science Quarterly, 16*, 146–154.

Paille, M., & Pilkington, F. B. (2002). The global context of nursing: A human becoming perspective. *Nursing Science Quarterly, 15*, 165–170.

Parse, R. R. (1974). *Nursing fundamentals.* Flushing, NY: Medical Examination.

Parse, R. R. (1981). *Man-living-health: A theory of nursing.* New York: Wiley.

Parse, R. R. (1987). *Nursing science: Major paradigms, theories, and critiques.* Philadelphia: W. B. Saunders.

Parse, R. R. (1990). Parse's research methodology with an illustration of the lived experience of hope. *Nursing Science Quarterly, 3*, 9–17.

Parse, R. R. (1992). Human becoming: Parse's theory of nursing. *Nursing Science Quarterly, 5*, 35–42.

Parse, R. R. (1994a). Laughing and health: A study using Parse's research method. *Nursing Science Quarterly, 7*, 55–64.

Parse, R. R. (1994b). Quality of life: Sciencing and living the art of human becoming. *Nursing Science Quarterly, 7*, 16–21.

Parse, R. R. (Ed.). (1995). *Illuminations: The human becoming theory in practice and research.* New York: National League for Nursing Press.

Parse, R. R. (1996). Reality: A seamless symphony of becoming. *Nursing Science Quarterly, 9,* 181–183.

Parse, R. R. (1997a). The human becoming theory: The was, is, and will be. *Nursing Science Quarterly, 10,* 32–38.

Parse, R. R. (1997b). The language of nursing knowledge: Saying what we mean. In J. Fawcett & I. M. King (Eds.), *The language of theory and metatheory* (pp. 73–77). Indianapolis, IN: Sigma Theta Tau International Center Nursing Press.

Parse, R. R. (1998a). *The human becoming school of thought.* Thousand Oaks, CA: Sage.

Parse, R. R. (1998b). On true presence. *Illuminations, 7*(3), 1.

Parse, R. R. (1999a). *Hope: An international human becoming perspective.* Sudbury, MA: Jones and Bartlett.

Parse, R. R. (1999b). Nursing: The discipline and the profession. *Nursing Science Quarterly, 12,* 275.

Parse, R. R. (2001). *Qualitative inquiry: The path of sciencing.* Sudbury, MA: Jones and Bartlett.

Parse, R. R. (2003a). *Community: A human becoming perspective.* Sudbury, MA: Jones and Bartlett.

Parse, R. R. (2003b). The lived experience of feeling very tired: A study using the Parse research method. *Nursing Science Quarterly, 16,* 319–325.

Parse, R. R. (2004). A human becoming teaching-learning model. *Nursing Science Quarterly, 17,* 33–35.

Parse, R. R. (2005). The human becoming modes of inquiry: Emerging sciencing. *Nursing Science Quarterly, 18,* 297–300.

Parse, R. R. (2006). Research findings evince benefits of nursing theory–guided practice. *Nursing Science Quarterly, 19,* 87.

Parse, R. R. (2007a). Hope in "Rita Hayworth and Shawshank Redemption": A human becoming hermeneutic study. *Nursing Science Quarterly, 20,* 148–154.

Parse, R. R. (2007b). The humanbecoming school of thought in 2050. *Nursing Science Quarterly, 20,* 308.

Parse, R. R. (2008a, June). *The humanbecoming family model.* Paper presented at the Institute of Humanbecoming, Pittsburgh, PA.

Parse, R. R. (2008b). *The humanbecoming leading-following model. Nursing Science Quarterly, 21*(4), 369–375.

Parse, R. R. (2008c). A humanbecoming mentoring model. *Nursing Science Quarterly, 21,* 195–198.

Parse, R. R. (2008d). Nursing knowledge development: Who's to say how? *Nursing Science Quarterly, 21,* 101.

Parse, R. R. (2008e). Truth for the moment: Personal testimony as evidence. *Nursing Science Quarterly, 21,* 45–48.

Parse, R. R. (2009a). The humanbecoming family model. *Nursing Science Quarterly, 22,* 305-309.

Parse, R. R. (2009b). Knowledge development and programs of research. *Nursing Science Quarterly, 22,* 5–6.

Parse, R. R. (2009c). Mixed methods or mixed meanings in research? *Nursing Science Quarterly, 22,* 101.

Parse, R. R. (2010). Human dignity: A humanbecoming ethical phenomenon. *Nursing Science Quarterly, 23,* 257–262.

Parse, R. R. (2011a). Humanbecoming leading-following: The meaning of holding up the mirror. *Nursing Science Quarterly, 24,* 169-171.

Parse, R. R. (2011b). The humanbecoming modes of inquiry: Refinements. *Nursing Science Quarterly, 24,* 11–15.

Parse, R. R. (2011c). What people want from professional nurses. *Nursing Science Quarterly, 24,* 93.

Parse, R. R. (2012a). New humanbecoming conceptualizations and the humanbecoming community model: Expansions with sciencing and living the art. *Nursing Science Quarterly, 25,* 44–52.

Parse, R. R. (2012b). "The things we make, make us" *Nursing Science Quarterly, 25,* 125.

Parse, R. R. (2013a). Living quality: A humanbecoming phenomenon. *Nursing Science Quarterly, 26*(2), 111–115.

Parse, R. R. (2013b). "What we've got here is failure to communicate": The meaning of the term *nursing perspective. Nursing Science Quarterly, 26,* 5–7.

Parse, R. R., Coyne, B. A., & Smith, M. J. (1985). *Nursing research: Qualitative methods.* Bowie, MD: Brady.

Parse, R. R. (2014). *The humanbecoming paradigm: a transformational worldview.* Pittsburgh, PA: Discovery International Publications.

Quiquero, A., Knights, D., & Meo, C. O. (1991). Theory as a guide to practice: Staff nurses choose Parse's theory. *Canadian Journal of Nursing Administration, 4*(1), 14–16.

Rasmusson, D. L. (1995). True presence with homeless persons. In R. R. Parse (Ed.), *Illuminations: The human becoming theory in practice and research* (pp. 105–113). New York: National League for Nursing Press.

Rasmusson, D. L., Jonas, C. M., & Mitchell, G. J. (1991). The eye of the beholder: Parse's theory with homeless individuals. *Clinical Nurse Specialist, 5*(3), 139–143.

Ricoeur, P. (1976). *Interpretation theory: Discourse and the surplus of meaning.* Fort Worth, TX: Texas Christian University Press.

Ricoeur, P. (1981). *Hermeneutics and human sciences* (J. B. Thompson, trans.). Paris: Cambridge.

Rogers, M. E. (1992). Nursing science and the space age. *Nursing Science Quarterly, 5,* 27–34.

Santopinto, M. D. A., & Smith, M. C. (1995). Evaluation of the human becoming theory in practice with adults and children. In R. R. Parse (Ed.), *Illuminations: The human becoming theory in practice and research* (pp. 309–346). New York: National League for Nursing Press.

Smith, M. K. (2002). Human becoming and women living with violence. *Nursing Science Quarterly, 15,* 302–307.

Smith, S. M. (2012). The lived experience of doing the right thing: A Parse method study. *Nursing Science Quarterly, 25,* 82–89.

Stanley, G. D., & Meghani, S. H. (2001). Reflections on using Parse's theory of human becoming in a palliative care setting in Pakistan. *Canadian Nurse, 97,* 23–25.

Margaret Newman's Theory of Health as Expanding Consciousness

Chapter 16

MARGARET DEXHEIMER PHARRIS

Introducing the Theorist
Overview of the Theory
Applications of the Theory
Practice Exemplar
Summary
References

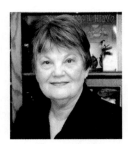

Margaret A. Newman

I don't like controlling,
manipulating other people.
I don't like deceiving, withholding,
or treating people as subjects or objects.
I don't like acting as an objective non-person.
I do like interacting authentically, listening,
understanding, communicating freely.
I do like knowing and expressing myself in
mutual relationships.

—MARGARET NEWMAN (1985)

Introducing the Theorist

Nurses who base their practice on Margaret Newman's theory of health as expanding consciousness (HEC) focus on being fully present to meaning and patterns in the lives of their patients. Newman (2005) stated, "[O]ne does not practice nursing *using* the theory, but rather the theory becomes a way of being with the client—a way of offering clients an opportunity to know and be known and to find their way" (p. xiv). Through their relationship with a nurse who understands the theory of HEC and attends to the evolving pattern of what is meaningful in their lives, patients are able to realize a previously undiscovered path for action. Just as patients' health predicaments are situated within the evolving pattern of complex relationships and events in their lives, so too, Newman's theory has evolved within the context of the meaningful relationships and events of her life.

After graduating from Baylor University, Newman returned to Memphis to work and to care for her mother, who had been diagnosed a few years earlier with amyotrophic lateral sclerosis (ALS), a degenerative neurological disease that progressively diminishes the movement of all muscles except those of the eyes. The process of caring for her mother over a 5-year period was transformative. Not knowing the trajectory of the disease, Newman learned to live day by day, fully immersed in the present (Newman, 2008b). Newman (2008a) stated she learned that "each day is precious and that the time of one's life is contained in the *present*" (p. 225).

Caring for her mother provided Newman with two additional significant realizations.

279

The first was that simply having a disease does not make a person unhealthy. Although Newman's mother's life was *confined* by the disease, her life was not *defined* by it. In other words, she could experience health and wholeness in the midst of having a chronic and progressive disease. The second important realization was that time, movement, and space are in some way interrelated with health, which can be manifested by increased connectedness and quality of relationships.

These early seeds of the HEC theory found fertile ground in 1959 when Newman entered nursing school at the University of Tennessee (UT) in Memphis. Her mother died 2 weeks before the beginning of the fall semester. Newman knew she could not go back to her previous life; the experience with her mother had deeply changed her.

After graduating from UT's baccalaureate nursing program, Newman stayed on at UT as a clinical instructor. The next year she went to the University of California, San Francisco (UCSF), to obtain her master's degree in medical–surgical nursing. When she graduated from UCSF in 1964, Newman was recruited back to Memphis to become the director of the Clinical Research Center. After directing the Clinical Research Center for 2½ years, Newman decided to pursue doctoral studies in nursing at New York University (NYU), where she would be able to study with Martha Rogers. In her doctoral work at NYU, Newman began studying movement, time, and space as parameters of health; however, she did so out of a logical positivist scientific paradigm. She designed an experimental study that manipulated participants' movements and then measured their perception of time (Newman, 1971, 1982). Her results showed a changing perception of time across the life span, with people's subjective sense of time increasing with age in such a way that time expanded for them (Newman, 1987). Although her work seemed to support what she later would term *health as expanding consciousness*, at the time Newman felt the method precluded direct application to shape nursing practice, which was what most interested her (Newman, 1997a).

After receiving her PhD in 1971, Newman joined the NYU faculty. While there, Newman published a seminal article in *Nursing Outlook* on nursing's theoretical evolution (Newman, 1972) and with colleague Florence Downs coauthored two editions of a book on research in nursing (Downs & Newman, 1977). Newman's early career in academia was centered on articulating the knowledge of the discipline and how it was developed.

In 1977, Newman joined the faculty at Penn State University as the professor-in-charge of graduate studies. At that time, she was invited to speak at a theory conference to be held in New York in 1978. It was in that address that she first clearly articulated her theory of health. The transcript of her talk was published as a chapter in a book she wrote about theory development in nursing (Newman, 1979), which was one of the first books published on the subject. Newman also organized a Nursing Theory Think Tank. She was also a member of a group of nurse theorists facilitated by Sister Callista Roy to discern how to organize nursing diagnoses so that they would be rooted in the knowledge of the discipline of nursing. This group presented papers in 1978 and 1980 to the North American Nursing Diagnosis Association. In 1982, they presented an organizing framework they had developed for nursing diagnoses called patterns of unitary man (humans).

In 1984, Newman took a position as nurse theorist at the University of Minnesota. As part of her theory development work, she conducted a pilot study of pattern identification. She invited Richard Cowling from Case Western and Jim Vail from the Army Nurse Corps to collaborate with her. Newman was at that time also a consultant to the Army Nurse Corps.

While at the University of Minnesota, Newman published two editions of her book, *Health as Expanding Consciousness* (Newman, 1986, 1994a), which attracted international attention. She conducted a series of lectures and dialogues in New Zealand in 1985 and in Finland in 1987 on health as expanding consciousness and nursing knowledge development.

Shortly after retiring from her position at the University of Minnesota, Margaret Newman returned to Memphis, Tennessee, where she continues to work on nursing knowledge development through her writing and by dialoguing with students and scholars from around the world.

Honors awarded to Dr. Newman include being named a Fellow of the American Academy of Nursing and a New York University Distinguished Scholar in Nursing. She has received Sigma Theta Tau International's Founders Award for Excellence in Nursing Research and the E. Louise Grant Award for Nursing Excellence from the University of Minnesota. She has been honored as an outstanding alumna by both the University of Tennessee and New York University. In 2008, Dr. Newman was named a Living Legend by the American Academy of Nursing.[1]

Overview of the Theory

As previously described, the seeds for the theory of HEC were planted in Margaret Newman's childhood and experience of caring for her mother as a young adult. Newman's undergraduate studies at the UT, master's studies at the UCSF, and doctoral studies at NYU also greatly influenced her quest for exploring and articulating the knowledge of the discipline of nursing. Reading and reflecting on the philosophical work of scholars from various disciplines—mainly Bentov (1978), Bohm (1980), Johnson (1961), Prigogene (1976), Rogers (1970), and Young (1976)—stretched Newman's view of the possibilities of nursing, and thus enriched the theory of HEC. Work and dialogue with colleagues and students further explicated the theory.

Academic and Philosophical Influences on the Theory

During her time at the University of California, San Francisco, Newman explored how nurses could respond to patients in a meaningful way

during short time spans. Newman's interest in attending to what is meaningful to the patient was influenced by Ida Jean Orlando's deliberative nursing approach. Inspired by Orlando's theoretical work, Newman began making deliberative observations about patients and reflecting what she observed back to the patient. The specific attention stimulated patients to respond by talking about what was meaningful in their unique circumstances.

In a publication of the results of her exploration of this approach to nursing during short time spans, Newman (1966) recounted walking into the room of a patient who had been in the hospital for some time. The patient was reading the newspaper, and Newman noticed that the woman was reading the want ads. Newman simply stated, "Reading the want ads, huh?" and waited for a response. The woman, who had been diagnosed with a chronic lung problem, worked in a factory that exuded toxic fumes, and she would no longer be able to work there. She was deeply concerned about her future. What ensued through their dialogue was a breakthrough for the patient, whose health-care predicament was couched in the larger context of her potential loss of income. Newman asked the woman if she had discussed this with her physician, and the woman responded that she had not discussed it with anyone. When Newman asked why not, the woman replied that no one had asked her about it. Once the meaning of her illness was understood within the context of her entire life, not just her physical state, a path toward health became apparent for the patient. This process of focusing on meaning in patients' lives to understand where the current health predicament fits in the whole of people's lives has endured as central to HEC.

Newman's theoretical insights evolved as she delved into the works of Martha Rogers and Itzhak Bentov, while at the same time reflecting back on her own experience (Newman, 1997b). Several of Martha Rogers's assumptions became central in enriching Margaret Newman's theoretical perspective (Newman, 1997b). First and foremost, Rogers saw health and illness not as two separate realities, but rather as a unitary process. This was congruent with Margaret Newman's earlier experience with her mother and with her patients. On a very deep level, Newman knew that people can experience health even when they are physically or mentally ill. Health is not the opposite of illness, but rather health and illness are both manifestations of a greater whole. One can be very healthy in the midst of a terminal illness.

Second, Rogers argued that all of reality is a unitary whole and that each human being exhibits a unique pattern. Rogers (1970) saw energy fields to be the fundamental unit of all that is living and nonliving, and she posited that there is interpenetration between the fields of person, family, and environment. Person, family, and environment are not separate entities but rather are an interconnected, unitary whole (Rogers, 1990). Finally, Rogers saw the life process as showing increasing complexity. These assumptions from Rogers's theory, along with the work of Itzhak Bentov (1978), helped to enrich Margaret Newman's (1997b) conceptualization of health and eventually the articulation of her theory. Bentov viewed life as a process of expanding consciousness, which he defined as the informational capacity of the system and the quality of interactions with the environment.

Basic Assumptions of the Theory of Health as Expanding Consciousness

Reflecting on these theoretical works helped Newman prepare for her *Toward a Theory of Health* presentation at the 1978 nursing theory conference in New York City. It was at that conference that the theory of health as expanding consciousness was first formally explicated. In her address (Newman, 1978) and in a written overview of the address (Newman, 1979), Newman outlined the basic assumptions that were integral to her theory at that time. Drawing on the work of Martha Rogers and Itzhak Bentov and on her own experience and insight, she proposed that:

• Health encompasses conditions known as disease or pathology, as well as states where disease is not present.

• Disease/pathology can be considered a manifestation of the underlying pattern of the person.
• The pattern of the person manifesting itself as disease was present before the structural and functional changes of disease.
• Removal of the disease/pathology will not change the pattern of the individual.
• If becoming "ill" is the only way a person's pattern can be manifested, then that is health for the person.
• Health is the expansion of consciousness (Newman, 1979).

Newman's presentation drew thunderous applause as she ended with, "[t]he responsibility of the nurse is not to make people well, or to prevent their getting sick, but to assist people to recognize the power that is within them to move to higher levels of consciousness" (Newman, 1978).

Although Margaret Newman never set out to become a nursing theorist, in that 1978 presentation in New York City, she articulated a theory that resonated with what was meaningful in the practice of nurses in many countries throughout the world. Nurses wanted to go beyond combating diseases; they wanted to accompany their patients in the process of discovering meaning and wholeness in their lives. Margaret Newman's proposed theory served as a guide for them to do so; it offered a new way of looking at the essence of nursing practice.

Developing the Theory of HEC

After identifying the basic assumptions of the theory of HEC, the next step was to focus on how to test the theory with nursing research and how the theory could inform nursing practice. Newman began to concentrate on the following:

• The mutuality of the nurse–client interaction in the process of pattern recognition
• The uniqueness and wholeness of the pattern in each client situation
• The sequential configurations of pattern evolving over time
• Insights occurring as choice points of action potential
• The movement of the life process toward expanded consciousness (Newman, 1997a)

To test the theory of HEC, which embraces reality as an undivided whole, Newman found that Western scientific research methodologies, which isolate particulate variables and analyze the relationships between them, were insufficient.

Newman saw a need to articulate that her work fell within a new paradigm of nursing. Like Martha Rogers (1970, 1990), Newman sees human beings as unitary and inseparable from the larger unitary field that combines person, family, and community all at once. Seeing change as unpredictable and transformative, she named the paradigm within which her work and the work of Martha Rogers are situated the unitary-transformative paradigm (Newman, Sime, & Corcoran-Perry, 1991). A nurse practicing within the unitary–transformative paradigm does not think of mind, body, spirit, and emotion as separate entities but rather sees them as manifestations of an undivided whole.

Newman's theory (1979, 1990, 1994a, 1997a, 1997b, 2008b) proposes that we cannot isolate, manipulate, and control variables to understand the whole of a phenomenon. The nurse and client form a mutual partnership to attend to the pattern of meaningful relationships and life experiences. In this way, a patient who has had a heart attack can understand the experience of the heart attack in the context of all that is meaningful in his or her life and, through the insight gained with pattern recognition, experience expanding consciousness. Newman's (1994a, 1997a, 1997b) methodology does not divide people's lives into fragmented variables but rather attends to the nature and meaning of the whole, which becomes apparent in the nurse–patient dialogue.

A nurse practicing within the HEC theoretical perspective possesses multifaceted levels of awareness and is able to sense how physical signs, emotional conveyances, spiritual insights, physical appearances, and mental insights are all meaningful manifestations of a person's underlying pattern. These manifestations also provide insight into the nature of the person's interactions with his or her environment. It takes disciplined study and reflection on practical experience applying the theory for nurses

to be able to see pattern as insight into the whole. Newman (2008b) states that practicing within a unitary paradigm requires a completely new way of seeing reality—it is like moving from seeing the Sun as revolving around Earth to realizing that it is actually Earth that revolves around the Sun.

Newman (1997a) asserted that knowledge emanating from the unitary–transformative paradigm is the knowledge of the discipline and that the focus, philosophy, and theory of the discipline must be consistent with each other and therefore cannot flow out of different paradigms. Newman (1997a) stated:

> The paradigm of the discipline is becoming clear. We are moving from attention on the other as object to attention to the we in relationship, from fixing things to attending to the meaning of the whole, from hierarchical one-way intervention to mutual process partnering. It is time to break with a paradigm of health that focuses on power, manipulation, and control and move to one of reflective, compassionate consciousness. The paradigm of nursing embraces wholeness and pattern. It reveals a world that is moving, evolving, transforming—a process. (p. 37)

Newman points the way for nurses to practice and conduct research within a unitary–transformative paradigm. In the unitary–transformative paradigm, the process of the nurse–patient partnership as integral to the evolving definition of health for the patient (Litchfield, 1993, 1999; Newman, 1997a) and is synchronous with participatory philosophical thought (Skolimowski, 1994) and research methodology (Heron & Reason, 1997).

When nurses view the world from a unitary perspective, they begin to see the nature of relationships and their meaning in an entirely new light. The work of Frank Lamendola and Margaret Newman (1994) with people with HIV/AIDS illustrates this. In a study they conducted, they found that the experience of HIV/AIDS opened participants to suffering and physical deterioration and at the same time introduced greater sensitivity and openness to themselves and others. Drawing on the work of cultural historian William Irwin Thompson, systems theorist Will McWhinney, and musician David Dunn, Lamendola and Newman, stated:

> They [Thompson, McWhinney, and Dunn] see the loss of membranal integrity as a signal of the loss of autopoetic unity analogous to the breaking down of boundaries at a global level between countries, ideologies, and disparate groups. Thompson views HIV/AIDS not simply as a chance infection but part of a larger cultural phenomenon and sees the pathogen not as an object but as heralding the need for living together characterized by a symbiotic relationship. (Lamendola & Newman, 1994, p. 14)

These authors pointed out that the AIDS epidemic has necessitated greater interconnectedness on the interpersonal, community, and global level. It has also called for a reconceptualization of the nature of the self and of treatment—inviting a new sense of harmonic integration within the immune system. Lamendola and Newman quoted Thompson (1989), who stated that we need to "learn to tolerate aliens by seeing the self as a cloud in a clouded sky and not as a lord in a walled-in fortress." This change in perspective helps nurses and patients move away from military metaphors in relationship to patients' bodies (i.e., *combating* disease, *waging battles* against *invading* cells, etc.) to focus instead on harmony and balance. Nursing care within a unitary perspective unveils meaning and opens the possibility for a new way of living for people with chronic conditions.

Applications of the Theory

Essential Aspects of Nursing Practice Within the HEC Perspective

Newman (2008b) synthesizes the basic assumptions of HEC in the following way:

• Health is an evolving *unitary pattern* of the whole, including patterns of disease.
• Consciousness is the *informational capacity* of the whole and is revealed in the evolving pattern.
• Pattern identifies the human–environmental process and is characterized by *meaning*. (p. 6)

Concepts important to nursing practice grounded in the theory of HEC include expanding consciousness, time, presence, resonance with the whole, pattern, meaning, insights as choice points, and the mutuality of the nurse–patient relationship.

Expanding Consciousness

Ultimate consciousness has been equated with love, which embraces all experience equally and unconditionally: pain as well as pleasure, failure as well as success, ugliness as well as beauty, disease as well as nondisease.
—M. A. NEWMAN (2003, p. 241)

Consciousness within the theory of HEC is not limited to cognitive thought. Newman (1994a) defined consciousness as the information of the system: the capacity of the system to interact with the environment. In the human system, the informational capacity includes not only all the things we normally associate with consciousness, such as thinking and feeling, but also all the information embedded in the nervous system, the immune system, the genetic code, and so on. The information of these and other systems reveals the complexity of the human system and how the information of the system interacts with the information of the environmental system (p. 33).

To illustrate consciousness as the interactional capacity of the person–environment, Newman (1994a) drew on the work of Bentov (1978), who presented consciousness on a continuum ranging from rocks on one end of the spectrum (which have little known interaction with their environment), to plants (which provide nutrients, give off oxygen, and draw carbon dioxide from the atmosphere) to animals (which can move about and interact freely), to humans (who can reflect and make in-depth plans regarding how they want to interact with their environment), and ultimately to spiritual beings on the spectrum's other end. Newman sees death as a transformation point, with a person's consciousness continuing to develop beyond the physical life, becoming a part of a universal consciousness (Newman, 1994a).

The *process* of expanding consciousness is characterized by the evolving pattern of the person–environment interaction (Newman, 1994a). The process of expanding consciousness is defined by Newman (2008b) as "a process of becoming more of oneself, of finding greater meaning in life, and of reaching new heights of connectedness with other people and the world" (p. 6). Nurses and their clients know that there has been an expansion of consciousness when there is a richer, more meaningful quality to their relationships. Relationships that are more open, loving, caring, connected, and peaceful are a manifestation of expanding consciousness. These deeper, more meaningful relationships may be interpersonal, or they may be relationships with the wider community or biosphere. Expanding consciousness is evident when people transcend their own egos, dedicate their energy to something greater than the individual self, and learn to build order against the trend of disorder. The process of expanding consciousness may look differently with changes in cognitive function; nurses must carefully discern patterns of meaning when this is the case. For example, when being present to people with dementia or to very young children, nurses realize that there is no past or future—there is only the present, and they must be fully present in the present on a deeper level than cognitive and verbal processes can take them (Newman, 2008b). People are best able to experience expanding consciousness when they are not chained to linear time.

Time and Presence

The time experienced
In a moment
Expands or diminishes
With consciousness.
If I am fully present
There is
No time.
Only consciousness.
—M. A. NEWMAN (2008A, P. 225)

Newman's earliest published work pointed to the ability of nurses to quickly and effectively attend to what is most important to patients and, by engaging patients in a dialogue about what is of utmost importance to them, to discern the patient's unique path toward health (Newman, 1966). Newman's latest work asserts that it is only when nurses move away from a sense of linear time to a more universal synchronization with the here and now that they can be truly present to patients in a meaningful and whole manner (Newman, 2008a). Newman stated:

> There is a need to get back to the natural cycles of the universe. The time of civilization (clock time and the Gregorian calendar) is not the same as the time of the rest of the biosphere, our living planet earth. Natural time is radial in nature, projecting from the center, and continuously moving in the direction of greater consciousness. (2008a, p. 227)

Newman asserted that the artificial time frame of clinic schedules and hospital shift work places nurses at odds with the natural rhythm of nurse–patient relationships, serves the needs of health systems administrations more than those of patients, and disrupts a meaningful nursing practice. She pointed out that the discipline of nursing has followed a trajectory from adherence to artificial linear time to the synchronization of time in interpersonal relationships, and now must move to the "instantaneous flow of information in each center of consciousness" and that "it is time to opt for practice that reflects this dimension" (Newman, 2008a, p. 227). When nurses must move out of a Western sense of time, they can be more fully present to patients.

Newman (2008b) asserted that it is only in relationship that people can fully come to know themselves. She drew on the work of T. D. Smith (2001), who suggested that "when the nurse considers the patient a *mystery to be engaged in* rather than a *problem to be solved,* the relationship is characterized by presence" (Newman, 2008b, p. 53). Newman further stated that "presence is enhanced by the nurse's openness and sensitivity to the other" and involves the nurse letting go of judgments of "good" or "bad" in relationship to patients' health behaviors.

When nurses are truly present to patients they concentrate more on intuitive knowing than on the gathering of facts and health-related data. They enter into a relaxed alertness and realize that transforming presence involves a keen awareness of their oneness with the patient (Newman, 2008b; Newman, Smith, Pharris, & Jones, 2008). Understanding the concept of resonance enables a transforming presence.

Resonating With the Whole

Newman (2008b) described resonance as the mechanism for acquiring essential information to guide nursing actions and to understand meaning in patients' lives. She stated, "This is an important distinction in the explication of nursing knowledge. Knowledge at the unitary, transformative level includes and transcends energy transfer at the sensorial level. It is *nonenergetic, nonlocal, and present everywhere*" (p. 35). She differentiated this information transfer from the transfer of sensory information (like heat and touch, which involve physical energy transfer) and suggests nurses continually rely on this information transfer when intuitive insights arise during the care of patients. Newman cautioned that "intellectualization breaks the field of resonance. If we analyze or evaluate an experience before we have resonated with it, the field is broken—the resonance is damped" (p. 37). "For instance, sometimes when we see familiar symptoms of a disease, we jump into a diagnostic conclusion and preclude receptivity to other data that would present a more complete picture. It assumes we are all the same" (p. 45). Resonance enables nurses to sense the unique situation and concerns of patients.

To resonate with patients and form open relationships, nurses must let go of personal judgments about patients and transcend cultural beliefs and values. In other words, the nurse needs to free himself or herself of all "should" and "ought to" attitudes and all personal preoccupations that might prevent total presence. Newman states there is no prescriptive way to sense the whole through resonance. She recommended that nurses pay attention to the client at the simplest level, begin with whatever presents itself, and assume that it is purposeful (Newman, 2008b).

Learning to resonate with patients involves relational engagement and reflection.

Most conventional education programs teach analytic processes attending to what is "logical." This leads students away from understanding the whole. Methods that involve empirical investigation assume that the whole comes after the parts; these methods tend to blind investigators to their relationship with the whole. Newman (2008b) drew on the work of Bohm (1980) to stress that "wholeness is what is real, with fragmentation as our response to fragmentary thought. The whole is irreducible and omnipresent" (p. 40). Newman (2008b) differentiated between the general and the universal. "Seeing comprehensively is concrete and holistic, whereas generalization is abstract and analytical; these ways of seeing go in opposite directions" (p. 47). Resonance is a way to sense into the whole through attention to one aspect or part of it, always with an eye on comprehending the whole. Resonance enables nurses to tap into the pattern of the whole.

Attention to Pattern and Meaning

Essential to Margaret Newman's theory is the belief that each person exhibits a distinct pattern, which is constantly unfolding and evolving as the person interacts with the environment. Pattern is information that depicts the whole of a person's relationship with the environment and gives an understanding of the meaning of the relationships all at once (Endo, 1998; Newman, 1994a). Pattern is characterized by meaning (Newman, 2008b) and is a manifestation of consciousness.

To describe the nature of pattern, Newman draws on the work of David Bohm (1980), who said that anything *explicate* (that which we can hear, see, taste, smell, touch) is a manifestation of the *implicate* (the unseen underlying pattern; Newman, 1997b). In other words, there is information about the underlying pattern of each person in all that we sense about them, such as their movements, tone of voice, interactions with others, activity level, genetic pattern, and vital signs. People can be identified from a distance by someone who knows them, just from the way in which they move. There is also information about their underlying pattern in all that they tell us about their experiences and perceptions, including stories about their life, recounted dreams, and portrayed meanings.

The HEC perspective sees disease, disorder, disconnection, and violence as an explication of the underlying implicate pattern of the person, family, and community. Reflecting on the meaning of these conditions can be part of the process of expanding consciousness (Newman, 1994a, 1997a, 1997b).

Pharris (1999) offered the example of a 16-year-old young man placed in an adult correctional facility after a murder conviction. This young man was constantly getting into fights and generally feeling lost. As he and the nurse researcher met over several weeks to gain insight into patterns of meaningful people and events in his life, the process seemed to be blocked, with no pattern emerging and little insight gained. He spoke of how he felt he had lost himself several years back when he went from being a straight-A student from a stable family to stealing cars, drinking, getting into fights, and eventually murdering someone. One week he walked into the room where the nurse was waiting, and his movements seemed more controlled and labored; he sat with his arms tightly cradling his bloated abdomen, and his chest was expanded as though he were about to explode. His palms were glistening with sweat. His face was erupting with acne. He talked as usual in a very detached manner, but his words came out in bursts. The nurse chose to give him feedback about what she was seeing and sensing from his body. She reflected that he seemed to be exerting a great deal of energy holding back something that was erupting within him. With this insight, he was quiet for a few minutes, and tears began rolling down his cheeks. Suddenly he began talking about a very painful family history of sexual abuse that had been kept secret for many years. It became obvious that the experience of covering up the abuse had been so all-encompassing that his pattern had been suppressed.

This young man had reached a point at which he realized his old ways of interacting with others were no longer serving him, and he chose to interact with his environment in a different way. By the next meeting, his movements had become smooth and sure, his complexion had cleared up, he was now able to reflect on his insights, and he no longer was involved in the chaos and fighting in his cell-block. He was able to let go of his need to control everything and was able to connect with the emotions of his childhood experiences; he was also able to cry for the first time in years.

In their subsequent work together, this young man and the nurse were able to distinguish between his implicate pattern, which had now become clear through their dialogue, and the impact that keeping the abusive experience a secret had had on him and on other members of his family. He was able to free himself of the shame he was carrying, which did not belong to him. Since that time, the young man has been able to transcend previous limitations and has become involved in several efforts to help others, both in and out of the prison environment. He has entered into several warm and loving relationships with family members and friends and has achieved academic success. This was evidence of expanding consciousness for the young man. He reflected that he wished he had had a nurse to talk with before "catching his case" (being arrested for murder). He had been seen by a nurse in the juvenile detention center, who performed a physical examination and gave him aspirin for a headache. A few days before the murder, he saw a nurse practitioner in a clinic who wrote a prescription for antibiotics and talked with him about safe sex. These interactions are explications of the pattern of the U.S. healthcare system and the increasingly task-oriented role that nursing is being pressured to take as juxtaposed with the transforming presence of a nurse whose practice is rooted in partnership that focuses on what is of utmost importance to the person (Jonsdottir, Litchfield, & Pharris, 2003, 2004).

The focus of nursing is on pattern and meaning. That which is underlying makes itself known in the physical realm. Nurses grounded in the theory of HEC are able to be in relationships with patients, families, and communities in such a way that insights arising in their pattern recognition dialogue shed light on an expanded horizon of potential actions (Litchfield, 1999; Newman, 1997a).

Insights Occurring as Choice Points of Action Potential

The disruption of disease and other traumatic life events may be critical points in the expansion of consciousness. To explain this phenomenon, Newman (1994a, 1997b) drew on the work of Ilya Prigogine (1976), whose theory of dissipative structures asserts that a system fluctuates in an orderly manner until some disruption occurs, and the system moves in a seemingly random, chaotic, disorderly way until at some point it chooses to move into a higher level of organization (Newman, 1997b). Nurses see this all the time—the patient who is lost to his work and has no time for his family or himself, and then suddenly has a heart attack, which leaves him open to reflecting on how he has been using his energy. Insights gained through this reflection give rise to transformation and decisions about where energy will be spent; and his life becomes more creative, relational, and meaningful. Nurses also see this in people diagnosed with a terminal illness that causes them to reevaluate what is really important, attend to it, and then to state that for the first time they feel as though they are really living. The expansion of consciousness is an innate tendency of humans; however, some experiences and processes precipitate more rapid transformations. Nurse researchers working within the theory of HEC have clearly demonstrated how nurses can create a mutual partnership with their patients to reflect on their evolving pattern and the points of transformation. Through this process, expanding consciousness is realized (Barron, 2005; Endo, Minegishi, & Kubo, 2005; Endo et al., 2000; Endo, Takaki, Nitta, Abbe, & Terashima, 2009; Flanagan, 2005, 2009; Hayes & Jones, 2007; Jonsdottir, 1998; Jonsdottir et al., 2003, 2004; Kiser-Larson, 2002; Lamendola, 1998; Lamendola & Newman, 1994; Litchfield, 1993, 1999, 2005; Moch, 1990; Musker, 2008; Neill, 2002a, 2002b; Newman, 1995; Newman & Moch, 1991; Noveletsky-Rosenthal, 1996; Pharris, 2002, 2005, 2011; Pharris & Endo, 2007; Picard, 2000, 2005; Pierre-Louis, Akoh, White & Pharris, 2011; Rosa, 2006; Ruka, 2005; Tommet, 2003; Yang, Xiong, Vang, & Pharris, 2009).

Newman (1999) pointed out that nurse–client relationships often begin during periods of disruption, uncertainty, and unpredictability in patients' lives. When patients are in a state of chaos because of disease, trauma, loss, or other causes, they often cannot see their past or future clearly. In the context of the nurse–patient partnership, which centers on the meaning the patient gives to the health predicament, insight for action arises, and it becomes clear to the patient how to get on with life (Jonsdottir et al., 2003, 2004; Litchfield, 1999; Newman, 1999). Litchfield (1993, 1999) explained this as experiencing an expanding present that connects to the past and creates an extended horizon of action potential for the future.

Endo (1998), in her work in Japan with women with cancer; Noveletsky-Rosenthal (1996), in her work in the United States with people with chronic obstructive pulmonary disease; and Pharris (2002), in her work with U.S. adolescents convicted of murder, found that it is when patients' lives are in the greatest states of chaos, disorganization, and uncertainty that the HEC nursing partnership and pattern recognition process is perceived as most beneficial to patients (Fig. 16-1).

Many nurses who encounter patients in times of chaos strive for stability; they feel they have to *fix* the situation, not realizing that this disorganized time in the patient's life presents an opportunity for growth. Newman (1999) states:

> The "brokenness" of the situation is only a point in the process leading to a higher order. We need to join in partnership with clients and dance their dance, even though it appears arrhythmic, until order begins to emerge out of chaos. We know, and we can help clients know, that there is a basic, underlying pattern evolving even though it might not be apparent at the time. The pattern will be revealed at a higher level of organization. (p. 228)

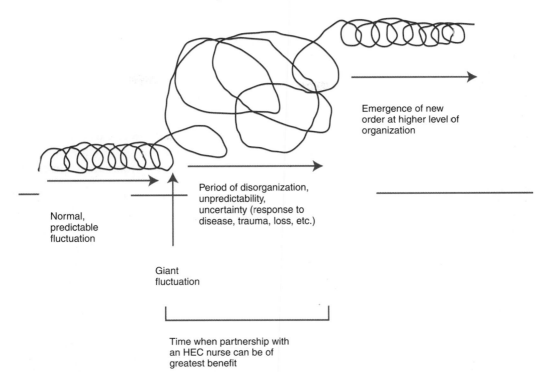

Fig 16 • 1 Prigogine's theory of dissipative structures applied to health as expanding consciousness (HEC) nursing.

The disruption brought about by the presence of disease, illness, and traumatic or stressful events creates an opportunity for transformation to an expanded level of consciousness (Newman, 1997b, 1999) and represents a time when patients most need nurses who are attentive to that which is most meaningful. Newman (1999, p. 228) stated, "Nurses have a responsibility to stay in partnership with clients as their patterns are disturbed by illness or other disruptive events." This disrupted state presents a *choice point* for the person to either continue going on as before, even though the old rules are not working, or to shift into a new way of being. To explain the concept of a *choice point* more clearly, Newman drew on Arthur Young's (1976) theory of the evolution of consciousness.

Young suggested that there are seven stages of binding and unbinding, which begin with total freedom and unrestricted choice, followed by a series of losses of freedom. After these losses come a choice point and a reversal of the losses of freedom, ending with total freedom and unrestricted choice. These stages can be conceptualized as seven equidistant points on a V shape (Fig. 16-2). Beginning at the uppermost point on the left is the first stage, *potential freedom*. The next stage is *binding*. In this stage, the individual is sacrificed for the sake of the collective, with no need for initiative because everything is being regulated for the individual. The third stage, *centering*, involves the development of an individual identity, self-consciousness, and self-determination. "Individualism emerges in the self's break with authority" (Newman, 1994b). The fourth stage, *choice*, is situated at the base of the V. In this stage, the individual learns that the old ways of being are no longer working. It is a stage of self-awareness, inner growth, and transformation. A new way of being becomes necessary. Newman (1994b) described the fifth stage, *decentering*, as being characterized by a shift from the development of self (individuation) to dedication to something greater than the individual self. The person experiences outstanding competence; his or her works have a life of their own beyond the creator. The task is

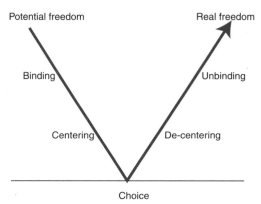

Fig 16 • 2 Young's spectrum of the evolution of consciousness.

transcendence of the ego. Form is transcended, and the energy becomes the dominant feature—in terms of animation, vitality, a quality that is somehow infinite. In this stage, the person experiences the power of unlimited growth and has learned how to build order against the trend of disorder (pp. 45–46).

Newman (1994b) stated that few experience the sixth stage, *unbinding,* or the seventh stage, *real freedom,* unless they have had these experiences of transcendence characterized by the fifth stage. It is in the moving through the choice point and the stages of decentering and unbinding that a person moves on to higher levels of consciousness (Newman, 1999). Newman proposed a corollary between her theory of health as expanding consciousness and Young's theory of the evolution of consciousness in that we "come into being from a state of potential consciousness, are bound in time, find our identity in space, and through movement we learn 'the law' of the way things work and make choices that ultimately take us beyond space and time to a state of absolute consciousness" (Newman, 1994b, p. 46).

The Mutuality of the Nurse–Client Interaction in the Process of Pattern Recognition

We come to the meaning of the whole not by viewing the pattern from the outside, but by entering into the evolving pattern as it unfolds.
—M. A. Newman

Nursing within the HEC perspective involves being fully present to the patient without judgments, goals, or intervention strategies. It involves *being with* rather than *doing for.* It is caring in its deepest, most respectful sense with a focus on what is important to the patient. The nurse–patient interaction becomes like a pure reflection pool through which both the nurse and the patient achieve a clear picture of their pattern and come away transformed by the insights gained.

To illustrate the mutually transforming effect of the nurse–patient interaction, Newman (1994a) offers the image of a smooth lake into which two stones are thrown. As the stones hit the water, concentric waves circle out until the two patterns reach one another and interpenetrate. The new pattern of their interaction ripples back and transforms the two original circling patterns. Nurses are changed by their interactions with their patients, just as patients are changed by their interactions with nurses. This mutual transformation extends to the surrounding environment and relationships of the nurse and patient.

In the process of doing this work, it is important that the nurse sense his or her own pattern. Newman states:

We have come to see nursing as a process of relationship that coevolves as a function of the interpenetration of the evolving fields of the nurse, client, and the environment in a self-organizing, unpredictable way. We recognize the need for process wisdom, the ability to come from the center of our truth and act in the immediate moment. (Newman, 1994b, p. 155)

Sensing one's own pattern is an essential starting point for the nurse. In her book *Health as Expanding Consciousness,* Newman (1994a, pp. 107–109) outlines a process of focusing to assist nurses as they begin working in the HEC perspective. It is important that the nurse be able to practice from the center of his or her own truth and be fully present to the patient. The nurse's consciousness, or pattern, becomes like the vibrations of a tuning fork that resonate at a centering frequency, and the client has the opportunity to resonate and tune to that clear frequency during their interactions (Newman, 1994a; Quinn, 1992). The nurse–patient relationship ideally continues until the patient finds his or her own rhythmic vibrations without the need of the stabilizing force of the nurse–patient dialogue. Newman (1999) points out that the partnership demands that nurses develop tolerance for uncertainty, disorganization, and dissonance, even though it may be uncomfortable. It is in the state of disequilibrium that the potential for growth exists. She states, "The rhythmic relating of nurse with client at this critical boundary is a window of opportunity for transformation in the health experience" (Newman, 1999, p. 229).

Relevance of HEC Across Cultures

Margaret Newman's theory of health as expanding consciousness is being used throughout the world, but it has been more quickly embraced and understood by nurses from indigenous and Eastern cultures, who are less bound by linear, three-dimensional thought and physical concepts of health and who are more immersed in the metaphysical, mystical aspect of human existence. Increasingly, however, HEC is being enthusiastically embraced by nurses in industrialized nations who are finding it difficult to nurse in the modern technologically driven and intervention-oriented health-care system, which is dependent on diagnosing and treating diseases (Jonsdottir et al., 2003, 2004). Practicing from an HEC perspective involves a holistic approach, which places what is meaningful to patients back into the center of the nurse's focus and what is meaningful to students back into the center of the focus of nurse educators. This person-centered approach has wide appeal across cultures.

HEC Research as Praxis

Margaret Newman's early research (1966, 1971, 1972, 1976, 1982, 1986, 1987) added to an understanding of the interrelatedness of time, movement, space, and consciousness as manifestations of health. Newman's further reflection on these studies in light of work she did at Walter Reed Hospital with Richard Cowling and John Vail related to pattern recognition,

revealed the need to look at health as expanding consciousness using a research methodology that acknowledges, understands, and honors the undivided wholeness of the human health experience. Newman, Cowling, and Vail's study participants were nurses at Walter Reed Hospital. Newman described one of the interviews she conducted as Vail and Cowling watched from another room. Newman asked the nurse to describe meaningful events in her life and Newman diagrammed the unfolding trajectory of the nurse's life. When they met the next day to reflect the sequential patterns Newman had identified, the nurse was able to see that experiences she had previously viewed as being extremely negative (e.g., a divorce), actually were stepping stones to expanded possibilities; she was suddenly able to view her life in a new way. The nurse researchers and participants were excited about the insights they gained. The pattern recognition research method was a powerful nursing practice process that shed light on theory—research, theory, and practice each illuminated and developed the other two. Newman went on to develop her pattern recognition nursing research method in which theory, practice, and research are one undivided process, each aspect shedding greater light on the other two.

Newman realized a need to *step inside* to view the whole from within—which is simply a metaphorical process since the researcher has been integrally within the whole all along. Newman's pattern recognition method cleared away the murky waters surrounding research, theory, and practice and what previously appeared to be three separate islands, became clearly visible as mountaintops on one undivided piece of land, newly emerged but always there as an undivided whole. HEC research as praxis unfolded uniquely in various countries and settings as nurse researcher-practitioner-theorists engaged in partnerships with individuals, families, and communities to understand patterns of meaning.

Focusing on the Process of Health Patterning and the Nurse–Patient Partnership

Merian Litchfield (1993) from New Zealand was the first researcher to apply the theory of health as expanding consciousness to a nursing partnership with families. Litchfield (1993, 1999, 2005) has led the way in focusing on the process of the nursing partnership with patients and families. In her first study, Litchfield (1993) described health patterning as "a process of nursing practice whereby, through dialogue, families with researcher as practitioner, recognize pattern in the life process providing opportunity for insight as the potential for action; a process by which there may be increased self-determination as a feature of health" (p. 10). Litchfield (1993) described her research as a "shared process of inquiry through which participants are empowered to act to change their circumstances" (p. 20). Through her research over several years with families with complex health predicaments requiring repeated hospitalizations, Litchfield (1993, 1999, 2005) found that she could not stand outside of the process of recognizing pattern to observe a fixed health pattern of the family. She saw the pattern as continuously evolving dialectically in the dialogue within the nursing partnership. The findings are literally created in the participatory process of the partnership (Litchfield, 1999). For this reason, Litchfield did not use diagrams to reflect pattern because she thought they would imply that the pattern is static rather than continually evolving. As the family reflects on the pattern of their interactions with each other and the environment, insight into action may involve a transformative process, with the same events being seen in a new light. Family health is seen as a function of the nurse–family relationship. Many of the families in partnership with Litchfield (1999, 2005) gained insight into their own predicaments in such a way that they required less interaction and service from traditional health-care services, and thus a cost saving in such services was realized.

Exploring Pattern Recognition as a Nursing Intervention

Emiko Endo (1998) explored HEC pattern recognition as a nursing intervention in Japan with women living with ovarian cancer. She asked, "When a person with cancer has an opportunity to share meaning in the life process

within the nurse–client relationship, what changes may occur in the evolving pattern?" Attending to the flow of meaningful thoughts for each participant and building on the previous work of Litchfield (1993), Endo found four common phases of the process of expanding consciousness for all participants: client–nurse mutual concern, pattern recognition, vision and action potential, and transformation. Participants differed in the pace of evolving movement toward a turning point and in the characteristics of personal growth at the turning point. The characteristics of growth ranged from assertion of self, to emancipation of self, to transcendence of self. Reflecting on her experience, Endo (1998) put forth that pattern recognition is "not intended to fix clients' problems from a medical diagnostic standpoint, but to provide individuals with an opportunity to know themselves, to find meaning in their current situation and life, and to gain insight for the future" (p. 60).

Endo et al. (2000) conducted a similar study with Japanese families in which the wife-mother was hospitalized because of a cancer diagnosis. Families found meaning in their patterns and reported increased understanding of their present situation. In the pattern recognition process, most families reconfigured from being a collection of separated individuals to trustful, caring relationships as a family unit, showing more openness and connectedness. The researchers concluded that pattern recognition as a nursing intervention was a "meaning-making transforming process in the family–nurse partnership" (p. 604).

HEC-Inspired Practice

Patricia Tommet (2003) used the HEC hermeneutic dialectic methodology to explore the pattern of nurse–parent interaction in families faced with choosing an elementary school for their medically fragile children. She found a pattern of *living in uncertainty* in the families during the intense period of disruption and disorganization after the birth of their medically fragile child through the first few years. After 2 to 3 years, the families exhibited a pattern of *order in chaos* where they learned how to live in the present, letting go of the way they lived in the past. Tommet found that "families changed from being passive recipients to active participants in the care of their children" (p. 90) and that the "experience of their children's birth and life transformed these families and through them, transformed systems of care" (p. 86). Tommet demonstrated insights gained in family pattern recognition and concluded that a nurse–parent partnership could have a more profound impact on these families, and hence the services they use, during the first 3 years of their children's lives.

Working with colleagues in New Zealand, Litchfield undertook a pilot project that included 19 families in a predicament of strife (Litchfield & Laws, 1999). The goal of the pilot project, which built on Litchfield's previous work (1993, 1999), was to explore a model of nurse case management incorporating the use of a family nurse who understands the theory of health as expanding consciousness. In the context of a family–family nurse partnership, the unfolding pattern of family living was attended to. Family nurses shared their stories of the families with the research group, who reflected together on the families' changing predicaments and the whole picture of family living in terms of how each family moved in time and place. Subsequent visits with the families focused on recognition of pattern and potential for action. The family nurse mobilized relief services if necessary and orchestrated services as needs emerged in the process of pattern recognition. The research group found that families became more open and spontaneous through the process of pattern recognition, and their interactions evidenced more focus, purposefulness, and cooperation. In analyzing costs of medical care for one participating family, it was estimated that a 3% to 13% savings could be seen by employing the model of family nursing, with greater savings being possible when family nurses are available immediately after a family disruption takes place (Litchfield & Laws, 1999). Based on Litchfield's work with families with complex health predicaments, the government funded a large demonstration project to support family nurses who would be able to nurse from unitary-transformative perspective and partner with families without having predetermined goals and outcomes that the families and nurses must achieve. These nurses are free to focus on family health as defined and experienced by the families themselves.

Endo and colleagues (Endo, Minegishi, & Kubo, 2005; Endo, Miyahara, Suzuki, & Ohmasa, 2005) in Japan have expanded their work to incorporate the pattern recognition process at the hospital nursing unit level. After engaging the professional nursing staff in reading and dialogue about the theory of HEC, nurses were encouraged to incorporate the exploration of meaningful events and people into their practice with their patients. Nurses kept journals and came together to reflect on the experience of expanding consciousness in their patients and in themselves. Endo, Miyahara, Suzuki, and Ohmasa (2005) concluded:

> Retrospectively it was found through dialogue in the research/project meetings that in the usual nurse–client relationships, nurses were bound by their responsibilities within the medical model to help clients get well, but in letting go of the *old rules*, they encountered an amazing experience with clients' transformations. The nurses' transformation occurred concomitantly, and they were free to follow the clients' paths and incorporate all realms of nursing interventions in everyday practice into the unitary perspective. (p. 145)

Jane Flanagan (2005, 2009) transformed the practice of presurgical nursing by developing the preadmission nursing practice model, which is based on HEC. The nursing practice model shifted from a disease focus to a process focus, with attention being given to the nurses knowing their patients and what is meaningful to them so that the surgery experience could be put in proper context and appropriate care provided. Nursing presurgical visits were emphasized. Flanagan reported that the nursing staff members were exuberant to be free to be nurses once again, and patients frequently stopped by to comment on their preoperative experience and evolving life changes.

Similarly, Susan Ruka (2005) made HEC pattern recognition the foundation of care at a long-term-care nursing facility, transforming the nursing practice and the sense of connectedness among staff, families, and residents: Each became more peaceful, relaxed, and loving.

Application of HEC at the Community Level

Pharris (2002, 2005) attempted to understand a community pattern of rising youth homicide rates by conducting a study with incarcerated teens convicted of murder. The youth in the study reported the pattern recognition process to be transformative, and expanding consciousness was visible in changed behaviors, increased connectedness, and more loving attention to meaningful relationships. The experience of the young men demonstrated that alterations in movement, time, and space inherent in the prison system can intensify the process of expanding consciousness. When the experiences of meaningful events and relationships were compared across participants, the pattern of disconnection with the community became evident. People from various aspects of the community (youth workers, juvenile detention staff, emergency hospital staff, pediatric nurses and physicians, social workers, educators, etc.) were engaged in dialogues reflecting on the youths' stories and the community pattern. Insights transformed community responses to young people at risk for violent perpetration. System change ensued.

Pharris (2005) and colleagues extended the community pattern recognition process through partnerships within a multiethnic community interested in understanding and transforming patterns of racism and health disparities. They engaged women and girls from all walks of life in the community in dialogue about their experiences of health, well-being, and racism. Findings were woven into a spoken word narrative that was presented in various forms (performances at meetings and gatherings, through community television and radio, and showing of DVD recordings) to members of the community so that meaningful dialogue could ensue. The process of reflecting on the community pattern generated insight into the nature of the community and what actions could be taken to dismantle racism and enhance health and well-being.

In a related study comparing the evolving patterns of Hmong women living in the United States with diabetes, Yang et al. (2009) found that the women's blood sugars rose and fell with their experiences of trauma, loss, separation, and isolation. Women in the study described their lives in Laos where they walked up and down hills carrying large bags of rice on their backs, picked fresh fruits and vegetables that grew near their homes, and engaged in myriad interactions with family and friends in the community. Then they described their life in the United States where they sit alone at home all day watching television in a language they do not understand and where they are fearful to walk outside and are driven by their sons and daughters to the grocery store, where they buy food wrapped in plastic. Dialogue on these findings, which were presented by two Hmong students as a play at a community dinner for Hmong women living with diabetes, shed light on needed individual, family, and community actions so that Hmong women living with diabetes could lead happy and healthy lives.

Similarly, Pierre-Louis et al. (2011) conducted an HEC study with African American women with diabetes. Pattern recognition revealed that blood sugars rose and fell with stress, depression, and trauma and that spiritual strength, mentors, and sister friends help to balance energy demands. Findings were woven into a spoken-word performance by the Black Story Tellers Alliance to engage African American women who have diabetes in action planning so that health can flourish in their lives.

Pavlish and Pharris (2012) published a book on community-based collaborative action research, which is rooted in Newman's theory and provides a framework for nurses to engage communities—whether hospital units, refugee camps, small towns, or groups of people—in a process of pattern recognition and action research to promote human flourishing.

Sharon Falkenstern (2003, 2009) found the community pattern to emerge as significant when she studied the process of HEC nursing with families with a child with special healthcare needs. She emphasized the importance of nursing partnership with families as they struggle to make sense of their experiences and try to discern how to get on with their lives. The evolving pattern of the families in Falkenstern's study illuminated the social and political forces on families from the educational, disabilities support, and health-care systems, as well as community patterns of caring, prejudice, and racism. Falkenstern summarized her experience of using HEC with families with children with special health-care needs in the following way:

My experience with this study has rekindled my passion for nursing. I felt affirmed that in the world of managed health care and educational cutbacks, a movement is growing to recapture the essence and value of nursing. While there is still much to be done for nursing within the political realm of health care, each nurse can control where and how they choose to practice. Especially, I realized that a nurse can experience joy and renewed energy by choosing to practice nursing within health as expanding consciousness. (2003, p. 232)

The pattern of the community is visible in the stories of individuals and families. Nurses can play an important role in engaging communities in dialogue as these stories are shared and their meaning reflected on. Methods that engage communities in dialogue about the meaning of patterns of health hold great potential. For example, if an HEC nurse were to take on the task of engaging nurses at the national level in a dialogue about what is meaningful in their practice, expanding consciousness would be manifest as the profession reorganizes at a higher level of functioning, with resultant health-care systems change. In the process, the population would no doubt experience a fuller, more equitable, and deeper sense of health, interconnectedness, and meaning.

Readers who are interested in learning more about Margaret Newman's theory of health as expanding consciousness are referred to an integrative review by Dr. Marlaine Smith (2011) and to Dr. Newman's website: healthasexpandingconsciousness.org

Practice Exemplar

Sandra is an adult nurse practitioner working in a community clinic in an urban area of the United States; she is about to enter the room of Gloria, a new patient with diabetes and hypertension. Gloria was referred by Anna, a physician colleague who felt that Gloria was "noncompliant," as evidenced by her uncontrolled hypertension and hemoglobin A1c levels that consistently hovered around 10. Anna felt that Gloria needed more care than she could provide for her.

Sandra's graduate program in nursing was based on the theory of health as expanding consciousness; the faculty paid attention to knowing her and what was meaningful to her in her educational and vocational journey. She experienced a relationship-based education process where the teacher is seen as "a catalyst to help students become who they will become rather than be 'trained'" and the learning process is a "dance between content and resonance" (Newman, 2008b, p. 75). Sandra felt known

and loved by the faculty. She had ample experience performing problem-solving approaches through the medical paradigm that leads to diagnoses, yet she realized that her nursing actions were best guided by a dialogue focused on understanding Gloria's physical health within the context of her life situation. She knew that the focus of her care for Gloria would arise out of their dialogue; she could not prescribe or predetermine the best care for Gloria.

Before entering the room where Gloria is waiting, Sandra consciously attends to freeing herself of any personal preoccupations or expectations of what might happen. She wants to fully attend to Gloria and sense what is of greatest importance to her right now, knowing that this will guide Sandra's nursing actions so that they can be of most benefit to Gloria. Sandra is confident that she will get a sense of this not only by asking questions and listening deeply but also through intuitive hunches that will arise through her resonant presence with Gloria.

Continued

Practice Exemplar cont.

On entering the room, Sandra warmly greets Gloria and concentrates on what she is sensing from Gloria's presence. She sits down next to Gloria in a relaxing and open manner. What most strongly calls Sandra's attention is that Gloria is wringing her hands, which are sweaty; and her muscles seem very tense.

After pausing for a moment, Sandra chooses to reflect back to Gloria what she sees. "Your muscles seem tense, like you might be anxious about something. How has life been going for you?" Gloria looks at Sandra, curious that Sandra is interested in her life. She responds, "Well, things have been hard." Sandra responds, "Hmm, tell me about that." Gloria explains that it has been difficult to take care of the two children she provides day care for. She says she doesn't have the energy but needs the money to pay her rent, which leaves her very little money to buy food, and she cannot afford her medications.

Sandra assures Gloria that the clinic has a plan that will provide her with her medications and that she will see that this is taken care of today—that she will go home with adequate medications. She tells Gloria that she would like to learn a little more about what has been meaningful in her life and asks her to describe meaningful events. Sandra uses the examination table paper to draw a diagram of what Gloria tells her. In very little time, Sandra has sketched a diagram of the flow of important events in Gloria's life. She learns that when immigrating to the United States from Africa, Gloria suffered intense abuse and was separated from her family and friends. She has children in the United States who constantly call her to babysit their children and to help them out. Gloria has also experienced intimate partner violence, and her current economic stress and depression have flowed from this experience. Gloria lives in a small apartment in a neighborhood where she would need to walk 2 miles to get to a store that sells fresh fruits and vegetables. She tells Sandra she is hesitant to leave her apartment.

Sandra reflects back to Gloria that she sees all of Gloria's energy going out to others and none coming back to her. She has gone from being very active to only moving around within her apartment. Tears run down Gloria's cheeks as she listens to Sandra's reflection. "That is so true!" They talk about sources of support, nurturance, and energy. Gloria identifies a woman in her building whose company she enjoys. They talk about the possibility of the two women walking to the supermarket together and simply getting together to talk. They identify a neighborhood women's walking group, which might be a source of support. They also talk about a women's group at the local library, but Gloria seems hesitant.

During the course of their conversation, Sandra has tried to clear herself of her own concerns, yet, as they talk, she keeps thinking about an experience of racism she witnessed at that library. She decides that it is important information and shares the story with Gloria. This provokes an outpouring of emotion from Gloria as she recounts her experiences of racism. They discuss how distorting these experiences are and how to move through them. They talk about how blood sugar and pressure respond to these situations and ways in which Gloria can best cope.

Sandra does all of the things for Gloria that her medical colleagues would do. She also discusses the services of the social worker, dietitian, and psychologist at the clinic so that Gloria can choose what might be most helpful to her at this time. Gloria hugs Sandra as she leaves, saying that she feels so much better, and adding, "You are a very good nurse!" Gloria leaves with a greater understanding of herself, of what is meaningful to her, and what actions she might take. Sandra is left with the same enhanced understanding of herself and her practice.

Sandra tucks the diagram they have drawn into a folder so that it can be elaborated on at subsequent visits. Sandra knows that Gloria's experience of health and well-being will evolve and that she can serve as a catalyst, witnessing and engaging in dialogue about the meaning of the pattern of Gloria's evolving health. Sandra will continue to focus on what she senses as meaningful to Gloria and engage in a relationship centered on Gloria's unfolding pattern of health. Hemoglobin A1c levels and blood pressure readings are only one aspect of that pattern.

As Sandra engages with more and more patients with similar predicaments, she gets a sense of the community pattern of health. She brings her insight to the clinic staff meetings where a rich dialogue about community health ensues. Sandra joins the CEO for a dialogue with the clinic's community board of directors to offer their insights. Through the subsequent dialogue, the board of directors and CEO commit themselves to ensuring that health-care providers have sufficient time to attend to

patients in a holistic manner, sponsoring community forums on racism and how to deal with it, embedding a mental health practitioner in the medical clinic, partnering with a community recreational facility so that patients have a safe place to exercise, encouraging community microeconomic enterprises for women, working with a community coop to provide an affordable source of nutritious food in the immediate neighborhood, and lobbying for health-care financing reform.

The circle of dialogue continues for Sandra. Her attention is on pattern and meaning in the evolving health of her patients and the community. She trusts that health is inherently present in her patients and the community and that reflection on what is meaningful is a catalyst for its evolving pattern. With this realization, Sandra is able to return home where she can be fully present to her family.

Summary

Margaret Newman's theory of health as expanding consciousness calls nurses to focus on that which is meaningful in their practice and in the lives of their patients. It attends to the evolving pattern of interactions with the environment for individuals, families, and communities. It is a theory that is relevant across practice settings and cultures. It informs and guides nursing practice, health-care administration, and education. The theory of HEC presents a philosophy of *being with* rather than simply *doing for*. It involves a different way of knowing—of resonating with patients, students, and health-care colleagues.

Nurses grounded in the theory of health as expanding consciousness bring to the patient encounter all that they have learned in school and in practice, yet they begin with a sense of nonknowing to take in what is most meaningful to the patient. Nurses attend to the patient's definition of health and see it in

the context of the patient's expression of meaningful relationships and events. The focus is not on predetermined outcomes mandated by the health system or on *fixing* the patient but rather on partnering with the patient in his or her experience of health. Rather than simply using technological tools and following prescribed clinical pathways, nurses offer their own transforming presence, knowing that the direction of their interaction with patients will arise out of the relationship's focus on the patient's evolving experience of health. Nurses realize that the process of expanding consciousness involves transcendence and new possibilities as people age or encounter a challenging life event. As nurses come to understand the meaning of patterns in the lives of individuals, families, and communities, they gain insights that inform population level dialogue for health policy transformation.

Newman (2008b) stated:

This theory asserts that every person in every situation, no matter how disordered and hopeless it may seem, is part of a process of expanding consciousness—a process of becoming more of oneself, of finding greater meaning in life, and of reaching new heights of connectedness with other people and the world. (p. 6)

Acknowledgments

The author thanks St. Catherine University for sabbatical support and scholarly research funding to review the Margaret A. Newman archives housed at the University of Tennessee and to interview Dr. Newman. That work has informed this chapter and her life. She also thanks Dr. Newman for editing this chapter and adding the section, "Losing Our Senses, Finding Our Selves," which includes her current thinking related to gerotrancendence and health as expanding consciousness and can be accessed in the electronic supplement to this chapter. This section can be found in the online supplementary materials for the chapter at: http://davisplus.fadavis.com

References

Barron, A. M. (2005). Suffering, growth, and possibility: Health as expanding consciousness in end-of-life care. In C. Picard & D. Jones (Eds.), *Giving voice to what we know: Margaret Newman's theory of health as expanding consciousness in research, theory, and practice* (pp. 43–52). Boston: Jones and Bartlett.

Bentov, I. (1978). *Stalking the wild pendulum.* New York: E. P. Dutton.

Bohm, D. (1980). *Wholeness and the implicate order.* London: Routledge & Kegan Paul.

Connor, M. (1998). Expanding the dialogue on praxis in nursing research and practice. *Nursing Science Quarterly, 11*(2), 51–55.

Downs, F. S., & Newman, M. A. (1977). *A source book on nursing research* (2nd ed.). Philadelphia: F. A. Davis.

Endo, E. (1998). Pattern recognition as a nursing intervention with Japanese women with ovarian cancer. *Advances in Nursing Science, 20*(4), 49–61.

Endo, E., Minegishi, H., & Kubo, S. (2005). Creating action research teams: A praxis model of care. In C. Picard & D. Jones (Eds.), *Giving voice to what we know: Margaret Newman's theory of health as expanding consciousness in research, theory, and practice* (pp. 143–152). Boston: Jones and Bartlett.

Endo, E., Miyahara, T., Suzuki, S., & Ohmasa, T. (2005). Partnering of researcher and practicing nurses for transformative nursing. *Nursing Science Quarterly, 18*(2), 138–145.

Endo, E., Nitta, E., Inayoshi, M., Saito, R., Takemura, K., Minegishi, H., et al. (2000). Pattern recognition as a caring partnership in families with cancer. *Journal of Advanced Nursing, 32*(3), 603–610.

Endo, E., Takaki, M., Nitta, N., Abe, K., & Terashima, K. (2009). Indentifying patterns in partnership with students who want to quit smoking. *Journal of Holistic Nursing, 27*(4), 256–265.

Falkenstern, S. K. (2003). *Nursing facilitation of expanding consciousness in families who have a child with special health care needs.* Unpublished doctoral thesis, Pennsylvania State University, University Park, PA.

Falkenstern, S. K., Gueldner, S. H., & Newman, M. A. (2009). Health as expanding consciousness with families with a child with special healthcare needs. *Nursing Science Quarterly, 22*(3), 267–279.

Flanagan, J. (2005). Creating a healing environment for staff and patients in a pre-surgery clinic. In: C. Picard & D. Jones (Eds.), *Giving voice to what we know: Margaret Newman's theory of health as expanding consciousness in research, theory, and practice* (pp. 53–64). Boston: Jones and Bartlett.

Flanagan, J. (2009). Patient and nurse experiences of theory-based care. *Nursing Science Quarterly, 22*(2), 160–172.

Hayes, M. O., & Jones, D. (2007). Health as expanding consciousness: Pattern recognition and incarcerated mothers, a transforming experience. *Journal of Forensic Nursing, 3*(2), 61–66.

Heron, J., & Reason, P. (1997). A participatory inquiry paradigm. *Qualitative Inquiry, 3*(3), 274–294.

Johnson, D. E. (1961). The significance of nursing care. *American Journal of Nursing, 61*(11), 63–66.

Jonsdottir, H. (1998). Life patterns of people with chronic obstructive pulmonary disease: Isolation and being closed in. *Nursing Science Quarterly, 11*(4), 160–166.

Jonsdottir, H., Litchfield, M., & Pharris, M. D. (2003). Partnership in practice. *Research and Theory for Nursing Practice, 17*(3), 51–63.

Jonsdottir, H., Litchfield, M., & Pharris, M. D. (2004). The relational core of nursing practice. *Journal of Advanced Nursing, 47*(3), 241–250.

Kiser-Larson, N. (2002). Life pattern of native women experiencing breast cancer. *International Journal for Human Caring, 6*(2), 61–68.

Lamendola, F. (1998). *Patterns of the caregiver experiences of selected nurses in hospice and HIV/AIDS care.* Unpublished doctoral thesis, University of Minnesota, Minneapolis.

Lamendola, F., & Newman, M. A. (1994). The paradox of HIV/AIDS as expanding consciousness. *Advances in Nursing Science, 16*(3), 13–21.

Litchfield, M. C. (1993). *The process of health patterning in families with young children who have been repeatedly hospitalized.* Unpublished master's thesis, University of Minnesota, Minneapolis.

Litchfield, M. (1999). Practice wisdom. *Advances in Nursing Science, 22*(2), 62–73.

Litchfield, M. C. (2005). The nursing praxis of family health. In: C. Picard & D. Jones (Eds.), *Giving voice to what we know: Margaret Newman's theory of health as expanding consciousness in research, theory, and practice* (pp. 73–83). Boston: Jones and Bartlett.

Litchfield, M., & Laws, M. (1999). Achieving family health and cost-containment outcomes. In: E. L. Cohen & V. De Back (Eds.), *The outcomes mandate: Case management in health care today* (pp. 306–314). St. Louis, MO: C. V. Mosby.

Moch, S. D. (1990). Health within the experience of breast cancer. *Journal of Advanced Nursing, 15,* 1426–1435.

Moss, R. (1991). *The I that is we.* Millbrae, CA: Celestial Arts.

Musker, K.M. (2008). Life patterns of women transitioning through menopause: A Newman research study. *Nursing Science Quarterly, 21*(4), 330-342.

Neill, J. (2002a). Transcendence and transformation in the life patterns of women living with rheumatoid arthritis. *Advances in Nursing Science, 24*(4), 27–47.

Neill, J. (2002b). From practice to caring praxis through Newman's theory of health as expanding consciousness: A personal journey. *International Journal for Human Caring, 6*(2), 48–54.

Newman, M. A. (1966). Identifying and meeting patients' needs in short-span nurse-patient relationships. *Nursing Forum, 5*(1), 76–86.

Newman, M.A. (1971). Time estimation in relation to gait tempo. *Perceptual and Motor Skills, 34,* 359–366.

Newman, M. A. (1972). Nursing's theoretical evolution. *Nursing Outlook, 20*(7), 449–453.

Newman, M. A. (1976). Movement tempo and the experience of time. *Nursing Research, 25,* 173–179.

Newman, M. A. (1978). *Nursing theory.* (Audiotape of an address to the 2nd National Nurse Educator Conference in New York.) Chicago: Teach'em, Inc.

Newman, M. A. (1979). *Theory development in nursing.* Philadelphia: F. A. Davis.

Newman, M. A. (1982). Time as an index of expanding consciousness with age. *Nursing Research, 31,* 290–293.

Newman, M. A. (1986). *Health as expanding consciousness.* St. Louis, MO: C. V. Mosby.

Newman, M. A. (1987). Aging as increasing complexity. *Journal of Gerontological Nursing, 12,* 16–18.

Newman, M. A. (1990). Newman's theory of health as praxis. *Nursing Science Quarterly, 3,* 37–41.

Newman, M. A. (1994a). *Health as expanding consciousness* (2nd ed.). Boston: Jones and Bartlett (NLN Press).

Newman, M. A. (1994b). Theory for nursing practice. *Nursing Science Quarterly, 7*(4), 153–157.

Newman, M. A. (1995). *A developing discipline.* Boston: Jones and Bartlett (formerly, New York: National League for Nursing Press).

Newman, M. A. (1997a). Experiencing the whole. *Advances in Nursing Science, 20*(1), 34–39.

Newman, M. A. (1997b). Evolution of the theory of health as expanding consciousness. *Nursing Science Quarterly, 10*(1), 22–25.

Newman, M. A. (1999). The rhythm of relating in a paradigm of wholeness. *Image: Journal of Nursing Scholarship, 31*(3), 227–230.

Newman, M. A. (2003). A world with no boundaries. *Advances in Nursing Science, 26*(4), 240–245.

Newman, M. A. (2005). Preface. In C. Picard & D. Jones (Eds.), *Giving voice to what we know: Margaret Newman's theory of health as expanding consciousness in research, theory, and practice* (pp. xxiii–xxvi). Sudbury, MA: Jones and Bartlett.

Newman, M. A. (2008a). It's about time. *Nursing Science Quarterly, 21*(3), 225–227.

Newman, M. A. (2008b). *Transforming presence: The difference that nursing makes.* Philadelphia: F. A. Davis.

Newman, M. A., & Moch, S. D. (1991). Life patterns of persons with coronary heart disease. *Nursing Science Quarterly, 4,* 161–167.

Newman, M. A., Sime, A. M., & Corcoran-Perry, S. A. (1991). The focus of the discipline of nursing. *Advances in Nursing Science, 14*(1), 1–6.

Newman, M. A., Smith, M. C., Pharris, M. D., & Jones, D. (2008). The focus of the discipline revisited. *Advances in Nursing Science, 31*(1), E16–E27.

Noveletsky-Rosenthal, H. T. (1996). *Pattern recognition in older adults living with chronic illness.* Unpublished doctoral thesis, Boston College, Chestnut Hill, MA.

Pavlish, C. P. & Pharris, M. D. (2012). *Community-based collaborative action research: A nursing approach.* Sudbury, MA: Jones and Bartlett.

Pharris, M. D. (1999). *Pattern recognition as a nursing intervention with adolescents convicted of murder.* Unpublished doctoral thesis, University of Minnesota, Minneapolis.

Pharris, M. D. (2002). Coming to know ourselves as community through a nursing partnership with adolescents convicted of murder. *Advances in Nursing Science, 24*(3), 21–42.

Pharris, M. D. (2005). Engaging with communities in a pattern recognition process. In C. Picard & D. Jones (Eds.), *Giving voice to what we know: Margaret Newman's theory of health as expanding consciousness in research, theory, and practice* (pp. 83–94). Boston: Jones and Bartlett.

Pharris, M. D. (2011). Margaret A. Newman's theory of health as expanding consciousness. *Nursing Science Quarterly, 24*(3), 193–194.

Pharris, M. D., & Endo, E. (2007). Flying free: The evolving nature of nursing practice guided by the theory of health as expanding consciousness. *Nursing Science Quarterly, 20*(2), 136–140.

Picard, C. (2000). Pattern of expanding consciousness in mid-life women: Creative movement and the narrative as modes of expression. *Nursing Science Quarterly, 13*(2), 150–158.

Picard, C. (2005). Parents of persons with bipolar disorder and pattern recognition. In C. Picard & D. Jones (Eds.), *Giving voice to what we know: Margaret Newman's theory of health as expanding consciousness in research, theory, and practice* (pp. 133–141). Boston: Jones and Bartlett.

Pierre-Louis, B., Akoh, V., White, P. & Pharris, M. D. (2011). Patterns in the lives of African American women with diabetes. *Nursing Science Quarterly, 24*(3), 227–236.

Prigogine, I. (1976). Order through fluctuation: Self-organization and social system. In Jantsch, E., & Waddington, C. H. (Eds.), *Evolution and consciousness* (pp. 93–133). Reading, MA: Addison-Wesley.

Quinn, J. F. (1992). Holding sacred space. The nurse as healing environment. *Holistic Nursing Practice, 6*(4), 26–36.

Rogers, M. E. (1970). *An introduction to the theoretical basis of nursing.* Philadelphia: F. A. Davis.

Rogers, M. E. (1990). Nursing science and the space age. *Nursing Science Quarterly, 5*(1), 27–34.

Rosa, K. C. (2006). A process model of healing and personal transformation in persons with chronic skin wounds. *Nursing Science Quarterly, 19*, 349–358.

Ruka, S. (2005). Creating balance, rhythm and patterns in people with dementia living in a nursing home. In C. Picard & D. Jones (Eds.), *Giving voice to what we know: Margaret Newman's theory of health as expanding consciousness in research, theory, and practice* (pp. 59–104). Boston: Jones and Bartlett.

Skolimowski, H. (1994). *The participatory mind.* London: Arkana.

Smith, M. C. (2011). Integrative review of research related to Margaret Newman's theory of health as expanding consciousness. *Nursing Science Quarterly, 24*(3), 256–272.

Smith, T. D. (2001). The concept of nursing presence: State of the science. *Scholarly Inquiry for Nursing Practice: An International Journal, 15*(4), 299–322.

Thompson, W. I. (1989). *Imaginary landscape: Making worlds of myth and science.* New York: St. Martin's Press.

Tommet, P. (2003). Nurse-parent dialogue: Illuminating the evolving pattern of families with children who are medically fragile. *Nursing Science Quarterly, 16*(3), 239–246.

Yang, A., Xiong, D., Vange, E., & Pharris, M.D. (2009). *Hmong American women living with diabetes. Journal of Nursing Scholarship, 41*(2), 139–148.

Young, A. M. (1976). *The reflexive universe: Evolution of consciousness.* San Francisco, CA: Robert Briggs Associates.

Grand Theories about Care or Caring

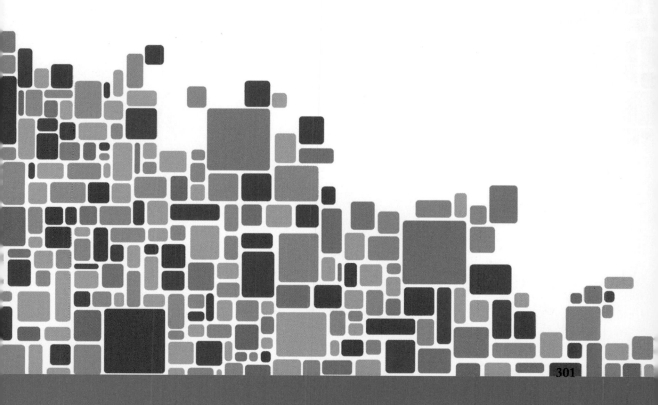

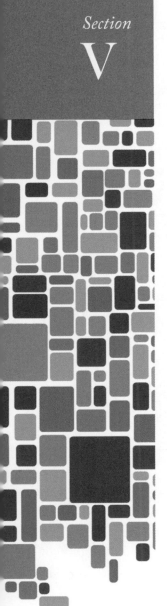

Grand Theories about Care or Caring

Three of the grand theories in this book focus on the phenomenon of care or caring in nursing. These theorists describe care or caring as the central domain of the discipline of nursing. Rather than place these in either the interactive–integrative or unitary–transformative paradigm, we situated them in a category of their own.

Madeleine Leininger's *theory of cultural care diversity and universality* is covered in Chapter 17. The theory is described, and practice applications of the theory are provided. Leininger was the first to define care as the essence of nursing; she asserted that care or nurturance can be understood only within cultural contexts.

Jean Watson's work can be conceptualized as a philosophy, grand theory, or middle-range theory, depending on the lens of the nurse working with the theory. Watson's theory is composed of the ten caritas processes, the transpersonal caring relationship, the caring occasion, and caring–healing modalities. Watson's theory draws from a spiritual dimension affirming that transpersonal caring is connecting and embracing the spirit or soul of another. She shares examples of how her theory is being advanced and applied as a model for practice through the Watson Caring Science Institute and the International Caritas Consortium.

The premise of Anne Boykin and Savina Schoenhofer's theory of *nursing as caring* is that the focus of nursing is the person living and growing in caring. The theory encompasses coming to know the other as caring, hearing and answering calls for caring, and nurturing the growth of the other as caring person. This theory has transformed, and is currently transforming, care in a variety of settings.

Chapter 17

Madeleine Leininger's Theory of Culture Care Diversity and Universality

Hiba Wehbe-Alamah

Introducing the Theorist
Overview of the Theory
Applications of the Theory
Summary
Practice Exemplar
References

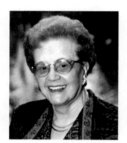

Madeleine M. Leininger

Introducing the Theorist

Madeleine M. Leininger (1925–2012) founded the worldwide field of transcultural nursing, the International Transcultural Nursing Society, and the *Journal of Transcultural Nursing.* Dr. Leininger obtained her initial nursing education at St. Anthony School of Nursing in Denver, Colorado. She earned her undergraduate degree from Mt. St. Scholastic College in Atchison, Kansas; her master's degree in psychiatric and mental health nursing from the Catholic University of America; and her PhD in social and cultural anthropology at the University of Washington (Boyle & Glittenberg Hinrichs, 2013). Dr. Leininger served as dean at the Universities of Washington and Utah, where she helped initiate and direct the first doctoral programs in nursing and facilitated the development of master's degree programs in nursing at American and overseas institutions. Recognized as a Living Legend by the American Academy of Nursing and a distinguished fellow by the Australian Royal College of Nursing, she served as a professor emerita in the College of Nursing at Wayne State University and adjunct professor at the University of Nebraska College of Nursing. Dr. Leininger passed away at her home in Omaha, Nebraska, at the age of 87 on August 10, 2012.

In the span of her prolific career, Madeleine Leininger published 35 books, wrote approximately 3,000 articles (some of which were never published), and gave more than 5,000 presentations or public lectures throughout the United States and abroad, in addition to contributing to numerous books and videos (Boyle & Glittenberg Hinrichs, 2013). Some of her well-known books include *Basic Psychiatric*

Concepts in Nursing (Leininger & Hofling, 1960); *Caring: An Essential Human Need* (1981); *Care: The Essence of Nursing and Health* (1984); *Care: Discovery and Uses in Clinical and Community Nursing* (1988); *Ethical and Moral Dimensions of Care* (1990d); and *Culture Care Diversity and Universality: A Theory of Nursing* (1991a, 2006a). *Nursing and Anthropology: Two Worlds to Blend* (1970) was the first book to bring together nursing and anthropology. The first book on transcultural nursing was *Transcultural Nursing: Concepts, Theories, and Practices* (1978, 1995, 2002). Her book *Qualitative Research Methods in Nursing* (1985, 1998) was the first published qualitative research methods book in nursing. In 1989, Dr. Leininger founded the *Journal of Transcultural Nursing,* the first transcultural nursing journal in the world.

Dr. Leininger conducted the first field study of the Gadsup Akuna of the Eastern Highlands of New Guinea in the early 1960s and went on to study more than cultures. She developed the first nursing research method called *ethnonursing,* used by scholars in nursing and other disciplines. She initiated the idea of worldwide certification of nurses prepared in transcultural nursing. Today, Basic (undergraduate) and Advanced (graduate) certifications are available through the Transcultural Nursing Society.

Overview of the Theory

One of Dr. Leininger's most significant and unique contributions was the development of her *culture care diversity and universality theory,* also known as the culture care theory (CCT), which she introduced in the early 1960s to provide culturally congruent and competent care (Leininger, 1991b, 1995, 2006a; McFarland, 2010). She believed that transcultural nursing care could provide meaningful, therapeutic health and healing outcomes. As she developed the theory, she identified transcultural nursing concepts, principles, theories, and research-based knowledge to guide, challenge, and explain nursing practices. This was a significant innovation in nursing and has helped open the door to new

scientific and humanistic dimensions of caring for people of diverse and similar cultures.

The theory of culture care diversity and universality was developed to establish a substantive knowledge base to guide nurses in discovery and use of transcultural nursing practices. During the post–World War II period, Dr. Leininger realized nurses would need transcultural knowledge and practices to function with people of diverse cultures worldwide (Leininger, 1970, 1978). Many new immigrants and refugees were coming to the United States, and the world was becoming more multicultural.

Leininger held that caring for people of many cultures was a critical and essential need, yet nurses and other health professionals were not prepared to meet this global challenge. Instead, nursing and medicine were focused on using new medical technologies and treatment regimens. They concentrated on biomedical study of diseases and symptoms. Shifting to a transcultural perspective was a major but critically needed change.

This part of the chapter presents an overview of the theory of culture care diversity and universality, along with its purpose, goals, assumptions, theoretical tenets, predicted hunches, related general features, and newest features. The next part of the chapter discusses applications of the knowledge in clinical and community settings. For a more in-depth discussion of the theorist's perspectives, consult the primary literature on the theory (Leininger, 1970, 1981, 1989a, 1989b, 1990a, 1990b, 1991a, 1995, 1997a, 1998, 2002, 2006a; McFarland, 2010).

Factors Leading to the Theory

Dr. Leininger's major motivation for the development of the CCT was the desire to discover unknown or little-known knowledge about cultures and their core values, beliefs, and needs. The idea for the CCT came to her while she was a clinical child nurse specialist in a child guidance home in a large Midwestern city (Leininger, 1970, 1991a, 1995, 2006a). From her focused observations and daily nursing experiences with the children in the home, she became aware that they were from many cultures, differing in their behaviors, needs, responses, and care expectations. In the home were youngsters who were Anglo American, African American, Jewish American, Appalachian, and many other cultures. Their parents responded to them differently, and their expectations of care and treatment modes were different. The reality was a shock to Leininger because she was not prepared to care for children of diverse cultures. Likewise, nurses, physicians, social workers, and health professionals in the guidance home were also not prepared to respond to such cultural differences.

It soon became evident that she needed cultural knowledge to be helpful to the children. Her psychiatric and general nursing care knowledge and experiences were inadequate. She decided to pursue doctoral study in anthropology. While in the anthropology doctoral program, she discovered a wealth of potentially valuable knowledge that would be helpful from a nursing perspective. To care for children of diverse cultures and link such knowledge into nursing knowledge and practice was a major challenge. It was essential to incorporate new cultural knowledge that went beyond the traditional physical and emotional needs of clients. Leininger was concerned about whether such learning would be possible, given nursing's traditional norms and orientation toward medical knowledge.

At that time, she questioned what made nursing a distinct and legitimate profession. She declared in the mid-1950s that care is (or should be) the essence and central domain of nursing. However, according to Leininger, many nurses resisted this idea because they thought care was unimportant, too feminine, too soft, and too vague and that it would never explain nursing and be accepted by medicine (Leininger, 1970, 1977, 1981, 1984). Nonetheless, Leininger firmly held to the claim and began to teach, study, and write about care as the essence of nursing, its unique and dominant attribute (Leininger, 1970, 1981, 1988, 1991a, 2006a). From both anthropological and nursing perspectives, she held that care and caring were basic and essential human needs for human growth, development,

and survival (Leininger, 1977, 1981, 2006a). She argued that what humans need is human caring to survive from birth to old age, when ill or well. Nevertheless, care needed to be specific and appropriate to cultures.

Her next step in the theory was to conceptualize selected cultural perspectives and transcultural nursing concepts derived from anthropology. She developed assumptions of culture care to establish a knowledge base for the new field of transcultural nursing. Synthesizing or interfacing culture care into nursing was a real challenge. (Leininger, 1976, 1978, 1990a, 1990b, 1991a, 2006a). Findings from the theory could provide the knowledge to care for people of different cultures. The idea of providing care was largely taken for granted or assumed to be understood by nurses, clients, and the public (Leininger, 1981, 1984). Yet the meaning of "care" from the perspective of different cultures was unknown to nurses and did not appear in the literature before the establishment of Leininger's theory in the early 1960s. Care knowledge had to be discovered with cultures.

Leininger (1981, 1988, 1990a, 1991a, 1995) maintained that before her work, there were no theories explicitly focused on care and culture in nursing environments, let alone research studies to explicate care meanings and phenomena in nursing. Theoretical and practical meanings of care in relation to specific cultures had not been studied, especially from a comparative cultural perspective. Leininger saw the urgent need to develop a whole new body of culturally based care knowledge to support transcultural nursing care. Shifting nurses' thinking and attitudes from medical symptoms, diseases, and treatments to that of knowing cultures and caring values and patterns was a major task. But nursing needed an appropriate theory to discover care, and Leininger held that her theory was "the only theory focused on developing new knowledge for the discipline of transcultural nursing" (Leininger, 2006a, p. 7). Essential features of the CCT and the ethnonursing research method were developed and/or revisited throughout Leininger's life (Leininger, 2006a, 2011).

Rationale for Transcultural Nursing: Signs and Need

The rationale for change in nursing in America and elsewhere (Leininger, 1970, 1978, 1984, 1989a, 1990a, 1995) was based on the following observations:

1. There were global migrations and interactions of people from virtually every place in the world due to modern electronics, transportation, and communication. These people needed sensitive and appropriate care.
2. There were signs of cultural stresses and cultural conflicts as nurses tried to care for clients from diverse Western and non-Western cultures.
3. There were cultural indications of consumer fears and resistance to health personnel as they used new technologies and treatment modes that did not fit their clients' values and lifeways.
4. There were signs that some clients from different cultures were angry, frustrated, and misunderstood by health personnel owing to ignorance of the clients' cultural beliefs, values, and expectations.
5. There were signs of misdiagnosis and mistreatment of clients from diverse cultures because health personnel did not understand the culture of the client.
6. There were signs that nurses, physicians, and other professional health personnel were becoming quite frustrated in caring for clients from unfamiliar cultures. Culture care factors were largely misunderstood or neglected.
7. There were signs that consumers of different cultures, whether in the home, hospital, or clinic, were being treated in ways that did not satisfy them and this influenced their recovery.
8. There were many signs of intercultural conflicts and cultural pain among staff that led to tensions.
9. There were very few health personnel of diverse cultures caring for clients.
10. Nurses were beginning to work in foreign countries in the military or as missionaries, and they were having great difficulty understanding and providing appropriate caring for clients of diverse cultures. They complained that they did not understand the peoples' needs, values, and lifeways.

Although anthropologists were clearly experts about cultures, many did not know what to do with patients, nor were they interested in nurses' work, in nursing as a profession, or in the study of human care phenomena in the early 1950s. Most anthropologists in those early days were far more interested in medical diseases, archaeological findings, and in physical and psychological problems of culture. For these reasons and many others, it was clearly evident in the 1960s that people of different cultures were not receiving care congruent with their cultural beliefs and values (Leininger, 1978, 1995). Nurses and other health professionals urgently needed transcultural knowledge and skills to work efficiently with people of diverse cultures.

Leininger therefore took a leadership role in the new field she called *transcultural nursing*. She defined transcultural nursing as an area of study and practice focused on cultural care (caring) values, beliefs, and practices of particular cultures. The goal was to provide culture-specific and congruent care to people of diverse cultures (Leininger, 1978, 1984, 1995, 2006a). The central purpose of transcultural nursing was to use research-based knowledge to help nurses discover care values and practices and use this knowledge in safe, responsible, and meaningful ways to care for people of different cultures. Today the CCT has led to a wealth of research-based knowledge to guide nurses and other health professionals in the care of clients, families, and communities of different cultures or subcultures.

Major Theoretical Tenets

In developing the theory of culture care diversity and universality, Leininger identified several predictive tenets or premises as essential for nurses and others to use.

Diversities and Commonalities

A principal tenet was that diversities and similarities (or commonalities) in culture care expressions, meanings, patterns, and practices would be found within cultures. This tenet challenges nurses to discover this knowledge so that nurses could use cultural data to provide therapeutic outcomes. It was predicted there would be a gold mine of knowledge if nurses were patient and persistent to discover care values and patterns within cultures, a dimension that had been missing from traditional nursing. Leininger maintained that human beings are born, live, and die with their specific cultural values and beliefs, as well as with their historical and environmental context, and that care is important for their survival and well-being. Leininger predicted that discovering which elements of care were culturally universal and which were different would drastically revolutionize nursing and ultimately transform health-care systems and practices (Leininger, 1978, 1990a, 1990b, 1991a, 2006a).

Worldview and Social Structure Factors

Another major tenet of the theory was that worldview and social structure factors—such as technology, religion (including spirituality and philosophy), kinship (family ties), cultural values, beliefs, and lifeways, political and legal factors, economic and educational factors, as well as ethnohistory, language expressions, environmental context, and generic and professional care—influence ways individuals, families, groups, and/or communities consider and deal with health, well-being, illness, healing, disabilities, and death (Leininger, 1995, 2006a). This broad and multifaceted view provides a holistic perspective for understanding people and grasping their world and environment within a historical context. Data from this holistic research-based knowledge guides nurses in caring for the health and well-being of the individual or to help disabled or dying clients from different cultures. Social structural factors influencing care of people from different cultures provide new insights for culturally congruent care. Systematic study by nurse researchers rather than superficial knowledge of culture is required to provide culturally congruent care. These factors, together with the history of cultures and knowledge of their environmental factors, were discovered to create

the theory and to bring forth new insights and new knowledge. These data disclose ways that clients can stay well and prevent illnesses. Indeed, to meet the theory's goal of making decisions that provide culturally congruent care, holistic cultural knowledge must be discovered (Leininger, 1991a, 2006a).

Discovering cultural care knowledge requires entering the cultural world to observe, listen, and validate ideas. Transcultural nursing is an immersion experience, not a "dip in and dip out" experience. No longer can nurses rely only on fragments of medical and psychological knowledge. Nurses must become aware of the social structure, cultural history, language use, and the environment in which people live to understand cultural care expressions. Thus, nurses need to understand the philosophy of transcultural nursing, the culture care theory, and ways to discover culture knowledge. Transcultural nursing courses and programs are essential to provide the necessary instruction and mentoring.

Professional and Generic Care

Another major and predicted tenet of the theory is that differences and similarities exist between the practices of two kinds of care: professional (etic) and generic (emic, traditional, indigenous, or "folk"; Leininger, 1991a, 2006a; McFarland, 2010). These differences influence the health, illness, and well-being of clients. Elucidating these differences identify gaps in care, inappropriate care, and also beneficial care. Such findings influence the recovery (healing), health, and well-being of clients of different cultures. Marked differences between generic and professional care ideas and actions lead to serious client–nurse conflicts, potential illnesses, and even death (Leininger, 1978, 1995). Such differences must be identified and resolved.

Three Modalities

Leininger identified three ways to attain and maintain culturally congruent care (Leininger, 1991a, 2006a; McFarland, 2010). The three modalities postulated are (1) culture care preservation and/or maintenance, (2) culture care accommodation and/or negotiation, and

(3) culture care restructuring and/or repatterning (Leininger, 1991a, 1995, 2006a). These three modes were very different from traditional nursing practices, routines, or interventions. They are focused on ways to use theoretical data creatively to facilitate congruent care to fit clients' particular cultural needs. To arrive at culturally appropriate care, the nurse has to draw on fresh culture care research and discovered knowledge from the people along with theoretical data findings. The care is tailored to client needs. Leininger believed that routine interventions would not always be appropriate and could lead to cultural imposition, tensions, and conflicts. Nurses need to shift from relying on routine interventions and from focusing on symptoms to employing care practices derived from the clients' culture and from the theory. They need to use holistic care knowledge from the theory as opposed to relying solely on medical data. Most important of all, they need to use both generic and professional care findings. This was a new challenge but a rewarding one for the nurse and the client if thoughtfully done, as it fosters nurse–client collaboration. Examples of the use of the three modalities can be found in several published sources (Leininger, 1995, 1999, 2002; McFarland et al., 2011; Wehbe-Alamah, 2008a, 2011) and are presented in the next part of this chapter.

Use of Leininger's theory has led to the discovery of new kinds of transcultural nursing knowledge. Culturally based care can prevent illness and maintain wellness. Methods for helping people throughout the life cycle, from birth to death, have been discovered. Cultural patterns of caring and health maintenance along with environmental and historical factors are important. Most important, the use of Leininger's theory has helped uncover significant cultural differences and similarities.

Theoretical Assumptions: Purpose, Goal, and Definitions of the Theory

This section discusses some of the major assumptions, definitions, and purposes of the theory. The theory's overriding purpose is to discover, document, analyze, and identify the cultural and care factors influencing humans in health, sickness, and dying and to thereby advance and improve nursing practices.

The theory's goal is to discover generic (folk) and professional care beliefs, expressions, and practices that could be incorporated into collaborative plans of care designed to provide culturally appropriate, safe, beneficial, and satisfying care to people of diverse or similar cultures, to promote their health and well-being, and to assist them in facing death or disabilities. Thus, the ultimate and primary goal of the theory is to provide culturally congruent care that is tailor-made for the lifeways and values of people (Leininger, 1991a, 1995, 2006a; McFarland, Mixer, Wehbe-Alamah, & Burke, 2012).

Theory Assumptions

Leininger postulated several theoretical assumptions, or basic beliefs, designed to assist researchers exploring Western and non-Western cultures (Leininger, 1970, 1977, 1981, 1984, 1991a, 1997b, 2006a):

1. Care is the essence and the central dominant, distinct, and unifying focus of nursing.
2. Humanistic and scientific care are essential for human growth, well-being, health, survival, and to face death and disabilities.
3. Care (caring) is essential to curing or healing, for there can be no curing without caring. (This assumption was held to have profound relevance worldwide.)
4. Culture care is the synthesis of two major constructs that guide the researcher to discover, explain, and account for health, well-being, care expressions, and other human conditions.
5. Culture care expressions, meanings, patterns, processes, and structural forms are diverse; but some commonalities (universalities) exist among and between cultures.
6. Culture care values, beliefs, and practices are influenced by and embedded in the worldview, social structure factors (e.g., religion, philosophy of life, kinship, politics,

economics, education, technology, and cultural values) and the ethnohistorical and environmental contexts.

7. Every culture has generic (lay, folk, naturalistic, mainly emic) and usually some professional (etic) care to be discovered and used for culturally congruent care practices.

8. Culturally congruent and therapeutic care occurs when culture care values, beliefs, expressions, and patterns are explicitly known and used appropriately, sensitively, and meaningfully with people of diverse or similar cultures.

9. The three modes of care offer therapeutic ways to help people of diverse cultures.

10. Qualitative research paradigmatic methods offer important means to discover largely embedded, covert, epistemic, and ontological culture care knowledge and practices.

11. Transcultural nursing is a discipline with a body of knowledge and practices to attain and maintain the goal of culturally congruent care for health and well-being (Leininger, 2006a, pp. 18–19).

Orientational Theory Definitions

To encourage discovery of qualitative knowledge, Leininger used orientational (not operational) definitions for her theory, to allow the researcher to discern previously unknown phenomena or ideas. Orientational terms allow discovery and are usually congruent with the client lifeways. They are important in using the qualitative ethnonursing discovery method, which is focused on how people understand and experience their world using cultural knowledge and lifeways (Leininger, 1985, 1991a, 1997b, 1997c, 2002, 2006a). The following are select examples:

1. *Culture:* The learned, shared, and transmitted values, beliefs, norms, and lifeways of a particular group that guides their thinking, decisions, and actions in patterned ways and often intergenerationally (Leininger, 2006a, p. 13).

2. *Care:* Those assistive, supportive, and enabling experiences or ideas toward others with evident or anticipated needs to ameliorate or improve a human condition or lifeway. Caring refers to actions, attitudes, and practices to assist or help others toward healing and well-being (Leininger, 2006a, p. 12). Care is both an abstract and a concrete phenomenon.

3. *Culture care:* Subjectively and objectively learned and transmitted values, beliefs, and patterned lifeways that assist, support, facilitate, or enable another individual or group to maintain well-being and health, to improve their human condition and lifeway, or to deal with illness, handicaps, or death (Leininger, 1991a, p. 47).

4. *Culture Care Diversity:* The differences or variabilities among human beings with respect to culture care meanings, patterns, values, lifeways, symbols, or other features related to providing beneficial care to clients of a designated culture (Leininger, 2006a, p. 16).

5. *Culture Care Universality:* The commonly shared or similar culture care phenomena features of human beings with recurrent meanings, patterns, values, lifeways, or symbols that serve as a guide for caregivers to provide assistive, supportive, facilitative, or enabling people care for healthy outcomes (Leininger, 2006a, p. 16).

6. *Professional (etic) care:* Formal and explicit cognitively learned professional care knowledge and practices obtained generally through educational institutions. They are taught to nurses and others to provide assistive, supportive, enabling, or facilitative acts for or to another individual or group in order to improve their health, prevent illnesses, or to help with dying or other human conditions (Leininger, 2006a, p. 14).

7. *Generic (emic) care:* The learned and transmitted lay, indigenous, traditional, or local folk knowledge and practices to provide assistive, supportive, enabling, and facilitative acts for or toward others with evident or anticipated health needs in order to improve well-being or to help with dying or other human conditions (Leininger, 2006a, p. 14).

8. *Culture care preservation and/or maintenance:* Those assistive, supportive, facilitative, or enabling professional acts or
decisions that help cultures to retain,
preserve, or maintain beneficial care beliefs and values or to face handicaps and
death (Leininger, 2006a, p. 8).

9. *Culture care accommodation and/or negotiation:* Those assistive, accommodating, facilitative, or enabling creative provider care
actions or decisions that facilitate adaptation to or negotiation with others for culturally congruent, safe, and effective care
for their health, well-being, or to deal with
illness or dying (Leininger, 2006a, p. 8).

10. *Culture care repatterning and/or restructuring:* Those assistive, supportive, facilitative, or enabling professional actions and
mutual decisions that help people to re-
order, change, modify, or restructure
their lifeways and institutions for better
(or beneficial) health-care patterns, practices, or outcomes (Leininger, 2006a,
p. 8). These patterns are mutually established between caregivers and receivers.

11. *Ethnohistory:* The past facts, events, instances, and experiences of human beings,
groups, cultures, and institutions that
occur over time in particular contexts
that help explain past and current lifeways
about culture care influencers of health
and well-being or the death of people
(Leininger, 2006a, p. 15).

12. *Environmental context:* The totality of
an event, situation, or particular experience that gives meaning to people's
expressions, interpretations, and social
interactions within particular geophysical,
ecological, spiritual, sociopolitical, and
technological factors in specific cultural
settings (Leininger, 2006a, p. 15).

13. *Worldview:* The way people tend to look
out on their world or their universe to
form a picture or value stance about life
or the world around them (Leininger,
2006a, p. 15).

14. *Cultural and social structure factors:* religion
(spirituality); kinship (social ties); politics;
legal issues; education; economics; technology; political factors; philosophy of

life; and cultural beliefs and values with
gender and class difference. The theorist
has predicted that these diverse factors
must be understood as they directly or
indirectly influence health and well-being
(Leininger, 2006a, p. 14).

15. *Culturally congruent care:* Culturally based
care knowledge, acts, and decisions used
in sensitive and knowledgeable ways to
appropriately and meaningfully fit the
cultural values, beliefs, and lifeways of
clients for their health and well-being,
or to prevent illness, disabilities, or death
(Leininger, 2006a, p. 15).

The Sunrise Enabler: A Conceptual Guide to Knowledge Discovery

Leininger developed the sunrise enabler
(Fig. 17-1) to provide a holistic and comprehensive conceptual picture of the major factors
influencing culture care diversity and universality (Leininger, 1995, 1997b; Leininger &
McFarland, 2002, 2006). The model can be a
valuable visual guide to elucidating multiple
factors that influence human care and lifeways
of different cultures. The enabler serves as a
cognitive guide for the researcher to reflect on
different predicted influences on culturally
based care.

The sunrise enabler can also be used as a
valuable aid in cultural and health-care assessment of clients. As the researcher uses the
model, the different factors alert him or her to
find culture care phenomena. Gender, sexual
orientation, race, class, and biomedical conditions are studied as part of the theory. These
determinants tend to be embedded in the
worldview and social structure and take time
to recognize. Care values and beliefs are usually
lodged into environment, religion, kinship,
and daily life patterns.

The nurse can begin the discovery at any
place in the enabler and follow the informant's
ideas and experiences about care. If one starts
in the upper part of the enabler, one needs to
reflect on all aspects depicted to obtain holistic
or total care data. Some nurses start with
generic and professional care then look at how
religion, economics, and other influences affect
these care modes. One always moves with the

CULTURE CARE

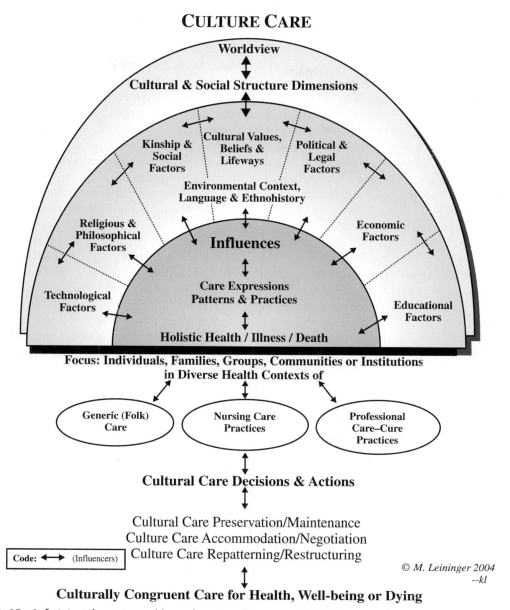

Fig 17 • 1 Leininger's sunrise enabler to discover culture care. (©*M. Leininger 2004.*)

informants', rather than the researcher's, interest and story. Flexibility in using the enabler promotes a total or holistic view of care.

The three transcultural care decisions and actions (in the lower part of the figure) are very important to keep in mind. Nursing decisions and actions are studied until one realizes the care needed. The nurse discovers with the informant the appropriate decisions, actions, or plans for care. Throughout this discovery

process, the nurse holds his or her own etic biases in check so that the informant's ideas will come forth, rather than the researcher's. Transcultural nurses are mentored in ways to withhold their biases or wishes and to enter the client's worldview.

The nurse begins the study by making explicit a specific *domain of inquiry*. For example, the researcher may focus on a domain of inquiry such as "culture care of Mexican

American mothers caring for their children in their home." Every word in the domain statement is important and studied with the sunrise enabler and the theory tenets. The nurse or researcher may have hunches about the domain and care, but until all data have been studied with the theory tenets, she or he cannot prove them. Informants' viewpoints, experiences, and actions are fully documented. Generally, informants select what they like to talk about first, and the nurse/researcher accommodates their interest or stories about care. During in-depth study of the domain of inquiry, all areas of the sunrise enabler are identified and confirmed with the informants. The informants become active participants throughout the discovery process in such a way as to feel comfortable and willing to share their ideas.

The real challenge is to focus care meanings, beliefs, values, and practices related to informants' cultures so that subtle and obvious differences and similarities about care are identified among key and general informants. The differences and similarities are important to document with the theory. If informants ask about the researcher's views, the latter must be carefully and sparsely shared. The researcher keeps in mind that some informants may want to please the researcher by talking about professional medicines and treatments. Professional ideas, however, often cloud or mask the client's real interests and views. If this occurs, the researcher must be alert to such tendencies and keep the focus on the informant's ideas and on the domain of inquiry studied. The informant's knowledge is always kept central to the discovery process about culture care, health, and well-being. If the researcher finds some factors unfamiliar, such as kinship, economics, and political and other considerations depicted in the model, the researcher should listen attentively to the informant's ideas. Obtaining insight into the informant's emic (insider's) views, beliefs, and practices is central to studying the theory (Leininger, 1985, 1991a, 1995, 1997b; Leininger & McFarland, 2002, 2006).

Throughout the study and use of the theory, the meanings, expressions, and patterns of culturally based care are important. The nurse/researcher listens attentively to informants' accounts about care and then documents the ideas. What informants know and practice about care or caring in their culture is significant. Documenting ideas from the informants' emic viewpoint is essential to arrive at accurate culturally based care. Unknown care meanings, such as the concepts of protection, respect, love, and many other care concepts, need to be teased out and explored in depth, as they are the key words and ideas in understanding care. Such care meanings and expressions are not always readily known; informants ponder care meanings and are often surprised that nurses are focused on care instead of medical symptoms. Sometimes informants may be reluctant to share ideas about social structure, religion, and economics or politics, as they fear these ideas may not be accepted or understood by health personnel. Generic folk or indigenous knowledge often has rich care data and needs to be explored. Generic care ideas need to be appropriately integrated into the three transcultural modes of decisions and actions for culturally congruent care outcomes. Generic and professional care are integrated so that the clients benefit from both types of care.

The sunrise enabler was developed with the idea to "let the sun enter the researcher's mind" and discover largely unknown care factors of cultures. Letting the sun "rise and shine" is important and offers fresh insights about care practices. A recent metasynthesis of 24 doctoral dissertations using Leininger's CCT and the ethnonursing research method led to the discovery of interpretive and explanatory culture care findings, new theoretical formulations, and evidence-based recommendations to guide nursing practice (McFarland et al., 2011).

Newest Addition to the Theory

In the summer of 2011, Dr. Leininger introduced *collaborative care* as a new care construct, which she offered as the next phase in the evolutionary development of CCT. She maintained that diverse cultural values, beliefs, expressions, actions, and practices within a family, a group, an institution, or other unit may present with situations in which conflicts may arise. She proposed collaborative care as a means or a strategy to resolve differences and provide culturally congruent care.

Leininger defined the collaborative care approach as those values, meanings, expressions, and actions by informants that reveal a desire and a plan to work with others in order to identify, attain, and maintain health and well-being and to resolve conflicts. This care construct has been published by McFarland and Wehbe-Alamah (McFarland & Wehbe-Alamah, 2015).

Current Status of the Theory

Currently, the theory of culture care diversity and universality continues to be studied and used in many schools of nursing within the United States and in other countries, such as Lebanon, Jordan, Saudi Arabia, Taiwan, China, Japan, and Finland (Leininger & McFarland, 2002, 2006; Wehbe-Alamah & McFarland; 2012). Interdisciplinary health personnel are becoming increasingly aware of transcultural nursing concepts that help them in their work. Several disciplines including dentistry, medicine, social work, and pharmacy have reported using the culturally congruent care theory or teaching it in their programs (McFarland, 2011).

The theory of culture care will remain of global interest and significance as nurses and other health-care professionals continue to explore cultures and their care needs and practices worldwide. Transcultural nursing concepts, principles, theory, and findings must become fully incorporated into professional areas of teaching, practice, consultation, and research. When this occurs, one can anticipate true transcultural health practices and concomitant benefits. Unquestionably, the theory will continue to grow in relevance and use as our world becomes more intensely multicultural. Nurses and other health professionals are expected to provide culturally congruent care to people of diverse cultures. The theory, along with many transcultural nursing concepts, principles, and research findings, will continue to prove indispensable.

Applications of the Theory

The purpose of this part of the chapter is to present the implications for nursing practice of the CCT and related ethnonursing research findings. Many nursing theories are rather abstract and do not focus on how practicing nurses might use the research findings related to a theory. However, with the CCT, along with the ethnonursing method, there is a built-in means for discovering and confirming data with informants in order to make practical nursing actions and decisions meaningful and culturally congruent (Leininger, 2002).[1]

Leininger purposefully avoided using the phrase *nursing intervention* because this term often implies to clients from different cultures that the nurse is imposing his or her (etic) views, which may not be helpful. Instead, the term *nursing actions and decisions* was used, but always with the clients helping to arrive at whatever actions or decisions were planned and implemented. The care modes fit with the clients' or peoples' lifeways and are both therapeutic and satisfying for them. The nurse can draw on scientific and evidence-based nursing, medical, and other knowledge with each care mode.

Data collected from the upper and lower parts of the sunrise enabler provide culture care knowledge for the nurse and other researchers to discover and establish useful ways to provide quality care practices. Active participatory involvement with clients is essential to arrive at culturally congruent care with one or all of the three action modes to meet clients' care needs in their particular environmental contexts. The use of these modes in nursing care is one of the most creative and rewarding features of transcultural and general nursing practice with clients of diverse cultures. Using Leininger's care modes in clinical practice shows respect to clients' beliefs, values, and expressions and establishes a partnership between health-care

---

[1]For additional information about the Ethnonursing Research Method please go to bonus chapter content available at FA Davis http://davisplus.fadavis.com

providers and clients to ensure safe, beneficent, and culturally congruent care (McFarland & Eipperle, 2008).

It is most important (and a shift in nursing) to carefully focus on the holistic dimensions, as depicted in the sunrise enabler, to arrive at therapeutic culture care practices. All the factors in the sunrise enabler must be considered to arrive at culturally congruent care. These include worldview; technological, religious, kinship, political–legal, economic, and educational factors; cultural values and lifeways; environmental context, language, and ethnohistory; and generic (folk) and professional care practices (Leininger, 2002, 2006a). Care generated from the CCT will become safe, congruent, meaningful, and beneficial to clients only when the nurse in clinical practice becomes fully aware of and explicitly uses knowledge generated from the theory and ethnonursing method, whether in a community, home, or institutional context. The CCT, used with the ethnonursing method, is a powerful means for exploring new directions and practices in nursing. Incorporating culture-specific care into client care is essential to the practice of professional care and to licensure as registered nurses. Culture-specific care is the safe means to ensure culturally based holistic care that fits the client's culture—a major challenge for nurses and other health-care professionals who practice and provide services in all health-care settings.

The Use of Culture Care Research Findings

Over the past 5 decades, Dr. Leininger and other research colleagues have used the CCT and the ethnonursing method to focus on the care meanings and experiences of 100 cultures (Leininger, 2002). They discovered 187 care constructs in Western and non-Western cultures between 1989 and 1998 (Leininger, 1998a, 1998b). Leininger listed the 11 most dominant constructs of care in priority ranking, with the most universal or frequently discovered first: respect for/about, concern for/about; attention to (details)/in anticipation of; helping–assisting or facilitative acts; active helping; presence (being physically there);

understanding (beliefs, values, lifeways, and environmental); connectedness; protection (gender related); touching; and comfort measures (Leininger, 2006b; McFarland, 2002). These care constructs are the most critical and important universal or common findings to consider in nursing practice, but care diversities will also be found and must be considered. The ways in which culture care is applied and used in specific cultures will reflect both similarities and differences among and within different cultures.

Next, two ethnonursing studies are reviewed with focus on the findings, which have implications for nursing practice.

Culture Care of Traditional Syrian Muslims in the Midwestern United States

In 2005, the theory of culture care diversity and universality and the ethnonursing research method were used to guide a study of the culture care of traditional Syrian Muslims in the Midwestern United States (Wehbe-Alamah, 2008b, 2011). The domain of inquiry for this ethnonursing study was the generic and the professional care meanings, beliefs, and practices related to health and illness of traditional Syrian Muslims living in several urban communities in the Midwestern United States. The purpose of this study was to discover, describe, and analyze the effect of worldview, cultural context, technological, religious, political, educational, and economic factors on the traditional Syrian Muslims' generic and professional care meanings, beliefs, and practices. The goal was to provide practicing nurses and other health-care providers with knowledge that can be turned into care actions and decisions that facilitate the provision of culturally congruent care to traditional Syrian Muslims living in similar contexts (Wehbe-Alamah, 2011).

Findings from this study revealed that the worldview of traditional Syrian Muslims is deeply embedded in the Islamic religion and the Syrian culture. Life is viewed as a test from God and a journey in which one must attempt to do as many good deeds as possible and to behave in a righteous way whether conducting business, taking care of housework, or engaging in any other regular daily activity. Kinship and familial relationships are treasured. Socializing with family members and friends are considered important aspects of Syrian lifeway. Visitations and telephone conversations as well as Friday prayer congregations are major social activities for Syrians. In Syrian Muslim society, the man typically assumes the role of the breadwinner, whereas the woman takes on other responsibilities, such as managing the household and raising the children (Wehbe-Alamah, 2008b).

Some of the discovered traditional cultural beliefs and practices included modesty, generous hospitality, segregation of men and women during social events such as wedding parties and dinner invitations, wearing of a coat or *jilbab* over clothes for women when in public, caring for older family members within the home setting, as well as visiting, praying for, and cooking for the sick. Normal everyday actions were considered by many informants as acts of worship. Engaging in religious practices such as prayer and Qur'an recitation or memorization was reported as a source of physical, spiritual, emotional, and mental support by numerous informants. Religious beliefs were determined to play an important role in a person's decision-making involving abortion, sterilization, autopsy, organ donation, birth control, and other significant health issues (Wehbe-Alamah, 2008a).

Caring was described as being considerate of other people's feelings and respecting their beliefs. Empathy, sympathy, sensitivity, unselfishness, and understanding were other qualities used to describe caring. Caring can be expressed by checking on others, being available to them, offering them help, cooking healthy food, and keeping a clean body and a hygienic environment. Caring can additionally be exemplified by withholding a diagnosis and/or prognosis from a patient especially if an impending death was expected and by burying the dead with 24 hours of their passing. Caring attributes of nurses were identified as smiling, responding quickly to the needs of sick patients, loving the nursing profession and role, and respecting the patient's culture (Wehbe-Alamah, 2008b).

A plethora of generic or folk practices were discovered and included some that are beneficial to health and others with potentially harmful ramifications. One such example is the consumption of raw liver, which is rich in iron and is used to treat anemia or iron deficiency. Another example is treating head lice by pouring gasoline over the scalp and massaging it into the hair. Folk practices that are beneficial to health included eating in moderation, exercising, and taking vitamin C when treating a cold (Wehbe-Alamah, 2008b).

Such information can be turned into culturally congruent decisions and actions that can impact clinical practice through the application of Leininger's culture care modes. Accordingly, nurses and other health-care providers can preserve and/or maintain the cultural beliefs, expressions, and practices of traditional Syrian Muslims by respecting the need for modesty and segregation and assigning same-sex health-care providers whenever possible. The cultural belief and practice of visiting the sick can be accommodated by encouraging a large number of visitors within the hospital setting with the negotiation of having only a few visitors in the patient's room at a time. The harmful folk practices of using gasoline to treat head lice and consuming raw liver to treat anemia can be repatterned and/or restructured through education of ramifications and discussion of healthier alternatives.

Practice Exemplar

A Middle Eastern patient in labor identified as Mrs. Sarah Islam has just been admitted to the obstetrics floor. She is accompanied by her husband and is dressed in loose clothing that covers all of her body except for her face and hands. She belongs to the Muslim faith and wears a head cover. Her husband requests that only female health-care providers (HCPs) be assigned to his wife. The nurse provides culturally congruent care to this family using Leininger's culture care theory.

Continued

Practice Exemplar cont.

According to this theory, the worldview of every human being is affected by cultural and social structural dimensions, including but not limited to cultural values, beliefs, and lifeways, and kinship, social, and religious factors. Therefore, professional nursing care must incorporate an understanding of these beliefs and practices. As a result, the nurse proceeds by conducting a cultural assessment to identify important needs and prohibitions that need to be addressed in the plan of care. The nurse begins by explaining that she would like to ask questions to learn about how to best care for the client and her family. The cultural assessment reveals the following:

• Modesty and privacy are important values to Mrs. and Mr. Islam and should be preserved whenever possible, according to cultural and religious teachings. The couple explains that this can be achieved by assigning same-sex HCPs and by preventing male individuals from entering the patient's room without first obtaining permission to do so.
• Pork-derived products including gelatin are prohibited in Islam and therefore should be excluded from diet and medications. The couple explains that Jello and gelatin-encapsulated medications contain gelatin and should be avoided.
• A special prayer needs to be whispered by the father in the newborn's ears after birth. The couple requests that the newborn be handed to the father as soon as possible after birth to facilitate this practice.
• Visitation by family members and friends is to be expected following birth. The couple informs you that they expect at least 30 visitors.
• Smoking the water pipe is a common cultural practice and is often carried in the presence of children. Mr. Islam smokes the water pipe twice a day.

Having identified important cultural and religious values, practices, needs, and prohibitions, the nurse proceeds to develop a culturally congruent plan of care using Leininger's Culture care modes:

Culture care preservation and/or maintenance:

• The nurse includes a note in the electronic health record about identified cultural and religious values, practices, needs, and prohibitions. This will assist with continuity of culturally congruent care.
• The nurse is female; therefore she is able to care for Mrs. Islam.
• The nurse places a sign at Mrs. Islam door that reads: "No males allowed without permission."
• The obstetrician and all nursing staff attending the birth are informed about the important practice of handing the newborn to the father within minutes of birth. The father recites the prayer in the baby's ears. The nurse attends the birth and ensures that this happens.

Culture care accommodation and/or negotiation:

• The nurse arranges for kitchen staff to provide vegetarian Jello versus animal-derived Jello.
• The nurse arranges for medications to be ordered or dispensed in tablet versus gelcap format.
• The nurse negotiates with the family to have visitors come at different times, wait in waiting room, and visit in numbers of 2 or 3 at a time.

Culture care restructuring and/or repatterning:

• The nurse educates the client and her husband about dangers associated with smoking and secondhand smoking inhalation implications to the newborn. She advises the discontinuation of this practice. (Alternatively, the nurse negotiates with Mr Islam to only smoke outdoors and cut down to once a day.)

Upon discharge, Mr. and Mrs. Islam thank you, the nurse, for providing them with the best care they have ever received in a Western health-care setting.

■ Summary

The purpose of the CCT and the ethnonursing method is to discover culture care knowledge and to combine generic and professional care. The goal is to provide culturally congruent nursing care using the three modes of nursing actions and decisions that are meaningful, safe, and beneficial to people of similar and diverse cultures worldwide (Leininger, 1991b, 1995, 2006a). The clinical use of the three major care modes (culture care preservation and/or maintenance; culture care accommodation and/or negotiation; and culture care repatterning and/or restructuring) by nurses to guide nursing judgments, decisions, and actions is essential in order to provide culturally congruent care that is beneficial, satisfying, and meaningful to the people nurses serve. The studies presented here substantiate that the three modes are care-centered and are based on the use of generic care (emic) knowledge along with professional care (etic) knowledge obtained from research using the CCT along with the ethnonursing method. This chapter has reviewed only a small selection of the culture care findings from ethnonursing research studies conducted over the past 5 decades. There is a wealth of additional findings of interest to practicing nurses who care for clients of all ages from diverse and similar cultural groups in many different institutional and community contexts around the world. More in-depth culture care findings, along with the use of the three modes, can be found in the *Journal of Transcultural Nursing* (1989–2013), in the *Online Journal of Cultural Competence in Nursing and Healthcare* (www.OJCCNH.org) and in the numerous books and articles written by Dr. Madeleine Leininger and researchers using her theory and method. Nurses in clinical practice can refer to research studies and doctoral dissertations conceptualized within the CCT for additional detailed nursing implications for clients from diverse cultures (Leininger & McFarland, 2002; McFarland et al., 2011).

The theory of culture care diversity and universality is one of the most comprehensive yet practical theories to advance transcultural and general nursing knowledge with concomitant ways for practicing nurses to establish or improve care to people. Nursing students and practicing nurses have remained the strongest advocates of the CCT (Leininger, 2002). The theory focuses on a long-neglected area in nursing practice—culture care—that is most relevant to our multicultural world.

The theory of culture care diversity and universality is depicted in the sunrise enabler as a rising sun. This visual metaphor is particularly apt. The future of the CCT shines brightly indeed because it is holistic and comprehensive; and it facilitates discovering care related to diverse and similar cultures, contexts, and ages of people in familiar and naturalistic ways. The theory is useful to nurses and nursing as well as to professionals in other disciplines such as physical, occupational, and speech therapy, medicine, social work, and pharmacy. Healthcare practitioners in other disciplines are beginning to use this theory because they also need to become knowledgeable about and sensitive and responsible to people of diverse cultures who need care (Leininger, 2002; McFarland, 2011).

References

Boyle, J., & Glittenberg Hinrichs, J. (2013). Madeleine Leininger, PhD, LHD, RN, FRCA, FAAN: A remembrance. *Journal of Transcultural Nursing, 24*(1), 5.

Leininger, M. (1970). *Nursing and anthropology: Two worlds to blend.* New York: Wiley.

Leininger, M. (1976). Transcultural nursing presents an exciting challenge. *The American Nurse, 5*(5), 6–9.

Leininger, M. (1977). Caring: The essence and central focus of nursing. *Nursing Research Foundation Report, 12*(1), 2–14.

Leininger, M. (1978). *Transcultural nursing: Concepts, theories, and practices.* New York: Wiley.

Leininger, M. (1981). *Caring: An essential human need.* Thorofare, NJ: Slack.

Leininger, M. (1984). *Care: The essence of nursing and health.* Thorofare, NJ: Slack.

Leininger, M. (1985). *Qualitative research methods in nursing* (pp. 33–73). Orlando, FL: Grune & Stratton.

Leininger, M. (1988). *Care: Discovery and uses in clinical and community nursing.* Detroit, MI: Wayne State University Press.

Leininger, M. (1989a). Transcultural nursing: Quo vadis (where goeth the field)? *Journal of Transcultural Nursing, 1*(1), 33–45.

Leininger, M. (1989b). Transcultural nurse specialists and generalists: New practitioners in nursing. *Journal of Transcultural Nursing, 1*(1), 4–16.

Leininger, M. (1990a). Transcultural nursing: A worldwide necessity to advance nursing knowledge and practices. In J. McCloskey & H. Grace, (Eds.), *Current issues in nursing.* St. Louis, MO: C. V. Mosby.

Leininger, M. (1990b). Culture: The conspicuous missing link to understand ethical and moral dimensions of human care. In M. Leininger (Ed.), *Ethical and moral dimensions of care.* Detroit, MI: Wayne State University Press.

Leininger, M. (1990d). *Ethical and moral dimensions of care.* Detroit, MI: Wayne State University Press.

Leininger, M. (1991a). *Culture care diversity and universality: A theory of nursing.* New York: National League for Nursing Press.

Leininger, M. (1991b). The theory of culture care diversity and universality. In M. Leininger (Ed.), *Culture care diversity and universality: A theory of nursing* (pp. 5–68). New York: National League for Nursing Press.

Leininger, M. (1995). *Transcultural nursing: Concepts, theories, research, and practice.* Columbus, OH: McGraw-Hill College Custom Series.

Leininger, M. (1997a). Overview and reflection of the theory of culture care and the ethnonursing research method. *Journal of Transcultural Nursing, 8*(2), 32–51.

Leininger, M. (1997b). Overview of the theory of culture care with the ethnonursing research method. *Journal of Transcultural Nursing, 8*(2), 32–53.

Leininger, M. (1997c). Transcultural nursing research to transform nursing education and practice: 40 years. *Image: Journal of Nursing Scholarship, 29*(4), 341–347.

Leininger, M. (1998a). *Qualitative research methods in nursing.* Dayton, OH: Greyden Press

Leininger, M. (1998b). Special research report: Dominant culture care (emic) meanings and practice findings from Leininger's theory. *Journal of Transcultural Nursing, 9*(2), 44–47.

Leininger, M. (2002). Part I: The theory of culture care and the ethnonursing research method. In M. M. Leininger & M. R. McFarland (Eds.), *Transcultural nursing: concepts, theories, and practice* (3rd ed., pp. 71–98). Sudbury, MA: Jones and Bartlett.

Leininger, M. (2006a). Culture care diversity and universality theory and evolution of the ethnonursing method. In M. M. Leininger & M. R. McFarland (Eds.). *Culture diversity & universality: A worldwide nursing theory* (2nd ed., pp. 1–41). Sudbury, MA: Jones and Bartlett.

Leininger, M. (2006b). Ethnonursing: A research method with enablers to study the theory of culture care. In M. M. Leininger & M. R. McFarland (Eds.). *Culture diversity & universality: A worldwide nursing theory* (2nd ed., pp. 43–81). Sudbury, MA: Jones and Bartlett.

Leininger, M. (2009). *It is time to celebrate, reflect and look into the future.* Retrieved on January 9, 2013, from the Transcultural Nursing Society website at: http://www.tcns.org/Foundress.html

Leininger, M. (2011). Leininger's reflection on the ongoing father protective care research. *The Online Journal of Cultural Competence in Nursing and Healthcare, 1*(2), 1–13. http://www.ojccnh.org/1/2/index.shtml

Leininger, M., & Hofling, C. (1960). *Basic psychiatric concepts in nursing.* Philadelphia: Lippincott.

Leininger, M. M., & McFarland, M. R. (Eds). (2002). *Transcultural nursing: Concepts, theories, and practice* (3rd ed.). New York: McGraw-Hill.

Leininger, M., & McFarland, M. (2002). *Transcultural nursing: Concepts, theories, research, and practice* (3rd ed.). New York: McGraw-Hill. Chinese Complex Translation Copyright 2007 by Wu-nan Book, Inc. (Book translated into Chinese).

Leininger, M. M., & McFarland, M. R. (Eds.) (2006). *Culture diversity & universality: A worldwide nursing theory* (2nd ed.). Sudbury, MA: Jones and Bartlett.

McFarland, M. R. (2002). Part II: Selected research findings from the culture care theory. In M. M. Leininger & M. R. McFarland (Eds.), *Transcultural nursing: Concepts, theories, and practice* (3rd ed., pp. 99–116). New York: McGraw-Hill.

McFarland, M. R. (2010). Madeleine Leininger: Culture care theory of diversity and universality. In A. M. Tomey & M. R. Alligood (Eds.), *Nursing theorists and their work* (7th ed., pp. 454–479, with revisions from 2006 ed.). St. Louis, MO: Elsevier

McFarland, M. R. (2011).*The culture care theory and a look to the future for transcultural nursing.* Keynote address presented at the 37th Annual Conference of the International Society of Transcultural Nursing, Las Vegas, NV.

McFarland, M. R., & Eipperle, M. K. (2008). Culture care theory: A proposed practice theory guide for nurse practitioners in primary care settings. *Contemporary Nurse: A Journal for the Australian Nursing Profession, 28*(1–2), 48–63.

McFarland, M. R., Mixer, S. J., Wehbe-Alamah, H., & Burk, R. (2012). Ethnonursing: A qualitative research method for all disciplines. *Online International Journal of Qualitative Methods, 11*(3), 259–279. University of Alberta, Canada.

McFarland, M. R., & Wehbe-Alamah, H. B. (2015). The theory of culture care diversity and universality. In McFarland and Wehbe-Alamah (Eds), *Culture care diversity and universality: A worldwide nursing theory* (3rd ed., Ch 1, pp. 1-31). Sudbury, MA: Jones and Bartlett.

McFarland, M., Wehbe-Alamah, H., Wilson, M., & Vossos, H. (2011). Synopsis of findings discovered within a descriptive meta-synthesis of doctoral dissertations guided by the Culture Care Theory with use of the ethnonursing research method. *Online Journal of Cultural Competence in Nursing and Healthcare, 1*(2), 24–39. Retrieved from http://www.cultural-competence-project.org/ojccnh/1(2).shtml

Wehbe-Alamah, H. (2008a). Bridging generic and professional care practices for Muslim patients through the use of Leininger's culture care modes. *Contemporary Nurse, 28*(1–2), 83–97.

Wehbe-Alamah, H. (2008b). *Culture care of Syrian Muslims in the Midwestern USA: The generic and professional health care beliefs, expressions, and practices of Syrian Muslims and implications to practice.* Saarbrucken, Germany: VDM Verlag Dr. Muller

Wehbe-Alamah, H. (2011). The use of culture care theory with Syrian Muslims in the Mid-western United States. *Online Journal of Cultural Competence in Nursing and Healthcare, 1*(3), 1–12. Retrieved from http://www.cultural-competence-project.org/ojccnh/1(3).shtml

Wehbe-Alamah, H., & McFarland, M. (2012). *The Taiwanese cultural experience.* Podium presentation at the 38th Annual Conference of the Transcultural Nursing Society. Orlando, Florida.

Jean Watson's Theory of Human Caring

Chapter 18

JEAN WATSON

Introducing the Theorist
Overview of the Theory
Applications of the Theory
Practice Exemplar by Terri Woodward
Summary
References

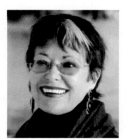

Jean Watson

Introducing the Theorist

Dr. Jean Watson is distinguished professor emerita and dean of nursing emerita at the University of Colorado Denver, where she served for more than 20 years and held an endowed Chair in Caring Science for more than 16 years. She is founder of the original Center for Human Caring at the University of Colorado Health Sciences, is a Living Legend in the American Academy of Nursing, and served as president of the National League for Nursing. Dr. Watson founded and directs the nonprofit Watson Caring Science Institute, dedicated to furthering the work of caring, science, and heart-centered *Caritas* Nursing, restoring caring and love for nurses' and health-care clinicians' healing practices for self and others.

Watson earned undergraduate and graduate degrees in nursing and psychiatric–mental health nursing and holds a doctorate in educational psychology and counseling from the University of Colorado at Boulder. She is a widely published author and is the recipient of several awards and honors, including an international Kellogg Fellowship in Australia; a Fulbright Research Award in Sweden; and 10 honorary doctoral degrees, including seven from international universities in Sweden, the United Kingdom, Spain, Japan, and British Colombia and Montreal, Quebec, Canada.

Dr. Watson's original book on caring was published in 1979. Her second book, *Nursing: Human Science and Human Care,* was written while on sabbatical in Australia and reflects the metaphysical and spiritual evolution of her thinking. A third book, *Postmodern Nursing and Beyond,* moves beyond theory to reflect the

321

ontological foundation of nursing as an overarching framework for transforming caring and healing practices in education and clinical care (Watson, 1999). Additional empirical and clinical caring research foci developments include the first and second editions of the book on caring instruments, *Assessing and Measuring Caring in Nursing and Health Sciences* (2002, 2008b), which offers a critique and collation of more than 20 instruments for assessing and measuring caring. Her *Caring Science as Sacred Science* makes a case for a deep moral–ethical, spirit-filled foundation for caring science and healing based on infinite love and an expanding cosmology. Watson's 2008(a) theoretical work, *Nursing: The Philosophy and Science of Caring, Revised New Edition,* revisits and reworks her first book, *Nursing: The Philosophy and Science of Caring* (1979, reprinted 1985), bringing the original publication up to date to include all the changes made during the past 30 years. This latest update introduces *Caritas* nursing as the culmination of a caring science foundation for professional nursing. A coauthored educational book, *Creating a Caring Science Curriculum: Emancipatory Pedagogies* by Marcia Hills and Watson, was published in 2011 followed by two additional coauthored research and measurement books, *Measuring Caritas. International Research on Caritas as Healing* (Nelson & Watson, 2011) and *Caring Science, Mindful Practice: Implementing Watson's Human Caring Theory* (Sitzman & Watson, 2014).

The Watson Caring Science Institute is developing educational, clinical, and administrative–leadership and research models that seek to sustain and deepen authentic caring–healing practices for self and other, transforming practitioners and patients alike. The *caring science* model, integrating *Caritas* with the science of the heart in collaboration with the Institute of HeartMath (www.heartMath.com), deepens intelligent heart-centered caring. All of Watson's latest publications and innovative educational partnerships, activities, new programs, speaking calendar, and directions and developments, including information about a nontraditional doctorate in caring science as sacred science can be found on the website: www.watsoncaringscience.org.

Overview of the Theory

The *theory of human caring* was developed between 1975 and 1979 while I was teaching at the University of Colorado. It emerged from my own views of nursing, combined and informed by my doctoral studies in educational, clinical, and social psychology. It was my initial attempt to bring meaning and focus to nursing as an emerging discipline and distinct health profession that had its own unique values, knowledge, and practices, and its own ethic and mission to society. The work was also influenced by my involvement with an integrated academic nursing curriculum and efforts to find common meaning and order to nursing that transcended settings, populations, specialty, and subspecialty areas.

From my emerging perspective, I make explicit that nursing's values, ethic, philosophy, knowledge, and practices of human caring require language order, structure, and clarity of concepts and worldview underlying nursing as a distinct discipline and profession. The theory goes beyond the dominant physical worldview and opens to subjective, intersubjective, and inner meaning, underlying healing processes and the life world of the experiencing person. This original (Watson, 1979) language framed this orientation that required unique caring–healing arts. The human caring processes were named the "10 carative factors," which complemented conventional medicine but stood in stark contrast to "curative factors." At the same time, this emerging philosophy and theory of human caring sought to balance the cure orientation of medicine, giving nursing its unique disciplinary, scientific, and professional standing with itself and its public.

The early work has continued to evolve dynamically from the original writings of 1979, 1981, 1985, and the 1990s to a more updated view of 10 caritas processes, to caring science as sacred science, and to a unitary global consciousness for leadership. My work now makes connections between human caring, healing, and even peace in our world, with nurses as *caritas peacemakers* when they are practicing human caring for self and others. This shift moves to more explicit metaphysical/spiritual focus on transpersonal caring moment, post-modern critiques, to metaphysical—from theory to ontological paradigm for caring science. A broad, evolving unitary caring science worldview underlies the fluid evolution of the theory and the philosophical-ethical foundation for this work.

Major Conceptual Elements

The major conceptual elements of the original (and emergent) theory are as follows:

- Ten carative factors (transposed to ten caritas processes)
- Transpersonal caring moment
- Caring consciousness/intentionality and energetic presence
- Caring–healing modalities

Other dynamic aspects of the theory that have emerged or are emerging as more explicit components include:

- Expanded views of self and person (unitary oneness; embodied spirit)
- Caring–healing consciousness and energetic heart-centered presence
- Human–environmental field of a caring moment
- Unitary oneness worldview: unbroken wholeness and connectedness of all
- Advanced caring–healing modalities/ nursing arts as a future model for advanced practice of nursing qua nursing (consciously guided by one's nursing ethical–theoretical–philosophical orientation)

Caring Science as Sacred Science

The emergence of the work is a more explicit development of *caring science* as a deep moral–ethical context of infinite and cosmic love. As soon as one is more explicit about placing the human and caring within their science model, it automatically forces a relational unitary worldview and makes explicit caring as a moral ideal to sustain humanity across time and space; one of the gifts and the raison d'être of nursing in the world, but yet to be recognized within and without. Nevertheless, a caring-science orientation is necessary for the survival of nursing as well as humanity at this crossroads in human evolution.

This view takes nursing and healing work beyond conventional thinking. The latest orientation is located within the ageless wisdom traditions and perennial ingredients of the discipline of nursing, while transcending nursing. Caring science as a model for nursing allows nursing's caring–healing core to become both discipline-specific and transdisciplinary. Thus, nursing's timeless, ancient, enduring, and most noble contributions come of age through a caring-science orientation—scientifically, aesthetically, ethically, and practically.

Ten Carative Factors

The original work (Watson, 1979) was organized around 10 carative factors as a framework for providing a format and focus for nursing phenomena. Although *carative factors* is still the current terminology for the "core" of nursing, providing a structure for the initial work, the term *factor* is too stagnant for my sensibilities today. I have extended carative to *caritas* and *caritas processes* as consistent with a more fluid and contemporary movement of these ideas and with my expanding directions.

Caritas comes from the Latin word meaning "to cherish and appreciate, giving special attention to, or loving." It connotes something that is very fine; indeed, it is precious. The word *caritas* is also closely related to the original word *carative* from my 1979 book. At this time, I now make new connections between carative and caritas and without hesitation use them to invoke love, which caritas conveys. This usage allows love and caring to come together for a new form of deep, transpersonal caring. This relationship between love and caring connotes inner healing for self and others, extending to nature and the larger universe, unfolding and evolving within a cosmology that is both metaphysical and transcendent with the coevolving human in the universe. This emerging model of transpersonal caring moves from carative to *caritas*. This integrative expanded perspective is postmodern in that it transcends conventional industrial, static models of nursing while simultaneously evoking both the past and the future. For example, the future of nursing is tied to Nightingale's sense of "calling," guided by a deep sense of commitment and a covenantal ethic of human service, cherishing our phenomena, our subject matter, and those we serve.

It is when we include caring and love in our work and in our life that we discover and affirm that nursing, like teaching, is more than just a job; it is also a life-giving and life-receiving career for a lifetime of growth and learning. Such maturity and integration of past with present and future now require transforming self and those we serve, including our institutions and our profession. As we more publicly and professionally assert these positions for our theories, our ethics, and our practices—even for our science—we also locate ourselves and our profession and discipline within a new, emerging cosmology. Such thinking calls for a sense of reverence and sacredness with regard to life and all living things. It incorporates both art and science, as they are also being redefined, acknowledging a convergence among art, science, and spirituality. As we enter into the transpersonal caring theory and philosophy, we simultaneously are challenged to relocate ourselves in these emerging ideas and to question for ourselves how the theory speaks to us. This invites us into a new relationship with ourselves and our ideas about life, nursing, and theory.

Original Carative Factors

The original carative factors served as a guide to what was referred to as the "core of nursing" in contrast to nursing's "trim." *Core* pointed to those aspects of nursing that potentiate therapeutic healing processes and relationships—they affect the one caring and the one being cared for. Further, the basic core was grounded in what I referred to as the philosophy, science, and art of caring. Carative is that deeper and larger dimension of nursing that goes beyond the "trim" of changing times, setting, procedures, functional tasks, specialized focus around disease, and treatment and technology. Although the "trim" is important and not expendable, the point is that nursing cannot be defined around its trim and what it does in a given setting and at a given point in time. Nor can nursing's trim define and clarify

its larger professional ethic and mission to society—its raison d'être for the public. That is where nursing theory comes into play, and transpersonal caring theory offers another way that both differs from and complements that which has come to be known as "modern" nursing and conventional medical–nursing frameworks.

The 10 carative factors included in the original work are the following:

1. Formation of a humanistic–altruistic system of values.
2. Instillation of faith–hope.
3. Cultivation of sensitivity to one's self and to others.
4. Development of a helping–trusting, human caring relationship.
5. Promotion and acceptance of the expression of positive and negative feelings.
6. Systematic use of a creative problem-solving caring process.
7. Promotion of transpersonal teaching–learning.
8. Provision for a supportive, protective, and/or corrective mental, physical, societal, and spiritual environment.
9. Assistance with gratification of human needs.
10. Allowance for existential–phenomenological–spiritual forces. (Watson, 1979, 1985)

Although some of the basic tenets of the original carative factors still hold and indeed are used as the basis for some theory-guided practice models and research, what I am proposing here, as part of my evolution and the evolution of these ideas and the theory itself, is to transpose the carative factors into "clinical caritas processes."

From Carative Caritas Processes

As carative factors evolved within an expanding perspective and as my ideas and values have evolved, I now offer the following translation of the original carative factors into caritas processes, suggesting more open ways in which they can be considered.

1. Formation of a humanistic–altruistic system of values *becomes* the practice of loving

kindness and equanimity within the context of caring consciousness.

2. Instillation of faith–hope *becomes* being authentically present and enabling and sustaining the deep belief system and subjective life world of self and one being cared for.

3. Cultivation of sensitivity to one's self and to others *becomes* cultivation of one's own spiritual practices and transpersonal self, going beyond ego self, opening to others with sensitivity and compassion.

4. Development of a helping–trusting, human caring relationship *becomes* developing and sustaining a helping–trusting, authentic caring relationship.

5. Promotion and acceptance of the expression of positive and negative feelings *becomes* being present to, and supportive of, the expression of positive and negative feelings as a connection with deeper spirit of self and the one being cared for (authentically listening to another's story).

6. Systematic use of a creative problem-solving caring process *becomes* creative use of self and all ways of knowing as part of the caring process; to engage in the artistry of caring-healing practices (creative solution seeking becomes caritas coach role).

7. Promotion of transpersonal teaching-learning *becomes* engaging in genuine teaching-learning experience that attends to unity of being and meaning, attempting to stay within others' frames of reference.

8. Provision for a supportive, protective, and/or corrective mental, physical, societal, and spiritual environment *becomes* creating a healing environment at all levels (a physical and nonphysical, subtle environment of energy and consciousness, whereby wholeness, beauty, comfort, dignity, and peace are potentiated).

9. Assistance with gratification of human needs *becomes* assisting with basic needs, with an intentional caring consciousness, administering "human care essentials," which potentiate wholeness and unity of being in all aspects of care; sacred acts of basic care; touching embodied spirit and evolving spiritual emergence.

10. Allowance for existential–phenomenological–spiritual forces *becomes* opening and attending to spiritual-mysterious and existential dimensions of one's own life-death; soul care for self and the one being cared for. "Allowing for miracles."

What differs in the caritas process framework is that a decidedly spiritual dimension and an overt evocation of love and caring are merged for a new unitary cosmology for this millennium. Such a perspective ironically places nursing within its most mature framework and is consistent with the Nightingale model of nursing—yet to be actualized but awaiting its evolution. This direction, while embedded in theory, goes beyond theory and becomes a converging paradigm for nursing's future.

Thus, I consider my work more a philosophical, ethical, intellectual blueprint for nursing's evolving disciplinary/professional matrix, rather than a specific theory per se. Nevertheless, others interact with the original work at levels of concreteness or abstractness. If the theory is "read" at the carative factor level, it can be interpreted as a middle-range theory. If the theory is "read" at the transpersonal unitary caring science/transpersonal caring consciousness level, the theory can be interpreted as a grand theory located within the unitary–transformative context.

The caring theory has been and increasingly is being used nationally and internationally as a guide for educational curricula, clinical practice models, methods for research and inquiry, and administrative directions for nursing and health-care delivery.

Reading the Theory

The "theory" can be "read" as a philosophy, an ethic, a paradigm, an expanded science model, or a theory. If read as a theory, it can be "read" as a grand theory within the unitary–transformative paradigm when understood at the transpersonal, energetic-field level of caritas-universal love and evolving consciousness.

It can be "read" as middle-range theory when read at the carative factors/caritas process level, which provides the structure and language of the theory, as both middle range and specific. When used in clinical settings, the theory helps nurses to frame their experiences around the caritas processes to sustain the caring-science focus, as well as developing language systems, including computerized documentation systems, to document and study caring within a designated language system (Rosenberg, 2006, p. 55). The middle-range focus is also congruent with clinical caring research projects, utilizing the caring language of carative/caritas. Indeed, many of the more formalized caring assessment tools are based on the language of this structure. Several multisite research projects are now underway using consistent caring assessment tools, such as Duffy's Caring Assessment Tool and the Nelson, Watson, and Inova Health Instrument Caring Factor Survey (Persky, Nelson, Watson, & Bent, 2008). The latest *Watson Caritas Patient Score* is being used in multisite clinical studies as an international research project. (For more information, go to www.watsoncaringscience.org.) In addition, most of the current caring-science assessment tools may be seen in *Assessing and Measuring Caring in Nursing and Health Sciences*, 2nd ed. (Watson, 2008b).

Heart-Centered Transpersonal Caring Moment: Caritas Field

Whether the "theory" is read at different levels, used as a language system for documentation, used as a guide for professional nursing practice models, or used as the focus of multisite or individual clinical caring research studies, the essence of the lived theory is in the transpersonal caring moment. The caring moment can be located within any caring occasion, as a concept within middle-range or even prescriptive or practice-level theory.

However, the caring moment is most evident within the transpersonal caritas energetic field model, in that one's consciousness, intentionality, energetic heart-centered presence is radiating a field beyond the two people or the situation, affecting the larger field. Thus, nurses can become more aware, more awake, more conscious of manifesting/radiating a caritas field of love and healing for self and others, helping to transform self and system. For more comprehensive understanding of this work, see *Nursing: The Philosophy and Science of Caring* (revised 2nd ed.; Watson, 2008a). Indeed, the latest research based on the science of the heart has demonstrated that the loving heart-centered person is radiating love that can be measured several feet beyond themselves, affecting the subtle environment of all. Moreover, this research affirms that the heart is actually sending more messages to the brain, rather than the other way around. For more information, please visit www.heartMath .com; www.heartMath.org

This work posits a unitary oneness worldview of connectedness of all; it embraces a value's explicit moral foundation and takes a specific position with respect to the centrality of human caring, "caritas," and universal love as an ethic and ontology. It is also a critical starting point for nursing's existence, broad societal mission, and the basis for further advancement for caring–healing practices. Nevertheless, its use and evolution are dependent on "critical, reflective practices that must be continuously questioned and critiqued in order to remain dynamic, flexible, and endlessly self-revising and emergent" (Watson, 1996, p. 143).

Transpersonal Caring Relationship

The terms *transpersonal* and *transpersonal caring relationship* are foundational to the work. *Transpersonal* conveys a concern for the inner life world and subjective meaning of another who is fully embodied. But the transpersonal also energetically goes beyond the ego self and beyond the given moment, reaching to the deeper connections to spirit and with the broader universe. Thus, a transpersonal caring relationship moves beyond ego self and radiates to spiritual, even cosmic, concerns and connections that tap into healing possibilities and potentials. Transpersonal caring is both immanent, fully physical and embodied physically, while also paradoxically transcendent, beyond physical self.

Transpersonal caring seeks to connect with and embrace the spirit or soul of the other through the processes of caring and healing and being in authentic relation in the moment.

Such a transpersonal relationship is influenced by the caring consciousness and intentionality and energetic presence of the nurse as she or he enters into the life space or phenomenal field of another person and is able to detect the other person's condition of being (at the soul or spirit level). It implies a focus on the uniqueness of self and other and the uniqueness of the moment, wherein the coming together is mutual and reciprocal, each fully embodied in the moment, while paradoxically capable of transcending the moment, open to new possibilities.

The transpersonal caritas consciousness nurse seeks to "see" the spirit-filled person behind the patient, behind the colleague, behind the disease or the diagnosis or the behavior or personality one may not like and connect with that spirit-filled individual who exists behind the illusion. This is heart-centered caritas practice guided by the very first caritas process: cultivation of loving kindness and equanimity with self and other, allowing for development of more caring, love, compassion, and authentic caring moments.

Transpersonal caring calls for an authenticity of being and becoming, an ability to be present to self and others in a reflective frame. The transpersonal nurse has the ability to center consciousness and intentionality on caring, healing, and wholeness, rather than on disease, illness, and pathology.

Transpersonal caring competencies are related to ontological development of the nurse's human caring literacy and ways of being and becoming. Thus, "ontological caring competencies" become as critical in this model as "technological curing competencies" to the conventional modern, Western techno-cure nursing-medicine model, which is now coming to an end.

Within the model of transpersonal caring, clinical caritas consciousness is engaged at a foundational ethical level for entry into this framework. The nurse attempts to enter into and stay within the other's frame of reference for connecting with the inner life world of meaning and spirit of the other. Together, they join in a mutual search for meaning and wholeness of being and becoming, to potentiate

comfort measures, pain control, a sense of well-being, wholeness, or even a spiritual transcendence of suffering. The person is viewed as whole and complete, regardless of illness or disease (Watson, 1996, p. 153).

Assumptions of the Transpersonal Caring Relationship

The nurse's moral commitment, intentionality, and caritas consciousness exist to protect, enhance, promote, and potentiate human dignity, wholeness, and healing, wherein a person creates or cocreates his or her own meaning for existence, healing, wholeness, and living and dying.

The nurse's will and consciousness affirm the subjective-spiritual significance of the person while seeking to sustain caring in the midst of threat and despair—biological, institutional, or otherwise. This honors the I–Thou relationship versus an I–It relationship (Buber, 1923/1996).

The nurse seeks to recognize, accurately detect, and connect with the inner condition of spirit of another through authentic caritas (loving) presencing and being centered in the caring moment. Actions, words, behaviors, cognition, body language, feelings, intuition, thought, senses, the energy field, and so on—all contribute to the transpersonal caring connection. The nurse's ability to connect with another at this transpersonal spirit-to-spirit level is translated via movements, gestures, facial expressions, procedures, information, touch, sound, verbal expressions, and other scientific, technical, esthetic, and human means of communication into nursing human art/acts or intentional caring-healing modalities.

The caring–healing modalities within the context of transpersonal caring/caritas consciousness potentiate harmony, wholeness, and unity of being by releasing some of the disharmony, the blocked energy that interferes with the natural healing processes. As a result, the nurse helps another through this process to access the healer within, in the fullest sense of Nightingale's view of nursing.

Ongoing personal–professional development and spiritual growth and personal spiritual practice assist the nurse in entering into this deeper level of professional healing practice, allowing the nurse to awaken to the transpersonal condition of the world and to actualize more fully "ontological competencies" necessary for this level of advanced practice of nursing. Valuable teachers for this work include the nurse's own life history and previous experiences, which provide opportunities for focused studies, as the nurse has lived through or experienced various human conditions and has imagined others' feelings in various circumstances. To some degree, the necessary knowledge and consciousness can be gained through work with other cultures and the study of the humanities (art, drama, literature, personal story, narratives of illness journeys) along with an exploration of one's own values, deep beliefs, relationship with self and others, and one's world. Other facilitators include personal-growth experiences such as psychotherapy, transpersonal psychology, meditation, bioenergetics work, and other models for spiritual awakening. Continuous growth is ongoing for developing and maturing within a transpersonal caring model. The notion of health professionals as wounded healers is acknowledged as part of the necessary growth and compassion called forth within this theory/philosophy.

Caring Moment/Caring Occasion

A caring occasion occurs whenever the nurse and another come together with their unique life histories and phenomenal fields in a human-to-human transaction. The coming together in a given moment becomes a focal point in space and time. It becomes transcendent, whereby experience and perception take place, but the actual caring occasion has a greater field of its own, in a given moment. The process goes beyond itself yet arises from aspects of itself that become part of the life history of each person, as well as part of a larger, more complex pattern of life (Watson, 1985, p. 59; 1996, p. 157).

A caring moment involves an action and a choice by both the nurse and the other. The moment of coming together presents the two with the opportunity to decide how to be in the moment in the relationship—what to do with and in the moment. If the caring moment is transpersonal, each feels a connection with the other at the spirit level; thus, the moment transcends time and space, opening up new possibilities for healing and human connection at a deeper level than that of physical interaction. For example:

> [W]e learn from one another how to be human by identifying ourselves with others, finding their dilemmas in ourselves. What we all learn from it is self-knowledge. The self we learn about . . . is every self. IT is universal—the human self. We learn to recognize ourselves in others . . . [it] keeps alive our common humanity and avoids reducing self or other to the moral status of object. (Watson, 1985, pp. 59–60)

Caring (Healing) Consciousness

The dynamic of transpersonal caring (healing) within a caring moment is manifest in a field of consciousness. The transpersonal dimensions of a caring moment are affected by the nurse's consciousness in the caring moment, which in turn affects the field of the whole. The role of consciousness with respect to a holographic view of science has been discussed in earlier writings (Watson, 1992, p. 148) and includes the following points:

- The whole caring–healing–loving consciousness is contained within a single caring moment.
- The one caring and the one being cared for are interconnected; the caring-healing process is connected with the other human(s) and with the higher energy of the universe.
- The caring–healing–loving consciousness of the nurse is communicated to the one being cared for.
- Caring–healing–loving consciousness exists through and transcends time and space and can be dominant over physical dimensions.

Within this context, it is acknowledged that the process is relational and connected. It transcends time, space, and physicality. The process is intersubjective with transcendent possibilities that go beyond the given caring moment.

Implications of the Caring Model

The caring model or theory can be considered a philosophical and moral/ethical foundation for professional nursing and is part of the central focus for nursing at the disciplinary level. A model of caring includes a call for both art and science. It offers a framework that embraces and intersects with art, science, humanities, spirituality, and new dimensions of mind–body–spirit medicine and nursing evolving openly as central to human phenomena of nursing practice.

I emphasize that it is possible to read, study, learn about, and even teach and research the caring theory. However, to truly "get it," one has to experience it personally. The model is both an invitation and an opportunity to interact with the ideas, to experiment with and grow within the philosophy, and to live it out in one's personal and professional lives.

Applications of the Theory

The ideas as originally developed, as well as in the current evolving phase (Watson, 1979, 1985, 1999, 2003, 2005, 2008, 2011), provide us with a chance to assess, critique, and see where or how, or even if, we may locate ourselves within a framework of caring science/caritas as a basis for the emerging ideas in relation to our own theories and philosophies of professional nursing and/or caring practice. If one chooses to use the caring-science perspective as theory, model, philosophy, ethic, or ethos for transforming self and practice, or self and system, the following questions may help (Watson, 1996, p. 161):

- Is there congruence between the values and major concepts and beliefs in the model and the given nurse, group, system, organization, curriculum, population needs, clinical administrative setting, or other entity that is considering interacting with the caring model to transform and/or improve practice?
- What is one's view of "human"? And what does it mean to be human, caring, healing, becoming, growing, transforming, and so on? For example, in the words of Teilhard de Chardin (1959): "Are we humans having a spiritual experience, or are we spiritual beings having a human experience?" Such thinking in regard to this philosophical question can guide one's worldview and help to clarify where one may locate self within the caring framework.
- Are those interacting and engaging in the model interested in their own personal evolution? Are they committed to seeking authentic connections and caring–healing relationships with self and others?
- Are those involved "conscious" of their caring *caritas* or noncaring consciousness and intentionally in a given moment at an individual and a systemic level? Are they interested and committed to expanding their caring consciousness and actions to self, other, environment, nature, and wider universe?
- Are those working within the model interested in shifting their focus from a modern medical science–technocure orientation to a true heart-centered authentic caring–healing–loving model?

This work, in both its original and evolving forms, seeks to develop caring as an ontological–epistemological foundation for a theoretical–philosophical–ethical framework for the profession and discipline of nursing and to clarify its mature relationship and distinct intersection with other health sciences. Nursing caring theory–based activities as guides to practice, education, and research have developed throughout the United States and other parts of the world. The caring/caritas model is consistently one of the nursing caring theories used as a guide in Magnet Hospitals in the United States and found to be culturally consistent with nursing in many other cultures, nations, and countries. Nurses' reflective-critical practice models are increasingly adhering to a caring ethic and ethos as the moral and scientific foundation for a profession that is coming of age for a new global era in human history.

Latest Developments

The Watson Caring Science Institute (WCSI) was established in 2007 as a nonprofit foundation. The following statements define and describe the goals, missions, and purposes of the International Caritas Consortium (ICC) and the WCSI as two interrelated entities. The general goals and objectives of the WCSI are to steward and serve the ICC in its activities and more specifically to:

• Transform the dominant model of medical science to a model of caring science by reintroducing the ethic of caring and love, necessary for healing.
• Deepen the authentic caring–healing relationships between practitioner and patient to restore love and heart-centered human compassion as the ethical foundation of health care.
• Translate the model of caring–healing/ caritas into more systematic programs and services to help transform health care one nurse, one practitioner, one educator, and one system at a time.
• Ensure caring and healing for the public, reduce nurse turnover, and decrease costs to the system.

International Caritas Consortium Charter

The main purposes of the unfolding and emerging ICC (Watson, 2008a, pp. 278–280) are as follows:

1. To explore diverse ways to bring the caring theory to life in academic and clinical practice settings by supporting and learning from each other
2. To share knowledge and experiences so that we might help guide self and others in the journey to live the caring philosophy and theory in our personal and professional lives.

The consortium gatherings, sponsored by systems implementing caring theory in practice:

• Provide an intimate forum to renew, restore, and deepen each person's and each system's commitment and authentic practices of human caring in their personal/ professional life and work.
• Learn from each other through shared work of original scholarship, diverse forms of caring inquiry, and modeling of caring–healing practices.

• Mentor self and others in using and extending the theory of human caring to transform education and clinical practices.
• Develop and disseminate caring science models of clinical scholarship and professional excellence in the various settings in the world.

Activities for Caritas Consortium Gatherings

• Provide a safe forum to explore, create, and renew self and system through reflective time out.
• Share ideas, inspire each other, and learn together.
• Participate in use of appreciative inquiry in which each member is facilitative of each other's work, each participant learning from others.
• Create opportunities for original scholarship and new models of caring science–based clinical and educational practices.
• Generate and share multisite projects in caring theory/caring science scholarship.
• Network for educational and professional models of advancing caring–healing practices and transformative models of nursing.
• Share unique experiences for authentic self-growth within the caring science context.
• Educate, implement, and disseminate exemplary experiences and findings to broader professional audiences through scholarly publications, research, and formal presentations.
• Envision new possibilities for transforming nursing and health care.

Because of the many national and international developments and sincere desire for authentic change, new projects using caring science, caritas theory, and the philosophy of human caring are now underway in many systems. The WCSI and the ICC are examples of individuals and representatives of systems convening (in these cases, once a year) to deepen and sustain what is referred to as caritas nursing—that is, bringing caring and love and heart-centered human-to-human practices back into our personal life and work world (Watson, 2008a).

Caring Indicators and Programs

Although these earlier-named systems are identified as sponsors of the growing ICC, examples of how these systems are implementing the theory are captured through identified acts and processes depicting such transformative changes.

Caring theory-in-action reflects transformative processes that are representative of actions taking place in many of the systems in the ICC and other systems guided by caring science and caring theory. The following are examples of such caring-in-action indicators:

- Make human caring integral to the organizational vision and culture through new language and documentation of caring, such as posters.
- Introduce and name new professional caring practice models, leading to new patterns of delivery of caring/care (e.g., Attending Caring Nursing Project, Patient Care Facilitator Role, the 12-Bed Hospital).
- Create conscious intentional meaningful rituals—for example, hand washing is for infection control but may also be a meaningful ritual of self-caring—energetically cleansing, blessing, and releasing the last situation or encounter, and being open to the next situation.
- Selectively use of caring–healing modalities for self and patients (e.g., massage, therapeutic touch, reflexology, aromatherapy, calmative essential oils, sound, music, arts, a variety of energetic modalities).
- Dim the unit lights and have designated "quiet time" for patients, families, and staff alike to soften, slow down, and calm the environment.
- Create healing spaces for nurses—sanctuaries for their own time out; this may include meditation or relaxation rooms for quiet time.
- Cultivate one's own spiritual heart-centered practices of loving kindness and equanimity to self and others.
- Intentionally pause and breathe, preparing the self to be present before entering patient's room.
- Use centering exercises and mindfulness practices, individually and collectively.
- Place magnets on patient's door with positive affirmations and reminders of caring practices.
- Explore documentation of caring language and integration in computerized documentation systems.
- Participate in multisite research assessing caring among staff and patients.
- Create healing environments, attending to the subtle environment or caritas field.
- Display healing objects, stones, or a blessing basket.
- Create Caritas Circles to share caring moments.
- Perform Caring Rounds at bedside with patients.
- Interview and select staff on the basis of a "caring" orientation. Asking candidates to describe a "caring moment."
- Develop of "caring competencies" using caritas literacy as guide to assess and promote staff development and ensure caring.

These and other practices are occurring in a variety of hospitals across the United States, often in Magnet hospitals or those seeking Magnet recognition, where caring theory and models of human caring are used to transform nursing and health care for staff and patients alike.

The names of other health-care clinical and educational systems incorporating caring theory into professional nursing practice models (many are Magnet hospitals or preparing to become Magnet hospitals) can be found at www.watsoncaringscience.org.

These identified system examples are exemplars of the changing momentum today and are guided by a shift toward an evolved consciousness. They rely on moral, ethical, philosophical, and theoretical foundations to restore human caring and healing and health in a system that has gone astray—educationally, economically, clinically, and socially. This shift is in a hopeful direction and is based on a grassroots transformation of nursing, one that emerging from the inside out. The dedicated leaders who are ushering in these changes serve as an inspiration for sustaining nursing and human caring for practitioners and patients alike.

Conclusion

Consistent with the wisdom and vision of Florence Nightingale, nursing is a lifetime journey of caring and healing, seeking to understand and preserve the wholeness of human existence across time and space and national/geographic boundaries, to offer heart-centered compassionate, informed knowledgeable human caring to society and humankind. This timeless view of nursing transcends conventional minds and mindsets of illness, pathology, and disease that are located in the physical body with curing as end goal, often at all costs. In nursing's timeless model, caring, kindness, love, and heart-centered compassionate service to humankind are restored. The unifying focus and process is on connectedness with self, other, nature, and God/the Life Force/the Absolute. This vision and wisdom is being reignited today through a blend of old and new values, ethics, and theories and practices of human caring and healing. These caritas consciousness practices preserve humanity, human dignity, and wholeness and are the very foundation of transformed thinking and actions.

Such a values-guided relational ontology and expanded epistemology and ethic is embodied in caring science as the disciplinary ground for nursing, now and in the future. The advancement of nursing theory, which includes both ideals and practical guidance, is increasingly evident as nursing makes its major contribution to health care and matures as a distinct caring–healing profession—one that balances and complements conventional, medical–institutional practices and processes. Nevertheless, much work remains to be done. New transformative, human-spirit–inspired approaches are required to reverse institutional and system lethargy and darkness. To create the necessary cultural change, the human spirit has to be invited back into our health-care systems. Professional and personal models are required that open the hearts of nurses and other practitioners. New horizons of possibilities have to be explored to create space whereby compassionate, intentional, heart-centered human caring can be practiced. Such authentic personal/professional practice models of caring science are capable of leading us, locally and globally, toward a moral community of caring. This community will restore healing and health at a level that honors and sustains the dignity and humanity of practitioners and patients alike.

The Watson Caring Science Institute is dedicated to create, conduct, and sponsor Caring Science/Caritas education, training, and support to serve the current and future generations of health-care professionals globally (www.watsoncaringscience.org; WCSI, 4405 Arapahoe Avenue, Suite 100, Boulder, CO 80303).

Practice Exemplar

Practice Exemplar by Terry Woodward, RN, MSN.

October 2002 presented the opportunity for 17 interdisciplinary health-care professionals at the Children's Hospital in Denver, Colorado, to participate in a pilot study designed to (1) explore the effect of integrating caring theory into comprehensive pediatric pain management and (2) examine the Attending Nurse Caring Model® (ANCM) as a care delivery model for hospitalized children in pain. A 3-day retreat launched the pilot study. Participants were invited to explore transpersonal human caring theory (caring theory) as taught and modeled by Dr. Jean Watson, through experiential interactions with caring–healing modalities. The end of the retreat opened opportunities for participants to merge caring theory and pain theory into an emerging caring-healing praxis.

Returning from the retreat to the preexisting schedules, customs, and habits of hospital routine was both daunting and exciting. We had lived caring theory, and not as a remote and abstract philosophical ideal; rather, we had experienced caring as the very core of our true selves, and it was that call that had led us into the health-care professions. Invigorated by the retreat, we returned to our 37-bed acute care inpatient pediatric unit, eager to apply caring theory to improve pediatric pain management. Our experiences throughout the retreat had accentuated caring as our core value. Caring theory could not be restricted to a single area of practice.

Wheeler and Chinn (1991) define praxis as "values made visible through deliberate action" (p. 2). This definition unites the ontology, or the essence, of nursing to nursing actions, to what nurses do. Nursing within acute care inpatient hospital settings is practiced dependently, collaboratively, and independently (Bernardo, 1998). Bernardo described dependent practice as energy directed by and requiring physician orders, collaborative practice as interdependent energy directed toward activities with other health-care professionals, and independent practice as "where the meaningful role and impact of nursing may evolve" (p. 43). Our vision of nursing practice was based in the caring paradigm of deep respect for humanity and all life, of wonder and awe of life's mystery, and the interconnectedness from mind–body–spirit unity into cosmic oneness (Watson, 1996). Gadow (1995) described nursing as a lived world of interdependency and shared knowledge, rather than as a service provided. Caring praxis within this lived world is a praxis that offers "a combination of action and reflection . . . praxis is about a relationship with self, and a relationship with the wider community" (Penny & Warelow, 1999, p. 260). Caring praxis, therefore, is collaborative praxis.

Collaboration and cocreation are key elements in our endeavors to translate caring theory into practice. They reveal the nonlinear process and relational aspect of caring praxis. Both require openness to unknown possibilities, both honor the unique contributions of self and other(s), and both acknowledge growth and transformation as inherent to life experience. These key elements support the evolution of praxis away from predetermined goals and set outcomes toward authentic caring–healing expressions. Through collaboration and

cocreation, we can build on existing foundations to nurture evolution from what is to what can be.

Our mission—to translate caring theory into praxis—had strong foundational support. Building on this supportive base, we committed our intentions and energies toward creating a caring culture. The following is not intended as an algorithm to guide one through varied steps until caring is achieved but is rather a description of our ongoing processes and growth toward an ever-evolving caring praxis. These processes are cocreations that emerged from collaboration with other ANCM participants, fellow health professionals, patients and families, our environment, and our caring intentions.

First Steps

One of our first challenges was to make the ANCM visible. Six tangible exhibits were displayed on the unit as evidence of our commitment to caring values. First, a large, colorful poster titled "CARING" was positioned at the entrance to our unit. Depicting pictures of diverse families at the center, the poster states our three initial goals for theory-guided practice: (1) create caring–healing environments, (2) optimize pain management through pharmacological and caring–healing measures, and (3) prepare children and families for procedures and interventions. Watson's clinical caritas processes were listed, as well as an abbreviated version of her guidelines for cultivating caring–healing throughout the day (Watson, 2002). This poster, written in caring theory language, expressed our intention to all and reminded us that caring is the core of our praxis.

Second, a shallow bowl of smooth, rounded river stones was located in a prominent position at each nursing desk. A sign posted by the stones identified them as "Caring–Healing Touch Stones," inviting one to select a stone as "every human being has the ability to share their incredible gift of loving–healing. These stones serve as a reminder of our capacity to love and heal. Pick up a stone, feel its smooth

Continued

cool surface, let its weight remind you of your own gifts of love and healing. Share in the love and healing of all who have touched this stone before you and pass on your love and healing to all who will hold this stone after you."

Third, latched wicker blessing baskets were placed adjacent to the caring–healing touch stones. Written instructions invited families, visitors, and staff to offer names for a blessing by writing the person's initials on a slip of paper and placing the paper in the basket. Every Monday through Friday, the unit chaplain, holistic clinical nurse specialist (CNS), and interested staff devoted 30 minutes of meditative silence within a healing space to ask for peace and hope for all names contained within the baskets.

Fourth, signs picturing a snoozing cartoon-styled tiger were posted on each patient's door announcing "Quiet Time." Quiet time was a midday, half-hour pause from hospital hustle-bustle. Lights in the hall were dimmed, voices hushed, and steps softened to allow a pause for reflection. Staff members tried not to enter patient rooms unless summoned.

Fifth, a booklet was written and published to welcome families and patients to our unit, to introduce health team members, unit routines, available activities, and define frequently used medical terms. This book emphasized that patients, parents, and families are members of the health team. A description of our caring attending team was also included.

Sixth and most recently, the unit chaplain, child-life specialist, and social worker organized a weekly support session called "Goodies and Gathering," offered every Thursday morning. It was held in our healing room—a conference room painted to resemble a cozy room with a beautiful outdoor view and redecorated with comfortable armchairs, soft lighting, and plants. Goodies and Gathering extended a safe retreat within the hospital setting. Offering 1 hour to parents and another to staff, these professionals provided snacks to feed the body, a sacred space to nourish emotions, and their caring presence to nurture the spirit.

Attending Caring Team (ACT)

To honor the collaborative partnership of our ANCM participants, to include patients and families as equal partners in the health-care team, and to open participation to all, we adopted the name Attending Caring Team (ACT). The acronym ACT reinforces that our actions are opportunities to make caring visible. Care as the core of praxis differs from the centrality of cure in the medical model. To describe our intentions to others, we compiled the following "elevator" description of ACT, a terse, 30-second summary that rendered the meaning of ACT in the time frame of a shared elevator ride:

The core of the Attending Caring Team (ACT) is caring-healing for patients, families, and ourselves. ACT cocreates relationships and collaborative practices between patients, families and health care providers. ACT practice enables health care providers to redefine themselves as caregivers rather than taskmasters. We provide Health Care not Health Tasks.

Large signs were professionally produced and hung at various locations on our unit. These signs served a dual purpose. The largest, posted conspicuously at our threshold, identified our unit as the home of the Attending Caring Team. Smaller signs, posted at each nurse's station, spelled out the above ACT definition, inviting everyone entering our unit to participate in the collaborative cocreation of caring–healing.

Giving ourselves a name and making our caring intentions visible contributed to establishing an identity, yet may be perceived as peripheral activities. For these expressions to be deliberate actions of praxis, the centrality of caring as our core value was clearly articulated. Caring theory is the flexible framework guiding our unit goals and unit education and has been integrated into our implementation of an institutional customer-service initiative.

Unit goals are written yearly. Reflective of the broader institutional mission statement, each unit is encouraged to develop a mission

Practice Exemplar cont.

statement and outline goals designed to achieve that mission. In 2003, our mission statement was rewritten to focus on provision of quality *family-centered care,* defined as "an environment of caring-healing recognizing families as equal partners in collaboration with all health care providers." One of the goals to achieve this mission literally spelled out *caring.* We promote a caring-healing environment for patients, families, and staff through:

• Compassion, competence, commitment
• Advocacy
• Respect, research
• Individuality
• Nurturing
• Generosity

Education

Unit educational offerings were also revised to reflect caring theory. Phase classes, a 2-year curriculum of serial seminars designed to support new hires in their clinical, educational, and professional growth, now include a unit on self-care to promote personal healing and support self-growth. The unit on pain management was expanded to include use of caring–healing modalities. A new interactive session on the caritas processes was added that asks participants to reflect on how these processes are already evident in their praxis and to explore ways they can deepen caring praxis both individually and collectively as a unit. The tracking tool used to assess a new employee's progress through orientation now includes an area for reflection on growing in caring competencies. In addition to changes in phase classes, informal "clock hours" were offered monthly. Clock hours are designed to respond to the immediate needs of the unit and encompass a diverse range of topics, from conflict resolution, debriefing after specific events, and professional development, to health treatment plans, physiology of medical diagnosis, and in-services on new technologies and pharmacological interventions. Offered on the unit at varying hours to accommodate all work

shifts, clock hours provide a way for staff members to fulfill continuing educational requirements during workdays.

Customer Service to Covenantal

In the practice of human caring as a formal theory and practice model, there is a philosophical shift from a customer-service mindset to viewing nursing and human caring as a covenant with humanity to sustain human caring in the world.

Within this exemplar, caring theory has provided depth to an institutional initiative to use FISH philosophy to enhance customer service (Lundin, Paul, & Christensen, 2000). Imported from the Pike Place Fish Market in Seattle, FISH advocates four premises to improve employee and customer satisfaction: presence, make their day, play, and choose your attitude. Briefly summarized, FISH advocates that when employees bring their full awareness through presence, focus on customers to make their day, invoke fun into the day through appropriate play, and through conscious awareness choose their attitude, work environments improve for all. When the four FISH premises are viewed from the perspective of transpersonal caring, they become opportunities for authentic human-to-human connectedness through I–Thou relationships. The merger of caring theory with FISH philosophy has inspired the following activities. A parade composed of patients, their families, nurses, and volunteers—complete with marching music, hats, streamers, flags, and noisemakers—is celebrated two to three times a week just before the playroom closes for lunch. This flamboyant display lasts less than 5 minutes but invigorates participants and bystanders alike. In addition to being vital for children and especially appropriate in a pediatric setting, play unites us all in the life and joy of each moment. When our parade marches, visitors, rounding doctors, and all others on the unit pause to watch, wave, and cheer us on. A weekly bedtime story is read in our healing room. Patients are invited to bring

Continued

Practice Exemplar cont.

their pillows and favorite stuffed animal or doll and come dressed in pajamas. Night- and day-shift staff members have honored one another with surprise beginning-of-the-shift meals, staying late to care for patients and families, and refusing to give off-going report until their on-coming coworkers had eaten. Colorful caring stickers are awarded when one staff member catches another in the ACT of caring, being present, making another's day, playing, and choosing a positive attitude. These acts are authentic and not performed as hospitality acts and within the customer mindset; rather, they are a professional covenant nursing has with humanity around the world.

ACT Guidelines

Placing caring theory at the core of our praxis supports practicing caring–healing arts to promote wholeness, comfort, harmony, and inner healing. The intentional conscious presence of our authentic being to provide a caring–healing environment is the most essential of these arts. Presence as the foundation for cocreating caring relationships has led to writing ACT guidelines. Written in the doctor order section of the chart, ACT guidelines provide a formal way to honor unique families' values and beliefs. Preferred ways of having dressing changes performed, most helpful comfort measures, home schedules, and special needs or requests are examples of what these guidelines might address. ACT members purposefully use the word *guideline* as opposed to *order* as more congruent with cocreative collaborate praxis and to encourage critical thinking and flexibility. Building practice on caring relationships has led to an increase in both the type and volume of care conferences held on our unit. Previously, care conferences were called as a way to disseminate information to families when complicated issues arose or when communication between multiple teams faltered and families were receiving conflicting reports, plans, and instructions. Now these conferences are offered proactively as a way to coordinate team efforts and to ensure we are working toward the families' goals. Transitional conferences provide an opportunity to coordinate continuity of care, share insight into the unique personality and preferences of the child, coordinate team effort, meet families, provide them with tours of our unit, and collaborate with families. Other caring–healing arts offered on our unit are therapeutic touch, guided imagery, relaxation, visualization, aromatherapy, and massage. As ACT participants, our challenge is to express our caring values through every activity and interaction. Caring theory guides us and manifests in innumerable ways. Our interview process, meeting format, and clinical nurse specialist (CNS) role have been transfigured through caring theory. Our interview process has transformed from an interrogative three-step procedure into more of a sharing dialogue. We are adopting another meeting style that expresses caring values.

Our unit director had the foresight to budget a position for a CNS to support the cocreation of caring praxis. The traditional CNS roles—researcher, clinical expert, collaborator, educator, and change agent—have allowed the integration of caring theory development into all aspects of our unit program. The CNS role advocates self-care and facilitates staff members to incorporate caring-healing arts into their practice through modeling and hands-on support. In addition to providing assistance, searching for resources, acting as liaison with other health-care teams, and promoting staff in their efforts, the very presence of the CNS on the unit reinforces our commitment to caring praxis.

Conclusion

We continue to work toward incorporating caring ideals in every action. Currently, we are modifying our competency-based guidelines to emphasize caring competency within tasks and skills. Building relationships for supportive collaborative practice is the most exciting and most challenging endeavor we are now facing as old roles are reevaluated in light of cocreating caring-healing relationships.

Practice Exemplar cont.

Watson and Foster (2003) described the potential of such collaboration:

The new caring–healing practice environment is increasingly dependent on partnerships, negotiation, coordination, new forms of communication pattern and authentic relationships. The new emphasis is on a change of consciousness, a focused intentionality toward caring and healing relationships and modalities, a shift toward a spiritualization of health vs. a limited medicalized view. (p. 361)

Our ACT commitment is to authentic relationships and the creation of caring–healing environments.

Summary

Nursing's future and nursing in the future will depend on nursing maturing as the distinct health, healing, and caring profession that it has always represented across time but has yet to fully actualize. Nursing thus ironically is now challenged to stand and mature within its own caring science paradigm, while simultaneously having to transcend it and share with others. The future already reveals that all health-care practitioners will need to work within a shared framework of caring–healing relationships and human–environmental energetic field modalities. Practitioners of the future pay attention to consciousness, intentionality, energetic human presence, transformed mind–body–spirit medicine, and will need to embrace healing arts and caring practices and processes and the spiritual dimensions of care much more completely.

Thus, nursing is at its own crossroad of possibilities, between worldviews and paradigms. Nursing has entered a new era; it is invited and required to build on its heritage and latest evolution in science and technology but must transcend itself for a new future, yet to be known. However, nursing's future holds promises of caring and healing mysteries and models yet to unfold, as opportunities for offering compassionate caritas services at individual, system, societal, national, and global levels for self, for profession, and for the broader world community. Nursing has a critical role to play in sustaining caring in humanity and making new connections between caring, love, healing, and peace in the world.

References

Bernardo, A. (1998). Technology and true presence in nursing. *Holistic Nursing Practice, 12*(4), 40–49.

Buber, M. (1996). *I and Thou* (W. Kaufmann, Trans.). New York, NY: Touchstone. (Original work published 1923)

de Chardin, P. (1959). *The phenomenon of man.* New York, NY: Harper & Row Publishers, Inc.

Gadow, S. (1995). Narrative and exploration: Toward a poetics of knowledge in nursing. *Nursing Inquiry, 2,* 211–214.

Hills, M. & Watson, J. (2011). *Creating a caring curriculum. Emancipatory pedagogies* (a Caring Science Library Series with Springer/Watson Caring Science Institute). New York: Springer.

Lundin, S. C., Paul, H., & Christensen, J. (2000). *Fish! A remarkable way to boost morale and improve results.* New York: Hyperion.

Nelson, J., & Watson, J. (2011). *Measuring caritas. International research on caritas as healing* (a Caring Science Library Series with Springer/Watson Caring Science Institute). New York: Springer.

Penny, W., & Warelow, P. J. (1999). Understanding the prattle of praxis. *Nursing Inquiry, 6*(4), 259–268.

Persky, G., Nelson, J.W., Watson, J., & Bent, K. (2008). Profile of a nurse effective in caring. *Nursing Administration Quarterly, 32*(1), 15–20.

Rosenberg, S. (2006). Utilizing the language of Jean Watson's caring theory within a computerized documentation system. *CIN: Computers, Informatics, Nursing, 24*(1), 53–56.

Sitzman, K., & Watson, J. (2014). *Caring science, mindful practice: implementing Watson's human caring theory.* New York: Springer.

Swanson, K. M. (1991). Empirical development of a middle range nursing theory. *Nursing Research, 40*(3), 161–166.

Vivinus, M., & Nergaard, B. (1990). *Ever yours, Florence Nightingale.* Cambridge, MA: Harvard University Press.

Watson, J. (1979). *Nursing. The philosophy and science of caring.* Boston: Little Brown. Reprinted 1985. Boulder, CO: University Press of Colorado.

Watson, J. (1985). *Nursing: Human science and human care.* Norwalk, CT: Appleton Century. Reprinted 1988, 1999, 2007. New York: National League for Nursing Press; Sudbury, MA: Jones and Bartlett.

Watson, J. (1996). Watson's theory of transpersonal caring. In P. H. Walker & B. Newman (Eds.), *Blueprint for use of nursing models: Education, research, practice and administration.* New York: National League for Nursing Press.

Watson, J. (1999). *Postmodern nursing and beyond.* New York: Churchill Livingstone.

Watson, J. (2001). Post-hospital nursing: Shortage, shifts and scripts. *Nursing Administration Quarterly, 25*(3), 77–82.

Watson, J. (2002). Intentionality and caring-healing consciousness: A practice of transpersonal nursing. *Holistic Nursing Practice, 16*(4), 12–19.

Watson, J. (2003). *Assessing and measuring caring in nursing and health sciences.* New York: Springer.

Watson, J. (2005). *Caring science as sacred science.* Philadelphia: F. A. Davis.

Watson, J. (2008a). *Nursing: The philosophy and science of caring* (rev. 2nd ed. with Caritas Meditation CD). Boulder, CO: University Press of Colorado; www.upcolorado.com

Watson, J. (2008b). *Assessing and measuring caring in nursing and health sciences* (2nd ed.). New York: Springer.

Watson, J. (2011). *Human caring science. A theory of nursing.* Boston: Jones and Bartlett.

Watson, J., & Foster, R. (2003). The Attending Nurse Caring Model®: Integrating theory, evidence and advanced caring-healing therapeutics for transforming professional practice. *Journal of Clinical Nursing, 12,* 360–365.

Wheeler, C. E., & Chinn, P. L. (1991). *Peace and power: A handbook of feminist process* (3rd ed.). New York: National League for Nursing Press.

Bibliography

For complete listing of all Watson's calendar, program, publications, videos of presentations, audio readings and other media, go to: www.watsoncaringscience.org. Also see videos on YouTube.

Selected Journal Articles

Fawcett, J. (2002). The nurse theorists: 21st century updates—Jean Watson. *Nursing Science Quarterly, 15*(3), 214–219.

Fawcett, J., Watson, J., Neuman, B., & Hinton-Walker, P. (2001). On theories and evidence. *Journal of Nursing Scholarship, 33*(2), 121–128.

Quinn, J., Smith, M., Swanson, K., Ritenbaugh, C., & Watson, J. (2003). The healing relationship in clinical nursing: Guidelines for research. *Journal of Alternative Therapies, 9*(3), A65–79.

Watson, J. (1988). Human caring as moral context for nursing education. *Nursing and Health Care, 9*(8), 422–425.

Watson, J. (1988). New dimensions of human caring theory. *Nursing Science Quarterly, 1*(4), 175–181.

Watson, J. (1990). The moral failure of the patriarchy. *Nursing Outlook, 28*(2), 62–66.

Watson, J. (1998). Nightingale and the enduring legacy of transpersonal human caring. *Journal of Holistic Nursing, 16*(2), 18–21.

Watson, J. (2000). Leading via caring–healing: The four-fold way toward transformative leadership. *Nursing Administration Quarterly* (25th Anniversary Edition), *25*(1), 1–6.

Watson, J. (2000). Reconsidering caring in the home. *Journal of Geriatric Nursing, 21*(6), 330–331.

Watson, J. (2000). Via negativa: Considering caring by way of non-caring. *Australian Journal of Holistic Nursing, 7*(1), 4–8.

Watson, J. (2001). Post-hospital nursing: Shortages, shifts, and scripts. *Nursing Administrative Quarterly, 25*(3), 77–82. Available online at http://www.dartmouth.edu/~ahechome/workforce.html, then click "The Nursing Shortage."

Watson, J. (2002). Guest editorial: Nursing: Seeking its source and survival. *ICU NURS WEB J 9,* 1–7. www.nursing.gr/J.W.editorial.pdf

Watson, J. (2002). Holistic nursing and caring: A values based approach. *Journal of Japan Academy of Nursing Science, 22*(2), 69–74.

Watson, J. (2002). Intentionality and caring-healing consciousness: A theory of transpersonal nursing. *Holistic Nursing Journal, 16*(4), 12–19.

Watson, J. (2002). Metaphysics of virtual caring communities. *International Journal of Human Caring, 6*(1).

Watson, J. (2003). Love and caring: Ethics of face and hand. *Nursing Administrative Quarterly, 27*(3), 197–202.

Watson, J., & Foster, R. (2003). The attending nurse caring model: Integrating theory, evidence and advanced caring-healing therapeutics for transforming professional practice. *Journal of Clinical Nursing, 12,* 360–365.

Watson, J., & Smith, M. C. (2002). Caring science and the science of unitary human beings: A transtheoretical discourse for nursing knowledge development. *Journal of Advanced Nursing, 37*(5), 452–461.

Watson, J. (1994). A frog, a rock, a ritual: An eco-caring cosmology. In: E. Schuster & C. Brown (Eds.), *Caring and environmental connection.* New York: National League for Nursing Press.

Watson, J. (1996). Artistry and caring: Heart and soul of nursing. In D. Marks-Maran & P. Rose (Eds.), *Reconstructing nursing: Beyond art & science* (pp. 54–63). London: Bailliére Tindall.

Watson, J. (1996). Poeticizing as truth on nursing inquiry. In J. Kikuchi, H. Simmons, & D. Romyn, D. (Eds.), *Truth in nursing inquiry* (pp. 125–139). Thousand Oaks, CA: Sage.

Watson, J. (1996). Watson's theory of transpersonal caring. In P. H. Walker & B. Neuman (Eds.), *Blueprint for use of nursing models: Education, research, practice, & administration* (pp. 141–184). New York: National League for Nursing Press.

Watson, J. (1999). Alternative therapies and nursing practice. In J. Watson (Ed.), *Nurse's handbook of alternative and complementary therapies.* Springhouse, PA: Springhouse.

Watson, J., & Chinn, P. L. (1994). Art and aesthetics as passage between centuries. In P. L. Chinn & J. Watson (Eds.), *Art and aesthetics in nursing* (pp. xiii–xviii). New York: National League for Nursing Press.

Audiovisual or Media Productions

CD: Jean Watson: A caring moment. Care for the Journey CD. www.nursing.ucdenver.edu/caring

CD: Caritas meditation. Jean Watson. Four meditations with music by Gary Malkin. In J. Watson, 2008). *Nursing: The philosophy and science of caring.* (rev. ed.). Boulder, CO: University Press of Colorado.

Watson FITNE. (1997). *The nurse theorists portraits of excellence. Jean Watson: A theory of caring* [video and CD]. To obtain, go to: www.fitne.net.

Watson, J. (1988). *The Denver nursing project in human caring* [videotape]. University of Colorado Health Science Center, School of Nursing, Denver, CO. Contact: ellen.janasko@ucdenver.edu.

Watson, J. (1988). *The power of caring: The power to make a difference* [videotape]. Center for Human Caring Video, University of Colorado Health Sciences Center, School of Nursing, Denver, CO. Contact: ellen.janasko@ucdenver.edu

Watson, J. (1989). *Theories at work* [videotape]. New York: National League for Nursing. In conjunction with University of Colorado Health Science Center/School of Nursing Chair in Caring Science. Contact ellen.janasko@ucdenver.edu

Watson, J. (1994). *Applying the art and science of human caring,* Parts I and II [videotape]. New York: National League for Nursing. In conjunction with the University of Colorado Health Science Center/School of Nursing, Chair in Caring Science. Contact: Ellen. janasko@ucdenver.edu.

Watson, J. (1999). *A meta-reflection on nursing's present* [audiotape]. American Holistic Nurses Association. Boulder, CO: SoundsTrue Production.

Watson, J. (1999). *Private psalms. A mantra and meditation for healing* [CD]. Music by Dallas Smith and Susan Mazer. To obtain: www.watsoncaringscience.org

Watson, J. (2000). *Importance of story and health care.* Second National Gathering on Relationship-Centered Caring, Fetzer Institute Conference, Florida.

Watson, J. (2001). *Creating a culture of caring* [audiotape]. At the Creative Healthcare Management 9th Annual Meeting, Minneapolis, MN.

Watson, J. (2001, September). *Reconnecting with spirit: Caring and healing our living and dying.* International Parish Nursing Conference, Westberg Symposium. Available at https://watsoncaringscience.org/about-us/jean-bio/nationalinternational-presentations/

Theory of Nursing as Caring

ANNE BOYKIN AND SAVINA O. SCHOENHOFER

Chapter 19

Introducing the Theorists
Nursing as Caring: An Overview
Applications of the Theory
Practice Exemplar
Summary
References

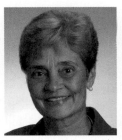 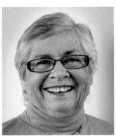

Anne Boykin   *Savina O. Schoenhofer*

Introducing the Theorists

Anne Boykin

Anne Boykin is Professor Emerita and past Dean of the Christine E. Lynn College of Nursing at Florida Atlantic University. She is Director of the College's Anne Boykin Institute for the Advancement of Caring in Nursing. This institute provides global leadership for nursing education, practice, and research grounded in caring; promotes the valuing of caring across disciplines; and supports the caring mission of the college. She has demonstrated a long-standing commitment to the advancement of knowledge in the discipline, especially regarding the phenomenon of caring.

Positions she has held within the International Association for Human Caring include: president-elect (1990–1993), president (1993–1996), and member of the nominating committee (1997–1999). As immediate past president, she served as co-editor of the journal *International Association for Human Caring* from 1996 to 1999.

Her scholarly work is centered in caring as the grounding for nursing. This is evidenced in her coauthored book, *Nursing as Caring: A Model for Transforming Practice* (Boykin & Schoenhofer, 1993, rev. ed. 2001a), and the book *Living a Caring-based Program* (Boykin, 1994). The latter book illustrates how caring grounds all aspects of a nursing education program. Dr. Boykin has also authored numerous book chapters and articles. She is currently retired and serves as a consultant locally, regionally, nationally, and internationally on the topic of caring-based health-care transformations.

Dr. Boykin is a graduate of Alverno College in Milwaukee, Wisconsin; she received her master's degree from Emory University in Atlanta, Georgia, and her doctorate from Vanderbilt University in Nashville, Tennessee.

Savina O. Schoenhofer

Savina O'Bryan Schoenhofer began her initial nursing study at Wichita State University, where she earned undergraduate degrees in nursing and psychology and graduate degrees in nursing and counseling. She completed a PhD in educational foundations/administration at Kansas State University in 1983. In 1990, Schoenhofer cofounded *Nightingale Songs,* an early venue for communicating the beauty of nursing in poetry and prose. In addition to her work on caring, she has written on nursing values, primary care, nursing education, support, touch, personnel management in nursing homes, and mentoring. Her career in nursing has been significantly influenced by three colleagues: Lt. Col. Ann Ashjian (Ret.), whose community nursing practice in Brazil presented an inspiring model of nursing; Marilyn E. Parker, PhD, a faculty colleague who mentored her in the idea of nursing as a discipline, the academic role in higher education, and the world of nursing theories and theorists; and Anne Boykin, PhD, who introduced her to caring as a substantive field of nursing study.

Schoenhofer coauthored the book, *Nursing as Caring: A Model for Transforming Practice* (1993, 2001a) with Boykin. Boykin and Schoenhofer, together with Kathleen Valentine, coauthored the book, *Health Care System Transformation for Nursing and Health Care Leaders: Implementing a Culture of Caring* (2013).

Nursing As Caring: Overview

This chapter is intended as an overview of the *theory of nursing as caring*, a general theory, framework, or disciplinary view of nursing. A general theory or framework of nursing presents an abstract, integrated, comprehensive picture of nursing as a practiced discipline. The theory of nursing as caring offers a view that permits a broad, encompassing understanding of any and all situations of nursing practice (Boykin & Schoenhofer, 1993, 2001a). This theory serves as an organizing framework for nursing scholars in the various roles of practitioner, researcher, administrator, teacher, and developer.

Initially, we present the theory in its most abstract form, addressing assumptions and key themes. We then illustrate the meaning of the theory of nursing as caring through exemplars in the role dimensions of nursing care, nursing education, nursing administration and nursing research.

Nursing as Caring: Historical Perspective

The theory of nursing as caring is an outgrowth of the curriculum development work in the Christine E. Lynn College of Nursing at Florida Atlantic University, where both authors were among the faculty group revising the caring-based curriculum for initial program accreditation. When the revised curriculum was in place, each of us recognized the potential and even the necessity of continuing to develop and structure ideas and themes toward a comprehensive expression of the meaning and purpose of nursing as a discipline and a profession. The point of departure was the acceptance that *caring is the end, rather than the means, of nursing, and that caring is the intention of nursing, rather than merely its instrument.* This work led to the statement of focus of nursing as "nurturing persons living caring and growing in caring."

Further work to identify foundational assumptions about nursing clarified the idea of the nursing situation, a shared lived experience in which the caring between nurse and nursed enhances personhood, with personhood understood as living grounded in caring. The clarified focus and the idea of the nursing situation are the key themes that draw forth the meaning of the assumptions underlying the theory and permit the practical understanding of nursing as both a discipline and a profession. As critique of the theory and study of nursing situations progressed, the notion of nursing being primarily concerned with health was seen as limiting, and we now understand nursing to be concerned with human living.

Three bodies of work significantly influenced the initial development of nursing as caring. Roach's (1987/2002) basic thesis that caring is the human mode of being was incorporated into the most basic assumption of the theory. We view Paterson and Zderad's (1988) existential phenomenological theory of humanistic nursing as the historical antecedent of nursing as caring. Seminal ideas from humanistic nursing such as "the between," "call for nursing," "nursing response," and "personhood" serve as substantive and structural bases for our conceptualization of nursing as caring. Mayeroff's (1971) work, *On Caring*, provided a language that facilitated the recognition and description of the practical meaning of caring in nursing situations. Roach's (1987/2002) five Cs (described in detail later) of caring expand on that basic language. In addition to the work of these thinkers, both authors are long-standing members of the community of nursing scholars whose study focuses on caring and are supported and undoubtedly influenced in many subtle ways by the members of this community and their work.

Fledgling forms of the theory of nursing as caring were first published in 1990 and 1991, with the first complete exposition of the theory presented at a conference in 1992 (Boykin & Schoenhofer, 1990, 1991; Schoenhofer & Boykin, 1993), followed by the publication of *Nursing as Caring: A Model for Transforming Practice* in 1993 (Boykin & Schoenhofer, 1993), which was revised with the addition of an epilogue in 2001 (Boykin & Schoenhofer, 2001a).

Assumptions and Key Themes of Nursing as Caring

Assumptions

Certain fundamental beliefs about what it means to be human underlie the theory of nursing as caring. The following assumptions reflect a particular set of values that provide a basis for understanding and explicating the meaning of nursing and are key to understanding the practical meaning of the theory of nursing as caring.

- Persons are caring by virtue of their humanness.

- Persons are whole and complete in the moment.
- Persons are caring, moment to moment.
- Personhood is a way of living grounded in caring.
- Personhood is enhanced through participation in nurturing relationships with caring others.
- Nursing is both a discipline and a profession.

Key Themes

Caring
Caring is an altruistic, active expression of love and is the intentional and embodied recognition of value and connectedness. Caring is not the unique province of nursing. However, as a discipline and a profession, nursing uniquely focuses on caring as its central value, its primary interest, its focus for scholarship, and the direct intention of its practice. "As an expression of nursing, *caring is the intentional and authentic presence of the nurse with another who is recognized as person living caring and growing in caring*" (Boykin & Schoenhofer, 2001a, p. 13). The full meaning of caring cannot be restricted to a definition but is illuminated in the experience of caring and in dynamic reflection on that experience.

Focus and Intention of Nursing
Disciplines as identifiable entities or "branches of knowledge" grow from the holistic "tree of knowledge" as need and purpose develop. A discipline is a community of scholars with a particular perspective on the world and on what it means to be in the world. The disciplinary community represents a value system that is expressed in its unique focus on knowledge and practice. The *focus of nursing*, from the perspective of the theory of nursing as caring, is *person living caring and growing in caring*. The general *intention of nursing* as a practiced discipline is *nurturing persons living caring and growing in caring*.

Nursing Situation
The practice of nursing, and thus the practical knowledge of nursing, lives in the context of person-with-person caring. The *nursing situation* involves particular values, intentions, and actions of two or more persons choosing to live a nursing relationship. *Nursing situation* is

understood to mean the shared lived experience in which caring between nurse and nursed enhances personhood. Nursing is created in the "caring between." All knowledge of nursing is created and understood within the nursing situation. Any single nursing situation has the potential to illuminate the depth and complexity of nursing knowledge. Nursing situations are best communicated aesthetically to preserve the lived meaning of the situation and the openness of the situation as text. Storytelling, poetry, graphic arts, dance, and other expressive modes effectively represent the lived experience of nursing and allowing for reflection and creativity in advancing understanding.

Personhood

Personhood is understood to mean living grounded in caring. From the perspective of the theory of nursing as caring, personhood is the universal human call. A profound understanding of personhood communicates the paradox of person-as-person and person-in-communion all at once.

Direct Invitation

The concept of *direct invitation* was briefly introduced in the epilogue of the 2001 revised edition of nursing as caring (Boykin & Schoenhofer, 2001a). It evolved from a convergence of ontology and aesthetics as a way to more effectively communicate nursing as caring in practice.

The context for understanding *direct invitation* is the *nursing situation. Direct invitation* communicates clearly that the core service of nursing is to offer caring and to invite the one nursed to share that which matters most to them in that moment. It is through this invitation that the *call for nursing* is heard and *nursing responses* are created. *Direct invitation* establishes an openness between the nurse and one nursed and strengthens the *caring between.*

Call for Nursing

"A call for nursing is a call for acknowledgment and affirmation of the person living caring in specific ways in the immediate situation" (Boykin & Schoenhofer, 2001a, p. 13). *Calls for nursing* are calls for nurturance through personal expressions of caring. Calls for nursing originate within persons as they live caring

uniquely, expressing personally meaningful dreams and aspirations for growing in caring. Calls for nursing are individually relevant ways of saying, "Know me as caring person in the moment and be with me as I try to live fully who I truly am." Intentionality and authentic presence open the nurse to hearing calls for nursing. Because calls for nursing are unique situated personal expressions of that which matters to the person nursed, they cannot be predicted, as in a "diagnosis." Nurses develop sensitivity and expertise in hearing calls through intention, experience, study, and reflection in a broad range of human situations.

Nursing Response

As an expression of nursing, "caring is the intentional and authentic presence of the nurse with another who is recognized as living caring and growing in caring" (Boykin & Schoenhofer, 2001a, p. 13). The nurse enters the nursing situation with the intentional commitment of knowing the other as caring person, and in that knowing, acknowledging, affirming, and celebrating the person as caring. The *nursing response* is a specific expression of caring nurturance to sustain and enhance the one nursed in ways that matter as he or she lives caring and grows in caring in the situation of concern. *Nursing responses* to calls for caring evolve as nurses clarify their understandings of calls through presence and dialogue. *Nursing responses* are uniquely created for the moment and cannot be predicted or automatically applied as preplanned protocols. Sensitivity and skill in creating unique and effective ways of communicating caring are developed through intention, experience, study, and reflection in a broad range of human situations.

The "Caring Between"

The *caring between* is the source and ground of nursing. It is the loving relation into which nurse and nursed enter and which they cocreate by living the intention to care. Without the loving relation of the *caring between,* unidirectional activity or reciprocal exchange can occur, but nursing in its fullest sense does not occur. It is in the context of the *caring between* that personhood is enhanced, each expressing self as caring and recognizing the other as caring person.

Dance of Caring Persons

The relational model for organizational design involving nursing is analogous to the dancing circle, the *dance of caring persons*. What this circle represents is the commitment of each dancer to understand and support the study of the discipline of nursing. Core dimensions of caring illustrated in the dance of caring persons model include the following:

• Acknowledgment that all persons have the capacity to care by virtue of their humanness
• Commitment to respect for person in all institutional structures and processes
• Recognition that each participant in the enterprise has a unique valuable contribution to make to the whole and is present in the whole
• Appreciation for the dynamic though rhythmic nature of the dance of caring persons, enabling opportunities for human creativity

Persons making up the dance of caring persons in any given situation involving nursing are the one nursed and family, nurses and other health-care workers, administrative and support staff, and relevant corporate, governmental, and social communities. Regardless of the role, the "responsibility of all is to recognize, value, and celebrate the unique ways caring is lived by colleagues, as well as to support each other in the growth of caring" (Pross, Hilton, Boykin, & Thomas, 2011, p. 28).

Lived Meaning of Nursing as Caring

Abstract presentations of assumptions and themes lay the groundwork and provide an orienting point. However, the lived meaning of nursing as caring can best be understood by the study of a nursing situation. The following poem is one nurse's expression of the meaning of nursing, situated in one particular experience of nursing and linked to a general conception of nursing.

I CARE FOR HIM
My hands are moist,
My heart is quick,
My nerves are taut,
He's in the next room,
I care for him.
The room is tense,
It's anger-filled,
The air seems thick,
I'm with him now,
I care for him.
Time goes slowly by,
As our fears subside,
I can sense his calm,
He softens now,
I care for him.
His eyes meet mine,
Unable to speak,
I feel his trust,
I open my heart,
I care for him.
It's time to leave.
Our bond is made,
Unspoken thoughts,
But understood,
I care for him!
—J. M. COLLINS (1993)

Each encounter—each nursing experience—brings with it the unknown. In reflection, Jim Collins shares a story of practice that illuminates the opportunity to live and grow in caring. In the nursing situation that inspired this poem, the nurse and nursed live caring uniquely. Initially, the nurse experiences the familiar human dilemma, aware of separateness while choosing connectedness as he responds to a yet unknown call for nursing: ["My] hands are moist,/my heart is quick/my nerves are taut . . . I care for him." As he enters the situation and encounters the patient as person, he is able to "let go" of his presumptive knowing of the patient as "angry." The nurse enters with the guiding perspective that all persons are caring. This allows Nurse Jim to see past the "anger-filled" room and to be "with him" (Stanza 2). As they connect through their humanness, the beauty and wholeness of one nursed is uncovered and nurtured. By living caring moment to moment, hope emerges and fear subsides. The nurse issues a direct invitation as "I open my heart" (Stanza 4) to hear that which matters most in the moment. Through this experience, both nurse and nursed live and grow in their understanding and expressions of caring.

In the first stanza, the nurse prepares to enter the nursing relationship with the formed intention of offering caring in authentic presence. Perhaps he has heard a report that the person he is about to encounter is a "difficult patient" and this is a part of his awareness; however, his nursing intention to care reminds him that he and his patient are, above all, caring persons. In the second stanza, the nurse enters the room, experiences the challenge that his intention to nurse has presented, and responds to the call for authentic presence and caring: "I'm with him now,/I care for him." Patterns of knowing are called into play as the nurse brings together intuitive, personal knowing, empirical knowing, and the ethical knowing that it is right to offer care, creating the integrated understanding of aesthetic knowing that enables him to act on his nursing intention (Boykin, Parker, & Schoenhofer, 1994; Carper, 1978). Mayeroff's (1971) caring ingredients of courage, trust, and alternating rhythm are clearly evident.

Clarity of the call for nursing emerges as the nurse begins to understand that this particular man in this particular moment is calling to be known as a uniquely caring person, a person of value, worthy of respect and regard. The nurse listens intently and recognizes the unadorned honesty that sounds angry and demanding and is a personal expression of a heartfelt desire to be truly known and worthy of care. The nurse responds with steadfast presence and caring, communicated in his way of being and of doing. The caring ingredient of hope is drawn forth as the man softens and the nurse takes notice.

In the fourth stanza, the "caring between" develops and personhood is enhanced as dreams and aspirations for growing in caring are realized: "His eyes meet mine . . . I open my heart." In the last stanza, the nursing situation is completed in linear time. But each one, nurse and nursed, goes forward newly affirmed and celebrated as caring person, and the nursing situation continues to be a source of living caring and growing in caring.

Assumptions Underlying Nursing as Caring in the Context of the Nursing Situation

In Collins's (1993) poem, the power of the basic assumption that all persons are caring by virtue of their humanness enabled the nurse to find the courage to live his intentions. The idea that persons are whole and complete in the moment permits the nurse to accept conflicting feelings and to be open to the nursed as a person, not merely as an entity with a diagnosis and superficially understood behavior. The nurse demonstrated an understanding of the assumption that persons live caring from moment to moment, striving to know self and other as caring in the moment with a growing repertoire of ways of expressing caring. Personhood, a way of living grounded in caring that can be enhanced in relationship with caring other, comes through in that the nurse is successfully living his commitment to caring in the face of difficulty and in the mutuality and connectedness that emerged in the situation. The assumption that nursing is both a discipline and a profession is affirmed as the nurse draws on a set of values and a developed knowledge of nursing as caring to actively offer his presence in service to the nursed.

Nursing practice guided by the theory of nursing as caring entails living the commitment to know self and other as living caring in the moment and growing in caring. Living this commitment requires intention, formal study, and reflection on experience. Mayeroff's (1971) caring ingredients offer a useful starting point for the nurse committed to knowing self and other as caring persons. These ingredients include knowing, alternating rhythm, honesty, courage, trust, patience, humility, and hope. Roach's (1992) five Cs—commitment, confidence, conscience, competence, and compassion—provide another conceptual framework that is helpful in providing a language of caring. Coming to know self as caring is facilitated by:

• Trusting in self; freeing self up to become what one can truly become, and valuing self.

• Learning to let go, to transcend—to let go of problems, difficulties, in order to remember the interconnectedness that enables us to know self and other as living caring, even in suffering and in seeking relief from suffering.

• Being open and humble enough to experience and know self to be at home with one's feelings.

• Continuously calling to consciousness that each person is living caring in the moment and we are each developing uniquely in our becoming.

• Taking time to fully experience our humanness, for one can only truly understand in another what one can understand in self.

• Finding hope in the moment. (Schoenhofer & Boykin, 1993, pp. 85–86)

Applications of the Theory

Nursing Practice

The nursing as caring theory, grounded in the assumption that all persons are caring, has as its focus a general call to nurture persons as they live caring uniquely and grow as caring persons. The challenge for nursing, then, is not to discover what is missing, weakened, or needed in another but to come to know the other as caring person and to nurture that person in situation-specific, creative ways. We no longer understand nursing as a "process" in the sense of a complex sequence of predictable acts resulting in some predetermined desirable end product. Nursing, we believe, is inherently a process, in the sense that it is always unfolding and guided by intention.

An everyday understanding of the meaning of caring is obviously challenged when the nurse is presented with someone for whom it is difficult to care. "Difficult to care" situations are those that demonstrate the extent of knowledge and commitment needed to nurse effectively. In these extreme (although not unusual) situations, a task-oriented, non–discipline-based concept of nursing may be adequate to

ensure the completion of certain treatment and surveillance techniques. Still, in our eyes, that is an insufficient response—it certainly is not the nursing we advocate. The theory of nursing as caring calls on the nurse to reach deep within a well-developed knowledge base that has been structured using all available patterns of knowing, grounded in the obligations inherent in the commitment to know persons as caring. These patterns of knowing may develop knowledge as intuition; scientifically quantifiable data emerging from research; and related knowledge from a variety of disciplines, ethical beliefs, and many other types of knowing. All knowledge held by the nurse that may be relevant to understanding the situation at hand is drawn forward and integrated into practice in particular nursing situations (aesthetic knowing). Although the degree of challenge presented from situation to situation varies, the commitment to know self and other as caring persons is steadfast.

All persons are caring, even when not all chosen actions of the person live up to the ideal to which we are all called by virtue of our humanness. In discussions of hypothetical situations involving child molesters, serial killers, and even political figures who have attempted mass destruction and racial annihilation, certain ethical systems permit and even call for making judgments. However, when such a person presents to the nurse for care, the nursing ethic of caring supersedes all other values. The theory of nursing as caring asserts that it is *only* through recognizing and responding to the other as a caring person that nursing is created and personhood enhanced in that nursing situation. Caring effectively in "difficult-to-care" situations is the most challenging prospect a nurse can face. It is only with sustained intention, commitment, study, and reflection that the nurse is able to offer nursing in these situations. Falling short in one's commitment does not necessitate self-deprecation nor warrant condemnation by others; rather, it presents an opportunity to care for self and other and to grow in personhood. Making real the potential of such an opportunity calls for seeing with clarity, reaffirming commitment, and engaging in study and reflection, individually and in concert with caring others.

To know the other as caring, the nurse must find some basis for respectful human connection with the person. Does this mean that the nurse must like everything about the person, including personal life choices? Perhaps not; however, the nurse as nurse is not called on to judge the "other," only to care for the other. A concern with judging or censuring another's actions is a distraction from the real purpose for nursing—that is, coming to know the other as caring person, as one with dreams and aspirations of growing in caring, and responding to calls for caring in ways that nurture personhood, that matter to the one nursed.

Nurses are frequently heard to say they have no time for caring, given the demands of the role (Boykin & Schoenhofer, 2000). All nursing roles are lived out in the context of a contemporary environment, and the environment for practice, administration, education, and research is fraught with many challenges. Some of these challenges are the following:

• technological advancement and proliferation that can promote routinization and depersonalization on the part of the caregiver as well as the one seeking care;
• demands for immediate and measurable outcomes that favor a focus on the simplistic and the superficial;
• organizational and occupational configurations that tend to promote fragmentation and alienation; and
• economic focus and profit motive ("time is money") as the apparent prime institutional value.

Nurses express frustration when evaluating their own caring efforts against an idealized, rule-driven conception of caring. Practice guided by the theory of nursing as caring reflects the assumption that caring is created from moment to moment and does not demand idealized patterns of caring. Caring in the moment (and from moment to moment) occurs when the nurse is living a committed intention to know and nurture the other as caring person (Boykin & Schoenhofer, 2000). No predetermined ideal amount of time or form

of dialogue is prescribed. Simple examples of living this intention to care follow.

When the nurse goes first *to the person*, rather than going directly to the IV or the monitor, it becomes clear that the use of technology is one way the nurse expresses caring *for the person* (Schoenhofer, 2001). In proposing his model of machine technologies and caring in nursing, Locsin (1995, 2001) distinguishes between mere technological competence and technological competence as an intentional expression of caring in nursing. Simply avowing an intention to care is not sufficient; the committed intention to care is supported by serious study of caring and ongoing reflection if nurses are to communicate caring effectively from moment to moment. As Locsin (1995, p. 203) so aptly stated:

> as people seriously involved in giving care know, there are various ways of expressing caring. Professional nurses will continue to find meaning in their technological caring competencies, expressed intentionally and authentically, to know another as a whole person. Through the harmonious coexistence of machine technology and caring technology the practice of nursing is transformed into an experience of caring.

Another example of living the commitment to care is witnessed in caring for the unconscious person. How is this commitment lived? It requires that all ways of knowing be brought into action. The nurse must make self as caring person available to the one nursed. The fullness of the nurse as caring person is called forth. This requires use of Mayeroff's caring ingredients: the alternating rhythm of knowing about the other and knowing the other directly through authentic presence and attunement; the hope and courage to risk opening self to one who cannot communicate verbally, patiently trusting in self to understand the other's mode of living caring in the moment; honest humility as one brings all that one knows and remains open to learning from the other. The nurse attuned to the other as person might for example experience the vulnerability of the person who lies unconscious from surgical anesthetic or traumatic injury. In that vulnerability, the nurse recognizes that the one nursed is living caring in humility, hope, and trust. Instead of responding to the vulnerability, merely "taking care of" the other, the nurse practicing nursing as caring might respond by honoring the other's humility, by participating in the other's hopefulness, by steadfast trustworthiness. Creating caring in the moment in this situation might come from the nurse resonating with past and present experiences of vulnerability. Connected to this form of personal knowing might be an ethical knowing that power as a reciprocal of vulnerability can develop undesirable status differential in the nurse–patient role relationship. As the nurse sifts through myriad empirical data, the most significant information emerges—this is a *person* with whom I am called to care. Ethical knowing again merges with other pathways as the nurse forms the decision to go beyond vulnerability and engage the other as caring person, rather than as helpless object of another's concern. Aesthetic knowing comes in the praxis of caring, in living chosen ways of honoring humility, joining in hope, and demonstrating trustworthiness in the moment (Schoenhofer & Boykin, 1993, pp. 86–87).

A third example of living the intention to care is evidenced in postmortem care. "Nurses speak of caring for their deceased patients as nursing those who have gone and who are still in some way present" (Boykin & Schoenhofer, 2001a, p. 19). Nurses who practice in end-of-life situations offer genuine presence, continue to feel the human connection to the person who has recently died and to the family circle that is part of that person's life, and recognize postmortem care as truly nursing. One nurse was moved by the beauty of post-mortem nursing care offered by her colleagues in the operating room and shared this poetic expression of connectedness.

> *Journey's End*
> *The chaos has stopped,*
> *The journey from birth to death has ceased,*
> *Your body lies on the OR table, alone,*
> *We cluster at the end of the room,*
> *Making the necessary phone calls,*
> *Starting the paperwork,*
> *Telling the young resident:*

> *"Yes, you must complete the paperwork." And*
> *"Go talk to the family now,"*
> *Then we turn back to you*
> *And begin our reverent and loving care:*
> *Covering your wound, removing the lines,*
>   *cleansing your body,*
> *One of us says, "We are being good nurses,"*
> *And another quips back, "It's because we are*
>   *old nurses,"*
> *And we laugh*
> *(But we know we will teach the young ones*
>   *how to do this too),*
> *We place you on a stretcher (not the gruesome*
>   *morgue gurney)*
> *And take you to the viewing room,*
> *One of us goes and brings your family to you,*
> *Murmuring comfort, "We are so sorry for*
>   *your loss."*
> *After a few minutes, we leave*
> *And return to the OR*
> *To take care of another patient.*

—Florence N. Cooper, RN

The nurse practicing within the caring context described here will most often be interfacing with the health-care system in two ways: first, communicating nursing so that it can be understood; second, articulating nursing service as a unique contribution within the system in such a way that the system itself grows to support nursing. Recognizing these system relationships as aspects of the dance of caring persons involving the nursed and family and encompassing all who are part of the system is crucial for creating the kind of environment in which caring is expressed effectively and perceived as growth-promoting.

Nursing Administration

From the viewpoint of nursing as caring, the nurse administrator makes decisions through a lens in which the focus of nursing is on nurturing persons living caring and grow in caring. All activities in the practice of nursing administration are grounded in a concern for creating, maintaining, and supporting an environment in which calls for nursing are heard and nurturing responses are given. From this point of view, the expectation arises that nursing administrators participate in shaping a culture that evolves from the values articulated within nursing as caring and recognized as the dance of caring persons.

Although often perceived to be "removed" from the direct care of the nursed, the nursing administrator is intimately involved in multiple nursing situations simultaneously, hearing calls for nursing and participating in responses to these calls. As calls for nursing are known, one of the unique responses of the nursing administrator is to enter the world of the nursed either directly or indirectly, to understand special calls when they occur, and to assist in securing the resources needed by each nurse to nurture persons living and growing in caring (Boykin & Schoenhofer, 1993). All administrative activities should be approached with this goal in mind. Here, the nurse administrator reflects on the obligations inherent in the role in relation to the nursed. The presiding moral basis for determining right action is the belief that all persons are caring. Frequently, the nurse administrator may enter the world of the nursed through the stories of colleagues who are assuming another role, such as that of nurse manager. Policy formulation and implementation allow for the consideration of unique situations. The nursing administrator assists others within the organization to understand the focus of nursing and to secure the resources necessary to achieve the goals of nursing.

Nursing Education

From the perspective of nursing as caring, all nursing structures and activities should reflect the fundamental assumption that persons are caring by virtue of their humanness. This view applies in nursing education as in practice and administrative role engagement. Other assumptions and values reflected in the education program include knowing the person as whole and complete in the moment and living caring uniquely; understanding that personhood is a way of living grounded in caring and is enhanced through participation in nurturing relationships with caring others; and, finally, affirming nursing as a discipline and profession.

The curriculum, the foundation of the education program, asserts the focus and domain of nursing as nurturing persons living caring and growing in caring; thus, all activities of the program of study are directed toward developing, organizing, and communicating nursing knowledge, that is, knowledge of nurturing persons living caring and growing in caring.

The dance of caring persons relational model is relevant for organizational design of nursing education, as well as for nursing practice. Participants in the dance of caring persons include administrators, faculty, colleagues, students, staff, community, and the nursed and their families. What the dance of caring persons represents in nursing education settings is the commitment of each dancer to understand and support the study of the discipline of nursing. The role of educational administrator in the circle is more clearly understood through reflection on the origin of the word. The term *administrator* derives from the Latin *ad ministrare,* to serve (according to *Webster's New World Dictionary of the American Language*; Guralnik, 1976). This definition connotes the idea of rendering service. Administrators within the circle are by the nature of their role obligated to ministering, to securing, and to providing resources needed by faculty, students, and staff to meet program objectives. Faculty, students, and administrators dance together in the study of nursing. Faculty support an environment that values the uniqueness of each person and sustains each person's unique way of living and growing in caring. This process requires trust, hope, courage, and patience. Because the purpose of nursing education is to study the discipline and practice of nursing, the nursed must be in the circle. The community created is that of persons living caring in the moment and growing in personhood, each person valued as special and unique. (Boykin & Schoenhofer, 1993, pp. 73–74)

In teaching nursing as caring, faculty assist students to come to know, appreciate, and celebrate self and "other" as caring persons. Students, as well as faculty, are in a continual search to discover greater meaning of caring as uniquely expressed in nursing. Examples of a nursing education program based on values similar to those of nursing as caring are illustrated in the book *Living a Caring-based Program* (Boykin, 1994).

Nursing Research and Development

The roles of researcher and developer in nursing take on a particular focus when guided by the theory of nursing as caring. The assumptions and focus of nursing explicated in the theory provide an organizing value system that suggests certain key questions and methods. Research questions lead to exploration and illumination of patterns of living caring personally (Schoenhofer, Bingham, & Hutchins, 1998) and in nursing practice (Schoenhofer & Boykin, 1998b). Dialogue, description, and innovations in interpretative approaches characterize research methods. Development of systems and structures (e.g., policy formulation, information management, nursing delivery, and reimbursement) to support nursing necessitates sustained efforts in reframing and refocusing familiar systems as well as creating novel configurations (Schoenhofer, 1995; Schoenhofer & Boykin, 1998a; Boykin, Schoenhofer, & Valentine, 2013).

The practicality of the theory of nursing as caring has been tested in various nursing practice settings. Nursing practice models have been developed in acute and long-term care settings. Research studies focused on designing, implementing and evaluating a theory-based practice model using nursing as caring on a telemetry unit of a for-profit hospital (Boykin, Schoenhofer, Smith, St. Jean, & Aleman, 2003); the emergency department of a community hospital (Boykin, Bulfin, Baldwin, & Southern, 2004; Boykin, Schoenhofer, Bulfin, Baldwin, & McCarthy, 2005); and the intensive care unit of a for-profit hospital (Dyess, Boykin, & Bulfin, 2013) have demonstrated that when nursing practice is intentionally focused on coming to know a person as caring and on nurturing and supporting those nursed as they live their caring, transformation of care occurs. Within these practice models based on nursing as caring, those nursed could articulate the "experience of being cared for"; patient and nurse satisfaction increased dramatically; nurse retention increased; and the environment for care became grounded in the values of and respect for person.

Touhy, Strews, and Brown (2005) described a project to transform an entire for-profit health-care organization by intentionally grounding it in nursing as caring. *Caring from the heart*—the model for interdisciplinary practice in a long-term care facility and based on the theory of nursing as caring—was designed through collaboration between project personnel and all stakeholders. Foundational values of respect and coming to know ground the model, which revolves around the major themes of responding to that which matters, caring as a way of expressing spiritual commitment, devotion inspired by love for others, commitment to creating a home environment, and coming to know and respect person as person (2005). The major building blocks of the nursing model for an acute care hospital and for a long-term care facility each reflect central themes of nursing as caring, but those themes are drawn out in ways unique to the setting and to the persons involved in each setting. The differences and similarities in these two practice models demonstrate the power of nursing as caring to transform practice in a way that reflects unity without conformity, uniqueness within oneness.

PRACTICE EXEMPLAR

Nursing administration, nursing practice, nursing education, and nursing research require a full understanding of nursing as nurturing persons living caring and growing in caring. This online supplemental resource for this chapter contains four practice exemplars, illustrating the use of the nursing as caring theory to guide practice in nursing administration, clinical simulation laboratory in nursing education, and nursing research.[1] The exemplars were drawn from the practice experience of the nurses who wrote them, and most illustrate stories of actual nursing situations. A nursing administration exemplar addresses health-care

---

[1]For additional practice exemplars please go to bonus chapter content available at FA Davis http://davisplus .fadavis.com

Continued

system leadership and caring. The nursing education exemplar illustrates the use of the simulation laboratory in teaching nursing from the perspective of nursing as caring. Two research exemplars are also provided online, one focusing on the development of a research approach compatible with nursing as caring, and a second addressing the use of nursing as caring as the nursing theoretical perspective underpinning a doctoral dissertation study. The following advanced practice nursing exemplar illuminates advanced nursing practice grounded in nursing as caring.

Advanced Nursing Practice Exemplar: Primary Care Clinic Grounded in Nursing as Caring

Two nurse practitioners, Kathi Voege Harvey, FNP, and Elizabeth Tsarnas, FNP, whose practice setting is a primary care clinic, shared their way of creating nursing as caring in a community-based program of nursing for persons living with diabetes.

Our primary care clinic serves the population of patients who are considered the underserved and fall within the lower socioeconomic level, including those individuals labeled by society as the working poor, uninsured, unemployed, illiterate, disabled, homeless, and recent migrants from many parts of the world. This vulnerable population creates greater challenges, yet we are empowered by our disciplinary view of the theory of nursing as caring to deliver quality and evidence-based health care to all who come.

Call for Nursing

As a result of our observation that individuals with diabetes struggled to incorporate a diabetic-friendly diet and exercise into their lifestyles, we developed a collaborative program that brought experts in nursing and fitness together in a world outside of the clinic setting. This innovative program supports participants in their endeavor to develop a new health-care plan through an exercise, education, and support-group curriculum. The first group to be formed was limited to women because the

lived experiences of some of the early participants were very "fragile" and dealt with personal issues such as domestic violence and depression. As these women's personhood and their struggle with obesity and diabetes emerged, we felt a need to protect them in this, their first venture of sharing. These women's lives had been grounded in caring, but circumstances seemingly beyond their control had affected their personhood. A safe, nurturing relationship with other caring individuals was needed to allow them to trust and grow again.

Nursing Situation

One of the champions of this program, named BP, a 42-year-old woman, was diagnosed with insulin-dependent diabetes 10 years ago. Because of the rapid progression of her disease process, she had bilateral arterial bypass surgery that resulted in limited mobility. BP took a 2-year sabbatical from our clinic and has recently returned. She had been without medications and supplies for months, which increased the neuropathic pain to her lower extremities. She also shared with us that she was under increased stress while preparing for her upcoming wedding. Our conversations would always include the importance of looking into the future at 10, 20, and 30 years to visualize the many disabilities she could develop within that time which would reduce her quality of life and how she could alter that future. Over the past several months, she has taken control of her disease by checking her sugars more often and regularly taking her insulin. She married a month ago and noticed that her husband, KP, had symptoms of diabetes. After checking his blood sugar, which consistently was very elevated, she brought him to the clinic to receive health care. Her enthusiasm for improving her heath was contagious, and she was excited that she could share her journey with her new husband.

Several weeks later, BP introduced us to her mother-in-law, SP, who has prediabetes and with whom BP, her new husband, and her young nephew were living. SP was feeling like she could not take control of her life, so she was referred to us for evaluation, and we invited her to join our group of women. One evening after a support group, which BP and her mother-in-law attended, we walked them to the front of the building where they met BP's husband, who had been exercising in the gym, and his nephew, who was only 12 years old and had been abandoned by his natural parents. As we introduced ourselves to this shy, very thin, 12-year-old young man, we engaged him in conversation so that we could come to know him. We learned that he had been made to come but was angry because he was too young to be in the gym. His grandmother had previously confided in us that he did not have any friends or participate in anything and that he was beginning to have anger outbursts. We identified yet another call for nursing and decided to explore possible sports or activities in which this young man would like to participate. After some investigation, we were able to include him in an adolescent "boot camp" that met at the same time as his family's exercise classes and also a soccer team right on the premises. As he experiences caring through nurturing with his family and us, it is our hope that his fears will subside and allow him to realize the beauty of his uniqueness and his boundless potential.

In this situation BP's nurturing lived experience enabled her to enhance her personhood and touch the lives of those she loved in a way that she had been touched. BP was living in caring and growing in caring, and the completeness she experienced empowered her to care for others, like her family, so that they too could be whole and complete in the moment.

Nursing Response

All persons are caring by virtue of their humanness. As nurses, we readily recognize calls for nursing that others might easily miss. Our personhood as nurses grounded in caring and equipped with the wisdom of knowledge about nurturing relationships and human well-being that we have pursued passionately through our advanced education arm us with the confidence to be intentionally and authentically present

with others in their situations of concern. We feel comfortable to respond to calls for nursing without preplanned protocols or preconceived solutions because we are responding uniquely to each situation with the "other" with the intention to communicate caring and commitment to work with them to achieve their goals.

Our nursing situation with the P family began with one member, who sought help to improve her health, which had been ravaged by diabetes. Over time, the loving relationship of "caring between" developed among BP, her nurse practitioners, her trainer, and her classmates. Boundaries of roles disappeared in this relationship, and BP began to experience wholeness and completeness in the moment that was so healing that she invited her family members into her dance of caring persons so that they, too, could experience well-being. We have all grown through this lived experience, and as nurse practitioners, our way of living grounded in caring has been reaffirmed.

Lived Meaning of Nursing As Caring

A patient first enters the doors of our free clinic appearing as an unopened rosebud with many thorns. The closed bud represents security and protection from the unknown. Many who have limited exposure to a health-care system enter our world with fear of what will be discovered and doubts about the competency of those giving something without cost. The thorns represent the patients' defense system if they should encounter threats to their safety. The rose petals gradually begin to open as the patient experiences each caring moment through the authentic presence of the nurse whose intention is to promote health and healing through physical, emotional, and spiritual discovery and restoration. After the rose completely opens and the thorns soften, the patient begins an acceptance process, and true healing begins. Each room within the clinic resembles a beautiful vase that is full of roses of all shapes, sizes, and colors, representing the uniqueness of each individual the nurse encounters. Others within the room help to achieve the same goals as the nurses and caregivers and represent oxygen,

Continued

Practice Exemplar cont.

sunlight, and water needed to foster growth and strength. Reflecting on the beauty and uniqueness of each rose prepares the nurse for a new unopened rosebud.

Ways of Knowing

Although we must be skilled in both science and clinical experience, the nurse is always nurturing and growing in caring to provide a new dimension of healing that allows us to enter the patient's world to experience and understand their needs in a way that is more than just a prescription or treatment modality. This story reinforces the requisite not only to have the knowledge to properly treat the disease process but also to offer encouragement through dialogue and physical availability to help patients engage in exercise, classroom instruction, and healthy behaviors that produce positive results in patient outcome measures.

Personally, as we listened to the stories of all of the participants in this program, we realized how lucky we were to experience this intensely caring bond between what once were patients and nurse practitioners and now were persons, whole and complete in the moment. We came to realize that our ability to care for others living with chronic illnesses was being viewed through a much more realistic lens. We had always known that changes in lifestyle to improve health outcomes were difficult to implement, no matter how much clinical sense they made. But dwelling in the moment with these women who were struggling to maintain well-being while life just kept happening and who were still able to lose weight, decrease their medications, and make difficult decisions about their lives as our "caring between" relationship evolved, made us realize that wherever we are, whatever we do, we never stop caring, and we never stop being nurses. As others who oversaw this pilot program began to express amazement at what we saw as nursing, we knew our secret was out: Others in the community were beginning to identify nursing as caring, and one by one they asked to join in the dance of caring persons.

The nurse administrator is subject to challenges similar to those of the practitioner and often walks a precarious tightrope between direct caregivers and corporate executives (Boykin & Schoenhofer, 2001b). The nurse administrator, whether at the executive or managerial level of the organization chart, is held accountable for "customer satisfaction" as well as for the "bottom line." Nurses who move up the executive ladder may be suspected of disassociating from their nursing colleagues on the one hand and of not being sufficiently cognizant of the harsh realities of fiscal constraint on the other hand. Administrative practice guided by the assumptions and themes of nursing as caring can enhance eloquence in articulating the connection between caregiver and institutional mission: the person seeking care. Nursing practice leaders who recognize their care role, indirect as it may be, are in an excellent position to act on their committed intention to promote caring environments. Participating in rigorous negotiations for fiscal, material, and human resources and for improvements in nursing practice calls for special skill on the part of the nurse administrator, skill in recognizing, acknowledging, and celebrating the other (e.g., CEO, CFO, nurse manager, or staff nurse) as a caring person. The nurse administrator who understands the caring ingredients (Mayeroff, 1971) recognizes that caring is neither soft nor fixed in its expression. A developed understanding of the caring ingredients helps the nurse administrator mobilize the courage to be honest with self and "other," to trust patience, and to value alternating rhythm with true humility while living a hope-filled commitment to knowing self and "other" as caring persons.

Health Care System Transformation for Nursing and Health Care Leaders: Implementing a Culture of Caring (Boykin, Schoenhofer, & Valentine, 2013) proposes practical strategies for total, integrated system transformation based on the tenets of the dance of caring persons and grounded in the assumptions of

Practice Exemplar cont.

nursing as caring. Many of the challenges of nurse managers and nurse administrators as well as those experienced by other health-care system leaders are currently being addressed by the Institute of Medicine, the Joint Commission, and other health policy groups. Solutions implied in the Hospital Consumer Assessment of Healthcare Providers and Systems are congruent with the values of nursing as caring and are amplified and given substance by specific assumptions and concepts of nursing as caring.

■ Summary

The theory of nursing as caring is grounded in assumptions that persons are caring by virtue of their humanness, that caring unfolds moment to moment, that personhood is living grounded in caring, and that personhood is enhanced in relationships with caring persons. From that basic philosophical perspective, the focus of nursing as a discipline and a professional practice is nurturing persons living caring and growing in caring. The nurse enters into the world of the other with the intention of knowing the other as person living caring and growing in caring. In authentic presence, the nurse offers a direct invitation to the one nursed to express what matters most in the situation. In nursing situations, shared lived experiences of caring, the nurse hears calls for caring and creates effective caring responses. In the caring between nurse and nursed, personhood is enhanced.

The theory of nursing as caring is used by practitioners and administrators of nursing services in a range of institutional and community-based nursing practice settings. The theory is also used to guide nursing education, nursing education administration and nursing research. More detailed information about the theory, an extensive bibliography, and examples of use of the theory are available at http://nursingascaring.com.

References

Boykin, A. (Ed.). (1994). *Living a caring-based program.* New York: National League for Nursing Press.

Boykin, A., Bulfin, S., Baldwin, J., & Southern, B. (2004). Transforming care in the emergency department. *Topics in Emergency Medicine, 26*(4), 331–336.

Boykin, A., Parker, M. E., & Schoenhofer, S. O. (1994). Aesthetic knowing grounded in an explicit conception of nursing. *Nursing Science Quarterly, 7,* 158–161.

Boykin, A., & Schoenhofer, S. O. (1990). Caring in nursing: Analysis of extant theory. *Nursing Science Quarterly, 3*(4), 149–155.

Boykin, A., & Schoenhofer, S. O. (1991). Story as link between nursing practice, ontology, epistemology. *Image, 23,* 245–248.

Boykin, A., & Schoenhofer, S. O. (1993). *Nursing as caring: A model for transforming practice.* New York: National League for Nursing Press.

Boykin, A., & Schoenhofer, S. O. (1997). Reframing outcomes: Enhancing personhood. *Advanced Practice Nursing Quarterly, 3*(1), 60–65.

Boykin, A., & Schoenhofer, S. O. (2000). Is there really time to care? *Nursing Forum. 35*(4), 36–38.

Boykin, A., & Schoenhofer, S. O. (2001a). *Nursing as caring: A model for transforming practice* (rev. ed.). Sudbury, MA: Jones & Bartlett.

Boykin, A., & Schoenhofer, S. O. (2001b). The role of nursing leadership in creating caring environments in health care delivery systems. *Nursing Administration Quarterly, 25*(3), 1–7.

Boykin, A., Schoenhofer, S., Bulfin, S., Baldwin, J., & McCarthy, D. (2005). Living caring in practice: The transformative power of the theory of nursing as caring. *International Journal for Human Caring, 9*(3), 15–19.

Boykin, A., Schoenhofer, S. O., Smith, N., St. Jean, J., & Aleman, D. (2003). Transforming practice using a caring-based nursing model. *Nursing Administration Quarterly, 27,* 223–230.

Boykin, A., Schoenhofer, S. O., & Valentine, K. (2013). *Health care system transformation for nursing and health care leaders: Implementing a culture of caring.* New York, NY: Springer Publishing Company.

Carper, B. A. (1978). Fundamental patterns of knowing in nursing. *Advances in Nursing Science, 1*(1), 13–24.

Collins, J. M. (1993). I care for him. *Nightingale Songs, 2*(4), 3. Retrieved form http://nursing.fau.edu/uploads/docs/451/Nightingale%20Songs%20vol%202%20no%204%20November%201993.pdf

Dyess, S. M., Boykin, A., & Bulfin, M. J. (2013). Hearing the voice of nurses in caring theory-based practice. *Nursing Science Quarterly, 26*(2), 167-173.

Finch, L. P., Thomas, J. D., Schoenhofer, S. O., & Green, A. (2006). Research-as-praxis: A mode of inquiry into caring in nursing. *International Journal for Human Caring, 10*(1), 28–33.

Gaut, D., & Boykin, A. (Eds.). (1994). *Caring as healing: Renewal through hope.* New York: National League for Nursing Press.

Guralnik, D. (Ed.). (1976). *Webster's new world dictionary of the American language.* Cleveland: William Collings & World.

Locsin, R. C. (1995). Machine technologies and caring in nursing. *Image, 27,* 201–203.

Locsin, R. C. (2001). *Advancing technology, caring, and nursing.* Westport, CT: Auburn House, Greenwood Publishing Group.

Mayeroff, M. (1971). *On caring.* New York: Harper & Row.

Orlando, I. (1961). *The dynamic nurse–patient–relationship: Function, process and principles.* New York: G. P. Putnam's Sons.

Paterson, J. G., & Zderad, L. T. (1988). *Humanistic nursing.* New York: National League for Nursing Press.

Pross, E., Hilton, N., Boykin, A., & Thomas, C. (2011). The dance of caring persons. *Nursing Management, 42*(10), 25–30.

Roach, M. S. (1987). *The human act of caring.* Ottawa, Canada: Canadian Hospital Association.

Roach, M. S. (1992). *The human act of caring: A blueprint for the health professions* (rev. ed.). Ottawa, Canada: Canadian Hospital Association Press.

Schoenhofer, S. O. (1995). Rethinking primary care: Connections to nursing. *Advances in Nursing Science, 17*(4), 12–21.

Schoenhofer, S. O. (2001). Infusing the nursing curriculum with literature on caring: An idea whose time has come. *International Journal for Human Caring, 5*(2), 7–14.

Schoenhofer, S. O., Bingham, V., & Hutchins, G. C. (1998). Giving of oneself on another's behalf: The phenomenology of everyday caring. *International Journal for Human Caring, 2*(1), 23–29.

Schoenhofer, S. O., & Boykin, A. (1993). Nursing as caring: An emerging general theory of nursing. In M. E. Parker (Ed.), *Patterns of nursing theories in practice* (pp. 83–92). New York: National League for Nursing Press.

Schoenhofer, S. O., & Boykin, A. (1998a). The value of caring experienced in nursing. *International Journal for Human Caring, 2*(3), 9–15.

Schoenhofer, S. O., & Boykin, A. (1998b). Discovering the value of nursing in high-technology environments: Outcomes revisited. *Holistic Nursing Practice, 12*(4), 31–39.

Touhy, T. A., Strews, W., & Brown, C. (2005). Expressions of caring as lived by nursing home staff, residents, and families. *International Journal for Human Caring, 9*(3), 31–37.

Middle-Range Theories

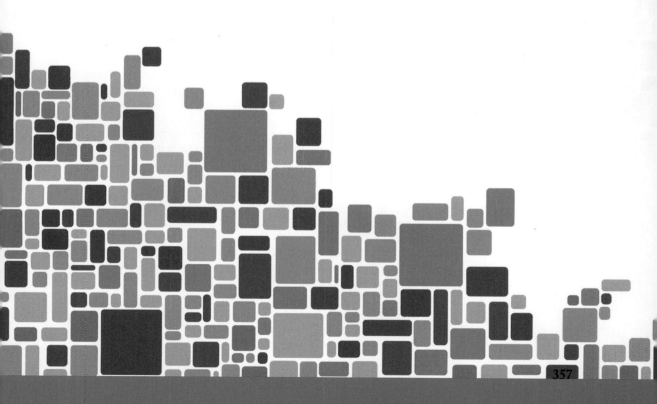

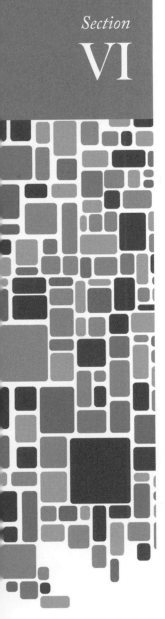

Middle-Range Theories

Twelve middle-range theories in nursing are presented in the final section. Each chapter is written by the scholars who developed the theory. Although we determine all to be at the middle range because of their more circumscribed focus on a phenomenon and more immediate relationship to practice and research, they still vary in level of abstraction.

Transitions are part of the human experience, and how we negotiate these transitions affects health and well-being. Afaf Meleis' transitions theory appears in Chapter 20. The theory includes the elaboration of transition triggers, properties of transitions, the conditions of change, and patterns of responses to transitions. Nursing interventions to promote a smooth passage during transitions are described.

Comfort is an important concept to nursing practice. Kolcaba's middle-range theory of comfort is presented in Chapter 21. She defines comfort as "to strengthen greatly" and identifies relief, ease, and transcendence as types of comfort, and physical, psychospiritual, environmental, and sociocultural as contexts in which comfort occurs.

Duffy's quality-caring model, described in Chapter 22, is being used in many health-care settings to address the issues of patient satisfaction, including patients' perceptions of not feeling cared for in the acute care environment. In this model the goal of nursing is to engage in a caring relationship with self and others to engender feeling "cared for."

Reed's theory of self-transcendence is presented in Chapter 23. The focus of the theory is on facilitating self-transcendence for the purpose of enhancing well-being. Reed defines self-transcendence as the capacity to expand the self-boundary intrapersonally (toward greater awareness of one's beliefs, values, and dreams), interpersonally (to connect with others, nature, and surrounding environment), transpersonally (to relate in some way to dimensions beyond the ordinary and observable world), and temporally (to integrate one's past and future in a way that expands and gives meaning to the present).

Smith and Liehr present story theory in Chapter 24. They posit that story is a narrative happening wherein a person connects with self-in-relation through nurse–person intentional dialogue to create ease. This theory has already been applied in a number of practice and research initiatives.

Parker and Barry's community nursing practice model has guided nursing practice in community settings in several countries. The model is represented by concentric circles with the nursing situation as core and connected with the outer spheres of influence in the community and environment.

Chapter 26 contains Locsin's theory of technological competency-caring. This theory dissolves the artificial and often assumed dichotomy between technology and caring, and asserts that technology is a way of coming to know the person as whole.

Ray and Turkel authored Chapter 27 on Ray's theory of bureaucratic caring. The theory uses a multidimensional, holographic model to facilitate the understanding of caring within complex healthcare environments.

In Chapter 28 Troutman-Jordan describes her theory of successful aging. The theory was informed by Roy's adaptation model and Tornstam's theory of gerotranscendence. Successful aging is characterized by living with meaning and purpose. Intrapsychic factors, functional performance and spirituality contribute to gerotranscendence and successful aging.

Elizabeth Barrett details her theory of power as knowing participation in change in Chapter 29. This middle range theory is derived from Rogers' science of unitary human beings. Barrett identifies the dimensions of power as: awareness, choices, freedom to act intentionally, and involvement in creating change.

In Chapter 30 Smith presents her theory of unitary caring. The theory evolved from viewing caring through the lens of Rogers' science of unitary human beings. The concepts of the theory are: manifesting intentions, appreciating pattern, attuning to dynamic flow, experiencing the Infinite and inviting creative emergence.

In Chapter 31 Swanson describes her trajectory and the process of developing of her middle-range theory of caring from research. The chapter provides insight to the evolution of theory. Swanson's theory of caring includes the concepts of knowing, being with, doing for, enabling, and maintaining belief.

Transitions Theory

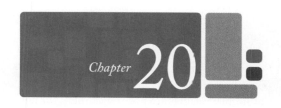

Chapter 20

AFAF I. MELEIS

Introducing the Theorist
Overview of the Theory
Application of the Theory
Practice Exemplar by Diane Gullett
Summary
References

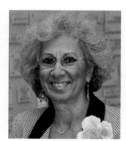

Afaf I. Meleis

Introducing the Theorist

Dr. Afif I. Meleis is a Professor of Nursing and Sociology and the former Margaret Bond Simon Dean of Nursing at the University of Pennsylvania School of Nursing and the former Director of the School's WHO Collaborating Center for Nursing and Midwifery Leadership. Before coming to Penn, she was a Professor on the faculty of nursing at the University of California Los Angeles and the University of California San Francisco for 34 years. She is a Fellow of the Royal College of Nursing in the United Kingdom, the American Academy of Nursing, and the College of Physicians of Philadelphia; a member of the Institute of Medicine, the George W. Bush Presidential Center Women's Initiative Policy Advisory Council, and the National Institutes of Health Advisory Committee on Research on Women's Health; a Board Member of the Consortium of Universities for Global Health; and cochair of the IOM Global Forum on Innovation for Health Professional Education and the Harvard School of Public Health-Penn Nursing-Lancet Commission on Women and Health. Dr. Meleis is also President Emerita and Counsel General Emerita of the International Council on Women's Health Issues and the former Global Ambassador for the Girl Child Initiative of the International Council of Nurses.

Dr. Meleis's research scholarship is focused on the theoretical development of the nursing discipline, structure and organization of nursing knowledge, transitions and health, and global immigrant and women's health. She is the originator of the *transitions theory*, a central concept of nursing phenomenon. This theory continues to be translated into policy, research, and evidence-based practice and better quality care in the 21st century.

She has mentored hundreds of students, clinicians, and researchers from around the world who, under her guidance, have achieved prominent leadership positions. She is the author of more than 175 articles in social sciences, nursing, and medical journals; more than 40 chapters; 7 books; and numerous monographs and proceedings. Her award-winning book, *Theoretical Nursing: Development and Progress*, now in its 5th edition (1985, 1991, 1997, 2007, 2012), is used widely throughout the world.

Overview of Transition Theory

A patient is admitted to the hospital; another is being discharged to a home, to a rehabilitation center, or to an assisted living facility; a third has just been diagnosed with a life-threatening disease; a fourth is preparing for an intrusive surgery; a fifth just got the news that her spouse has a long-term illness, and finally, a sixth is a new graduate from a nursing school beginning his first position as a nurse. What do they all have in common? Each of these scenarios is about the experience and responses of patients, families to health and illness situations; the experience of coping with changes from one phase, site, identity, position, role, or situation to another. The change event itself—whether it is birthing a baby, starting a new position, receiving a life-changing diagnosis, facing impending death, hospitalization, or surgery—is a turning point, but the *experience* is more fluid and longitudinal. The transition experience starts before the event and has an ending point that is fluid, that varies based on many variables. Understanding the nature of and responses to change, facilitating and supporting the experience and responding to it at different phases, and remaining or becoming healthy before, during or at the end of the event, wherever that elusive ending point is, is what transitions theory is about. This theory provides a framework to generate research questions and to serve as a guide to effective nursing care before, during, and after the transition.

Origins of the Theory

Three paradigms guided the development of transitions theory in more than 40 years of clinical research and theoretical work. The first is *role theory*, a dynamic and interactionist paradigm developed by Dr. Ralph Turner, whom I consider the father of interactive role theory. Role theory framed the type and nature of questions about how to help patients, clients, and families in their transition from one role to another, how to take on a new role, or change behaviors in a role. I wondered about the mechanisms and the processes that new mothers and fathers learned and negotiated as they become adept at performing the behaviors of parenting, at picking up the cues that differentiate the meaning of the different crying episodes or different patterns of sleep. From that theoretical heritage, I developed a framework for intervention that I called *role supplementation* (Meleis, 1975). This framework requires the nurse to accurately analyze the goals, sentiments, and behaviors necessary for the role he or she wishes to help the client develop. Such roles might include parenting roles, patient roles, or wellness roles. The desired outcome of applying role theory is the client's mastery of the role. Nurses help people acquire or change roles by modeling behaviors, allowing their clients to rehearse roles, and providing them with support while they are developing these roles.

A second paradigm that influenced the development of transitions theory is the *lived experience*, which contrasts the perceived views with the received views. As we, in nursing, began questioning what we know and how we know it, it became apparent that other ways of knowing (Carper, 1978) that complement and, perhaps, transcend empirical knowing. This personal, experiential knowing is by its nature subjective. It is more holistic and encompassing, embedded in practice, and framed by history. On the basis of the writing of many illuminating nonnurse authors (Polanyi, 1962) and nurse authors (among them Benner, Tanner, & Chesla, 1996; Munhall, 1993; Sarvimaki, 1994), I described the perceived view (Meleis, 2012) and used it as a driving paradigm for the development of the concept of *transitions* (Chick & Meleis, 1986). This paradigm helped us focus on questions related to the nature and lived experience of the response to change and the experience of being in transition.

The third paradigm that informs transitions theory is that of feminist postcolonialism. The tenets of this paradigm encompass an epistemic system that questions power relationships in societies and institutions and that links societal and political oppressions that shape the responses to change events. This paradigm gave us a framework for understanding the experience of transition through the multiple lenses of race, ethnicity, nationality, and gender. Each of these qualities creates power differentials that must be considered if we truly want to understand how people experience and cope with transition and to provide preventive and therapeutic interventions to help them achieve health and wellness outcomes. Using a feminist postcolonialist framework helps us consider the conditions shaped by power inequities in a society or in institutions of healing (e.g., hospitals, nursing homes, community agencies) and how these power inequities can shape the allocation of resources as well as the provision of nursing care through transitions. The delineation of conditions surrounding the transition experience was illuminated by employing a feminist postcolonialist framework.

These three paradigms—roles theory, perceived views on lived experiences, and feminist postcolonialism—shaped the evolution of transitions theory through some 40 years of its development.

Assumptions of the Theory

- A human being's responses are shaped by interactions with significant others and reference groups.
- Change through health and illness events and situations trigger a process that begins at or before and extends beyond the event time.
- Whether aware or not aware, individuals and/or families experience a process triggered by changes with varied responses and outcomes.
- Outcomes of the experience of the transition are shaped by the nature of the experience.
- Preventative and therapeutic actions can influence outcomes.

- Individuals have the capacity to learn and enact new roles influenced by their environment..
- By producing critical and well-supported evidence, inequities in health care can be changed to more equitable systems of delivery.
- Gender, race, culture, heritage, and sexual orientation are contexts that shape people's experiences and outcomes of health–illness events as well as the health care provided.
- Nursing perspective is defined by humanism, holism, context, health, well-being, goals, and caring.
- Environment is defined as physical, social, cultural, organizational, and societal and influences experience, interventions, and outcomes.
- Individuals, families, and communities are partners in the care processes.

Concepts and Propositions of Transitions Theory

The transitions theory provides a framework to describe the experience of individuals who are confronting, living with, and coping with an event, a situation, or a stage in growth and development that requires new skills, sentiments, goals, behaviors, or functions. Transition is defined as "a passage from one life phase, condition, or status to another" (Chick & Meleis, 1986). It is a complex and multifaceted concept embracing several components, including process, time span, and perception.[1]

---

[1]This section of the chapter borrows heavily from the many publications about this theory, which evolved and was transformed by many mentees and collaborators over the years (Chick & Meleis, 1986; Schumacher & Meleis, 1994; Meleis, Sawyer, Im, et al., 2000; and Meleis, 2010). Without the partnerships, the co-authorship, and collaboration of many mentees, I would not have been able to develop transitions theory. It is an integration of all the previous writings about transition theory. Their influence is manifested in the many co-authored publications. Among my mentee collaborators are Drs. DeAnne Messias, Eun-Ok Im, Kathy Dracup, Linda Sawyer, Karen, Schumacher, Pat Jones, Norma Chick, Leslie Swendsen, and Patrician Tragenstein. While I acknowledge and respect the co-opted contributions of all my collaborators, the liberty I have taken in integrating the theory from all previous work is entirely my responsibility.

Transition Triggers

Four types of situations trigger a transition experience (Fig. 20-1). All are characterized by some type of change. Change is related to an external event while transition is an internal process (Chick & Meleis, 1986). The first trigger is a change in health or an illness situation that could initiate a diagnosis or an intervention process, particularly the kinds that require prolonged diagnostic procedures or treatment protocols, for example, cancer, schizophrenia, autism, diabetes, or Alzheimer's disease, among others. Each of these diagnoses is preceded by many unknowns, uncertainties about the processes that follow, and fears about consequences. They all also require new behaviors, resources, and coping strategies, and they involve sets of relationships, newly established, changed, or severed.

A second trigger is *developmental transitions*, which are exemplified by life phases as manifested by age (e.g., adolescence, aging, menopause) or by roles (e.g., mothering, fathering, marrying, divorcing). Developmental transitions influence the health and well-being of people and may or may not require interfacing with health-care professionals and the health-care system. Developmental phases and roles influence health and illness behaviors as well as inform the responses of individuals to such events as birthing, breastfeeding, among many others. These examples of developmental transitions are of interest to nursing because of the evidence in the literature that demonstrates how nurses deal with, what they write about and research, as well as how they care for individual health-care needs during the many phases in their development.

Similarly, the third change trigger for a transition is what we call *situational transitions*, all of which have health-care implications. These are exemplified by experiences and responses to situational changes such as the admission to or discharge from a hospital or rehabilitation institution, as well as the changes that a new graduate nurse experiences becoming a manager or an expert or that a student nurse learning the ropes of his or her first clinical rotation experiences at a new hospital.

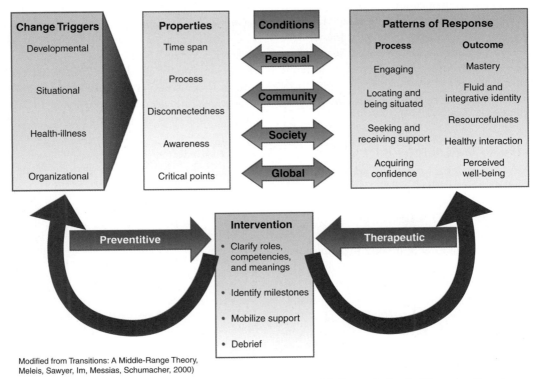

Modified from Transitions: A Middle-Range Theory, Meleis, Sawyer, Im, Messias, Schumacher, 2000)

Fig 20 • 1 Transitions: A middle-range theory. *Modified from Meleis, A.I., Sawyer, L., Im, E., Schumacher, K., and Messias D. (2000). Experiencing transitions: An emerging middle range theory.* Advances in Nursing Science, 23*(1), 12.*

The fourth type of change trigger that starts a process of transition is linked to organizational rules and functioning (Schumacher & Meleis, 1994). There are many examples of organizational transitions: the arrival of a new chief executive officer, chief nursing officer, or any other new leader; the implementation of electronic health records; a different system of care; use of new technology throughout an organization; or moving nursing practice to the community. The experience of transition here is for a whole organization as opposed to individuals or families.

Properties of Transition

Besides a triggering change event, transitions are characterized by properties that we described in 1986 (Chick & Meleis 1986; see Table 20-1). The first is a time span, which could begin from the moment an event or a situation comes to the awareness of an individual. It could be a symptom, a diagnosis, an emergency room visit, a flood, an earthquake, an accident, or a decision to undergo surgery. Unlike its beginning, the end of a transition is fluid. The end may be determined when a final goal is achieved, be it mastery of new roles, developing certain competencies, feeling a sense of well-being, or acquiring a desired quality of life.

Another property that defines transition is that it is a process. The change event itself is static, but the experience that ensues is a dynamic and fluid process. The distance between the beginning of this process and when it exactly ends may correspond with other similar processes or may be unique. Bridges (1980, 1991) characterized the process following change events as requiring at first an ending period followed by an experience of confusion or a neutral period followed by a period he calls the new beginning. That is when the process is completed.

Disconnectedness is an additional characteristic of transition. Whether the triggering change

is health related, developmental, situational, or organizational, one of the properties of the transition experience is a sense of impending or actual disconnectedness. A clear example is the implementation of electronic health records in a school or hospital. Those who will be experiencing the change will manifest responses that could reflect a level of disconnect from their current mode of recording patients' health data and maintaining continuity in patients' files. The transition experience reflects a disruption in a person's feeling of security associated with what is known and familiar. There is a sense of loss—of familiar signposts, reference points, or state of health—and a feeling of incongruity between past, present, and future expectations. Those who are responding to the change experience a discontinuity of regular patterns disrupted by the unfamiliar.

Another important property of transitions is awareness—awareness of the change event, of the situation, of triggers, and of the internal experience of transition. The difference between change and transition is the difference between external and internal experience. Perception, awareness, and the defining and redefining of the meaning of the change for the self and others are properties of a transition experience. They make transition dynamic, incorporating meaning and changing interpretation over a span of time.

The presence of milestones that may be turning points is yet another property of transitions. Identifying milestones is essential to understanding the phases in the transition experience as well as to identifying the appropriate assessment points and intervention points. The goals of transition theory are to describe triggers, to anticipate experience, to predict outcomes, and to provide guidelines for interventions.

Conditions of Change

Change triggers initiate a process with patterns of responses that are both observable and nonobservable behaviors and either functional or dysfunctional. These responses start from the moment a change trigger is anticipated and are influenced by personal, community, societal, or global conditions. Among the personal conditions are the meaning and the values attributed to the change and the context of it. A person's experience and responses are also influenced by the expectations of how self or others will react,

Table 20 • 1 Concepts

- Time
- Process
- Experiences
- Milestones
- Conditions

the level of knowledge and skills related to the change, and the belief about what is expected of those undergoing the change. Other personal conditions that influence the experience and responses are the level of planning and the level of existing health and well-being of the person, the family, the organization, the community, or the country at large (Schumacher & Meleis, 1994). In addition, the responses are mediated by the level of vulnerability and sense of marginalization those experiencing the transition find themselves in or are subjected to (Hall, Stevens, & Meleis, 1994; Stevens, Hall, & Meleis, 1994). Community conditions, such as support from partners and the availability of role models and resources, promote or inhibit effective healthy transitions. Community norms about and resources for dealing with sexism, homophobia, poverty, ageism, and nationalism also could promote or inhibit healthy experiences and outcomes of transitions. Global conditions that could influence the experience of transitions, including policies and mandates developed by international organizations, define how certain triggers are viewed and appear at the global consciousness. For example, the transition of the HIV/AIDS patient through the diagnosis and treatment process could be mediated by the global attention and resources that have been given to researchers, clinicians, and patients who have or are associated with the disease. There are vast differences between how infected individuals experienced the diagnosis and treatment of HIV/AIDS before the global attention to it and post–President's Emergency Plan for AIDS Relief aid offered by the Western world.

Patterns of Responses

How do individuals, families, and organizations respond to a change event? What questions should be asked to define and understand their responses? This is an area of knowledge that is ripe for systematic investigation. Many theories can describe responses. Among them are grief theories (Kübler-Ross, 1969) and crisis theories (Lindemann, 1979). We have proposed two sets of responses from a nursing perspective: process patterns and outcome patterns.

Process Patterns

Process patterns are measured by the degree of engagement in the particular change event as well as in the actions and intervention plans (Schumacher, Jones, & Meleis, 1999). Levels of engagement could be assessed through patterns of questions, types of responses, and the congruency between actions, sentiments, and goals of those who are experiencing the transition and those who are guiding and advising about these actions. Following directions, accuracy of perceived information, the consistency of meanings of the event, and the degree of involvement in all aspects of transition experience and actions related to the change event are indicators of engagement levels.

A second process pattern of response is called location and being situated (Meleis, Sawyer, Im, Schumacher, & Messias, 2000). Recognizing one's position in a complex system of relationships and being connected and able to interact with a web of different interactions is a pattern of response that should be examined to uncover the nature of responses to a transition trigger. How a person sees, initiates, and relates to teams of health professionals following a diagnosis of cancer or to a new immigrant's environment determines a pattern of response. How and when a person, a family, or a community confronted by a change trigger seek support from health-care providers, are indicators of the extent that they understand the needs and timeliness in seeking the support. It is also an indication of realizing their position within the health-care system.

Another process pattern is the level of confidence in handling the new, multiple, and sometimes conflicting demands on a person, family, or organization in the midst of attempting to deal with a triggering event. Similarly, the level of confidence may be determined by the individual's ability to identify priorities of needs and to outline different levels of actions or interventions. The actions could be as simple as describing from whom they should seek help to more complex self-care interventions.

Outcome Patterns

Although patterns in process responses are assessed at different points in dealing with a change trigger, outcome responses are assessed at a point determined to be at the end of the transition process. Five patterns of responses are defined as outcomes—mastery, fluid integrative identities, resourcefulness, healthy interactions, and perceived well-being (Meleis et al., 2000). Mastery includes role mastery, which is manifested by integrating the sentiment, goals, and behaviors in one's identity, and behaving with confidence, knowledge, and expertise. Examples are becoming a mother (Hattar-Pollara, 2010; Mercer, 2004; Shin & Whitetraut 2007), accepting hospice or end-of-life care (Larkin, Dierckx de Casterlé, & Schotsmans, 2007), or becoming adept at being at risk while continuing to function in other roles.

Mastery goes beyond roles, however, and includes mastery of one's environment as manifested in seeking and utilizing appropriate resources and co-opting supportive environmental conditions. Learning to cope with technology at home, living with it, and reformulating one's identity to incorporate it in one's daily repetitions is an example of this mastery (Fex, Gullvi, Ik, & Soderhamn, 2010).

Fluid and integrative identity is another outcome response pattern (Meleis et al., 2000). This pattern is characterized by the ability to swing back and forth between the multiple identities a person in transition experiences. Let's consider a person who must undergo kidney dialysis and who emerges from her dialysis session to assume other identities, without any one of the identities dominating her time and energy. A person with an integrative identity is able to live, function, and be well, despite the uncertainties and ambiguities of living with a chronic illness, a nagging pain, or a set of essential treatments. This pattern of outcome response is characterized by the ability to carry the sentiments, the goals, the actions, and the baggage of different ways of being (Messias, 1997). It is the ability to "navigate unknown waters" (Duggleby et al., 2010). One indicator for an outcome pattern of response is current compared with previous quality of life.

Another outcome pattern of response is healthy interactions and connections as manifested in maintaining relationships and or developing new connections or relationships that affirm the completion of a transition. Questions to be investigated are the extent to which caregivers burdened by extensive healthcare needs of patients with heart failure are able to develop relationships with health-care providers while maintaining meaningful supportive relationships in their lives. For example, telehealth can play a significant role in facilitating caregivers' abilities to meet the needs of heart failure patients by maintaining continuous communication with family and caregivers. Telenurses can then deliver the evidence-based professional consulting and supportive care based on technology that improves patients' self-care behaviors. These interventions can also alleviate caregivers' burdens and improve their health outcomes, allowing them time to meet their own needs (e.g., health or social needs; Chiang, Chen, Dai, & Ho, 2012).

These types of questions are important to answer because some research has demonstrated that the health of partners or caregivers is intertwined with that of seriously ill patients, that is, the more an illness affects the patient's physical and mental ability, the greater the impact this will have on the health of their partner or caregiver due to insurmountable stress, disruption in their relationships, and neglect of their own health. These unintended health consequences may be further exacerbated by the lack of social, emotional, or practical support the partner or caregiver experiences (Christakis & Allison, 2006). For this reason, having strong social networks in place during these periods of transition could play a significant role in promoting positive health outcomes for the caregiver, which would in turn positively affect the health of the patient. For major areas of investigation, see Table 20-2.

Intervention Framework

The goal of intervention within transitions theory is to facilitate and inspire healthy process and outcome responses. Nursing interventions that support healthy process behaviors as well as healthy outcome behaviors include the following: clarifying meanings, providing expertise, setting goals, modeling the role of others; providing resources, opportunities for rehearsal, access to reference groups and role models, and debriefing.

Clarifying Roles, Meanings, Competencies, Expertise, Goals, and Role Taking

Through interaction, dialogue, and interviews, the nurse probes for the values of the person

Table 20 • 2 **Major Areas of Investigation**

- Describe and interpret the different transition experiences and responses.
- Identify transition properties.
- Develop and test preventative and therapeutic interventions.
- Identify milestones and turning points associated with different change triggers.
- Describe and test determinants of process and outcome responses.
- Develop instruments and investigative tools for properties, conditions, processes, and outcome responses.
- Explore strategies to modify policies essential to mitigate, facilitate or inhibit healthy processes and outcome responses.

experiencing the transition process, as well as those of their significant others, and determines the meanings they attribute to the event and the different stages in the transition. Competencies and the extent to which the person is able to master each of the competencies are identified, as well as the ease in performing the competency and the level of engagement in learning or modifying the competency—be it testing blood sugar levels, bathing a baby, changing a nursing unit, or reaching out for new connections in a nursing home.

Similarly, observing, questioning or interviewing significant others—whether they are partners or friends—to determine levels of engagement and the extent of competency mastery is another significant component of a program for intervention during transition process, especially at critical milestones. Significant others or reference groups to be included in the assessment or the intervention are those whose viewpoints are used as a frame of reference. Roles, whether they are new ones, at-risk ones, or those that may be lost, are formed and imputed through a process of definition and redefinition. Similarly, new competencies are acquired through a process of teaching, learning, rehearsing, modeling, and reinforcement by those who are in the support or network systems (Petch, 2009; Swendsen, Meleis, & Jones, 1978; van Staa, 2010).

Identifying Milestones and Using Critical Points

A *critical point* is the time when questions tend to arise about a care trajectory or when signs and symptoms tend to manifest themselves. It is a

point when healing progresses or there is a relapse, a point when infection, inflammation, distress, anxiety, noncompliance, or other conditions may begin appearing and when an appropriate intervention may advance the treatment and healing course. Care is maximized at such a point. A 6-week check-up for a postpartum mother has always been designated a critical point or a milestone, but this milestone is driven by the biomedical model as it relates to when the uterus reverts to its normal size. However, it is imperative to identify milestones from a nursing perspective when our goals are self-care, quality of life, role mastery, and managed care. Identifying milestones or turning points is essential in the trajectory of managing and facilitating transitions. This area of the theory invites research to provide evidence to identify and support those points where there is a need for intervention to enhance both a healthy transition process and outcomes. Biomedical driven goals are not inclusive of goals driven by a nursing perspective and holistic approach.

Providing Supportive Resources, Rehearsals, Reference Groups, and Role Models

Mobilizing partnerships, resources, and supportive groups is another component in intervention strategies. Clarifying roles, competencies, values, and abilities to understand what others are experiencing are important processes for facilitating a healthy transition and in achieving healthy outcomes at the termination of a transition. These may be accomplished by identifying a nurse as a go-to person for questions, observing patients who may have gone through a similar event, and being afforded opportunities to imagine, mentally enact, or actually practice what the person may encounter, do, or feel during the different phases of transition. Having a support group, rehearsing competencies, becoming in touch with feelings about events or competencies, visualizing different scenarios, and describing the different if–then situations may enhance healthy transitions and outcomes. We have called these processes *role modeling* and *role rehearsal*, as well as *defining and identifying reference groups* (Meleis, 1975; Meleis & Swendsen, 1978). An example of this type of intervention is an interdisciplinary mentoring program that the Hospital of the University of Pennsylvania implemented, which pairs nurses with medical students starting their first clinical rotations to facilitate the transitional adjustment of the medical students to their new environment. This program also highlights the important role nurses play in patient care, which fosters a sense of teamwork and collegiality between medical students and nurses from the beginning (Sapega, 2012).

Debriefing

Debriefing is a well-researched, core nursing intervention used at critical points during transition experiences. "Debriefing is defined as a process of communicating to others the experiences that a person or group encountered around a critical event" (Meleis, 2010, p. 457). It is a tool used in nursing to help a person come to terms with the transition experience and attain psychological well-being (Steele & Beadle, 2003). Nurses ask their patients questions after birthing, traumatic events, disasters, surgical procedures, during a new admissions process, and at discharge. The patient may recount his or her story emotionally, relate to it cognitively, describe it, interpret its meaning, reflect on it, or share feelings. The story usually includes the context, the before, the during, and the subsequent responses related to the experience. Nurses engage in dialogues with their patients about the events, ask questions, and provide patients and families with the opportunity to process the events and the aftermath. For example, a number of maternity units provide postnatal debriefing services for new

mothers. Postnatal debriefing is a psychological intervention that enables women to come to terms with their experience and promotes psychological well-being. Through postnatal debriefing, health-care professionals can identify the emotional and psychological needs of the patient and refer them to appropriate resources or other mental health specialists. This service gives new mothers the opportunity to ask questions, debrief about their experiences, describe their feelings, and receive information and reasons for care they have been provided or need (Steele & Beadle, 2003).

In addition to patients, nurses themselves, as well as other health-care providers, also benefit from debriefing. Hospitals have implemented debriefing, or critical incident stress management, programs to help their staff cope with stress and sorrow at work and to mitigate the impact of traumatic events. For example, Children's Memorial Hospital in Chicago launched a mentor program that matched new nursing graduates with seasoned nurses to help them cope with the stress and heartache of caring for sick children and interacting with distressed parents and family members. This program significantly reduced the high turnover rate among new nursing graduates that the hospital had been experiencing (Huff, 2006).

Applications of Transitions Theory
Research

Transitions theory has been used extensively as a theoretical framework in research all around the world to examine a broad spectrum of transition experiences resulting from health–illness, developmental, situational, and organizational transitions and the effect of these transitions on the health of individuals, families, and communities. It has been used to develop strategies and interventions to facilitate healthy transitions and has served as a conceptual basis and guide to

• understand and examine teenager's concerns as they transition through high school in the United States (Rew, Tyler, & Hannah, 2012).

- demonstrate in Taiwan that nurse-led transitional care combining telehealth care and discharge planning significantly alleviates family caregiver burden and stress and improves family function (Chiang et al., 2012).
- study the impact on self-care of people with heart failure and develop strategies to implement a therapeutic regimen in Portugal (Mendes, Bastos, & Paiva, 2010).
- explore in greater depth chronic obstructive pulmonary disease (COPD) patients' experiences during and after pulmonary rehabilitation in Norway (Halding & Heggdal, 2011).
- analyze Finnish women's hysterectomy experiences as a process of transition in their lives and describe representations of hysterectomy in Finnish women's and health magazines (Nykanen, Suominen, & Nikkonen, 2011).
- assess the cultural factors that may contribute to the low diagnosis rate of postpartum depression in Asian American (e.g., Asian Indian, Chinese, Filipina) mothers (Goyal, Wang, Shen, Wong, & Palaniappan, 2012).

These research studies demonstrate how transitions theory has supported and aided nurse researchers and scholars to describe the transition experiences and responses, confirm the components of the transition experience, and identify the essential properties of transition, including the critical points and events, to ultimately reach the goal of promoting healthy outcomes and easing transitions for their clients, families, and communities.

- As indicated by Kralik, Visentin, and van Loon (2006) in their comprehensive literature review of transitions theory, future research to advance knowledge about transitions should include longitudinal comparative and longitudinal cross sectional designs.
- In 2007, at the University of Pennsylvania, we established the New Courtland Center on Transitions and Health. Transitions theory provided the foundation for its theoretical basis. Driven by Dr. Mary Naylor's scholarship, a current focus of the center is on the transitional care model for the elderly population. Although independently developed on the East Coast of the United States as an

intervention using advanced practice nurses, the transitional care model reflects the components of transition theory (Naylor, 2002).

Practice

Transitions theory has been applied in practice by nurses to aid clients, families, and communities in preparing for, navigating through, and adapting to transition experiences to enhance health outcomes. The operationalization of transitions theory enhances nurses' understanding of patient and caregiver transitions and leads to the development of nursing therapeutics, interventions, and resources that are tailored to the unique experiences of clients and their families in order to promote successful, healthy responses to transition. As mentioned earlier in this chapter, the illness of patients can take a heavy toll on the health of their caregivers due to the stress, role transitions, disruption in relationships, and bereavement they may experience. Transitions theory has been used as a conceptual framework in practice to help health-care providers gain a holistic understanding of the caregiver's beliefs, views, unique experiences, and desired outcomes, which in turn enables nurses and health-care providers to allocate resources and implement interventions targeted to the caregivers' specific needs to optimize the health of both the patient and the caregiver (Blum & Sherman, 2010). It helps identify the barriers to, as well as facilitators of, the transition, unique to each individual patient and caregiver, which in turn enhances the nurses' or health-care providers' ability to effectively guide them through the transition experiences.

The conceptual underpinnings of transitions theory have also been used to analyze the transitions that intensive care unit (ICU) patients and their families encounter after they are discharged from ICU and the provision of nursing services needed for continuity of care. By digging deeper to fully comprehend the stress patients and families experience when being discharged from ICU, including their potential feelings of abandonment, unimportance, or ambivalence, nurses can better assist patients and families in the ICU transfer process and ensure the provision of optimum health-care services to continue care (Chaboyer, 2006).

Transitions theory has also been used to understand and characterize the personal experiences of perimenopausal and menopausal women. Findings from this research have been translated into practice in the clinical setting. Understanding women's personal experiences using transitions theory equips nurses to proactively educate women on what to expect before perimenopausal or menopausal symptoms begin, thus decreasing anxiety and confusion and instead "normalizing the experience" (Marnocha, Bergstrom & Dempsey, 2011).

Education

Transitions theory is used in graduate and undergraduate curricula in countries around the world. Universities that have integrated transitions theory in their nursing education programs include the University of Connecticut in Storrs and Clayton State University in Morrow, Georgia. Clayton State University has used transitions theory in its curriculum, and has made it central to their nursing program's philosophy. On its website, transitions theory is defined, and it is emphasized that "[n]egotiating successful transitions depends on the development of an effective relationship between the nurse and client. This relationship is a highly reciprocal process that affects both the client and nurse" (Clayton State University, 2012). With regard to the graduate curriculum in nursing at the university,

---

The culmination of graduate nursing education is the synthesis of advanced skills in order to provide excellent nursing care and to foster ongoing professional development in order to promote nursing research, ethical decision-making reflecting an appreciation of human diversity in health and illness among individuals, families, and communities experiencing life transitions. (Clayton State University, 2012)

At the University of California San Francisco (UCSF), I taught a graduate course on transitions and health to respond to an increasing educational demand of graduate students. Additionally, many doctoral students in nursing and other disciplines around the world, including Sweden and the United States, have used transitions theory as a basis for their doctoral dissertations.

Developing Situation-Specific Theories

Transitions theory continues to be further developed, tested, and refined to understand and describe the relationships among the major beliefs, patterns, and concepts of diverse groups of populations undergoing various types of transition experiences. A number of situation-specific theories have evolved from transitions theory. A situation-specific theory is a coherent representation and depiction of a set of concepts and their interrelationships to a set of outcomes related to health and illness experiences and responses, as well as to nursing actions to prevent the effects of illness or ameliorate the effects of interventions (Meleis, 2010). For example, a situation-specific theory explaining the menopausal symptom experiences of Asian immigrant women within the sociocultural contexts in the United States was grounded in transitions theory (Im, 2010). Others include *Transitions and Health: A Framework for Gerontological Nursing* (Schumacher, Jones, & Meleis, 1999) and *Situation-Specific Theory of Pain Experience for Asian American Cancer Patients* (Im, 2008).

Practice Exemplar by Diane Lee Gullett, MSN, MPH

The following Practice Exemplar is framed with Afaf Meleis' Transition Theory.

I met Wayne when I was volunteering as a nurse in a free clinic in New Orleans (N.O.) in 2012. He was a 26-year-old young man who appeared gaunt with dark circles under his eyes. Wayne presented with a chief complaint of insomnia, depression, nighttime sweating, and a lack of energy for the past 10 months. He informed me that the other practitioners he visited had given him medications for sleep and depression. He stated

Continued

these had been unsuccessful in relieving his symptoms. I asked Wayne if any blood work had been done. He suddenly became very anxious, stood up and began pacing the room, wringing his hands, looking at the floor, and refusing to make eye contact. He started for the door and told me he didn't need to have any blood drawn and that this was a mistake. I assured him that I would not draw any blood without his consent and gently asked him if he would be willing to stay and speak with me a bit further.

Nurse: Can you remember when you first started noticing your symptoms?

Wayne: I guess it was in August or maybe September.

Nurse: Thinking back can you remember any significant changes in your life at that time?

Wayne: You know, I have wracked my brain thinking about that. The only thing I can think of is that this was about the time Hurricane Katrina hit.

Nurse: Were you living in New Orleans (N.O.) when Hurricane Katrina hit the city?

Wayne: Yeah, I was starting my freshman year of college.

Nurse: Would you mind sharing some of your experiences about that time in your life with me?

(Intervention: Debriefing).

Wayne: I was a 19-year-old honors student (Condition: Personal). I had just moved to N.O. to major in international business 10 days before the storm (Change trigger: Situational). The apartment community where I lived was evacuated, so I was forced to leave the city and go to my stepfather's house in Arkansas (Property: Time span). I didn't understand the severity of the situation at the time, I mean I had never been through a hurricane before (Condition: Personal). I thought it would be an opportunity to get ahead with my schoolwork and visit with my family. I didn't take much, two pairs of pants and some books. I mean it never occurred to me that I would need more than that. You know you have to leave, so

you take what you think you need which you later realize isn't enough and isn't what you should have taken, but no one prepares you for that (Condition: Personal). I enrolled in classes at Louisiana State University in Baton Rouge 3 weeks after Katrina, since my old college wasn't offering classes at that time. I lasted 5 minutes. I went through the whole process and I just dropped out (Property: Milestone) immediately after doing it because I just couldn't wrap my mind around it.

Nurse: Could you explain a bit more about what you mean when you say you "couldn't wrap your mind around it." (Clarifying meaning)

Wayne: I, it, was everything from my social life, to what I was studying, to my financial situation. I was on this path of what I was going to do and when I came back, I just couldn't do it. I just, honestly, I just didn't care. It seemed like there were so many other more important things than worrying about my grades or what I was studying. I dropped out of school with a 1.5 GPA and decided to return to N.O. It was only about 3 months after Katrina and too soon. My thought process, though, was just I need to get my life back to normal, I need to get things to be the way that they were. Even 7 years later, they are not. It is, you acknowledge on some level, that it is never going to be the way that it was, but it's like your driving force, this need to get your life back to normal (Property: Process). And then you get the new normal, so it's not what you had before, it's not even close. It's not even, it's, I can't even describe how different it is.

Change Triggers

Hurricane Katrina serves as the situational change trigger for Wayne's transitioning experience. The hurricane generated situational changes including relocating to a new city, enrolling at a new college, and living in a new community. The nature of Wayne's transitional experience; however, must also be considered within the context of other possible change triggers. Wayne is simultaneously experiencing a developmental life phase change moving from late adolescence to early adulthood manifested in his role transition from high school student to independent college student. Limited worldly experience and youth are personal conditions that inhibit Wayne's ability to cope with the reality of the changes triggered by Hurricane Katrina. His inexperience is evident in his initial response to Hurricane Katrina as a mini-vacation for which he took only a few articles of clothing, never thinking he wouldn't be able to return to resume his college life or collect those things he held personally valuable. Wayne's inability to effectively reconcile his previous life with his new one inhibits a healthy outcome response leading to his failure to maintain his GPA and eventually dropping out of school. The nurse recognizes Hurricane Katrina as the situational change trigger that contextually situates Wayne's unique transition experience and serves as the foundation for mutual meaning making between the nurse and Wayne.

Nurse: *Could you tell me a little bit more about your feelings during that time and your 'need to get your life back to normal' (Clarifying meaning).*

Wayne: *I came back with no plan other than to try and resume my life, and without realizing that all of the things that were in my life before might not be there after (Property: Disconnectedness). That is, even down to grocery stores, you know for a long time you had to drive to the suburbs just to make groceries. Like, for example when my old apartment community reopened, I was adamant that I wanted to move back. I had to move back into that same apartment, and I did ultimately, but it wasn't the same. It wasn't physically the same because it had been gutted and then it wasn't the same because it wasn't the same circumstances, it wasn't the same people. So I did not realize, I just wanted to move back and continue my life, I didn't realize that the things that were part of my life may not be there like they*

were before (Property: Disconnectedness).

Nurse: *This must have been a very difficult time for you. How did you cope with all these changes in your life? (Intervention: Questioning)*

Wayne: *Things during the first year or two after I returned to the city are still a little hazy. I do remember totaling three cars within 2 weeks after returning to N.O., you know I don't know where my head was (Property: Critical point). I haven't been in an accident since. I haven't even had a speeding ticket, but literally within this period I totaled three cars. I can say speaking in honesty that you know for a long time after the storm that my way of dealing with my day to day life really was sex and drugs (Property: Critical point). What started with just every now and then became like weeks–long binges, and when you get involved with those things, it brings a completely new element into your life that you probably wouldn't have considered before. I mean, I will be the first to say I have done things since the storm that I never would have considered before. Such as certain substances, sexually, bath houses. . . . (Property: Critical point). I think it was an escape; it was because when you are high, when you are messed up, and you're not thinking about the things around you . . . you are not thinking at all really, you are just you know, you are getting away from all these pressures that are on your mind (Property: Awareness).*

Nurse: *What did you feel like you needed to escape from (Intervention: Clarifying meaning)?*

Wayne: *At the time, I had new financial struggles that I hadn't had before. Things like work, some family problems, and the way things were in the city. Everything was so different than it had been before Katrina (Conditions: Personal and Community).*

Properties of Transition

Properties of transition (i.e., time span, process, disconnectedness, awareness, and critical points)

Continued

assist the nurse in describing change triggers, specific milestones and ascertaining the different phases of a person's transition experience. This knowledge assists the nurse in identifying interventions and support mechanisms important in facilitating healthy transition experiences or recognizing those factors inhibiting healthy transitions. Wayne encounters the property of time span when he first becomes aware of Hurricane Katrina. The nurse recognizes Hurricane Katrina as an external trigger of change which in and of itself is static. Wayne's process of transition, on the other hand, signifies a dynamic internal change evident in his struggle to regain his old life, his inability to do so and his reluctance to accept the new normal. Disconnectedness manifests in Wayne's recognition of the disruption Hurricane Katrina brought to his familiar way of being in the world; from where he shopped, where he lived, who his friends were, and who he understood himself to be. He sincerely yearns to return to the familiar only to find his environment (personal, community, and societal conditions) irrevocably changed. The dynamic nature of awareness is reflected in Wayne's continual reinterpretation and willingness to find meaning in his experiences following Katrina. His story is filled with a sense of movement from trying to return to normal to acknowledging the "new normal" and from participating in risk-taking behaviors as coping strategies to recognizing these as ineffective. The nurse recognizes many turning points or milestones within Wayne's transition experience starting with his dropping out of school, crashing multiple cars, using drugs and alcohol, and engaging in unprotected sex. Without appropriate interventions, all of these played a role in inhibiting a healthy transition experience for Wayne.

Nurse: Did you have anyone who was able to support you or who you felt like you could go to for help during this time (Intervention: Assessing support systems)?

Wayne: I wasn't getting the support from my family because they couldn't relate, they . . . I suppose on some level they were like this sucks

but they couldn't at all understand what I was going through (Property: Disconnectedness). There weren't many people who stayed in the city and those who became my friends ended up being the wrong crowd. I mean the city was a disaster there was a curfew, military presence, no garbage pickup for months, no grocery stores, and certainly no counseling or places to go to for help (Condition: Community). It was as if those of us who stayed in the city were on our own. I think a lot of people were in bad shape. I remember hearing about a lot of people committing suicide.

Nurse: Do you think you made the wrong decision returning to N.O. so soon after Hurricane Katrina?

Wayne: Absolutely. You know, even now, if it were going to happen again, I couldn't, I would leave, I would leave my stuff, and I would not come back. It wasn't the experience itself, it was the after effect. And the way it affected my life. . . . I can't go back to trying to fit the pieces of my life back together or trying to resume a sense of normalcy that will never return because even though I know better now, while you intellectually know better, emotionally you are still going to be going through the processes (Process patterns: Engagement). There is nothing you can do about that, you can't control that. . . . I just can't do it. I am a pretty strong person, I always have been, but that was one time in my life that I can sincerely say I had a mental and emotional breakdown. It was what it was, and I can't do anything about that (Properties: Awareness).

Conditions of Change

There are multiple personal, community, and societal conditions influencing Wayne's patterns of response to Hurricane Katrina and are important for the nurse to recognize as part of his transition process. Personal conditions are those, which center on an individual's experience with the change trigger and other personal conditions that influence the well-being of the individual within the broader framework of family and community. Wayne's youth and lack

Practice Exemplar by Diane Lee Gullett, MSN, MPH cont.

of experience with natural disasters are personal conditions that influenced Wayne's responses to the situational change. Wayne naively returned to N.O. with the intent of getting his life back to normal only to be confronted with the reality of an irrevocably changed reality and his place in it. Wayne also expresses feelings of isolation when discussing his belief that others including his family could not relate to what he was going through. Wayne's lack of knowledge and skills, poor planning, and increased sense of marginalization reflect personal and community conditions that inhibited rather than facilitated a healthy transition experience. The limited level of existing community and social resources available within the city following Hurricane Katrina also inhibited Wayne's transition experience. Katrina created catastrophic conditions within the city that left a nonexistent social, political, and economic infrastructure. Employment, housing, medical care and mental health services were virtually nonexistent within the city. Wayne was not aware of the fact that he needed help during this time and states the reality of limited access to even basic services within the city. Community conditions including cultural and social norms were also dramatically altered by the catastrophic conditions that existed in the city. These conditions for a young person such as Wayne may have presented a loss of positive role-modeling essential to developing effective coping strategies following such a traumatic experience. Wayne admits to engaging in homosexual behavior, unprotected sex, doing drugs, and hanging out with the wrong crowd. Societal conditions stigmatizing homosexuality may have prohibited him from seeking support from his family or friends, further perpetuating his feelings of marginalization.

Nurse: Are you able to think about your future at all, envision what you want to do moving forward (Intervention: Visualizing different scenarios).

Wayne: One thing I can say moving forward, I have, I really want to get out of N.O. It's that still even today, it is such a major part

of, and I know I am not alone in this, your everyday mental process. Your life is separated into before Katrina and after Katrina. And you refer to things like that, on a daily basis your life before the storm and after the storm and you think about it every day. I can't imagine, I can't imagine living somewhere that you don't think about that, I can't imagine living somewhere where that is not a part of your daily process, it's not a part of your shared experience (Patterns of response: Locating).

Nurse: After listening to your story, it seems that the changes brought about by Hurricane Katrina greatly affected your life. I think some of the symptoms you described to me could be related to what you experienced during this very difficult time in your life. Speaking with others who have experienced similar circumstances may provide a way to express what you have been through. I know of a local support group not far from here that has some members who were also in college at the time that Hurricane Katrina hit. Would you be interested in attending one of these groups (Intervention: Mobilizing support)?

Wayne: I would like that. (Patterns of response: Receiving support) I feel better just talking with someone about all of this. Can I tell you something and you won't judge me (Patterns of response: Seeking support)?

Nurse: Of course. I want you to feel this is a safe environment and that I am not here to judge you.

Wayne: You know when I told you about the bathhouses; well it happened a lot and with men. I didn't use protection most of the time. I am so ashamed and so scared.

Nurse: Wayne, you do not need to be ashamed. A lot of young men and women experiment sexually throughout their lives, but it is important to practice safe sex. Can you tell me more about what you are scared of specifically (Intervention: Clarifying meaning)?

Wayne: I am scared that I may have AIDS. I took a home HIV test a couple of months ago, the kind that uses your saliva. It was

Continued

Practice Exemplar by Diane Lee Gullett, MSN, MPH cont.

positive, but I have been too afraid to do anything about it or tell anyone. I know, I am stupid, right (Properties: Critical point)?

Nurse: *No, I don't think you are stupid. I think you are rather brave for telling me and for making the decision to talk about this (Intervention: providing expertise).*

Wayne: *I feel relieved but really scared, that is the reason I was going to leave when you mentioned the blood test. I don't know what to do. It was my fault. I don't even remember most of it. I wasn't like this before Katrina, I don't know what has happened to me since then, I am a mess (Patterns of response: Being situated).*

Nurse: *I realize you are scared, but the first step is setting up a time for you to get an HIV blood test, if you feel you are okay with that (Intervention: Setting goals). I have the phone number of a local clinic, we can call together and schedule an appointment for you. There are counselors who will be there to support you through the process (Intervention: Providing resources). You will not be alone. Are you still engaging in unprotected sex with other partners or using drugs that place you or someone else at risk (Intervention: Providing expertise)?*

Wayne: *No, I haven't done any of those things in over a year. I stopped hanging out with that crowd and I don't have any desire to go back to doing any of those things (Patterns of response: Awareness).*

Nurse: *I believe it is important for you to explore your feelings and experiences before and after Hurricane Katrina in a safe environment. I think it would be helpful for you to meet with a counselor in addition to attending a couple of support groups. We can talk about your options and decide together how you would like to move forward, does that sound like a plan (Intervention: Mobilizing support and setting goals)? Are you close to anyone you feel would be supportive right now (Intervention: Assessing support systems)?*

Wayne: *I don't want anyone else to know about this for right now, if that is okay? I would prefer to see a counselor and maybe go to a*

support group but not with anyone else. Thank you so much for listening to me and for taking the time to help me.

Nurse: *You are welcome. Thank you for sharing your experience with me, for being brave enough to talk about what you are going through, for trusting me and allowing me to support you as you journey through this process.*

Patterns of Response

The nature of Wayne's transition experience can be gleaned through his dialogue with the nurse. Process patterns are assessed at different points during the transition experience while outcome patterns are assessed at a point determined to be at the end of the transition process. Wayne's responses indicate he is still engaged in the transition process despite the 7 years that had passed since Hurricane Katrina. He informs the nurse that he no longer hangs out with the wrong crowd or participates in risky behaviors such as unprotected sex. Wayne's willingness to stop engaging in risk-taking behaviors indicates a conscious choice to modify his behavior. Additionally, he opens up to the nurse about taking a home HIV test and decides to take a HIV blood test, indicating an active search for information by which to address his concerns. Both modifying his behavior and seeking out information suggests Wayne is actively involved or engaged in the process of transition. The nurse is aware that he is consistently comparing his actions using a before Katrina and after Katrina perspective as a way to create new meaning from his experience or 'locate' himself. He is attempting to understand his new way of being in the world by comparing it to his old way of being in the world. These comparisons also provide Wayne with a way of "situating" himself or a way to assist him with explaining why he engaged in the high-risk behaviors. The nurse inquires about Wayne's family and friends to determine his support system. Wayne indicates that he does not have a close relationship with either his family or friends at this time. He seeks support from the nurse by expressing his concerns and fears about the

Practice Exemplar by Diane Lee Gullett, MSN, MPH cont.

HIV testing. Additionally, he demonstrates a willingness to receive support by agreeing to attend groups and see a counselor. Acquiring confidence is usually a progressive movement in the transition process marked by increasing confidence in dealing with the triggering event. This is accomplished by developing strategies for prioritizing needs and developing a sense of wisdom generated through the lived experience. This can be seen in Wayne's decision to make an appointment to take an HIV blood test and seek support.

The nurse will assess for completion of the transition process when Wayne is able to demonstrate outcome responses including mastery, fluid and integrative identity, resourcefulness, health interactions, and perceived well-being. He may demonstrate mastery by integrating the skills he previously had in order to be an honors student in international business with the new skills he develops to positively cope with the changes brought about by Hurricane Katrina. A fluid and integrative identity may be assessed by asking Wayne to describe his previous quality of life compared with his current quality of life following intervention strategies. Wayne would demonstrate healthy interaction and thereby affirm the completion of his transition process by developing and maintaining meaningful and supportive relationships.

Intervention Framework

The goal of interventions is to facilitate and inspire healthy process and outcome responses. These interventions include clarifying roles, meanings, and expertise; identifying milestones; mobilizing support; and debriefing. The nurse dialogues and interacts with Wayne to clarifying his statements as a way of determining the meaning he attributes to Hurricane Katrina. This interaction also assists the nurse in determining where in the transition process Wayne is; for instance, the nurse is able to determine that Wayne remains in the process of transitioning his experience. Identifying the process Wayne uses to define and redefine his various roles

including his new one as a potentially HIV-positive patient; his at-risk ones, including partaking in drugs, alcohol, and unprotected sex; and his old ones as college student offer insight about his coping strategies and patterns of response. Milestones or critical points are periods of heightened vulnerability in which a person experiences difficulty with self-care. Although Wayne's story is rife with critical points, the one the nurse is most immediately concerned with is Wayne's symptoms of depression and his anxiety over taking an HIV blood test. Recognizing that Wayne has a limited support system, the nurse's interventions to address his feelings of depression are aimed at identifying a counselor and encouraging participation in reference or support groups. To address Wayne's anxiety and uncertainty over taking an HIV blood test the nurse provides supportive dialogue, expertise about where to get tested, offers to schedule an appointment at a local clinic, discusses the process of taking the test, and identifies a counselor. Debriefing serves to provide context and meaning about Wayne's experiences with Hurricane Katrina as a traumatic change trigger. The nurse uses clarifying questions and authentic presence to encourage Wayne to share his personal experiences, and in doing so, Wayne is able to find meaning in his experience.

Summary

Using authentic presence and awareness in this nursing situation created a space where Wayne and I could connect and develop a relationship grounded in trust and caring. This caring relationship provided an opportunity for Wayne to share his experiences, fears, and anxieties with me. A caring-based philosophy of nursing guided by Meleis's transitions theory served as the lens through which I was able to recognize Wayne's symptoms as critical points or milestones rather than medical diagnoses. I was also able to understand Hurricane Katrina as a major change trigger in Wayne's life, which guided my nursing interventions. Without this, Wayne could easily have left the clinic not

Continued

Practice Exemplar by Diane Lee Gullett, MSN, MPH cont.

receiving the care he needed, resulting in delayed testing for HIV, prolonged illness, and perhaps suicide. Through clarifying questions, I was able to gain insight into the meaning of Wayne's lived experience with Hurricane Katrina and identify his current and past coping strategies for adjusting to these changes. Not recognizing Katrina as a change trigger may have led me to assume Wayne's symptoms were a result of other factors in his life. Wayne has experienced multiple transitions in the 7 years since Hurricane Katrina, resulting in many unhealthy outcomes. His transition from living and attending school in N.O. to having to do the same in Baton Rouge resulted in him going from an honors student to a college dropout. His transition from living in N.O. before Katrina to living in N.O. after Katrina caused Wayne to have an emotional and mental breakdown. Without appropriate interventions or support, Wayne was unprepared for the reality of the multiple changes in his life following Hurricane Katrina. Wayne responded with ineffective coping strategies identified as milestones or critical points and included unprotected homosexual sex, using drugs and alcohol, and dropping out of school. These responses generated unhealthy outcomes manifested in Wayne's current complaints of depression, insomnia, lethargy, and possibly HIV. Recognizing Wayne's current symptoms as a critical point, I was able to develop appropriate nursing interventions. These included debriefing, providing resources, and setting goals. Contemporary approaches to disaster remain, dominated by biomedical models of care grounded in objective rather than subjective perspectives. This approach may work in the short term when the physical needs are paramount; however, when the needs of individuals transitioning a disaster extend beyond the physical, biomedical approaches will fail to address their more holistic needs. Preventing unhealthy outcomes such as those Wayne experienced will require a more holistic approach to nursing in disaster. Framing individual and collective responses to natural disaster using a nursing theoretical lens such as Meleis's transition theory serves as a foundation for generating disciplinary specific knowledge and research on nursing in disaster.

■ Summary

Transitions theory continues to be used to advance nursing knowledge about the experience and the responses of the many transitions that individuals, families, communities, and organizations encounter as well as the experiences, the responses, and the therapeutics that nurses use, translating the theory to policy, research, and evidence-based practice and better quality care in the 21st century. It is for its potential, its utility, and for the research programs that have and could emanate from it that we have defined nursing as "facilitating transitions to enhance a sense of well-being" (Meleis & Trangenstein, 1994).

References

Benner, P., Tanner, C., & Chesla, C. (1996). *Expertise in nursing practice: Caring, clinical judgment and ethics.* New York: Springer.

Blum, K., & Sherman, D. (2010). Understanding the experience of caregivers: A focus on transitions. *Seminars in Oncology Nursing, 26*(4), 243–258.

Bridges, W. (1980). *Making sense of life's changes: Transitions.* Menlo Park, CA: Addison-Wesley.

Bridges, W. (1991). *Managing transitions: Making the most of changes.* Menlo Park, CA: Addision, Wesley.

Carper, B. A. (1978). Fundamental patterns of knowing in nursing. *Advances in Nursing Science, 1*(1), 13–24.

Chaboyer, W. (2006). Intensive care and beyond: Improving the transitional experiences for critically ill patients and their families. *Intensive and Critical Care Nursing, 22*, 187–193.

Chiang, L., Chen, W., Dai, Y., & Ho, Y. (2012) The effectiveness of telehealth care on caregiver burden, mastery of stress, and family function among family caregivers of heart failure patients: A quasi-experimental study. *International Journal of Nursing Studies*.

Chick, N., & Meleis, A. I. (1986). Transitions: A nursing concern. In P. L. Chinn (Ed.), *Nursing research methodology* (pp. 237–257). Boulder, CO: Aspen.

Christakis, N. A., & Allison, P. D. (2006). Mortality after hospitalization of a spouse. *New England Journal of Medicine, 354*(7), 719–730.

Clayton State University. (2012). *Program philosophy—School of Nursing*. Retrieved from www.clayton.edu/health/nursing/philosophy

Duggleby, W., Penz, K., Goodridge, D., Wilson, D., Leipert, B., Berry, P., et al. (2010). The transition experience of rural older persons with advanced cancer and their families: A grounded theory study. *BMC Palliative Care, 9*, 5.

Fex, A., Gullvi, F., Ek, A., & Soderhamn, O. (2010). Health-illness transition among persons using advanced medical technology at home. *Scandinavian Journal of Caring Studies, 25*, 253–261.

Goyal, D., Wang, E., Shen, J., Wong, E., & Palaniappan, L. (2012). Clinically identified postpartum depression in Asian American mothers. *Journal of Obstetric, Gynecologic, and Neonatal Nursing (JOGNN), 41*(3), 408–416.

Halding, A., & Heggdal, K.(2011). Patients' experiences of health transitions in pulmonary rehabilitation. *Nursing Inquiry, 19*(4), 345–356.

Hall, J. M., Stevens, P. E., & Meleis, A. I. (1994). Marginalization: A guiding concept for valuing diversity in nursing knowledge development. *Advances in Nursing Science, 16*(4), 23–41.

Hattar-Pollara, M. (2010). Developmental transitions. In A. Meleis (Ed.), *Transitions theory: Middle-range and situation specific theories in nursing research and practice* (pp. 87–94). New York: Springer.

Huff, C. (2006). Emotional debriefing: Hospitals give staff new ways to cope with stress and sadness at work. *Hospitals and Health Networks, 80*(8), 38.

Im, E. (2008). The situation-specific theory of pain experience for Asian American cancer patients. *Advances in Nursing Science, 31*(4), 319–331.

Im, E. (2010). A situation-specific theory of Asian immigrant women's menopausal symptom experience in the U.S. *Advances in Nursing Science, 33*(2), 143–157.

Kralik, D., Visentin, K., & van Loon, A. (2006). Transition: A literature review. *Journal of Advanced Nursing, 55*(3), 320–329.

Kübler-Ross, E. (1969). *On death and dying*. New York: Touchstone.

Larkin, P. J., Dierckx de Casterlé, B., & Schotsmans, P. (2007). Transition towards end of life in palliative care: An exploration of its meaning for advanced cancer patients in Europe. *Journal of Palliative Care, 23*(2), 69–79

Lindemann, E. (1979). *Beyond grief: Studies in crisis intervention*. New York: Jason Aronson.

Marnocha, S. K., Bergstrom, M., & Dempsey, L. F. (2011). The lived experience of perimenopause and menopause. *Contemporary Nurse, 37*(2), 229–240.

Meleis, A. I. (1975). Role insufficiency and role supplementation: A conceptual framework. *Nursing Research, 24*, 264–271.

Meleis, A. I. (1985). *Theoretical nursing: Development and progress*. Philadelphia, PA: J.B. Lippincott Publishers.

Meleis, A. I. (1991). *Theoretical nursing: Development and progress* (2nd ed.). Philadelphia, PA: J. B. Lipincott Publishers.

Meleis, A. I. (1997). *Theoretical nursing: Development and progress* (3rd ed.). Philadelphia, PA: Lippincott Williams & Wilkins.

Meleis, A. I. (2007). *Theoretical nursing: Development and progress* (4th ed.). Philadelphia, PA: Lippincott Williams & Wilkins.

Meleis, A. I. (2010). *Transitions theory: Middle-range and situation-specific theories in nursing research and practice*. New York: Springer.

Meleis, A. I. (2012). *Theoretical nursing: Development and progress* (5th ed.). Philadelphia, PA: Lippincott Williams & Wilkins.

Meleis, A. I., Sawyer L., Im, E., Schumacher, K., & Messias, D. (2000). Experiencing transitions: An emerging middle range theory. *Advances in Nursing Science, 23*(1), 12–28.

Meleis, A. I., & Swendsen, L. (1978). Role supplementation: An empirical test of a nursing intervention. *Nursing Research, 27*, 11–18.

Meleis, A. I., & Trangenstein, P. A. (1994). Facilitating transitions: Redefinition of a nursing mission. *Nursing Outlook, 42*(6), 255–259.

Mendes, A. I., Bastos, F., & Paiva, A. (2010). The person with heart failure: Factors that facilitate/impede the health/disease transition. *Revista de Enfermagem Referência [Journal of Nursing Reference], III*(2), 7–16.

Mercer, R. T. (2004). Becoming a mother versus maternal role attainment. *Nursing Scholarship, 36*(3), 226–232.

Messias, D. K. H. (1997). *Narratives of transnational migration, work, and health: The lived experiences of Brazilian women in the United States*. Unpublished doctoral dissertation, School of Nursing, University of California, San Francisco.

Munhall, P. L. (1993). "Unknowing": Toward another pattern of knowing in nursing. *Nursing Outlook, 41*, 125–128.

Naylor, M. (2002). Transitional care of older adults. In P. Archbold & B. Stewart (Eds.), *Annual review of nursing research* (Vol. 20, pp. 127–147). New York: Springer.

Petch, A. (2009). *Managing transition: Support for individuals at key points of change*. Bristol: The Policy Press.

Polanyi, M. (1962) *Personal knowledge.* London: Routledge and Kegan Paul.

Rew, L., Tyler, D., & Hannah, D. (2012). Adolescents' concerns as they transition through high school. *Advances in Nursing Science, 35*(3), 205–221.

Sapega, S. (2012). Those first days in clinical. *Penn Medicine,* XXIII(3), 12–14

Sarvimaki, A. (1994). Science and tradition in the nursing discipline. *Scandinavian Journal of Caring Sciences, 8*(3), 137–142.

Schumacher, K., & Meleis, A. I. (1994). Transitions: A central concept in nursing. *Image: Journal of Nursing Scholarship, 26*(2), 119–127.

Schumacher, K. L., Jones, P. S., & Meleis, A. I. (1999). Helping elderly persons in transition: A framework for research and practice. In E. A. Swanson & T. Tripp-Reimer (Eds.), *Life transitions in the older adult: Issues for nurses and other health professionals* (pp. 1-26). New York: Springer.

Shin, H., & Whitetraut, R. (2007). The conceptual structure of transition to motherhood in the neonatal intensive care unit. *Journal of Advanced Nursing, 58*(1), 90–98.

Steele, A. M., & Beadle, M. (2003). A survey of postnatal debriefing. *Journal of Advanced Nursing, 43*(2), 130–136.

Stevens, P. E., Hall, J. M., & Meleis, A. I. (1992). Examining vulnerability of women clerical workers from five ethnic racial groups. *Western Journal of Nursing Research, 14*(6), 754–774.

Swendsen, L., Meleis, A. I., & Jones, D. (1978). Role supplementation for new parents: A role mastery plan. *The American Journal of Maternal Child Nursing, 3*, 84–91.

van Staa, A. (2010). *Book review: "Managing transition: Support for individuals at key points of change." International Journal of Integrated Care, 10*(22), 1–2.

Katharine Kolcaba's Comfort Theory

Chapter 21

KATHARINE KOLCABA

Introducing the Theorist
Overview of the Theory
Application of the Theory
Practice Exemplar
References
Appendix A

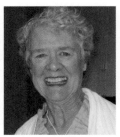

Katharine Kolcaba

Introducing the Theorist

Katharine Kolcaba was born and educated in Cleveland, Ohio. In 1965, she received a diploma in nursing and practiced part time for many years in the operating room, medical–surgical units, long-term care, and home care before returning to school. In 1987, she graduated with the first RN to MSN class at the Frances Payne Bolton School of Nursing, Case Western Reserve University (CWRU), with a specialty in gerontology. While attending graduate school, Kolcaba maintained a head nurse position on a dementia unit. In the context of that unit, she began theorizing about comfort.

After graduating with her master's degree in nursing, Kolcaba joined the faculty at the University of Akron (UA) College of Nursing, where her clinical expertise was gerontology and dementia care. She returned to CWRU to pursue her doctorate in nursing on a part-time basis while teaching full time. Over the next 10 years, she used course work from her doctoral program to further develop her theory. During that time, Kolcaba published a framework for dementia care (1992a), diagrammed the aspects of comfort (1991), operationalized comfort as an outcome of care (1992b), contextualized comfort in a middle range theory (1994), tested the theory in several intervention studies (Kolcaba & Fox, 1999; Kolcaba, 2003; Kolcaba, Dowd, Steiner, & Mitzel, 2004; Kolcaba, Tilton, & Drouin, 2006; Dowd, Kolcaba, Steiner, & Fashinpaur, 2007), and further refined the theory to include hospital-based outcomes (2001). She has an extensive series of publications to document each step in the process, most of which have been compiled in her book *Comfort Theory and Practice* (2003). Many publications and comfort assessments also are available on her website at www.TheComfortLine.com.

Kolcaba taught nursing at UA for 22 years and is now an associate professor emerita. Kolcaba still teaches her web-based theory course once a year, and she represents her own company, The Comfort Line, as a consultant. In this capacity, she works with health-care agencies and hospitals that choose to apply comfort theory on an institution-wide basis. She also is founder and member of her local parish nurse program and is a member of the American Nurses Association and Sigma Theta Tau. Kolcaba continues to work with students at all levels and with nurses who are conducting comfort studies. She resides in the Cleveland area with her husband, and near her two daughters, their children, and her mother. One other daughter resides in Chicago.

Overview of the Theory

In *comfort theory* (CT), comfort is a noun or an adjective and an outcome of intentional, patient/family focused, quality care. Despite everyone's familiarity with the idea of comfort, it is a complex term that has several meanings and usages in ordinary language. The use of comfort as a noun and an outcome is specific to CT and different from its alternative usages as a verb, adverb (as in comfortably), and process (Kolcaba, 1995). From the Oxford English Dictionary, Kolcaba learned that the original definition of comfort meant "to strengthen greatly." Her assumptions were that (1) the need for comfort is basic, (2) persons experience comfort holistically, (3) self-comforting measures can be healthy or unhealthy, and (4) enhanced comfort (when achieved in healthy ways) leads to greater productivity.

From the nursing literature, Kolcaba used three nursing theories to describe three distinct types of comfort (Kolcaba, 2003). *Relief* was synthesized from the work of Orlando (1961/1990), who stated that nurses relieved the needs expressed by patients. *Ease* was synthesized from the work of Henderson (1978), who described 13 basic functions of humans that needed to be maintained for homeostasis. *Transcendence* was derived from Paterson and Zderad (1976), who believed that patients could rise above their difficulties with the help of nurses. These types of comfort were consistent with usages in nursing textbooks.

The four contexts in which comfort is experienced by patients are physical, psychospiritual, sociocultural, and environmental and came from a further review of literature regarding holism in nursing (Kolcaba, 1991, 2003). When these four contexts of experience are juxtaposed with the three types of comfort, a taxonomic structure (TS), or grid, is created that covers the nursing meaning of comfort as a patient outcome. This TS, with definitions of each type and context of comfort, provides a map of the content of comfort so that nurses can use it to pattern their care for each patient and family member. Kolcaba's technical definition of the outcome of comfort is: The immediate experience of being strengthened when needs for relief, ease, and transcendence are addressed in four contexts of experience. Figure 21-1 contains the TS of comfort with the corresponding definitions of relief, ease, transcendence and the physical, psychospiritual, environmental, and sociocultural contexts.

Other uses of the TS of comfort are as follows: (1) for determining the existence and extent of unmet comfort needs in patients or family members; (2) for designing comforting interventions, which often can be "bundled" in a single patient interaction; and (3) for creating measurements of holistic comfort for documentation in practice and research; such measurements would be conducted before and after comfort interventions and/or interactions. A place to note the nature and time of the nursing intervention next to baseline and subsequent comfort measurements is essential in medical records. These strategies are discussed further in a later section of this chapter.

One way to think about the grid is that comfort is an umbrella outcome that entails relief from discomforts such as anxiety, pain, environmental stressors, and/or social isolation. Because the TS represents a holistic definition of comfort, the cells on the grid are interrelated; and as a whole, comfort interventions directed to one part of the grid have effects on all parts of the grid. Total comfort at any one time is also greater than the sum of its individual parts.

	Relief	Ease	Transcendence
Physical	Pain		
Psychospiritual	Anxiety		
Environmental			
Sociocultural			

Type of comfort:

Relief: the state of having a specific comfort need met.

Ease: the state of calm or contentment.

Transcendence: the state in which one can rise above problems or pain.

Context in which comfort occurs:

Physical: pertaining to bodily sensations, homeostatic mechanisms, immune function, etc.

Psychospiritual: pertaining to internal awareness of self, including esteem, identity, sexuality, meaning in one's life, and one's understood relationship to a higher order or being.

Environmental: pertaining to the external background of human experience (temperature, light, sound, odor, color, furniture, landscape, etc.)

Sociocultural: pertaining to interpersonal, family, and societal relationships (finances, teaching, health care personnel, etc.) Also to family traditions, rituals, and religious practices.

Adapted with permission from Kolcaba, K. & Fisher, E. A holistic perspective on comfort care as an advance directive. Crit Care Nurs Q,18(4):66-76, (c)1996. Aspen Publishers.

Fig 21 • 1 Taxonomic structure of comfort (or comfort grid).

Therefore, comfort interventions to treat anxiety also may reduce the dosage of analgesia needed for adequate pain relief. On a comfort continuum, the concept of *total comfort* (as much as can be expected given the circumstances) is at one extreme end, and *suffering* is at the other end.

Propositions of Comfort Theory

CT contains three intuitive parts that can be applied or tested separately or as a whole. The first part states that comforting interventions, when effective, result in increased comfort for recipients (patients and families), compared with a preintervention baseline. Increased comfort is the immediate desired outcome for this kind of care. Comfort interventions address basic human needs, such as rest, homeostasis, therapeutic communication, and viewing patients holistically. These comfort interventions are often nontechnical and complement delivery of technical care. Care providers, such as nurses, may also be considered recipients if the institution makes a commitment to improving comfort in its work setting (discussed later).

When comfort is not enhanced to the fullest extent possible, nurses consider intervening variables for possible explanations as to why comfort interventions did not work. Abusive homes, lack of financial resources, devastating diagnoses, or cognitive/psychological impairments may render ineffective the most appropriate interventions and comforting actions. The aspect of transcendence, however, guides nurses to help patients "rise above" or be inspired to achieve mutually determined goals regardless of life circumstances. Nurses who practice CT never give up "being with" and inspiring their patients. Thus, this focus on comfort is proactive, energized, intentional, and longed for by recipients of care in all settings.

The second part of CT states that increased comfort of recipients results in their being strengthened for their tasks ahead, which are called health-seeking behaviors (HSBs). HSBs are subsequent recipient goals and are negotiated between nurses and the recipients. In the practice of nursing administration, when the intended recipients are bedside nurses, HSBs are negotiated with nursing staff.

The third part of CT states that increased engagement in HSBs results in increased *institutional integrity* (InI). Enhanced InI strengthens the institution and its ability to gather evidence for best practices and best policies. Best practices and policies lead to quality care, which, in many ways, benefits the "bottom financial line" of the institution.

Kolcaba believes that nurses already know how and want to practice comforting care and that it can be easily incorporated into every nursing action. Many nurses deliver comforting care intuitively but do not document its total effects on patients as enhanced comfort. The explicit focus on and documentation of this type of holistic care is called comfort management and, as shown in the TS, includes more than relief of pain or anxiety. Thus, when nurses adopt CT as a professional practice model, they are using a simple pattern for individualized care that is efficient, creative, and satisfying to themselves and to recipients of their care. When enhanced comfort is documented, nurses can also demonstrate their real contributions to better institutional outcomes such as higher patient satisfaction, fewer readmissions, or shorter length of stay. The diagram of CT shows the relationships between these simple concepts (Fig. 21-2). Definitions of the concepts follow the diagram.

Theoretical Definitions for Diagram Concepts

In the context of comfort theory, **health-care needs** are defined as needs for comfort, arising from stressful health-care situations that cannot be met by recipients' traditional support systems. They include physical, psychospiritual, sociocultural, and environmental needs made apparent through monitoring and verbal or nonverbal reports, needs related to pathophysiological parameters, needs for education and support, and needs for financial counseling and intervention.

Comfort interventions are defined as intentional actions designed to address specific comfort needs of recipients, including physiological, social, cultural, financial, psychological, spiritual, environmental, and physical interventions. Within these contexts of experience, there are three types of comfort interventions (described later): technical, coaching, and comfort food for the soul.

Intervening variables are defined as interacting forces that influence recipients' perceptions of total comfort. These consist of variables such as past experiences, age, attitude, emotional state, support system, prognosis, finances, education, cultural background, and the totality of elements in recipients' experience. They are not easily influenced by nurses.

Comfort was defined technically earlier in this chapter. It is the state that is experienced immediately by recipients of comfort interventions. It entails the holistic experience of *being strengthened* through having comfort needs addressed.

The concept of **health-seeking behaviors** was developed by Dr. Rozella Schlotfeldt (1975) and represents the broad category of subsequent outcomes related to the pursuit of health. Schlotfeldt stated that HSBs could be internal or external. She was ahead of her time in thinking that a peaceful death could also be an HSB

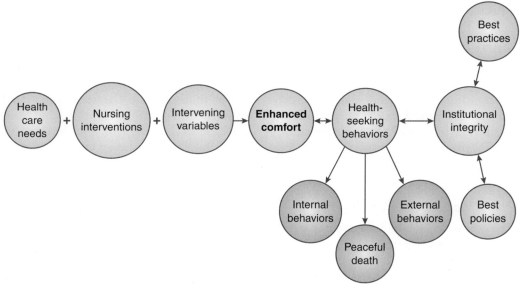

Fig 21 • 2 Conceptual framework for comfort theory.

(Schlotfeldt, 1975). Realistic HSBs are determined by recipients of care in collaboration with their health-care team.

Institutional integrity is defined as those corporations, communities, schools, hospitals, regions, states, and countries that possess qualities of being complete, whole, sound, upright, appealing, ethical, and sincere. When an institution displays this type of integrity, it can produce valuable evidence for best practices and best policies. **Best practices** are health-care interventions that produce the best possible patient and family outcomes based on empirical evidence. **Best policies** are institutional or regional policies, ranging from basic protocols for procedures and medical conditions to systems for access and delivery of health care. Best policies are also determined from empirical evidence.

As stated previously, the diagram and specific definitions for the concepts in CT provide a pattern and practical rationale for practicing comfort management. This kind of care is individualized, efficient, holistic, and therapeutic. Importantly, the nurturing aspect of nursing provides the altruistic motivation for practicing comfort management. It is the traditional mission and passion of nursing (Kolcaba, 2003; Morse, 1992). But the practical rationale is important at the institutional level because without administrative support for optimal staffing and employment practices, nurses often cannot give the kind of care that drew them to the profession.

For teaching and learning purposes, care plans based on CT are provided on Kolcaba's website and in her book (Kolcaba, 2003). One is for patients, and one is for patients and family members, as defined by the patient. (Note: For teaching and learning, it is not necessary to distinguish among relief, ease, and transcendence when assessing and intervening for unmet comfort needs.) Institutional outcomes can be included in the care plans even if these data are not accessible to students and beginning nurses (Kolcaba, 1995). These care plans can also be applied in home care and in long-term care.

Application of the Theory in Practice

As noted earlier, according to CT, there are three types of comforting interventions: technical, coaching, and comfort food for the soul. *Technical interventions* are those that are specified by other disciplines or by nursing protocols; they include medications, treatments, monitoring schedules, insertion of lines, and so forth. For patients, competency in the administration and documentation of technical interventions is the minimum expectation for nurses. *Coaching* consists of supportive nursing actions, active listening, referrals to other members of the health-care team, advocacy, reassurance, and so forth. *Comfort food for the soul* comprises those extra special, holistic, and more time-consuming nursing interventions such as back or hand massage, guided imagery, music or art therapy, a walk outside, or special arrangements for family members. The latter two types of interventions require considerably more expertise and confidence of nurses and are what patients most remember. And they are what Benner (1984) would ascribe to "expert" nurses.

However, most nurses focus on technical interventions first and, when time permits, implement coaching techniques. Interestingly, charting usually accounts only for technical interventions and the effects of analgesia; there are no places in traditional hospital records to record the more important healing interventions. But patients rarely remember the technical interventions; the important interventions to patients and their families are those that are not documented, such as coaching and comfort food for the soul, the most important work of expert nurses. Thus, there is a perpetual disconnect between legal charting and actions that patients want and need from their nurses and which we claim to be the essence of nursing. It is no wonder that, when pressed, nurses cannot describe the impact they make with patients and their families—coaching and comfort food interventions are not valued by administrators and are not even visible in patient care records. This can result in the value of nursing being understated or even invisible.

CT provides the language and rationale to once again claim and document essential nursing activities that are most beneficial to patients and family members in stressful health-care situations. It is also important to remember that the outcome of enhanced comfort is positive outcome and a true measure of quality care, rather than a measure of what quality care *is not*, such as the currently measured outcomes of nosocomial infections, falls, decubitus ulcers, medication errors, and failure to rescue. (Would *you* want to go to a hospital that was looking only at negative outcomes such as medication errors or "failures to rescue"?)

How to Be a Nurse

CT guides nurses to detect comfort needs of patients and families that are not being addressed and to develop interventions to meet those needs. Their caring actions are intuitive, but in this theory, caring is a comfort intervention in and of itself. CT describes how to care and how to BE a nurse, what is important to patients and families, and factors that facilitate healing. In addition, all technical nursing interventions are delivered in a comforting way.

Nurses and patients want to experience intentional and meaningful moments with each other and with family members, the kind that patients might call *wow moments*. ("Wow! I'll always remember that nurse.") Nurses usually sense when this happens, and these instances are sustaining, satisfying, and profound for them as well as for their patients. But nurses often fail to understand and share how the moment intentionally came to be created, especially if they practice without a theory. These special instances require appropriate theories to add both personal and disciplinary structure and meaning to such experiences (Chinn, 1998). CT is one such theory and can give structure to these experiences. CT states that the process of comforting a patient entails the *intention* to comfort, to be present, and to deliver comforting interventions based on the patient's and loved ones' unmet comfort needs (Kolcaba, 2003; Kolcaba online at http://www.thecomfortline.com/). If the patient needs time to voice concerns and questions, the nurse listens attentively and provides culturally appropriate encouragement and body language (a comforting intervention). The nurse knows exactly why and when to do this, because he or she is tuned into the whole person as patient and because the nurse wants to provide comfort, to soothe in times of distress and sorrow. Such an explanation of how to *be* a nurse is lacking in many other theories.

Institutional Advocacy

It is not enough for institution administrators to state that they want nurses and other care providers to practice comforting care—they need to implement documentation and reinforcement strategies to ensure this is done and to show that they value this kind of care. If administrators do not take on this responsibility, practicing nurses can be self-advocates and begin to document comforting interventions and their effects in narrative charting. Whether top-down and/or from the grassroots, the institutional ideal is for health-care institutions to provide ways in which comfort needs of patients and family members are routinely charted, beginning with baseline comfort levels. Comforting interventions are described and implemented, and comfort levels are reassessed and charted. Modifications to the interventions are made until comfort levels are sufficiently increased. Preferences of patients and families are honored wherever possible. In appropriate settings, comfort contracts (Appendix A) can be instituted and followed throughout a defined clinical situation such as surgery, labor and delivery, or an acute psychiatric episode.

According to CT, technical interventions should be documented as usual (often on a checklist including times), but methods of intentional caring also should be documented—in the same way that administration of pain medication is noted in two places. There are many suggestions for documentation on the instrument section at Kolcaba's website, including a verbal rating scale, a numeric diagram, comfort daisies for children, a comfort behaviors checklist for nonverbal or unresponsive patients, and several questionnaires about patient comfort for different research settings. These instruments can be downloaded from the website and used in practice and/or research, without permission because the website is in the public domain. The address is www.TheComfortLine.com.

In addition to providing methods for documentation of comfort needs and comforting measures, there are other ways that institutions can demonstrate their commitment to comfort management. These include building comfort management into orientation, in-service programs, performance reviews, and methods for nursing assignments (based in part on comfort needs of patients and family members).

Institutional Awards

Institutions have adopted CT to enhance nurses' work environments, such as in the quest for national recognition including Magnet Status, the Baldrich Award, and the Beacon Award. Many institutions discover that the application process for these types of awards is simplified when a professional practice model is adopted. The main benefit of doing so is that employees are on the "same page"—in the case of CT, comforting patients and family members in their own personalized styles and capacities. Moreover, and perhaps most important, administrative commitment to CT includes sufficient staffing levels in all departments to support this type of holistic health care. A large hospital system that adopted CT to undergird their application for Magnet Status and was successful in achieving Magnet Status shortly thereafter is Southern New Hampshire Medical Center (SNHMC; Kolcaba, Tilton, & Drouin, 2006).

When SNHMC decided to apply for Magnet Status, nurses from middle management formed a committee and reviewed several nursing theories. They chose CT because it most accurately reflected their values and goals. Kolcaba was contacted to arrange a consultative visit, which occurred after a sufficient time to prepare the other departments, including upper administrative levels, for the visit.

As part of this consultation, Kolcaba and the chief nursing officer visited all departments. They requested suggestions from the staff for ideas that would increase their comfort at work.

The many suggestions that were given came to be added to comfort "wish lists" on each unit. Another strategy adopted during this visit consisted of brief instructions about designing and implementing small "comfort studies" specific to each unit and to common clinical problems. The diagram of CT (see Fig. 21-2) defines the research process when comfort studies are undertaken, often a requirement for national awards. Any comforting intervention that is implemented by nurses, such as a "Comfort Cart" or hand massage demonstrate to evaluators how the practice model (CT) is implemented and that the nurses are conducting basic research. Strategies for publicizing the results of these studies as well as the institutional commitment to comfort management were also suggested.

The Meaning of Comfort Theory for Practice

Kolcaba routinely asks nurses and students in her audiences about their experiences during past hospitalizations, either as a patient or a family member. She asks if they remember any of their nurses, and if so, what do they remember? The stories that emerge are usually about nurses who demonstrated small, nontechnical, but very comforting acts of compassion and understanding. Examples of these interventions include the following: a brief back massage, helping a child make a phone call, sitting beside an anxious patient, making eye contact during an interaction, gently encouraging ambulation, listening attentively to role-change issues, holding a dying patient's hand, washing a patient's hair, making a family member comfortable during an overnight stay, and so forth. Patients remember these types of interventions for years after a stressful health-care episode because emotions run high and kind encounters are precious. Each is an example of a holistic comfort intervention that has greater positive effects on the patients' total comfort than could be imagined by the caregiver. These comforting interventions are examples of "wow moments" for receivers, and the exchange also renews the givers of such acts. Moreover, such comforting interventions can be delivered by any member of the health-care team or department within the context of their job description.

How Comfort Theory Lives in Practice

Best Practices

Currently, there is administrative interest in improving the "patient experience"—a factor that typically is measured by items on patient satisfaction instruments, the results of which are posted on public websites. The quality of the "patient experience," as rated by patients after a hospital stay, determines choices by insurance companies for future coverage of their enrollees. Often, these items are nursing sensitive, meaning that if nurses demonstrate simple comforting techniques, patients will respond favorably to those "patient experience" questions.

One administrative approach to enhancing the patient experience has been to implement scripting, in which members of the health-care team memorize specific prewritten statements to use during common patient encounters. An example is a standard script to be delivered on first introducing oneself to the patient such as, "Hello, I am Nurse Thomas, and I will be in charge of your care for today. If you need anything at all, please let me know." This approach may negate individualized care, the special needs of the patient and family, and the particular communication skills of the team member. And most patients can determine when such statements are prescripted, especially when they hear the same statements several times from different caregivers over the course of a hospital stay.

A different approach is to undergird all patient interactions with principles of CT, which caregivers learn in orientation and in-service programs. Principles of CT that are relevant to the patient experience are that (1) each interaction entails therapeutic use of self; (2) caregivers assess for comfort needs of patients and family members and design their interaction to meet those needs; (3) caregivers approach each patient and family member with the intent to comfort and make a personal, culturally appropriate connection; and (4) caregivers regularly reassess comfort of patients and family members and document comfort levels routinely. Using this approach facilitates individualized and efficient care and a more positive patient experience. Two

examples of how CT is being used to enhance the patient experience are at the Mount Sinai Hospital in New York City and at Kaiser Permanente Hospital in San Francisco.

Electronic Database

To support CT in practice, components have been incorporated into national electronic databases, such as the National Interventions Classification and the National Outcomes Classification systems (the Iowa Taxonomy) as well as the North American Nursing Diagnosis Association. Comforting interventions, comfort outcomes, and comfort diagnoses are included in these data systems, meaning that individualized comfort needs and the effectiveness of interventions to meet those needs can be charted electronically and entered into larger databases by a hospital system, at the local, state, region, or country level. Although there are at least 13 national databases for nursing, and others for medicine, when hospital systems select and contribute data to a mainstream system, documentation of patient care problems, interventions, and outcomes can be more widely compared, leading to more consistent and higher quality patient care practices. In this regard, an important feature of CT is the universality of its main concept, comfort. This is a word that is understood by all health-related disciplines and is translatable into most languages, as evident with the number of foreign language comfort instruments available on Kolcaba's website.

Best Policies

An example of how CT is used in practice is the creation of a policy for Comfort Management by the American Society of Peri-Anesthesia Nurses (ASPAN). This national association is composed of nurses who work in the following areas: ambulatory surgery, perioperative staging, operating room, postanesthesia recovery, and step-down. ASPAN decided collectively to apply CT in an explicit way throughout patients' surgical experiences. Kolcaba served as consultant and facilitator in this process.

First, they achieved national consensus about the development of Guidelines for Comfort

Management that would complement their existing Guidelines for Pain Management. The process proceeded with a survey of its membership about providing comfort to patients, then with a report of findings, then the conference about components of Comfort Management, and finally the composition of the guidelines (Kolcaba & Wilson, 2002; Wilson & Kolcaba, 2004).

The guidelines contain information about how to (1) perform a comfort assessment, (2) create a comfort contract with patients before surgery, (3) discover the interventions that patients and families use at home for specific discomforts, (4) use a checklist for comfort common management strategies, (5) document changes in comfort, and (6) implement pre- and post-testing for contact hours in comfort management. The completed Guidelines for Comfort Management are available on ASPAN's website (www.ASPAN.org). This is an example of a grassroots change (within a national association of nurses) that was disseminated to all perianesthesia settings and soon became a practice expectation. This example could be followed by any nursing specialty, at the macro level, or any patient care unit, at the micro level. The important point is that the model was initiated by nurses and is now an expectation that the Joint Commission reviews on recertification.

Practice Exemplar

When I received the night nurse's report about a new patient, Susan, I was told she was 55 years old, recovering from abdominal surgery where a large malignant tumor was discovered. This new diagnosis of cancer, and the subsequent cancer treatments to come, caused her to be very depressed. She was not eating and barely talking. I determined that I would try to get her to start eating and began a series of "comfort interventions."

I went into her room and introduced myself. Susan was crunched down in her bed, and her sheets were disheveled. I noticed her breakfast tray nearby, the cold scrambled eggs and everything else on the tray untouched. I asked her if she could eat or drink anything on the tray and she replied, "No." Her affect was flat and depressed, and she did not want to chat. My informal assessment concluded that her comfort needs were for improvements in the following: nutrition, mobility, positioning (physical needs); spirits and motivation (psychospiritual); social support, listening, understanding (sociocultural); and cleanliness of room, light and noise preferences, clean and tight linens (environmental).

I began implementing a comfort care plan automatically, asking Susan if anything at all might taste good to her? She weakly answered, "Maybe some cream of wheat." I told her I could order that. Then I asked if she could get into the chair so she could eat more easily. She agreed, and I helped her sit up. I adjusted the TV and shades in her room to her specifications, picked up tissues and trash, and put her call light at her fingertips. Already her affect improved a bit. I silenced the beeping IV pump . . . ahhhhh. "Are you comfortable?"

"Yes, I'm OK."

"Is there anything else I can do for you right now?"

"No." Telling her that I would return with the cream of wheat, I left the room, told a team member and the ward clerk that I would be in Susan's room, and asked them to try not to disturb us. I was going to help Susan eat some breakfast. I turned off my beeper, retrieved the cream of wheat, entered her room, and closed the door. We needed some uninterrupted time!

I sat down in front of her with the tray table between us, and I asked her if she needed help with the spoon. She nodded yes. I began spoon-feeding her the hot cereal with just the right amount of milk. Slowly, Susan began taking an interest in the cereal and me, asking me a few questions about myself as I did her. As we engaged in small talk, she continued to let me feed her, until the whole bowl was finished. "That tasted good," she said.

Continued

Practice Exemplar cont.

"I'm glad," I said. "You did very well. Now, I am going to see to my other patients and I'll look in on you again in about 15 minutes, which I was sure to do.

I had achieved two of the goals for my "plan" which was to (a) get Susan to start eating and (b) have her engage in conversation. I also gained a great deal of satisfaction from the encounter. I didn't realize it was a "Wow Moment" at the time, but for Susan it was. About

3 weeks later, I received a brief note from Susan who was now home. It is excerpted below:

It's your cream of wheat that started me back to recovery, but more than that, it was your tender loving care and time that I needed in my much weakened condition. It was quite an effort to raise my head to eat so I thank you and picture you feeding me very often in my mind. . . .Thank you for being a 'bedside nurse'!!

■ Summary

The midrange theory of comfort was first published in 1994 and has been tested repeatedly by nurse scientists since that time. Each test of the theory has supported the initial propositions, although many more tests need to be conducted on the relationships between patient/family goals and markers for institutional integrity. Instruments adapted and/or translated from the original General Comfort Questionnaire, the newer Comfort Behaviors Checklist, Comfort Daisies, and Verbal Rating Scale, and the General Comfort Questionnaire has been certified by AHRQ as a quality measure since 2003.

Comfort theory has also been applied frequently by health agencies and hospitals for the purpose of enhancing the work environment for staff and explicating a unifying theme for patient and family care. The theory is popular because it describes what expert nurses already know: One of the most important missions for nursing is *still* to bring comfort to our patients and families, no matter what their circumstances are. Comfort brings strength for those difficult health-care tasks that we must all face.

References

Benner, P. (1984). *From novice to expert.* Menlo Park, CA: Addison Wesley.

Chinn, P. L. (1998). Response to 'the comforting interaction": Developing a model of nurse-patient relationship. *Scholarly Inquiry for Nursing Practice, 11*(4), 345–347.

Dowd, T., Kolcaba, K., & Steiner, R. (2003). The addition of coaching to cognitive strategies: Interventions for persons with compromised urinary bladder syndrome. *Journal of Ostomy and Wound Management, 30*(2), 90–99.

Dowd, T., Kolcaba, K., Steiner, R., & Fashinpaur, D. (2007). Comparison of healing touch and coaching on stress and comfort in young college students. *Holistic Nursing Practice, 21*(4), 194–202.

Henderson, V. (1978). *Principles and practice of nursing.* New York: Macmillan.

Kolcaba, K. (1991). A taxonomic structure for the concept comfort. *Image: The Journal of Nursing Scholarship, 23*(4), 237–240.

Kolcaba, K. (1992a). The concept of comfort in an environmental framework. *Journal of Gerontological Nursing, 18*(6), 33–38.

Kolcaba, K. (1992b). Holistic comfort: Operationalizing the construct as a nurse-sensitive outcome. *ANS Advances in Nursing Science, 15*(1), 1–10.

Kolcaba, K. (1994). A theory of holistic comfort for nursing. *Journal of Advanced Nursing, 19*, 1178–1184.

Kolcaba, K. (1995). The art of comfort care. *Image: The Journal of Nursing Scholarship, 27*(4), 287–289.

Kolcaba, K. (2001). Evolution of the midrange theory of comfort for outcomes research. *Nursing Outlook, 49*(2), 86–92.

Kolcaba, K. (2003). *Comfort theory and practice: A vision for holistic health care and research* (pp. 113–124). New York: Springer.

Kolcaba, K., Dowd, T., Steiner, R., & Mitzel, A. (2004). Efficacy of hand massage for enhancing comfort of hospice patients. *Journal of Hospice and Palliative Care, 6*(2), 91–101.

Kolcaba, K., & Fox, C. (1999). The effects of guided imagery on comfort of women with early-stage breast cancer going through radiation therapy. *Oncology Nursing Forum, 26*(1), 67–71.

Kolcaba, K., Schirm, V., & Steiner, R. (2006). Effects of hand massage on comfort of nursing home residents. *Geriatric Nursing, 27*(2), 85–91.

Kolcaba, K., Tilton, C., & Drouin, C. (2006). Comfort theory: A unifying framework to enhance the practice environment. *Journal of Nursing Administration, 36*(11), 538–544.

Kolcaba, K., & Wilson, L. (2002). The framework of comfort care for perianesthesia nursing [with posttest for 1.2 contact hours]. *Journal of Perianesthesia Nursing, 17*(2), 102–114.

Morse, J. (1992) Comfort: The refocusing of nursing care. *Clinical Nursing Research. 1*(1), 91–106.

NQMC. (2014). National Quality Measures Clearinghouse, department of the *Agency for Healthcare Research and Quality.* 2014 Annual Verification Report.

Orlando, I. (1961/1990). *The dynamic nurse-patient relationship.* New York: National League for Nursing Press.

Paterson, J., & Zderad, L. (1976/1988). *Humanistic nursing.* New York: National League for Nursing Press.

Schlotfeldt, R. (1975). The need for a conceptual framework. In P. Verhonic (Ed.), *Nursing Research* (pp. 3–25). Boston: Little, Brown.

Wilson, L., & Kolcaba, K. (2004). Practical application of Comfort Theory in the perianesthesia setting. *Journal of PeriAnesthesia Nursing, 19*(3), 164–173.

Appendix A: Example of a Comfort Contract

Thank you for taking the time to complete the comfort contract. The purpose of this contract is to increase your comfort and pain management while you are hospitalized. Please rate your expectation of comfort from 0 to 10 (10 is highest) for each situation listed. Please use the comfort scale as directed for all items except when indicated otherwise and take your time and complete the following questions.

Developed by the following students at the University of Akron an distributed with their permission: Robert Bearss, Brent Ferroni, Ryan Hartnett, Kristy Kuzmiak, Brittney Stover, Spring 2006.

The Comfort Experience

1. I expect a comfort level of:
   a. _____ when the anesthesia wears off.
   b. _____ on postoperative day 1
   c. _____ on postoperative day 3 (when ambulating)
   d. _____ on postoperative day 5 (study conclusion day)
2. These interventions might assist to increase my comfort:
   Warming blanket (recovery room)
   Pet visitation
   Family visits (when anesthesia wears off)
   Music
   Cold washcloth
   Pillows—location: _____
   Massage
   Other _____
   (Circle All that Apply.)
3. In the past, I have required (small, moderate, large) amounts of pain medication to keep me comfortable.
4. I have had success with the following medications during my previous admissions to the hospital _____
5. The following medications I had taken have resulted in undesirable outcomes:

   _____

The undesirable outcomes have included:

_____
_____

Nursing Interventions

6. I prefer personal hygiene to be performed during the (morning, afternoon, evening).
7. I prefer my family to be present (all the time, occasionally, not at all) during my recovery.
8. I wish to have the following family member(s) present:_____.
9. I prefer to exclude the following persons from visiting my room_____.
10. I prefer to have a fan present in my room. (Yes/No)
11. I prefer updates regarding my status (only when asked, daily, not at all).

Extreme discomfort		Comfort				Extreme comfort		
1	2	3	4	5	6	7	8	9	10

Fig 21 • 3 Comfort scale.

Joanne Duffy's Quality-Caring Model©

JOANNE R. DUFFY

Introducing the Theorist
Overview of the Theory
Applications of the Model
Practice Exemplar
References

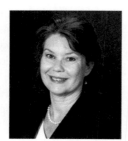

Joanne R. Duffy

Introducing the Theorist

Joanne R. Duffy, PhD, RN, FAAN, has had an extensive career encompassing clinical, administrative, and academic roles. Currently, she is the West Virginia University Hospitals Endowed Professor of Research and Evidence-based Practice and Interim Associate Dean for Research and PhD Education at the Robert C. Byrd Health Sciences Center, West Virginia University, Morgantown, WV, and is an Adjunct Professor at the Indiana University School of Nursing in Indianapolis, IN. She has directed four graduate nursing programs (critical care, care management, nursing administration, and a PhD program) and was a former Division Director of a school of nursing. She actively teaches nursing theory, research, and leadership in PhD, DNP, masters and honors programs, directs dissertations and scholarly projects, and interfaces with acute care health professionals and leaders to advance evidence-based practice. Dr. Duffy graduated from St. Joseph's Hospital School of Nursing in Providence, RI, completed her BSN at Salve Regina College in Newport, RI, and her master's and doctoral degrees at the Catholic University of America in Washington, DC.

Dr. Duffy has held clinical positions in intensive care, coronary care, and emergency services and is a cardiovascular clinical nurse specialist. She was an associate director of nursing at one urban hospital and two large academic medical centers, developed a Cardiovascular Center for Outcomes Analysis, and administrated a transplant center while simultaneously serving in academic appointments. Her special expertise in outcomes measurement has led to the focus of her work: maximizing health outcomes, particularly among older adults, through caring processes.

393

Dr. Duffy was the first to examine the link between nurse caring behaviors and patient outcomes and developed the caring assessment tool (including the newest version, the e-CAT) in multiple versions. She developed the middle-range quality-caring model© to guide professional practice and research, ultimately exposing the hidden value of nursing work. Dr. Duffy was the principal investigator on the national demonstration project, "Relationship-Centered Caring in Acute Care," has been the principal investigator for two caring-based intervention studies, and served as consultant to several multidisciplinary studies. Dr. Duffy was a consultant to the American Nurses Association (ANA) in the development and implementation of the National Database of Nursing Quality Indicators and the former chair of the National League for Nursing's Nursing Educational Research Advisory Council. Dr. Duffy is a Commonwealth Fund Executive Nurse Fellow, a recipient of several nursing awards, a Fellow in the American Academy of Nursing, a frequent guest speaker, and a former Magnet Appraiser. The first edition of her book, *Quality Caring in Nursing: Applying Theory to Clinical Practice, Education, and Research* received the AJN book of the year award in 2009. The second edition, *Quality Caring in Nursing and Health Systems: Implications for Clinical Practice, Education, and Leadership (2013),* focuses on caring relationships as the central organizing principle of health systems.

Overview of the Theory

The quality-caring model© was initially developed in 2003 to guide practice and research (Duffy & Hoskins, 2003). The seeds of the model were sown during discussions concerning nursing interventions, but it was informed from earlier work on caring (Duffy, 1992). While examining the outcomes variable of patient satisfaction in the late 1980s, Dr. Duffy uncovered that hospitalized patients who were dissatisfied often expressed, "Nurses just don't seem to care." This concern was corroborated in the literature and represented a clinical problem that significantly affected patients' perceptions of quality. Over time, Dr. Duffy

continued to study human interactions during illness, developing tools to measure caring (Duffy, 2002; Duffy, Brewer, & Weaver, 2014; Duffy, Hoskins, & Seifert, 2007) and studying the linkage between nurse caring and selected health-care outcomes (Duffy, 1992, 1993).

In 2002, it became apparent that there were few nursing theories that could guide the development of a caring-based nursing intervention while simultaneously speaking to the relationship between nurse caring and quality. As part of a research team, Drs. Duffy and Hoskins developed and tested the model in a group of heart failure patients (Duffy, Hoskins, & Dudley-Brown, 2005). Caring relationships were the core concept in this model and were believed to be integrated, although often hidden, in the daily work of nursing. This form of caring was considered different from the caring that occurs between family and friends because professional nurse caring requires specialized knowledge, attitudes, and behaviors that are specifically directed toward health and healing. Through this specialized knowledge, recipients feel "cared for," which was theorized as a positive emotion necessary for taking risks, feeling safe, learning new healthy behaviors, or participating effectively in decision making based on evidence. This sense of "feeling cared for" was considered an antecedent necessary to influence improved intermediate and terminal outcomes, particularly nursing-sensitive outcomes such as knowledge (including self-knowledge), safety, comfort, anxiety, adherence, human dignity, health, confidence, engagement, and positive experiences of care. Furthermore, the model was considered supportive to professional nursing because nurses themselves were theorized to benefit. Blending societal needs for measurable outcomes with the unique relationship-centered processes central to daily nursing practice represented a practical, postmodern approach.

The major purposes of the quality-caring model© at that time were to:

- Guide professional practice
- Describe the conceptual–theoretical–empirical linkages between quality of care and human caring
- Propose a research agenda that would provide evidence of the value of nursing

Because of the complexities of modern society, individuals, the health system, and the professionals who work in it, the Quality Caring Model© has evolved from its initiation in 2003. Since that time, the model has been revised twice (Fig. 22-1) to meet the demands of the multifaceted, interdependent, and global health system that "requires a more sophisticated workforce, one that understands the significance of systems thinking, whose practice is based on knowledge, multiple and oftentimes competing connections, and one that values relationships as the basis for actions and decision-making" (Duffy, 2009, p.192). In this revised version, the link between caring relationships and quality care is even more explicit, challenging the nursing profession to use caring relationships as the basis for daily practice. The revised model is considered a middle-range theory because it draws on others' work, is practical, and can be tested. It views quality as a dynamic, nonlinear characteristic that is influenced by caring

relationships. "Quality is not an endpoint per se, but a *process* of continuous learning and improvement . . . that treats patients as full partners . . . and is fully integrated into the work of health professionals" (Duffy, 2013, p. 31).

When caring relationships are the basis of nursing work, positive human connections are formed with patients and families that influence future interactions and positively influence intermediate health outcomes. Thus, caring is a *process* that involves a reciprocal relationship (characterized by caring factors) between human persons, whereby the positive emotion, "feeling cared for," is attained. It is this feeling of being "cared for" that matters in terms of enabling the conditions for *self-advancing systems*. As such, it is an essential performance indicator of quality nursing care. Caring relationships also are theorized to enhance interprofessional practice and benefit nurses themselves by maintaining congruence with professional values and contributing to meaningful work.

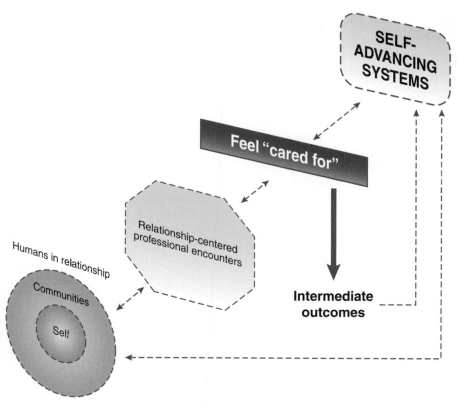

Fig 22 • 1 Revised quality-caring model©. *(From Duffy, J. [2013a]. Quality caring in nursing and health systems: Implications for clinicians, educators, and leaders [p. 34]. New York: Springer.)*

Concepts, Assumptions, and Propositions

In the latest revision of the quality-caring model©, there are four main concepts. The first is *humans in relationship.* This idea refers to the notion that humans are multidimensional beings with various characteristics that make them unique. Recognizing human characteristics, including how they differ and yet are the same, provides an understanding that influences human interactions and consequently, nursing interventions. Humans are also social beings connected to others through birth or in work, play, learning, worship, and local communities. It is through these connections that humans mature, enhance their communities, and advance.

Relationship-centered professional encounters consist of the independent relationship between the nurse and patient/family and the collaborative relationship that nurses establish with members of the health-care team. When these relationships are of a caring nature, the intermediate outcome of "feeling cared for" is generated. Embedded in this concept are the caring factors that are discussed in the next section. *Feeling cared for* is a positive emotion that signifies to patients and families that they matter. Caring relationships prompt this feeling, inciting persons', groups', and systems' capabilities to change, learn and develop, or self-advance. In other words, "feeling cared for" allows one to relax, feel secure, and get engaged in his or her health-care needs. It is an important antecedent to quality health outcomes, particularly those that are nursing-sensitive.

Patients and families who experience caring relationships from health-care providers are more apt to concentrate on their health, focus on learning about it, modify lifestyles, adhere to the recommendations and regimens, and actively participate in health-care decisions. They feel understood and more confident in their abilities. Over time, persons who experience caring interactions with health professionals progress or self-advance. *Self-advancing systems* is the final concept in this model. It is a phenomenon that emerges gradually over time and in space reflecting dynamic positive progress that enhances the systems' well-being. Self-advancing systems are stimulated by caring relationships, but the forward movement itself cannot be controlled directly; rather, it emerges over time, driven by caring connections. Self-advancing systems represent quality in the model because it is a dynamic concept that enhances an individual's or system's well-being.

The overall purposes of the revised quality-caring model© are to (1) guide professional practice and (2) provide a foundation for nursing research. It can also be used in nursing education (to guide curriculum development and facilitate caring student–teacher relationships) and in nursing leadership as a basis for human interactions and decision-making.

Assumptions of the revised quality-caring model© include the following:

- Humans are multidimensional beings capable of growth and change.
- Humans exist in relationship to themselves, others, communities or groups, nature (or the environment), and the universe.
- Humans evolve over time and in space.
- Humans are inherently worthy.
- Caring consists of processes that are used individually or in combination and often concurrently.
- Caring is embedded in the daily work of nursing.
- Caring is a tangible concept that can be measured.
- Caring relationships benefit both the carer and the one being cared for.
- Caring relationships benefit society.
- Caring is done "in relationship."
- Feeling "cared for" is a positive emotion.
- Professional nursing work is done in the context of human relationships. (Duffy, 2013, p. 33)

Propositions are those relational statements that tie model concepts to each other and in some instances can be the basis for hypothesis testing. Propositions of the quality-caring model© include the following:

Human caring capacity can be developed.
Caring relationships are composed of process or factors that can be observed.

Caring relationships require intent, specialized knowledge, and time.

Engagement in communities through caring relationships enhances self-caring.

Independent caring relationships between patients and health-care providers influence feeling "cared for."

Collaborative caring relationships among nurses and members of the health-care team influence feeling "cared for."

Caring relationships facilitate growth and change.

Feeling "cared for" is an antecedent to self-advancing systems.

Feeling "cared for" influences the attainment of intermediate and terminal health outcomes.

Self-advancement is a nonlinear, complex process that emerges over time and in space.

Self-advancing systems are naturally self-caring or self-healing.

Relationships characterized as caring contribute to individual, group, and system self-advancement (Duffy, 2013, p. 38)

Role of the Nurse

The overall role of the professional nurse in this model is to engage in caring relationships so that self and others feel "cared for" (Duffy, 2013, p. 33). Such actions positively influence intermediate and terminal health outcomes (self-advancement), including those that are nursing-sensitive.

The revised quality-caring model© specifically emphasizes the following responsibilities of professional nurses:

• Attain and continuously advance knowledge and expertise in caring processes.
• Initiate, cultivate, and sustain caring relationships with patients and families.
• Initiate, cultivate, and sustain caring relationships with other nurses and all members of the health-care team.
• Maintain an ongoing awareness of the patient/family point of view.
• Carry on self-caring activities, including personal and professional development.
• Integrate caring relationships with specific evidenced-based nursing interventions to positively influence health outcomes.

• Engage in continuous learning and practice-based research.
• Use the expertise of caring relationships embedded in nursing to actively participate in community groups.
• Contribute to the knowledge of caring and, ultimately, the profession of nursing using all forms of knowing.
• Maintain an open, flexible approach.
• Use measures of caring to evaluate nursing care. (Duffy, 2013, pp. 38–39)

Caring Relationships

There are four caring relationships essential to quality caring (Fig. 22-2). The first is the relationship with self. Because humans are multidimensional (comprising bio–psycho–social–cultural–spiritual components) that continuously interact in concert with the universe, their fundamental nature is integrated or whole. The many seemingly different parts relate to and depend on each other, generating an orientation of the self that represents a source of understanding often lost in the business of life. Individuals, particularly nurses, tend to go about their day habitually moving from one task to another without noticing their internal bodily processes, feelings, or connections with others. This externally driven focus separates individuals from those internal forces

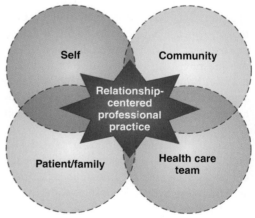

Fig 22 • 2 Four relationships necessary for quality caring. *(Copyright ©2013 J. Duffy. From Duffy, J. [2013a].* Quality caring in nursing and health systems: Implications for clinicians, educators, and leaders *[p. 53]. New York: Springer.)*

that hold a special knowledge of self. In nursing, professionals care for others and their families with ease, frequently "forgetting" to connect with self. Yet allowing oneself to slow down enough to access his or her own genuineness offers a clarity that is life enhancing. Some would say such inner awareness is necessary for authentic interaction and health (Davidson et al., 2003), whereas others (Siegel, 2007) believe it is necessary to adequately care for others. As human beings, professional nurses who are regularly "in touch" with themselves set up the conditions for self-caring, a state that offers a rich supply of energy and renewal.

In nursing, remaining self-aware is a necessary prerequisite for caring relationships because in knowing the self, it is possible to know others. Regular mindfulness activities such as prayer, meditation, quiet time, attention to physical health through regular exercise and proper nutrition, and creative activities, when performed in a conscious manner, promote insight. Likewise in the work environment, short pauses, consciously remembering to center on the person being cared for, attending to bodily needs such as nourishment and elimination, and even short time-outs ensure that the caring focus of nursing remains the priority. Reflective awareness by actively soliciting feedback about one's performance is another method of attaining self-knowledge that may offer professional nurses a boost in self-confidence or specific learning opportunities. Reflective analysis in which thoughts are actually documented in written or taped format and then analyzed for their subjective meanings can be used to inform clinical practice. Professional nurses need to acknowledge and reflect on the important work they do to value themselves and nursing, a precondition for caring relationships (Foster, 2004).

As the primary focus of nursing, patients and families who are ill are vulnerable and dependent on nurses for caring. Initiating, cultivating, and sustaining caring relationships with patients and families is an independent function of professional nursing that involves intention, choice, specific knowledge and skills, and time (Duffy, 2009). Intending to care depends on one's attitudes and beliefs; it shapes a nurse's choice and resulting behaviors, specifically whether "to care" for another. Such choice is a conscious decision that is required for effective caring relationships. Deep awareness of the self enhances caring intention and consequential behaviors become more positively focused toward the patient/family.

Collaborative relationships with members of the health-care team are essential to quality health care (Knaus, Draper, Wagner, & Zimmerman, 1986) and are depicted as an important relationship in the quality-caring model©. Nurses are already connected to one another by the work they do and with other members of the health team by the commonality of simultaneously providing services to patients and families. *But collaboration connotes mutual respect for the work of other health professionals and occurs best "in relationship."* Ongoing interaction is key to collaboration in order to seek the other's point of view, validate the work, share responsibilities, and evaluate the care. The quality-caring model© maintains that professional nurses have a responsibility for implementing collegial, caring interpersonal relationships with each other and members of the health-care team. Discussing specific clinical issues pertinent to patients, participating in joint rounds, improving quality or research projects, holding family conferences, and discharging rounds are all examples of positive collaboration that benefit not only patients and families but the health-care team as well. Affirming each other's unique contribution to patient care through genuine collaboration contributes to a healthy work environment that may increase work satisfaction.

Finally, caring for the communities nurses live and serve in reflects another caring relationship essential to the revised quality-caring model.© This relationship is predicated on the belief that humans interact with groups beyond the family to connect, share similar history and customs, and enhance the lives of each other. Engaging in communities provides professional nurses opportunities to use caring relationships as the basis for improving health or decreasing disease. Such activities contribute to the ongoing vitality of the community and enrich nurses' personal lives. The four relationships essential to quality caring, when well developed and practiced with knowledge of the caring factors, meets the needs of patients and families for quality health care.

The Caring Factors

Caring is not just a mindset or simple acts of kindness; rather, clinical caring requires knowledge (Mayerhoff, 1971) and skills, juxtaposed on caring values. Many have theorized about the qualities necessary for therapeutic relationships (Rogers, 1961; Yalom, 1975), but Watson (1979, 1985) identified 10 carative factors necessary for human caring in the patient–nurse relationship. Eight factors, reframed through research and clinical experience, are currently used to characterize caring in the quality-caring model©. These factors are specifically defined, facilitating the identification of specific cognitive and behavioral abilities necessary for caring relationships, and are as follows:

- Mutual problem-solving
- Attentive reassurance
- Human respect
- Encouraging manner
- Appreciation of unique meaning
- Healing environment
- Affiliation needs
- Basic human needs (Duffy, Hoskins, & Seifert, 2007)

The caring factors were initially derived from Watson's original work (Watson, 1979, 1985) but also are consistent with the intentions of other nursing theorists (Boykin & Schoenhofer, 1993; Henderson, 1980; Johnson, 1990; King, 1981; Leininger, 1981; Nightingale, 1992; Orem, 2001; Peplau, 1988; Roach, 1984; Roy, 1980; Swanson, 1991) and empirical research (Cossette, Cote, Pepin, Ricard, & D'Aoust, 2006; Boudreaux, Francis, & Loyacano, 2002; Campbell & Rudisill, 2006; Mangurten et al., 2006; Paul, Hendry, & Cabrelli, 2004; Wolf, Zuzelo, Goldberg, Crothers, & Jacobson, 2006). *Mutual problem-solving* refers to assisting patients and families to learn about, question, and participate in their health or illness. This is accomplished reciprocally and requires professional interaction that is informed and engaging. This factor recognizes that patients and families are the decision-makers in the health-care process and facilitating informed alternatives and adoption of their ideas is paramount.

Attentive reassurance refers to being available and offering a positive outlook to patients and families that helps them feel secure. Professional nurses who use this factor are able to "be with" their patients long enough to convey possibilities, focus on their unique needs, listen, and present some cheerful dialogue. *Human respect* implies valuing the human person of the other by acting in such a way that demonstrates that value. For example, calling a patient by his or her preferred name, performing tasks in a gentle manner, and maintaining eye contact show regard for the other. Using an *encouraging manner* or a supportive demeanor during interactions conveys confidence and is expressed both verbally and nonverbally. It is especially important to maintain uniformity between messages expressed and those implied by body language. *Appreciation of unique meanings* helps a patient feel understood because the nurse uses this factor to acknowledge what is significant to patients and families. In other words, nurses aim to see things from the patient's point of view and use his or her preferences and their sociocultural meanings in care. In this way, nurses tailor interventions to the patient's frame of reference. Cultivating a *healing environment*, including appealing surroundings, decreasing stressors (noise, lighting), ensuring patient privacy and confidentiality, and practicing in a safe manner are included in this factor. The particular norms and customs of a department in which a patient receives care also have an impact. This factor is especially important in acute care where adverse events remain a major source of harm, death, and disability for Americans (Fineberg, 2012). Ensuring that *basic human needs* are attended to during an illness (including the higher order needs; Maslow, 1954) has been a major role of the professional nurse that today is often delegated to unlicensed assistive personnel. Often this factor is blended with other nursing activities such as assessments, teaching and learning, and emotional support. Providing for basic human needs is an opportunity to further the development of caring relationships. Finally, appreciating the significance of *affiliation needs* refers to making sure that patients are not only allowed access to their families, but also that families are included in care decisions. Being open and approachable to families and keeping them informed is important to patients' well-being and should be a normal part of nursing care.

The caring factors are used "in relationship" with others and comprise the basis for the "knowledge and skills" required to practice according to the quality-caring model.© Using them is dependent on patient needs and the context of the situation. Not all factors are necessarily used at once; rather, the professional nurse uses his or her judgment to decide which are necessary for certain situations. When applied with expertise, these factors are theorized to positively affect recipients such that they feel "cared for." In fact, "feeling cared for" is a calming influence, allowing the patient to concentrate on the meaning of illness and the requirements for health and healing. Feeling cared for also sets up the conditions for future interactions with health professionals that sway eventual outcomes of care. "In other words, the patient's ability to progress is mediated somewhat by the feelings generated as a consequence of caring relationships" (Duffy, 2009, p. 72). Performing nursing in such a way that valuable time is spent predominantly in caring relationships with patients and families (i.e., using the caring factors) ensures that patients and families feel "cared for" and that health outcomes are positively impacted.

The caring factors are applicable to the other three relationships pertinent to the quality-caring model.© For example, collaborative relationships founded on the caring factors enhance teamwork and cooperation. As experts in caring, professional nurses are in a unique position to profoundly benefit the health-care system. Uniting caring knowledge and caring action(s) in relationships with self, patients and families, coworkers, and the community provides opportunities for creative innovations, improvements in practice, and a source of energy for future interactions. Furthermore, some nurses who practice this way describe richer work experiences that are naturally renewing (D'Antonio, 2008).

Applications of the Model
Clinical Practice

The quality-caring model© provides individual clinicians, teams of health professionals, educators, and leaders with a relationship-centric approach to health care. In doing so, it honors the interdependencies necessary for human advancement. For individual clinicians, it provides a "way of being with" patients and families (through the caring factors) that can be used to guide interventions, practice improvements, and ongoing learning about the self. For health-care teams, the model offers a way to relate to and engage with other health-care providers in care that is "best for the patient." The quality-caring model© offers health educators a caring pedagogy that honors caring relationships that are lived out through the behaviors of faculty members. In other words, teaching one "how to care" is dependent on the "caring milieu" generated by faculty members themselves who notice and share "caring moments," continuously reflect on the nature of nursing, and who use cognitive, psychomotor, and affective experiences to help students acquire the knowledge, skills, and attitudes of caring professionals. Likewise, relationship-centered leaders preserve the foundational caring patient–nurse relationship that gives nursing its identity, ensures ethical and legal services, and provides the nursing workforce with meaning.

In *Quality Caring in Nursing and Health Systems: Implications for Clinicians, Educators, and Leaders,* Duffy (2013a) highlights how many health systems are using the quality-caring model© to:

• Provide a foundation for patient-centered care
• Enhance interprofessional practice
• Facilitate staff-directed practice changes
• Redesign professional workflow
• Generate guiding principles for human resource practices
• Guide nurse residency programs
• Improve collective relational capacity
• Renew the meaning of nursing work
• Extend caring to others FIRST
• Build relationships with community groups

- Create a legacy of caring
- Sustain professionalism
- Revise nursing curricula
- Balance "doing" with "being"

Practice Improvement

Because caring relationships can be measured and their consequences assessed, the model affords an evaluation design for improvement of services. The quality-caring model© maintains that quality nursing care is based on the use of best evidence and asserts the nursing responsibility to engage in continuous learning, use measures of caring, and contribute to caring knowledge and practice-based research. Evaluation of nursing practice is an ongoing process that is tied to nurses' individual competency as well as the processes used in daily practice and their subsequent outcomes (both intermediate and terminal). Using the caring factors as the basis for competency statements or performance expectations from which individual nurses can complete self-evaluations, gather peer reviews, or be evaluated by their supervisors is a first step. A more comprehensive approach using the 360-degree method (Edwards & Ewen, 1996; London & Smither, 1995) provides assessments from the perspective of the one being evaluated (nurse self-evaluation), those being "cared for" (patients and families), the supervisor, and colleagues (other nurses, physicians, other members of the health-care team). This approach provides the one being evaluated with information about his/her performance from the perspective of recipients of his/her care. Thus, patients (those being "cared for") and colleagues (those within the health-care team) offer direct information about the nature of caring displayed by the nurse. Using these perspectives, the one being evaluated can reflect on this feedback, and then set personal goals for self-development, ultimately improving practice and benefitting themselves and others (self-advancement). The 360 degree approach to evaluating individual caring competence is thorough and relationship centered; it takes advantage of multiple sources and perspectives to provide important feedback about nursing practice.

Evaluating *processes* of care requires measuring the quality of caring relationships and using those data to efficiently revise practice. Although many performance improvement activities are conducted in today's health systems, few focus on the patient–provider relationship. The lack of focus on this relationship as a quality indicator, combined with performance reports that often do not represent the patient's perspective (Hudon, Fortin, Haggerty, Lambert, & Poitras, 2011), precludes practice improvement. Furthermore, RNs frequently do not receive performance information for 3 or 4 months or longer after patients are discharged.

Real-time patient feedback delivered directly to those providing care enhances performance improvement (Ayers et al., 2005; Nelson et al., 2008), and in the case of caring relationships, the patient's perspective, particularly at the point of care is crucial in its evaluation. To rapidly collect and disseminate patient feedback about caring relationships with nurses, the use of technology in the form of a bedside mobile device provides real-time data for use by RNs to revise their practice, providing routine evaluation of caring relationships *during the care process*. In a pilot study, Duffy and colleagues (2012) tested this approach in a sample of 86 hospitalized older adults using an electronic version of the 27-item Caring Assessment Tool (e-CAT; Duffy et al., 2014) and found it feasible and acceptable.

At the microsystems level, assessing nurse caring on a unit or departmental basis provides some evidence of how well the quality-caring model© is integrated into practice and points to performance improvement recommendations. Many tools exist that are available to assist this process (Watson, 2002). However, they vary in terms of how they define caring, the approach, how they are administered and scored, whose view they are obtaining (e.g., patients, nurses, or others), and validity and reliability. Only a few directly gather information from patients. This is an important component of assessment because the one being "cared for" is the direct source of knowledge and others' opinions may not be consistent. The revised *Caring Assessment Tool*© (CAT; Duffy, Hoskins et al., 2007, 2012), a 27-item instrument designed to capture patients' perceptions of nurse caring, has been used with success in several health-care institutions (Duffy, 2013). This tool has established validity and reliability and is available in English, Spanish, and Japanese. Using this tool provides an evaluation of nurse caring behaviors as perceived by patients that can be used for performance improvement and practice revisions.

Another instrument that was adapted from the CAT© is the Caring Assessment Tool for Administration (CAT-admin; Duffy, 2002). This tool is a 39-item questionnaire that assesses how nurses perceive nurse manager caring behaviors and has become important in the assessment of caring practice environments. Many other instruments exist to measure caring; however, ensuring that the conceptual base, population and setting, and perspective of the respondent are consistent with individual and organizational values is vital to successful evaluation.

Specific nursing-sensitive outcomes are likely to be influenced through use of the quality-caring model©, so knowledge about these is necessary to improve and accelerate its translation into practice. To extend the understanding and strengthen the evidence pertaining to caring relationships (specifically nurse caring) as a significant process indicator, tying it to outcomes indicators may better reflect the value of nursing. For example, hospitalized older adults frequently leave the hospital with poorer physical function than when admitted. This is a national problem with significant cost and clinical burden (Goodwin, Howrey, Zhang, & Kuo, 2011), not to mention the personal burden it places on patients and families. Measuring and reporting differences in functional status from admission to discharge for older adults on Quality-Caring units would add to the evidence base. Those with chronic illnesses, such as heart failure, cancer, and chronic obstructive pulmonary disease often are readmitted within 30 days of discharge, financially draining the US health system (Jackson, Trygstad, DeWalt, & DuBard, 2013). This burden may be lessened if nurses worked, through caring relationships, to engage and activate patients in their care before discharge. Patient engagement is a measurable intermediate outcomes indicator (Hibbard, Stockard, Mahoney,

& Tusler, 2004) that has been associated with decreased readmissions (Coulter, 2012) and reflects the relational aspect of nursing care, potentially raising positive regard for nursing's value.

Other nursing-sensitive intermediate outcomes indicators such as comfort, knowledge, dignity, optimistic mood, recovery time, adherence, contentment (versus anxiety), continence, cognition, empowerment, health-seeking behaviors, mobility, symptom control, and skin integrity are examples of affirming intermediate outcomes that could be used to demonstrate the effects of caring relationships. Many of these indicators have well-documented instruments that would easily translate to the clinical environment, rendering measurement and reporting feasible. Routinely using such existing tools may validate the effects of nurse caring on important intermediate outcomes and provide a basis for improvement.

Researching Caring Relationships

Effectively appraising research informs nursing practice by providing evidence that can guide nursing interventions. Unit-based journal clubs, nursing rounds, or even routine dialog can provide forums for such appraisal. With special attention to those studies that investigate aspects of caring relationships, nurses can help translate findings into practice and/or extend the research itself.

Because the quality-caring model© provides a set of concepts, assumptions, and propositions, questions generated from these theoretical ideas can provide the basis for research. For example, the proposition, "feeling 'cared for' influences the attainment of intermediate and terminal health outcomes" (Duffy, 2013a, p. 38) could be tested by linking the results of an instrument measuring caring with a set of specific patient outcomes. In fact, nurse researchers have investigated this and found some evidence that caring is linked to patient satisfaction, postoperative recovery, and decreased anxiety (Burt, 2007; Swan, 1998; Wolf, Zuzelo, Goldberg, Crothers, & Jacobson, 1998). Or consider the proposition, "relationships characterized as caring contribute to individual, group, and system self-advancement" (Duffy, 2013a, p. 38) might be tested by examining the relationship between adoption of a caring professional practice model and staff nurses' satisfaction with work.

Others have developed caring nursing interventions and used them to study effects on specific patient outcomes (Duffy et al., 2005; Erci et al., 2003). An example geared to optimizing patient-centered care for hospitalized older adults uses flexible education, rapid-cycle performance improvement, and facilitated group reflection to support busy RNs to use the caring factors in a complex environment (Duffy, 2013b). Such research adds to the knowledge base and offers implications for the improvement of nursing practice. Schools of nursing have used the caring factors to develop and test caring competencies of baccalaureate students longitudinally; and students themselves, particularly those in Doctor of Nursing Practice (DNP) programs, often use the quality-caring model© to guide their scholarly inquiries. Finally, nursing leaders study caring behaviors of nurse managers (using the CAT-adm) and evaluate implementation of the model organizationally using comparative designs of patient outcomes on implementation and control units.

Studying caring relationships is important to provide evidence of nursing's contribution to health-care and to advance the profession. Such evidence provides policymakers with documentation of nursing's value that may affect important decisions such as funding, job descriptions, promotion and advancement, and staffing. To that end, the quality-caring model© provides a foundation for continued research and model testing. Ensuring that results are disseminated quickly to the nursing community through publications and presentations is a nursing responsibility that can advance caring science.

Up until now, weaknesses in caring evaluation and research including the lag time behind new caring theories, the vagueness between findings and components of theory, measurement issues, and poorly designed studies with small and/or nonprobability samples have created gaps in caring knowledge. Linking caring to nursing-sensitive patient outcomes, improving existing caring instruments, designing caring-based interventions, educational caring, and cost–benefit analyses are urgently needed to provide evidence of nursing's value. Using rigorous methods, research that builds on the work of others and includes multiple patient populations and settings demonstrates the validity of caring theories and advances nursing practice.

Practice Exemplar

Mr. S is an 86-year-old man with chronic obstructive pulmonary disease (COPD) who lives with his daughter, her husband, and their three children. He has been living with the disease for 15 years and is mostly homebound. Mr. S has home oxygen, a wheelchair, and his own room on the second floor of the home equipped with a TV, DVD player, and books. He interacts with his grandchildren, who are teenagers, and relies on his daughter for activities of daily living. Mr. S lost his wife several years earlier to cancer and was a computer programmer before retirement. He was a two pack per day smoker who rarely exercised and had been in good health before his diagnosis. He communicates well verbally and uses an

intercom set up by his son-in-law when necessary. His breathing has been gradually getting worse (despite medications), and he produces quite a bit of sputum daily. He is easily fatigued and occasionally experiences wheezing. He takes both a short- and a long-acting bronchodilator and is on steroid therapy.

Mr. S has been noticing increasing insomnia lately with some nocturnal dyspnea and a cough. His pulmonary function studies have not changed, but his pulmonologist suggested that he consider elective lung volume reduction surgery (LVRS) to help him breathe better and avert an emergency. Mr. S subsequently entered a large teaching Magnet hospital at 7:30 a.m. one day to have this surgery

Continued

performed. He arrived in his wheelchair accompanied by his daughter. He was nervous about the procedure—not only because of the surgery itself but also because he knew he would most likely be in the intensive care unit afterward. That place scared him! The admitting office was busy, so the technician took his time gathering insurance information and then wheeled Mr. S down to the preop area. He sat in the wheelchair for 45 minutes until a nurse, who was busy on the phone, arrived. She introduced herself and stated that he should undress and get in bed so that she could begin her assessment. Mr. S's daughter assisted him, as she always does at home, and then placed him safely in the hospital bed. The nurse returned with a clipboard and began her assessment, collecting pertinent history. Then she began a physical assessment. Her resultant problem list consisted of two problems: shortness of breath due to COPD and sleep pattern disturbance. She told Mr. S a little about the upcoming surgery and asked his daughter to sign the consent papers. The anesthesiologist arrived to start the anesthesia, so Mr. S's daughter kissed him, and he was wheeled into the OR. Three hours later, he was in the recovery area, and when Mr. S's daughter saw her father, he was on a ventilator, with multiple IVs, and extremely agitated. He was able to take his own breaths but was obviously frightened. Because he was "tied down" to the bed rails, his daughter, who understood his anxiety, sat by his side and softly talked to him.

He used his hands to show her he felt like he couldn't breathe. The daughter, in turn, relayed this to the nurse, who asked her to tell him that this was a normal feeling after this surgery. Mr. S continued to experience anxiety, often coughing, and was eventually placed in the farthest bed so as to not disturb the other patients. Unfortunately, his daughter could not allay his concerns, and he continued to feel anxious and distressed.

It was 5:00 p.m., and Mr. S was doing well according to the nurses in the postanesthesia care unit (PACU); they began his discharge by searching for an intensive care unit (ICU) bed, but there were no available beds in this busy teaching hospital. Unfortunately, Mr. S had to stay in the PACU overnight until an ICU bed became available. Two other patients were also staying overnight. The PACU nurses were unhappy with this arrangement because it meant two of them would have to stay on call to staff the unit. They were overheard talking to each other, saying, "If I had wanted to work on a surgical floor, I wouldn't have applied to the PACU." Mr. S continued to display anxiety, often gagging and looking fearful with his eyes. His daughter could not help him because she didn't know enough about the procedure he had had to answer his questions. She thought maybe he was in pain, but he denied this. He continued to remain lying in the bed with his frightened look. The daughter asked the PACU nurses for help in figuring out what was wrong, but they saw that his vital signs, blood gases, and dressing were normal. One nurse decided to suction him, but there were few secretions. Her technique was rather rough; Mr. S grimaced with pain, and his daughter asked if it would always be this way. The nurse said it would get better with time and went over to talk to the other nurse. Mr. S remained anxious throughout the night while his daughter sat by his side. Neither of them slept. He was taken to the intermediate respiratory care unit at 8:30 a.m.

On this unit, Mr. S was cared for by a young nurse named Megan who had graduated 2 years earlier. Megan stopped briefly to focus herself and readjust her thoughts toward Mr. S before she entered his room. Taking a couple of slow deep breaths, Megan entered the room and quickly scanned the environment and the patient to notice anything significant. She introduced herself by name and then looked Mr. S in the eyes, smiled, and squeezed his hand lightly *(human respect)*. Then she asked what he would like to be called while he stayed with them and wrote that name on a board on the wall opposite his bed. Since he couldn't talk, Megan asked Mr. S's daughter to explain how she had been communicating with him; then Megan tried it with Mr. S to better understand his needs. Turns out, the daughter

Practice Exemplar cont.

was spelling words that were eventually incorporated into sentences.

Using the Quality Caring Model© as a frame of reference, Megan completed a physical assessment that included physiological, emotional, sociocultural, and spiritual components. Her goal was to use this opportunity to initiate a caring relationship with Mr. S and his family that could grow and be sustained throughout the hospitalization experience. Through this process, Megan came to know Mr. S as a retired software engineer who is widowed and lives with his married adult daughter and 3 grandchildren, is an avid reader of history, who was anxious and tired. She also learned he received his diagnosis of COPD 15 years earlier and had progressively become weaker, more breathless, and eventually homebound. Mr. S was taking multiple medications as well as O_2 therapy at home. His vital signs were good. Although he was slightly tachycardic with a heart rate of 112, his dressing was dry, and his back showed evidence of a beginning pressure ulcer at the coccyx region. Mr. S's daughter relayed her difficulty in caring for Mr. S while also working part time, raising three children, and maintaining a home. This family had not been on a vacation in several years. This physical assessment time provided Megan with the opportunity to understand the unique human being (Mr. S) in relationship to his family, his friends, and life role *(appreciation of unique meanings)* and to begin a relationship-centered professional encounter that was based on these findings.

She documented the results of the assessment in the computer, looking frequently at Mr. S so he could see her. The problem list Megan came up with included issues such as airway maintenance, anxiety, impaired communication, altered family processes, potential skin breakdown, inadequate knowledge, and inadequate coping. Then she sat down, and, using the caring factor *mutual problem-solving,* explained to Mr. S and his daughter what would happen on this unit, including how long they might stay, and how and when to contact her. She engaged them in the dialogue by inviting questions and asked them for guidance regarding Mr. S's normal routines. She relayed that she would be there all day and gave them her telephone number. Then she asked them what they knew about recovering from lung volume reduction surgery and listened attentively to their responses. She sat a little toward the patient and looked at him as he "talked." This took longer than usual because he was using letters to spell out words *(encouraging manner)*. She explained a little about living with COPD, but together they decided to wait until after they had some sleep to review care of the incision and other issues related to COPD. Megan assured Mr. S that he had the capacity to live well with this chronic disease, using examples of what she had already observed about the family *(attentive reassurance)*. Megan then asked the daughter if she wanted something to drink and made sure Mr. S was comfortable (pain free) as well. Then she offered him mouth care and turned him slightly to the side with a pillow behind his back. Megan closed the blinds and offered Mr. S's daughter a pillow and a reclining chair and let them sleep for 2 hours, as they had been up all night *(healing environment)*. She put a sign on the door reminding others that the patient was sleeping *(basic human needs and affiliation needs)*. For the first time in more than 24 hours, Mr. S was able to relax and shut his eyes, showing evidence of feeling "cared for."

Megan's professional encounter with this family was relaxed, genuine, and distinguished by the caring factors. With only 2 years' experience, she was competent in their use. Megan's focus and knowledge of herself provided the strength to meet this family's needs. During the time they were resting, Megan checked on them quietly and frequently *(healing environment)*. At one of these opportunities, Mr. S's daughter sought out Megan to relay her anxieties about taking Mr. S home. Megan listened and encouraged the daughter to adjust first to this new environment while she (Megan) would come back later to help them understand how to live with COPD *(affiliation needs)*.

During the next 2 days, Megan took care of Mr. S and spent time collaborating with Mr. S's

Continued

Practice Exemplar cont.

pulmonologist and surgeon on his care plan. She listed his problems, and when they came for rounds, Megan accompanied them, and they conversed about Mr. S's vital signs, his breathing (he had been extubated after 24 hours), incision, and secretions while also discussing some interventions Megan suggested based on her knowledge of his family situation, the patient's own routines, and their joint interactions. Including Mr. S in the discussions, they asked how he was feeling, and he communicated with Megan's help. During a conversation at the nurses' station, Megan and both physicians agreed that Mr. S could go home the next day with support. The surgeon relied on Megan's judgment about Mr. S's readiness for discharge because he had come to know her these last 2 years as a competent and caring nurse. Megan trusted her own recommendations; their encounter was collaborative and friendly.

Later that day, Megan returned with a written set of instructions about caring for chest incisions. She reviewed the instructions with both Mr. S and his daughter, answering questions, allowing the daughter and Mr. S to "practice." She used a positive approach, reassuring the daughter that she could do this and that she would be there in a couple of hours to review the procedure again *(attentive reassurance and encouraging manner)*. Megan then called the social worker and the home care team to get things rolling for discharge. Megan also took the daughter aside to discuss living and caring for an elderly man with COPD. She provided the daughter with referrals for a support group and a lung association program.

During report, Megan reviewed Mr. S's problem list and her recommended interventions to the oncoming nurse using the caring factors as a basis for the interaction. She felt good that Mr. S and his family were learning about his needs and pleased that she had relieved some of their anxiety. She said goodbye to all her patients and went to her weekly yoga class to unwind. The next morning, Megan had the same assignment and worked with Mr. S and his daughter to ensure their self-caring needs were met.

Although this "case" is typical in many acute care facilities, Mr. S is a unique individual who experienced two different nursing encounters. In the first instance, one might say that his physical needs were met, yet he was not affirmed as the one being treated (the nurses talked to his daughter about him), he was not adequately assessed by the preop nurse, he remained anxious for many hours postop, was isolated from others, didn't sleep, overheard professional nurses talking about not wanting to be there, was treated roughly, and was not turned for 12 hours despite the fact that he was immediately postop. On the intermediate care unit, the nurse used the caring factors to initiate and cultivate a caring relationship with him from admission. She used this relationship as the basis for care that included attention to his basic needs for sleep, comfort, and nutrition. Megan helped Mr. S understand his new situation and included his daughter, who was his caretaker. She was collaborative with the physicians and other nursing staff and positive in her demeanor. She referred to the patient as Mr. S and used her time appropriately to ensure that his transition to home would occur safely. In essence, this nurse saw the patient as a whole person, not a physical body after surgery, and used her caring knowledge and skills to build a relationship that generated trust and security. Through ongoing interaction, a connection developed between the nurse and patient that provided the insight necessary for effectively following the nursing process including specific interventions and evaluation. Although the tasks she performed were routine in nature, this nurse balanced doing with being caring. The caring relationship she established created a higher quality nursing care that benefited both the patient and the nurse.

Acknowledging the unique caring nature of nursing and demonstrating a professional commitment to it offers a way for nursing to help patients make sense of their illnesses. It also provides an opportunity for nursing to claim a unique place in the health-care system by generating evidence of the value of caring through high quality outcomes.

■ Summary

Practice-based knowledge is a hallmark of a profession; therefore, a strong alignment between a theory and the practice of it enhances its significance to society. Caring and quality in health care are implicitly tied together. Because humans exist in relation to others, caring relationships facilitate human advancement and the future interactions so necessary for excellent health care. Independent and collaborative caring relationships in health care contribute to patients' welfare in that they promote comfort, safety, consistent communication, and learning. Professional nurses who regularly relate to themselves and their communities are more equipped to engage in genuine independent and collaborative caring relationships with patients and families as well as advance their own self-caring. Spending time "in relationship" focuses attention on the patient versus the disease or task and generates a meaningful practice that is the basis for joy. In essence, the model benefits both patients and nurses as well as the profession and the health-care system. Theory-guided, evidence-based professional practice that is holistic and meaningful can make a profound impact on patient outcomes.

Implications of the revised quality-caring model© exist for educators to help students learn how to care. Transforming the learning environment with meaningful learning activities, clinical experiences, and frequent reflection on the salience of caring relationships helps students share meanings, elicit relevant data, listen, notice cues, establish rapport, and develop mutually caring interactions. Using evaluation techniques and frequent caring student–teacher interactions, nurse educators can greatly enhance learning outcomes. Clinical courses in which caring behaviors are valued and role-modeled by faculty are essential. Similarly, it is crucial that those nurses in leadership positions create caring–healing–protective environments for staff and patients in a cost-effective manner. Redesigning professional workflow so that its primary function is relationship centered and making decisions in a participatory manner are paramount to quality caring. Finally, showing evidence of nursing's foremost professional purpose (caring) through ordinary everyday caring actions blended with a culture of continuous inquiry creates novel possibilities for advancing the profession.

Example Institutions Using the Quality–Caring Model© for Professional Practice

Children's Mercy Hospital and Clinics, Kansas City, MO

Forsyth Medical Center, Winston-Salem, NC

Hannibal Medical Center, Hannibal, MO

Holy Cross Hospital, Silver Spring, MD

Johns Hopkins, Bayview, Baltimore, MD

Lakeland Regional Medical Center, Lakeland, FL

Lowell General Hospital, Lowell, MA

McLaren, Northern Michigan Medical Center, Petoskey, MI

M.D. Anderson Medical Center, Houston, TX

Methodist Hospital, Henderson, KY

Presbyterian Hospital, Charlotte, NC

Prince William Hospital, Manassas, VA

St. Joseph's Medical Center, Towson, MD

Swedish American Hospital, Rockford, IL

Texas Health Resources, Arlington, TX

Torrance Memorial Hospital, Torrance, CA

West Virginia University Hospitals, Morgantown, WV

References

Ayers, L. R., Beyea, S. C., Godfrey, M. M., Harper, D. C., Nelson, E. C., Batalden, P. B. (2005). Quality improvement learning collaborative. *Quality Management in Health Care, 14*(4), 234–247.

Boudreaux, E. C., Francis, J. L., & Loyacano, T. (2002). Family presence during invasive procedures and resuscitations in the emergency department: A critical review and suggestions for future research. *Annals of Emergency Medicine, 40*, 193–205.

Boykin, A., & Schoenhofer, S. (1993). *Nursing as caring: A model for transforming practice.* New York: National League for Nursing Press.

Burt, K. (2007). The relationship between nurse caring and selected outcomes of care in hospitalized older adults. *Dissertation Abstracts International* (UMI No. 3257620).

Campbell, P., & Rudisill, P. (2006). Psychosocial needs of the critically ill obstetric patient: The nurse's role. *Critical Care Nursing Quarterly, 29*(10), 77–80.

Cossette, S., Cote, J. K., Pepin, J., Ricard, N., & D'Aoust, L. X. (2006). A dimensional structure of nurse–patient interactions from a caring perspective: refinement of the Caring Nurse–Patient Interaction Scale (CNPI-Short Scale). *Journal of Advanced Nursing 55*(2), 198–214.

Coulter, A (2012). Patient Engagement—What Works? *Journal of Ambulatory Care Management, 35*(2), 80–89.

D'Antonio, M. (2008). Why I almost quit nursing. *Johns Hopkins Nursing, 6*(2), 34–35.

Davidson, R. J., Kabat-Zinn, J., Schumaker, J., Rosenkranz, M., Muller, D., & Santorelli, S. F. (2003). Alterations in brain and immune function produced by mindfulness meditation. *Psychosomatic Medicine, 65*(4), 564–570.

Duffy, J. (1992). Impact of nurse caring on patient outcomes. In D. A. Gaut (Ed.), *The presence of caring in nursing* (pp. 113–136). New York: National League for Nursing Press.

Duffy, J. (1993). Caring behaviors of nurse managers: Relationships to staff nurse satisfaction and retention. In D. Gaut (Ed.), *A global agenda for caring* (pp. 365–377). New York: National League for Nursing Press.

Duffy, J. (2002). Caring assessment tools and the CAT-admin version. In J. Watson (Ed.), *Instruments for assessing and measuring caring in nursing and health sciences* (pp. 131–148). New York: Springer.

Duffy, J. (2009). *Quality caring in nursing: Applying theory to clinical practice, education, and leadership.* New York: Springer Publishing.

Duffy, J., & Hoskins, L. (2003). The quality-caring model©: Blending dual paradigms, *Advances in Nursing Science, 26*(1), 77–88.

Duffy, J. (2013a). *Quality caring in nursing and health systems: Implications for clinicians, educators, and leaders.* New York, NY: Springer.

Duffy, J. (2013b). Theories focused on caring. In J. B. Butts & K. L. Rich (Eds.) *Philosophies and theories for advanced nursing practice* (pp. 507–524). Sudbury, MA: Jones & Bartlett Learning, LLC.

Duffy, J., Hoskins, L. M., & Dudley-Brown, S. (2005). Development and testing of a caring-based intervention for older adults with heart failure. *Journal of Cardiovascular Nursing, 20*(5), 325–333.

Duffy, J., Hoskins, L. M., & Seifert, R. F. (2007). Dimensions of caring: Psychometric properties of the caring assessment tool. *Advances in Nursing Science, 30*(3), 235–245.

Duffy, J., Brewer, B., & Weaver, M. (2014). Revision and Psychometric Properties of the Caring Assessment Tool. *Clinical Nursing Research, 23*(1), 80–93.

Duffy, J., Kooken, W., Wolverton, C., & Weaver, M. (2012). Evaluating patient-centered care: Feasibility of electronic data collection in hospitalized older adults. *Journal of Nursing Care Quality, 27*(4), 307–331.

Edwards, M., & Ewen, A. J. (1996). *360 degree feedback: The powerful new model for employee assessment & performance improvement.* New York: American Management Association.

Erci, B., Sayan, A., Tortumluoag, G., Kilic, D., Sahin, O., & Gungurmus, A. (2003). The effectiveness of Watson's caring model on the quality of life and blood pressure on patients with hypertension. *Journal of Advanced Nursing, 41*(2), 130–139.

Fineberg, H. V. (2012). Shattuck Lecture: A successful and sustainable health system—how to get there from here. *New England Journal of Medicine, 366*(11), 1020–1027.

Foster, R. (2004). Self-care: Why is it so hard? *Journal of Specialists in Pediatric Nursing, 9*(4), 85–94.

Goodwin, J. S., Howrey, B., Zhang, D., & Kuo, Y. F. (2011). Risk of continued institutionalization after hospitalization in older adults. *Journal of Gerontological Medical Science, 66*(12), 1321–1327.

Henderson, V. (1980). Nursing—yesterday and tomorrow. *Nursing Times, 76*, 905–907.

Hibbard, J. H., Stockard, J., Mahoney, E. R., & Tusler, M. (2004). Development of the Patient Activation Measure (PAM): Conceptualizing and measuring activation in patients and consumers. *Health Services Research, 39*(4 pt 1), 1005–1026.

Hudon, C., Fortin, M., Haggerty, J. L., Lambert, M., Poitras, M.E (2011). Measuring patients' perceptions of patient-centered care: A systematic review of tools for family medicine. *Annals Family Medicine, 9*(2), 155–164.

Institute of Medicine (2004). *Keeping patients safe: Transforming the work environment of nurses.* Washington, DC: author.

Jackson, C. T., Trygstad, T. K., DeWalt, D. A., & DuBard, C. A. (2013). Transitional care cut hospital readmissions for North Carolina Medicaid patients with complex chronic conditions. *Health Affairs, 32*(8), 1407–1415

Johnson, D. E. (1990). The behavioral system model for nursing. In M. E. Parker (Ed.), *Nursing theories in practice* (pp. 23–32). New York: National League for Nursing Press.

King, I. (1981). *A theory for nursing: Systems, concepts, process.* New York: Wiley.

Knaus, W. A., Draper, E. A., Wagner, D. P., & Zimmerman, J. E. (1986). An evaluation of outcome from intensive care in major medical centers. *Annals of Internal Medicine, 104*, 410–418.

Leininger, M. M. (1981). The phenomenon of caring: Importance of research and theoretical considerations.

In M. M. Leininger (Ed.), *Caring: An essential human need*. Thorofare, NJ: Slack.

London, M., & Smither, J. W. (1995). Can multisource feedback change perceptions of goal accomplishments, self evaluations, and performance-related outcomes? Theory based applications and directions for research. *Personnel Psychology, 48*, 803–839.

Mangurten, J., Scott, S., Guzzetta, C., Clark, A. P., Vinson, L., Sperry, J., et al. (2006). Effects of family presence during resuscitation and invasive procedures in a pediatric emergency department. *Journal of Emergency Nursing, 32*(3), 225–233.

Maslow, A. (1954). *Motivation and personality*. New York: Harper.

Mayerhoff, M. (1971). *On caring*. New York: Harper & Row.

Nelson, E. C., Godfrey, M. M., Batalden, P. B., Berry, S. A., Bothe, A. E., McKinley, K. E., et al. (2008). Clinical microsystems, part 1. The building blocks of health systems. *Joint Commission Journal of Quality Improvement, 34*(7), 367–378.

Nightingale, F. (1992). *Notes on nursing: What it is, and what it is not* (commemorative ed.). Philadelphia: Lippincott.

Orem, D. (2001). *Nursing concepts of practice* (6th ed.). Wilkes Barre, PA: Mosby.

Paul, F., Hendry, C., & Cabrelli, L. (2004). Meeting patient and relatives' information needs upon transfer from an intensive care unit: The development and evaluation of an information booklet. *Journal of Clinical Nursing, 13*, 396–405.

Peplau, H. E. (1988). *Interpersonal relations in nursing*. New York: Springer.

Roach, S. (1984). *Caring: The human mode of being: Implications for nursing—perspectives in caring* (Monograph 1). Toronto, CA: Faculty of Nursing, University of Toronto.

Rogers, C. (1961). On becoming a person: A therapist's view of psychotherapy. *Archives of General Psychiatry, 62*, 1377–1384.

Roy, C. (1980). The Roy adaptation model. In: J. P. Riehl & C. Roy (Eds.), *Conceptual models for nursing practice* (2nd ed., pp. 179–188). New York: Appleton-Century-Crofts.

Siegel, D. J. (2007). *The mindful brain*. New York: W. W. Norton.

Swan, B. (1998). Postoperative nursing care contributions to symptom distress and functional status after ambulatory surgery. *MEDSURG Nursing, 7*(3), 148–158.

Swanson, K. (1991). Empirical development of a middle range theory of caring. *Nursing Research, 40*, 161–166.

Watson, J. (1979). *Nursing: The philosophy and science of caring*. Boston: Little, Brown (2nd printing 1985). Boulder, CO: Colorado University Press.

Watson, J. (1985). *Nursing: Human science and human care*. New York: National League for Nursing Press.

Watson, J. (2002). *Instruments for assessing and measuring caring in nursing and health sciences*. New York: Springer.

Wolf, Z. R., Zuzelo, P. R., Goldberg, E., Crothers, R., & Jacobson, N. (2006). The Caring Behaviors Inventory for Elders: Development and psychometric characteristics. *International Journal for Human Caring, 10*(1), 49–59.

Yalom, I. D. (1975). *The theory and practice of group psychotherapy*. New York: Basic Books.

Pamela Reed's Theory of Self-Transcendence

Chapter *23*

PAMELA G. REED

Introducing the Theorist
Overview of the Theory
Applications of the Theory
Practice Exemplar
Summary
References

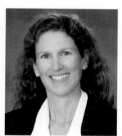

Pamela Reed

Introducing the Theorist

Pamela G. Reed is professor at the University of Arizona College of Nursing in Tucson. She received her academic degrees from Wayne State University in Detroit, Michigan: a BSN and an MSN with a double major in child & adolescent psychiatric–mental health nursing and nursing education, which prepared her both as a clinical nurse specialist and a nurse educator. In 1982, Dr. Reed received her PhD from Wayne State University, majoring in nursing research and theory with a minor in life span development and aging.

She promoted the study of spirituality as an area of scientific inquiry in nursing. Her research in spirituality, mental health and well-being, aging, and end-of-life was strongly influenced by the theoretical ideas of Martha Rogers and the life span developmentalists. Dr. Reed's theory of self-transcendence is based in part on her research and on her developmental perspective of well-being. The theory has been widely published and is used by many nurses in practice and research. In addition, Dr. Reed developed two widely used research instruments, the *Spiritual Perspective Scale* and the *Self-Transcendence Scale*.

Dr. Reed is a fellow in the American Academy of Nursing and is a member of a number of professional organizations including Sigma Theta Tau International, the American Nurses Association, and the Society of Rogerian Scholars. She serves on editorial review boards of numerous journals and as a contributing editor for *Applied Nursing Research* and *Nursing Science Quarterly*. Dr. Reed is coeditor of a nursing theory text, *Perspectives on Nursing Theory*, now in its 6th edition, and author, along with Nelma Shearer, of *Nursing Knowledge and Theory Innovation: Advancing the Science of Practice*.

411

Since January 1983, Dr. Reed has been on the University of Arizona faculty, where she teaches, writes, conducts research, and served as Associate Dean for Academic Affairs for 7 years. She has received many teaching awards from faculty and students. In addition to writing for research publications, she frequently writes about the philosophical and theoretical dimensions of nursing with a focus on practice-based knowledge development. She lives with her husband in the Sonoran desert of Tucson, Arizona, where her two daughters also reside.

Overview of the Theory

The focus of the theory is on facilitating the process of self-transcendence for the purpose of enhancing or supporting well-being. Theories from other sciences, such as psychology, also address self-transcendence. However, what distinguishes this particular theory as a *nursing* theory is its focus on well-being in the context of difficult health experiences. The theory proposes that people's capacity for self-transcendence is activated when they face life-threatening illness or undergo health-related changes that intensify awareness of vulnerability or mortality. This increase in self-transcendence is evident in expansion of self-boundaries in ways that foster well-being. Individuals have the capacity to expand their boundaries in healthy ways, but in serious illness or other health-related life crises, nurses and other professionals can be helpful in facilitating this process of self-transcendence. The scope of the theory has been extended beyond its original focus on later adulthood to address self-transcendence as a resource for well-being across the life span from adolescence to adulthood, with potential applications to childhood.

Foundations of the Theory

All theories are built on *assumptions* generally considered to be true as derived from widely accepted theory or empirical findings or as self-evident. Assumptions are not tested in research but instead serve as foundational ideas for the theory. Two major frameworks that originated in the mid-20th century and continue to be

relevant today motivated the theory of self-transcendence: Martha Rogers's (1970, 1980, 1990) conceptual system about the human–environment process and the life-span developmental science perspective articulated by Richard Lerner (e.g., 2002; Lerner, Lamb, & Freund, 2010), both of which are related to complexity science (e.g., Kauffman, 1995).

One philosophical assumption of self-transcendence theory is that humans undergo change that is developmental in nature (characterized by increasing complexity and organization) and as part of this innovative process, humans also possess inherent potential for healing, emotional growth, and well-being throughout the lifespan. This potential for well-being has been described by Reed (1997) most fundamentally as a *nursing process,* analogous to basic chemical processes of chemistry or the social processes of interest to sociologists. Self-transcendence is an example of a nursing process.

A second philosophical assumption is that humans, as open systems, impose conceptual boundaries on their "openness" to define their reality and provide a sense of identity and security. This assumption is based on ideas from life-span developmental psychology about the formation and differentiation of self across development. For example, theorists have identified the diffuse boundary between infant and parent, the increased sense of identity and self-consciousness in children and adolescents as they clarify their boundary between self and others, the increased differentiation of self and more secure sense of identity in middle adulthood, and the complex and expanded forms of connections to others and spirituality in later adulthood and end of life. This assumption was also influenced by Rogers's (1970, 1980) nursing science about perceived self-boundaries that may fluctuate during health-related life events. She proposed that humans are energy fields infinite in space and time, extending beyond the "discernible mass" we identify as the human body, and without boundaries.

Rogers (1994) used the term *pandimensionality* (revised from her former terms of four-dimensionality and multidimensionality) to describe the unbounded connections in the human–environment process and to challenge conventional distinctions between, for example, person and environment, living and dying. Her principle of *integrality* proposed a fundamental connectedness instead of these perceived boundaries. Her concept of *relative present* challenged conventional distinctions among past, present, and future to acknowledge both the individual's temporal perspectives and the discoveries in physics about space-time. So self-transcendence involves expanding and redefining self-boundaries during health events and is evident in connections to our inner life, to others, to natural and technological environments, and to imagined worlds. The theory is based on a pluralistic view of reality that accounts for the human capacity—as latent as it may be today—to expand self-boundaries in innovative ways.

The Theory: Concepts and Relationships

The theory of self-transcendence, like theories in general, is a compressed description of a phenomenon or process and does not catalog every instance of self-transcendence. A theory provides a coherent description of key concepts and their relationships, which researchers and practitioners can further specify for application to their unique situations. There are three major concepts in the theory: self-transcendence, vulnerability, and well-being.

Self-Transcendence

The core concept of the theory is self-transcendence. It refers to the capacity to expand self-boundaries in various ways that enhance well-being. For example, self-boundaries can expand intrapersonally (toward greater awareness of one's beliefs, values, and dreams), interpersonally (to connect with others, nature, and surrounding environment), transpersonally (to relate to dimensions beyond the ordinary, observable world), and temporally (to integrate one's past and future in a way that expands and gives meaning to the present). Other ways of expanding self-boundaries are possible. For example, in our increasingly technological world, expansion of self-boundaries may also involve

connectedness of self with nonliving entities such as symbolic objects, memories, machines, and prosthetics that influence well-being in profound ways.

One caveat in understanding the theory is that the term *self-transcendence* may evoke ideas about the mystical, supernatural, or other experiences that disconnect self from others or from the present. However, spiritual meanings associated with this theory refer more to terrestrial, everyday practices of spirituality that alter self-boundaries in meaningful ways to *connect* rather than *separate* a person from self, others, nature, and other aspects of our environment. Nevertheless, it may be important to acknowledge the unseen or the mystery in life.

With regard to assessment, the 15-item Self-Transcendence Scale (STS) was developed by Dr. Reed to measure self-transcendence in individuals who are either well or have health problems or other limitations due to illness or disability. The STS is used widely in research and may also be used by practicing nurses to better understand areas for assessing patients. The STS has been translated into several languages, including Spanish, Mandarin, and Korean.

Vulnerability

Vulnerability is a contextual concept in the theory and refers to an increased awareness of personal mortality. A wide variety of human experiences can increase this awareness, but of particular note are health-related events that are life threatening or that involve loss. Chronic and serious illness, disability, aging, bereavement, traumatic events, and facing end of life all are contexts of vulnerability and increased awareness of mortality.

For assessment, a variety of measures or questions can be used to assess a person's sense of vulnerability. Examples of areas to assess include perceived risk for illness, concerns about potential loss, and perspectives on living with a life-threatening illness.

Well-Being

Well-being is the third major concept in the theory. Well-being is defined broadly as a subjective feeling of health or wholeness as based on the person's own criteria at a given point in time. It involves an existential judgment by the individual and is influenced by one's history, culture, values, family and other significant relationships, and biophysical factors.

There are many measures for the assessment of well-being in nursing and other health and social sciences. This reveals the diversity of values about health and wellness. Examples of indicators of well-being that have been found to be significantly related to self-transcendence include life satisfaction, happiness, high morale in aging, self-care agency in chronic illness, sense of meaning in life, and specific indicators of mental health such as absence of depression, decreased anxiety, subjective well-being, and happiness.

Relationships Among the Concepts

Self-transcendence, as a nursing process, is linked logically with positive, health-promoting experiences. Self-transcendence can be a correlate if not a predictor of well-being. In addition, accumulated research findings support self-transcendence as a mediator of well-being during significant life events that increase sense of vulnerability. The model in Figure 23-1 depicts the three concepts and their relationships.

From the Rogerian-based assumption that human beings have potential for innovative expansion of self-boundaries, it was theorized

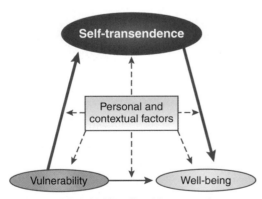

Fig 23 • 1 Model of Reed's self-transcendence nursing theory. *(Copyright ©2012 by Pamela G. Reed.)*

that vulnerability is related to increased self-transcendence. In other words, increased awareness of one's vulnerability or mortality can trigger positive, inner strengths—in this case self-transcendence, an idea long supported by experts on development at end of life (e.g., Becker, 1973; Corless, Germino, & Pittman, 1994; Erikson, 1986; Frankl, 1963; Marshall, 1996). Self-transcendence in turn may directly influence increased well-being. Self-transcendence may also function as a resource for well-being during increased vulnerability by mediating the relationship between increased vulnerability and well-being to help the person transform loss into a growth or healing experience of well-being.

Additional concepts in the theory are personal and contextual factors that can influence the relationships among vulnerability, self-transcendence, and well-being. Potential factors include age, gender, ethnicity, years of education, illness intensity, life history, social or spiritual support, and other factors concerning the person's social, cultural, and physical environment.

Applications of the Theory

Self-transcendence theory has applications in both research and practice. In research, the theory is used as a broad framework for exploring ideas about self-transcendence in qualitative studies and as a theoretical framework for examining specific relationships using quantitative measures. The theory has been studied for its practice applications with patients as well as among nurses, family caregivers, and other health-care providers, and healthy populations.

Research results support the significance of self-transcendence as a correlate or predictor of well-being across a variety of populations, particularly those experiencing serious illness or other challenging life situations.

Research

Examples of research applications include the following studies: clinical depression in older adults (Haugan & Innstrand, 2012; Reed, 1991;

Stinson & Kirk, 2006); bereavement (Chan, & Chan, 2011; Kausch & Amer, 2007); people diagnosed with HIV/AIDS (Coward, 1995; McCormick, Holder, Wetsel, & Cawthon, 2001; Ramer, Johnson, Chan, & Barrett, 2006; Sperry, 2011); chronic illness and loss in later life (Bickerstaff, Grasser, & McCabe, 2003; Gusick, 2008; Nygren et al., 2005); women with breast cancer (Coward, 2003; Farren, 2010; Matthews & Cook, 2009; Thomas, Burton, Quinn Griffin, & Fitzpatrick, 2010); liver and stem cell and transplant recipients (Bean & Wagner, 2006; Burns, Robb, & Haase, 2009; Williams, 2012); older adults both in the community and in nursing home (Haugan et al., 2012; McCarthy, 2011); and persons with dementia and other progressive or intractable diseases (Chen & Walsh, 2009; Iwamoto, Yamawaki, & Sato, 2011). Other research supports the significance of self-transcendence among caregivers of family members with dementia or other debilitating illness and at end-of-life (Acton, 2002; Guo, Phillips, & Reed, 2010; Kidd, Zauszniewski, & Morris, 2011; Kim, Reed, Hayward, Kang, & Koenig, 2011; Reed & Rousseau, 2007) and among nurses dealing with difficult caregiving situations (Hunnibell, Reed, Griffin, & Fitzpatrick, 2008; Palmer, Griffin, Reed, & Fitzpatrick, 2010). A literature search of the term *self-transcendence* using databases from nursing and other sciences (for example, CINAHL, BioMed Central, PsycInfo) will easily generate an up-to-date list of studies and clinically based articles on self-transcendence[1]. Also, see Reed (2013) for an extended list of references on self-transcendence.

---

[1] For additional practice exemplars please go to bonus chapter content available at FA Davis http://davisplus .fadavis.com

Practice

Practice applications summarized from this and other research indicate various self-transcendence strategies that expand self-boundaries. These approaches may be organized in terms of intrapersonal, interpersonal, and transpersonal approaches to boundary expansion. There may be overlap across these categories. Many of these activities also expand temporal boundaries by helping the person focus on the present.

Intrapersonal approaches help the person look inward to expand boundaries and integrate loss through self-knowledge and finding meaning or purpose in one's life. Examples of strategies that nurses may suggest for patients are meditation, self-reflection, and prayer; guided reminiscence and life review; self-talk, emotion or stress management, and relaxation strategies; artistic and other creative activities of self-expression, reading and writing poetry, music therapy, and journaling; and exercise and other physical activities.

Interpersonal activities that facilitate self-transcendence connect individuals to others through formal or informal means, including support groups, faith-based groups, or group psychotherapy; telephone or Internet-based interactions; volunteer work and other altruistic activities including those that allow one to be of help to others and to share one's wisdom. Of course, relationships with family and friends are central to the interpersonal dimension.

Transpersonal approaches for self-transcendence are designed to help the person connect with a power or purpose greater than self. The nurse's role in this process is often one of creating an environment or providing guidance that fosters approaches such as religious participation, spiritual exploration and expression, involvement in altruistic activities, and work on creative projects.

Practice Exemplar

This practice exemplar focuses on how to facilitate well-being outcomes through various strategies that support self-transcendence. The idea behind the interventions is that facilitating self-transcendence promotes positive mental health outcomes either by diminishing the negative effect that vulnerability has on well-being or more directly by enhancing those perspectives on life that increase emotional well-being.

Several years ago, Rose was diagnosed with emphysema. In her youth and through young adulthood, Rose had been a professional dancer on Broadway. But she now found that what were once the strongest parts of her body—her legs—were no longer able to carry her around with grace and ease. Her illness had advanced to the point that she required supplemental oxygen and a walker at home. This made it difficult for her to get out of the house as often as she desired. She lived alone, but her daughter, her family caregiver, visited her several times a week. Recently, Rose experienced a worsening of her physical symptoms and more difficulty breathing; so, with her daughter's encouragement, she moved closer to her daughter. Even though Rose's new apartment was more modern than her old house and her daughter could visit more often, Rose wasn't as happy in her new surroundings, and her daughter was concerned about her depressed mood during her frequent visits.

Their nurse worked together with Rose and her daughter to design a plan of care that not only tended to Rose's declining physical health needs and any other underlying problems but also focused on complex needs regarding her mental health and her emotional and social well-being. Self-transcendence theory provided a framework for practice to address these latter needs. The nurse acknowledged that Rose's worsening illness might be contributing to a heightened sense of vulnerability not only because it was life-threatening but also because it diminished the quality of certain areas of her life. The nurse operated from the basic assumption that nursing care could help activate Rose's inner strengths and potential to transcend some of the boundaries she was facing to attain a sense of well-being in the midst of vulnerability. And because the theory is a guide and not an exact recipe for intervention, using the theory increased the likelihood that the nurse, Rose, and her daughter together would discover important areas of self-transcendence unique to Rose's situation.

Intrapersonal

The nurse helped expand Rose's boundaries on an interpersonal level through a variety of interactions. Rose explained that she was a private person and didn't like to depend on others. The nurse's openness and empathy supported her in expressing her beliefs about quality of life, spiritual values, goals for herself, and dreams for her daughter's future. These insights were useful in making health-care and other decisions. Their discussions also helped Rose acknowledge and integrate difficult feelings into her life. Whether she resolved all of her concerns was not as important as acknowledging and accepting them for the time being. The nurse acknowledged Rose and her daughter's fears and losses along the way and supported their hope and faith that they could cope with, and maybe even grow from, the experience.

Interpersonal

Besides the fact that these objects confronted her with her mortality, Rose found it embarrassing that she had to use a walker and supplemental oxygen wherever she went. She perceived these items as foreign and undignified objects that announced her aging and disability to the world. Rose also missed her friends from her former home and especially missed her "mailbox neighbor" who also carried an oxygen tank. The nurse suggested that Rose participate in a pulmonary rehabilitation program, particularly a program-sponsored support group where she might gain friends among people who not only had similar illness experiences but who also, as Rose said, "looked like [her] too!" As Rose was able to expand her self-boundary to integrate assistive devices into her life, she became more

Practice Exemplar cont.

accepting of her illness and herself overall. Attending the support group also provided her opportunities to use her own experiences to help others. Sharing her wisdom with others was very gratifying to Rose and enhanced her well-being. The nurse also worked to ensure that Rose and her daughter would lead the health-care decisions and fully participate in health-care activities. She helped connect Rose and her daughter with resources to navigate the health-care system and address financial concerns. Information about the illness and self-care strategies helped demystify the health experience and regimen.

Transpersonal

Rose admitted that she was not particularly religious but found herself praying each morning and evening. The nurse was aware that religious beliefs held in youth can become important at the end of life, even if they had been eschewed during adulthood. The nurse acknowledged that Rose, like others, might find value in spiritual perspectives that connected her to some thing or some purpose larger than the individual. Even though she had difficulty believing in a life after death, the possibility offered some comfort and helped Rose integrate awareness about her own mortality and being separated from her family and friends. The nurse also guided Rose through a spiritual history of her life to uncover other sources of strength and perhaps make new discoveries about herself that she could draw from as time progressed.

Temporal

The illness initiated and intensified Rose's concerns about the future and fears about pain and mortality. The nurse explored these concerns with Rose in a realistic yet empathetic manner. A life review in which Rose reflected on her past, discussed anticipating the unknown, and then connected these insights to her present concerns provided a sense of meaning that she found emotionally satisfying. The nurse also facilitated Rose's fuller enjoyment in the present by encouraging positive experiences such as planning enjoyable activities, holding small celebrations, and taking pictures of important or memorable events. These activities generated a legacy and a gift that connected Rose's present to her family's future. Expanding her self-boundary to incorporate other temporalities gave Rose access to meaningful experiences that often sustained her across the trajectory of her illness. Also, simply reminding Rose to try to engage in positive self-talk was sometimes helpful in getting her through a difficult moment.

Rose's Self-Transcendence

Rose did not expect the nurse or her daughter to create self-transcendent experiences for her. But their support and guidance buttressed her own inner potential for healing through the illness experience. Transcending self-boundaries may require the support of others, even though there is the assumption that self-transcendence is a natural human capacity. Rose's openness to accepting help and guidance from the nurse was a first step in expanding her self-boundaries. By nurturing connections to her beliefs and values, her God, her support group friends, and to her daughter and nurse, Rose was able to expand her self-boundaries in ways that enhanced her well-being within the context of her incurable illness.

■ Summary

The theory of self-transcendence was built on the assumption that people may perceive self-boundaries but that they also have the capacity to expand or adjust these boundaries in positive ways, whether by bringing in new perspectives, revising old beliefs, reaching out to others, or connecting to something greater than oneself. The theory of self-transcendence acknowledges the tendency to construct a self-boundary as well as the capacity to transcend limiting views of self and the world in ways that reflect the pandimensional nature of living systems. The theory provides an approach to facilitating well-being in nursing practice by helping individuals expand their personal boundaries within their developmental and situational contexts.

The theory of self-transcendence comprises three key concepts: self-transcendence, well-being, and vulnerability. The theory's concepts were designed to be clear and measurable yet to be broad enough in scope to allow nurses the flexibility in using the theory across a variety of research and practice situations. Practitioners and researchers who use the theory can define the general concepts of vulnerability and well-being using more specific, measurable terms to make the theory applicable to their

specific group of patients or clinical practice setting.

In a general sense, the theory of self-transcendence is a *well-being theory* (Reed, 2008). The theory proposes that self-transcendence arises in contexts of vulnerability and facilitates well-being, either in directly increasing well-being or acting as a mediator in the relationship between vulnerability and well-being. Evidence to date indicates that self-transcendence interventions may diminish risks of vulnerability and increase sense of well-being during difficult health-related situations. Both practitioners and researchers can use the theory to build knowledge about facilitating human well-being across a variety of health experiences.

References

Acton, G. J. (2002). Self-transcendent views and behaviors: Exploring growth in caregivers of adults with dementia. *Journal of Gerontological Nursing, 28*(12), 22–30.

Bean, K. B., & Wagner, K. (2006). Self-transcendence, illness distress, and quality of life among liver transplant recipients. *The Journal of Theory Construction & Testing, 10*(2), 47–53.

Becker, E. (1973). *The denial of death.* New York: The Free Press.

Bickerstaff, K. A., Grasser, C. M., & McCabe, B. (2003). How elderly nursing home residents transcend losses of later life. *Holistic Nursing Practice, 17*(3), 159–165.

Burns, D. S., Robb, S. L., & Haase, J. E. (2009). Exploring the feasibility of a therapeutic music video intervention in adolescents and young adults during stem cell transplantation. *Cancer Nursing, 32*(5), 8–16.

Chan, W. C., & Chan, C. L. W. (2011). Acceptance of spousal death: The factor of time in bereaved older adults' search for meaning. *Death Studies, 35*, 147–162.

Chen, S., & Walsh, S. M. (2009). Effect of a creative-bonding intervention on Taiwanese nursing students' self-transcendence and attitudes toward elders. *Research in Nursing & Health, 32*, 204-216.

Corless, I. B., Germino, B. B., & Pittman, M. (1994). *Dying, death, and bereavement: Theoretical perspectives and other ways of knowing.* Boston: Jones and Bartlett.

Coward, D. (1995). Lived experience of self-transcendence in women with AIDS. *Journal of Obstetric, Gynecologic, and Neonatal Nursing, 24*, 314–318.

Coward, D. D. (2003). Facilitation of self-transcendence in a breast cancer support group: Part II. *Oncology Nursing Forum, 30 (2)*, 291–300.

Erikson, E. H. (1986). *Vital involvement in old age.* New York: Norton.

Farren, A.T., (2010). Power, uncertainty, self-transcendence, and quality of life in breast cancer survivors. *Nursing Science Quarterly, 23 (1)*, 63-71.

Frankl, V. E. (1963). *Man's search for meaning.* New York: Pocket Books.

Guo, G., Phillips, L., & Reed, P.G. (2010). End of life caregiver interactions with healthcare providers: Learning from the bad. *Journal of Nursing Care Quality, 25 (3 – July-Sept), 188-197.*

Gusick, G. M. (2008). The Contribution of Depression and Spirituality to Symptom Burden in Chronic Heart Failure, *Archives of Psychiatric Nursing, 22 (1)*, 53-55.

Haugan, G., & Innstrand, S. (2012). The effect of self-transcendence on depression in cognitively intact nursing home patients. *International Scholarly Research Network (ISRN) Psychiatry*, 2012, doi:10.5402/2012 /301325, 1-10.

Haugan,G., Rannestad, T., Hammervold, R., Gara°sen, H., & Espnes, G.A. (2012) Self-transcendence in cognitively intact nursing home patients: A resource for well-being. *Journal of Advanced Nursing*, DOI: 10.1111/j.1365-2648.2012.06106.

Hunnibell, L.S., Reed, P.G., Quinn-Griffin, M.Q., & Fitzpatrick, J.J. (2008). Self-transcendence and burnout in hospice and oncology nurses. *Journal of Hospice and Palliative Nursing, 10 (3)*, 172 – 179.

Iwamoto, R, Yamawaki, N., & Sato, T. (2011). Increased self-transcendence in patients with intractable diseases. *Psychiatry and Clinical Neurosciences, 65 (7)*, 638-647.

Kauffman, S. (1995). *At home in the universe: The search for laws of self-organization and complexity.* New York: Oxford University Press.

Kausch, K. D., & Amer, K. (2007). Self-transcendence and depression among AIDS memorial quilt panel makers. *Journal of Psychosocial Nursing, 45*(6), 45–53.

Kidd, L. I., Zauszniewski, J. A., & Morris, D. L. (2011). Benefits of a poetry writing intervention for family caregivers of elders with dementia. *Issues in Mental Health Nursing, 32*, 598–604.

Kim, S., Reed, P. G., Hayward, R. D., Kang, Y., & Koenig, H. G. (2011). Spirituality and psychological well-being: Testing a theory of family interdependence among family caregivers and their elders. *Research in Nursing & Health, 34*, 103–115.

Lerner, R. M. (2002). *Concepts and theories of human development* (3rd ed.). New York: Random House.

Lerner, R. M., Lamb, M. E., & Freund, A. M. (Eds.). (2010). *The handbook of life-span development: Social and emotional development.* Hoboken, NJ: Wiley.

Marshall, V. W. (1996). Death, bereavement, and the social psychology of aging and dying. In J. D. Morgan (Ed.), *Ethical issues in death, dying and bereavement* (pp. 57–75). Amityville, NY: Baywood.

Matthews, E. E., & Cook, P. F. (2009). Relationships among optimism, well-being, self-transcendence, coping, and social support in women during treatment for breast cancer. *Psycho-Oncology, 18*, 716–726.

McCarthy, V. L. (2011). A new look at successful aging: Exploring a mid-range nursing theory among older adults in a low-income retirement community. *The Journal of Theory Construction & Testing, 15*(1), 17–23.

McCormick, D. P., Holder, B., Wetsel, M. A., & Cawthon, T. W. (2001). Spirituality and HIV disease: An integrated perspective. *Journal of the Association of Nurses in AIDS Care, 12*(3), 58–65.

Nygren, B., Aléx, L., Jonsén, E., Gustafson, Y., Norberg, A., & Lundman, B. (2005). Resilience, sense of coherence, purpose in life and self-transcendence in relation to perceived physical and mental health among the oldest old. *Aging & Mental Health, 9*(4), 354–362.

Palmer, B., Quinn Griffin, M. T., Reed, P., & Fitzpatrick, J. J. (2010). Self-transcendence and work engagement in acute care staff registered nurses. *Critical Care Nursing Quarterly, 33*(2), 138–147.

Ramer, L., Johnson, D., Chan, L., & Barrett, M. T. (2006). The effect of HIV/AIDS disease progression on spirituality and self-transcendence in a multicultural population. *Journal of Transcultural Nursing, 17*(3), 280–289.

Reed, P. G. (1991). Self-transcendence and mental health in the oldest-old adults. *Nursing Research, 40*(1), 5–11.

Reed, P. G. (1997). Nursing: The ontology of the discipline. *Nursing Science Quarterly, 10*(2), 76–79.

Reed, P. G. (2008). Reed's theory of self-transcendence. *Nurse Theorists Portraits of Excellence* (Vol. 2). Athens, OH: Fitne Video.

Reed, P. G. (2013). Theory of self-transcendence. In M. Smith & P. Liehr, (Eds.), *Middle range theories for nursing* (3rd ed.). New York: Springer.

Reed, P. G., & Rousseau, E. (2007). Spiritual inquiry and well-being in life-limiting illness. *Journal of Spirituality, Religion, and Aging, 19*(4), 81–98.

Rogers, M. E. (1970). *An introduction to the theoretical basis of nursing.* Philadelphia: F. A. Davis.

Rogers, M. E. (1980). A science of unitary man. In J. Riehl & C. Roy (Eds.), *Conceptual models for nursing practice* (2nd ed., pp. 329–338). New York: Appleton-Century-Crofts.

Rogers, M. E. (1990). Nursing: Science of unitary, irreducible, human beings: Update 1990. In: E. A. M. Barrett (Ed.), *Visions of Rogers' science based nursing* (pp. 5–12). New York: National League for Nursing Press.

Rogers, M. E. (1994). The science of unitary human beings: Current perspectives. *Nursing Science Quarterly, 7*(1), 33–35.

Sperry, J. J. (2011). *The relationship of self transcendence, social interest, and spirituality to well-being in HIV/AIDS adults.* Unpublished doctoral dissertation, Florida Atlantic University.

Stinson, C. K., & Kirk, E. (2006). Structured reminiscence: An intervention to decrease depression and increase self-transcendence in older women. *Journal of Clinical Nursing, 15*(2), 208–218.

Thomas, J. C., Burton, M., Quinn Griffin, M. T., & Fitzpatrick, J. J (2010). Self-transcendence, spiritual well-being, and spiritual practices of women with breast cancer, *Journal of Holistic Nursing, 28*(2), 115–122.

Williams, B. J. (2012). Self-transcendence in stem cell transplantation recipients: A phenomenologic inquiry. *Oncology Nursing Forum, 39*(4), E41–E48.

Patricia Liehr and Mary Jane Smith's Story Theory

Chapter 24

PATRICIA LIEHR AND MARY JANE SMITH

Introducing the Theorists
Overview of the Theory
Applications of the Theory
Practice Exemplar
Summary
References

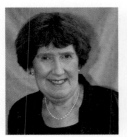

Patricia Liehr

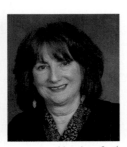

Mary Jane Smith

Introducing the Theorists

Patricia R. Liehr, PhD, RN, graduated from Ohio Valley Hospital School of Nursing in Pittsburgh, Pennsylvania. She completed her baccalaureate degree in nursing at Villa Maria College, her master's in family health nursing at Duquesne University, and her doctorate at the University of Maryland–Baltimore School of Nursing, with an emphasis on psychophysiology. She completed postdoctoral studies at the University of Pennsylvania as a Robert Wood Johnson Scholar. Dr. Liehr is currently a Professor of Nursing at the Christine E. Lynn College of Nursing at Florida Atlantic University. She has taught nursing theory to master's and doctoral students for nearly two decades.

Mary Jane Smith, PhD, RN, earned her bachelor's and master's degrees from the University of Pittsburgh and her doctorate from New York University. She has held faculty positions at the following nursing schools: University of Pittsburgh, Duquesne University, Cornell University-New York Hospital, and Ohio State University; and she is currently a Professor at West Virginia University School of Nursing. She has been teaching theory to nursing students for nearly three decades.

Overview of the Theory

Story theory evolved as the cocreators talked about their practice-research experience with pregnant teens and people recovering from a cardiac event (Smith & Liehr, 2014b). It was clear to the creators that health-promoting change was fostered when one's story of pregnancy or living through a cardiac event was embraced. It was as though acceptance of these health circumstances energized new directions for healing and health. Story theory was first published in 1999 (Smith & Liehr, 1999), and it has continued to be used, tested, and shaped for more than a decade (Smith & Liehr, 2014a).

Stories are integral to nursing practice. Practice decisions are informed both by physiological bodily responses and by the stories that infuse bodily responses with unique personal meaning. To focus on one without attention to the other contributes to less than optimal nursing care. There are times when either the physiological bodily responses or the story is foreground and the other is background; this foreground–background interplay dynamically emerges over the course of each nurse–person caring interaction. For instance, when a person comes into the emergency room with crushing chest pain and then suddenly becomes unconsciousness, numbers related to physiology are in the foreground. Heart rate, blood pressure, and respiratory rate guide critical immediate action. Within a short time, the nurse will want to begin to gather the story, including dimensions such as what the person was doing when the chest pain began, whether this has ever happened before, and what other life and health circumstances could have contributed to the chest pain. Stories are essential to even the most technology-driven nursing practice, and in some ways, the more technology-driven the practice, the more important the place of relevant health stories.

Our linear-thinking culture often places greater value on physiological bodily responses than stories. In fact, precious stories shared during nursing practice may be heard and disregarded or heard and acted on without another thought about the practice evidence generated. Practice stories are seldom chronicled, unfortunately lost to becoming part of the foundation of nursing practice evidence. The overall intent of this chapter is to describe story theory as a framework informing story-gathering and story analysis, thereby positioning story as a major thread of nursing practice evidence, contributing to substantive nursing knowledge.

This chapter first addresses the emergence of story, or narrative, as a topic of interest for health-care providers, including nurses. Then story theory is summarized, including the essential theory concepts (intentional dialogue, connecting with self-in-relation, creating ease) and discussion of ways that the theory comes alive in practice. Bringing the theory to life is described in the context of the theory method dimensions (complicating health challenge, developing story plot, movement toward resolving) aligned respectively with each theory concept. We discuss a seven-phase inquiry process for using the evidence from practice stories to grow the substantive knowledge of the discipline. Finally, an exemplar is used to highlight the potential of the theory for guiding practice through application of the seven-phase inquiry process.

Emergence of Story as a Topic of Interest

Story is not new to nursing. Nurse theorists (Boykin & Schoenhofer, 1991, 2001; Newman, 1999; Parse, 1981; Peplau, 1991; Watson, 1997) have called attention to the importance of listening to what matters since the time of Florence Nightingale, who implored nurses to stop chattering and begin listening (Nightingale, 1969). Others (Benner, 1984; Chinn & Kramer, 1999; Ford & Turner, 2001) have used the stories of practicing nurses to understand both the challenge and the essence of nursing practice. In a discussion of the importance of story for research with minority populations, Banks-Wallace (2002) discussed the therapeutic value of storytelling. Story sharing has also had a prominent place in research with elders (Heliker, 2007; Sierpina & Cole, 2004). It is often used by nurse researchers focused on the art of caring for people who have dementia (Crichton & Koch, 2007; Holm, Lepp, & Ringsberg, 2005; Keady, Williams, & Hughes-Roberts, 2007).

Recently, physicians have emphasized narrative medicine as both a way of learning clinical practice essentials and a way of approaching patients (Charon, 2006, 2012; Charon & Montello, 2002; Mehl-Medrona, 2007). Diamond, a psychotherapist, addressed the long history of using narrative, in forms such as personal testimony and letter writing, to treat alcoholism and addiction. In his book titled *Narrative Means to Sober Ends* (Diamond, 2000), he describes the spirit of narrative therapy: "Stories, not atoms, are the stuff that hold our lives and our world together" (p. 5). This view of stories resonates with the foundational assumptions of story theory and with a valuing of the important place of stories for health promotion. In *Narrative Medicine: The Use of History and Story in the Healing Process,* Mehl-Madrona (2007) approached the topic of narrative from a Native American perspective, distinguishing narrative medicine from conventional medicine and proceeding to share Native American stories that he described as maps for healing. The outside-the-discipline focus "confirms our beliefs about the significance of story and reminds us that this core dimension of nursing practice is now being recognized by other disciplines" (Smith & Liehr, 2014b, p. 229). Although we, the authors, do not equate story with narrative, we accept the place of narrative within the context of story. Story moves beyond narrative, intricately weaving remembered events, personal interpretations of the moment and hopes and dreams to create the "now" moment, guiding choices in the moment.

Story theory is one way to conceptualize an idea that has a long history in nursing and recently escalated attention from other disciplines. The authors believe that the structure of story theory creates possibilities for application and evaluation that are critical to the endeavor of building substantive disciplinary knowledge.

Foundations of the Theory

Story theory proposes that story is a narrative happening wherein a person connects with self-in-relation through nurse–person intentional dialogue to create ease (Smith & Liehr, 2014b). Ease emerges in the midst of accepting the whole story as one's own—a process of attentive embracing the complexity of one's situation. All nursing encounters occur within the context of story. The stories of the nurse, patient, family, and other health-care providers are woven together to create the tapestry of the moment— this is the whole story in the moment. Each time a nurse engages a patient about what matters most regarding a health challenge, story theory is applicable. By abandoning preexisting

assumptions, respecting the storyteller as the expert, and querying vague story directions, the nurse intentionally engages the other, enabling connecting with self-in-relation to create ease.

The theory is based on three assumptions that underpin the framework. The assumptions are that people (1) change as they interrelate with their world in a vast array of flowing connected dimensions, (2) live in an expanded present moment where past and future events are transformed in the here and now, and (3) experience meaning as a resonating awareness in the creative unfolding of human potential (Smith & Liehr, 2014b). These assumptions are consistent with a unitary–transformative "view of the world," an inherently complex view (Newman, Sime, & Corcoran-Perry, 1991), establishing a value structure that creates a foundation for the theory concepts.

The three concepts of the theory are intentional dialogue, connecting with self-in-relation, and creating ease (Fig. 24-1). The related method dimensions are complicating health challenge, developing story plot, and movement toward resolving. The nurse engages a person through intentional dialogue about a complicating health challenge, where connecting with self-in-relation ensues as the developing story plot surfaces through story sharing. As the storyteller makes explicit what may have been tacit (Polanyi, 1958), moments of ease accompany movement toward resolving the health challenge. Figure 24-1 depicts the theory model, indicating relationships among the theory concepts and related method dimensions.

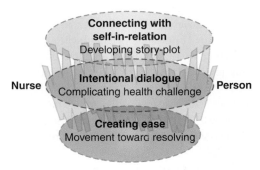

Fig 24 • 1 Story theory with method. *(Reprinted with permission of M. J. Smith and P. Liehr (2014). Story theory. Middle Range Theory for Nursing. New York: Springer, p. 234.)*

The current theory model spreads a "wave" across all concepts in the theory, expressive of the energy essential to story-sharing through intentional dialogue. The heavy dotted ellipse between nurse and person highlights nurse–person intentional dialogue, the core activity enabling connecting with self-in-relation and creating ease. There are three ellipses in the design of the model, mapping a vortex of a continually evolving process, encompassing all the theory concepts and associated method dimensions. The links between the essential elements of the model map the theory phenomenon as an energy-laden integrated whole.

Intentional Dialogue About a Complicating Health Challenge

Intentional dialogue is the central activity between nurse and person that brings story to life; it is querying emergence of a health challenge story in true presence (Smith & Liehr, 1999). True presence is a fully immersed way of being with another, where authenticity and mindfulness prevail. This purposeful engagement with another creates potential for embracing the whole story in the moment as the nurse summons the storyteller's narrative focusing on what matters most about a complicating health challenge (Smith & Liehr, 2014b). The complicating health challenge is a life circumstance in which life change generates uneasiness. Understanding the uneasiness refines the health challenge to enable meaningful nurse–person interaction. For instance, getting married could be both a joyful and an uneasy transition. In this case, the complicating health challenge may be articulated as the transition from being single to being married. What matters most to the anticipatory bride may be the uncertainty she is feeling in the midst of excited planning. This joyful–uneasy paradox will become the focus for the nurse using story theory to guide practice; the nurse will listen to the bride's complaint of stomach pain within the context of joy–uneasiness emerging in the transition to married life.

In another example, for a woman facing the complicating health challenge of a breast cancer diagnosis, it is possible that the thought of losing her breast matters most. However, what matters most could be the threat of a shortened life imposed by the cancer, the response of her husband to her changing body, or concern about who will care for her puppy while she is in the hospital. There is an endless list of possibilities known only to the person who is living the health challenge. The nurse can never assume to know what matters most about a health challenge regardless of the extent of experience in a particular practice environment. The nurse knows how to proceed only by querying what matters most about a complicating health challenge.

Connecting With Self-in-Relation Through Developing Story Plot

Connecting with self-in-relation occurs as reflective awareness on personal history (Smith & Liehr, 1999). It is an active process of recognizing self as related with others in a developing story-plot uncovered through intentional dialogue (Smith & Liehr, 2014b). To connect with self-in-relation, people see themselves not as isolated individuals but as existing and growing in a context, which includes awareness of other people and times, sensitivity to bodily expression, and a sense of history and future in the present moment. One way to gain insight into the story plot is to gather a health challenge story using a story-path approach. Story path begins with a focus on a present health challenge; then, moves to the past calling attention to the relationship between the past and the present challenge. The final phase of story-gathering, when using the story path approach, happens when the nurse asks about hopes and dreams related to the current health challenge. Sometimes this story path approach is visually depicted as the nurse and the story-sharer cocreate a picture of past-present-future along a horizontal line. When using story path, "the nurse encourages reckoning with a personal history by traveling to the past to arrive at the story beginning, moving through the middle, and into the future all in the present, thus going into the depths of the story to find unique meanings that often lie hidden in the ambiguity of puzzling dilemmas" (Smith & Liehr, 2014b, p. 231).

The story path is an expression of a developing story plot with high points, low points, and turning points. High points are times when things are going well by the storyteller's evaluation; low points are times when they are not going so well; and turning points are times when the story twists, sometimes subtly, sometimes dramatically, creating a shift in the forward view. Often, we and our colleagues have used a story-path approach to gather stories for research (Hain, 2007, 2008; Liehr, Nishimura, Ito, Wands, & Takahashi, 2011; Ramsey, 2012; Wands, 2013; Williams, 2007). The story path links present, past, and future (Liehr & Smith, 2000), beginning with the question, "What matters most to you right now about (the health challenge you are facing)?" This question is followed by one that queries the past, asking how it contributes to the present. Finally, hopes and dreams are elicited.

Figure 24-2 depicts a story path for Mary, a 29-year-old woman who has come to see the nurse practitioner for hypertension. Her blood pressure was recorded as 180/110 mm Hg on the primary care visit. The nurse has drawn a line on a sheet of paper and asked Mary to tell her where she is in her life path by marking the "present" on the line. Then she asks Mary what matters most in this present moment. Mary talks about her discomfort with her elevated blood pressure at her young age. She adds detail about her job as a project director for a research study while having just finished full-time study for her master's degree and now beginning work on her doctoral degree in psychology. Mary's home situation is "stabilized" by her husband John, whom she describes as mellow and the strongest supporter for "considering lifestyle changes to lower her high blood pressure." She tells the nurse that the only time her blood pressure is normal is on weekends, when she is away from work. She provides great detail about her work situation on this visit, describing work as an "out-of-control stress" environment aggravated by people who "seem to enjoy her stressful frenzy." Mary believes that work-related stress is the strongest contributor to her hypertension. The nurse clarifies with Mary, "So . . . are you saying that stress-induced high blood pressure is your pressing concern right now?" Mary says, "Yes." What matters most to Mary about the health challenge of hypertension on this visit is her stressful work life, which she feels unable to control. The nurse then moves to the past and asks Mary to identify situations and events on her story path that contributed to her current health challenge of stress-induced high blood pressure, and then to the future, asking her to note hopes and dreams related to the health challenge. Mary notes story-path events related to her father and identifies her desire to have a baby within the next 5 years. Each of these markings along the story path is discussed

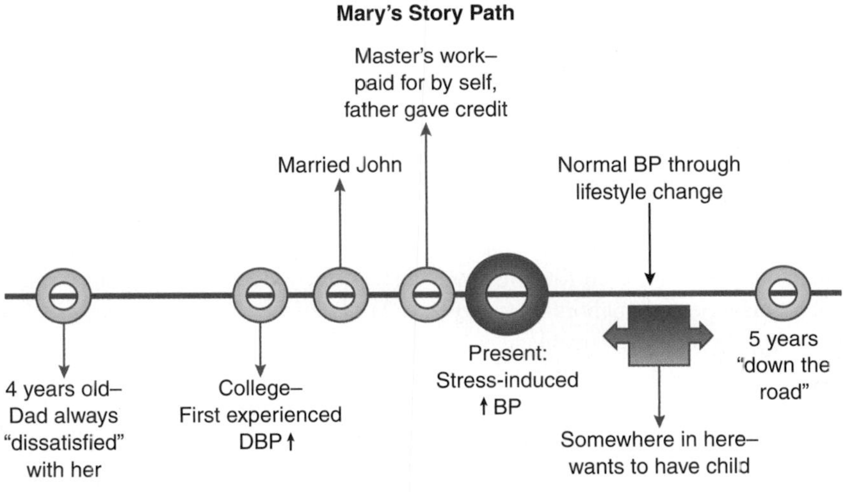

Fig 24 • 2 Mary's story path.

with the storyteller leading the way. The nurse makes notes on the story path so that both participants are engaged in the process, infusing the physiological indicator, a blood pressure of 180/110 mm Hg, with Mary's unique personal story.

Before ending any visit where story has been pulled into the foreground, it is important that the nurse ask if there is "anything else" about the health challenge that the storyteller wants to share to enhance understanding. What matters most about a health challenge may change from visit to visit, and any single visit may encompass more than one issue that matters the most. Detailed story paths include bits of evidence gleaned from what the storyteller emphasized. This evidence has the potential to guide nursing practice, including the next steps the nurse will take during this and upcoming visits.

Story path is just one approach to gathering the story in a practice setting. We have suggested others such as photographs, family trees, and pain diaries (Smith & Liehr, 2014b). There seems to be value in eliciting a story through a collaborative creation that enhances the telling and takes the story to a structure such as story path. The possible approaches for story gathering are limitless. The creative nurse will identify other unique approaches for querying what matters most about a health challenge. Coming to grips with what matters most about the health challenge one is facing is a process of embracing story, where paradoxically, embracing releases a person from story confines, engendering a sense of ease.

Creating Ease While Moving Toward Resolving

In the context of story theory, creating ease is defined as remembering disjointed story moments to experience flow in the midst of anchoring (Smith & Liehr, 1999) to an understanding of the whole story, even for only one "aha" moment. As a person anchors for a moment, embracing the comprehensible whole, flow ensues as easiness-with-self situated in a complex context. Ease is neither assured nor pervasive during story sharing. Sometimes it is elusive; sometimes it is experienced as only a moment in time. When story moments come together in a meaningful way for the person sharing a story, there is often some movement toward resolving the health challenge. Movement may be minuscule, or it may be a leap; it enables a shift in one's perspective usually accompanied by action to address what matters most about the health challenge.

Application of the Theory to Research

Story theory has been used to guide a story-centered intervention in a study of people with Stage 1 hypertension (Liehr et al., 2006). It has been used to guide structured data collection in qualitative studies with cancer patients (Williams, 2007), hemodialysis patients (Hain, 2008) and women suffering from migraine headaches (Ramsey, 2012). The story inquiry research method has also been used for story gathering and data analysis (Hain, Wands, & Liehr, 2011; Kelley & Lowe, 2012; Liehr et al., 2011; Wands, 2013). Details of the use of story theory for research can be found in the textbook *Middle Range Theory for Nursing* (Smith & Liehr, 2014a).

Application of the Theory

Application of the theory to nursing practice has occurred throughout discussion of the theory concepts, providing real-life examples that enable a move from conceptual to empirical. In the next section, we describe a seven-phase process that chronicles the development of nursing knowledge from evidence collected during nursing practice. Application to practice will surface as the exemplar of "transitioning to a nursing home" is described.

Practice Exemplar

Advancing Practice Scholarship Through Story Theory

We have proposed seven phases of inquiry for practicing nurses who want to develop practice evidence as a base for knowledge development (Smith & Liehr, 2005). The phases are as follows: (1) gather a story about what matters most about a health challenge; (2) compose a reconstructed story; (3) connect existing literature to the health challenge; (4) refine the name of the health challenge; (5) describe the developing story plot with high points, low points, and turning points; (6) identify movement toward resolving; and (7) collect additional stories about the health challenge (Smith & Liehr, 2014b). For the purposes of this chapter, we address all phases of the inquiry process except the last, which takes the nurse back to the practice environment to substantiate what emerged while completing the first six phases.

Phase one asks the practicing nurse to gather a story of what matters most about a health challenge. Querying what matters most about the health challenge is coming to know the unique perspective of the person sharing the story. To gather the story, the nurse could use a structured approach such as the story path, or story gathering could occur over time through attentive presence recognizing circumstance and life changes that are continually shaping one's story. Irrespective of how the nurse gathers the story, coming to know the other in true presence with mindful attention to what matters most culminates in a reconstructed story. The nurse in the following story queried the health challenge of transitioning to a nursing home environment for elders who had been living independently.

Phase two requires that the nurse compose a reconstructed story. A reconstructed story is a narrative creation with a beginning, a middle, and an end that weaves together the nurse's and the storyteller's perspective of the health challenge. The reconstructed story naturally incorporates what matters most about

the health challenge. The reconstructed story shared in this chapter was written by a nurse who cared for Elizabeth during the last months of her life in a nursing home. The nurse had practiced in this nursing home for 10 years, often witnessing the health challenge of transitioning from independent to nursing home living. The story gathering occurred over time, and story moments are synthesized as a reconstructed story to serve as an evidence base for understanding the independent living to nursing home living transition.

Elizabeth was an 88-year-old woman who enjoyed independent living in her bungalow with her husband of 65 years. She and her husband resided in the independent living component of a continuing care community. Elizabeth had a long history of atrial fibrillation, chronic heart failure, and diabetes; but she managed to remain independent, using a walker to get around. She attributed her independence to the devotion of her husband, who watched over her medication routine, diet, and the balance between her activity/rest patterns. At the end of January, Elizabeth began having difficulty moving her left leg, especially when she awoke in the morning. It seemed to her that her leg had fallen asleep due to positioning during the night. Then, one February morning, Elizabeth's lower leg was painful, cool to touch, and slightly discolored. Her husband called the community nurse, who immediately sent Elizabeth to the hospital, where a popliteal clot was found to be occluding the artery. Amputation was considered but rejected due to the complexity of Elizabeth's health situation. Clot-buster was dripped directly into Elizabeth's clot for 7 hours while she lay on her back and the clot dissolved. Elizabeth was relieved because she had always feared losing her leg after witnessing her grandmother's double amputation as a result of long-standing diabetes.

After 10 days in the hospital, Elizabeth returned to the nursing home component of her continuing care community, planning to

Continued

begin rehabilitation. Shortly after admission, she was diagnosed with the flu, delaying the start of rehabilitation. Once she began, the physical therapists referred to her as their "energizer bunny" because of her spirited approach to therapy. Throughout this time, it was very hard for Elizabeth to lift her left leg. No matter how hard she tried, she couldn't move it like she could move her right leg. Still, she was anticipating return to the bungalow to get on with everyday living with her husband. While Elizabeth was in the nursing home, her husband visited every day at mealtimes and when she was ready to go to sleep. She referred to these visits as the "best times of her day."

As part of the discharge plan, the physical therapists took Elizabeth to her bungalow to try out everyday activities. The difficulty moving her leg was magnified when she was in her usual environment, and the therapists began to think that she might not be able to return home. About the same time, Elizabeth began to have dramatic blood sugar swings that were accompanied by confusion and twitching that engaged all parts of her body. Her husband was anxious and looking for answers while she was consistently questioning: "What's going to happen to me now?" Her health challenge at this time was an arduous struggle to resume normal "independent" living in her bungalow with her husband, and what mattered most at this point was the unfamiliar, uncontrollable bodily experience and the uncertainty that ensued from unfamiliarity. The question "What's going to happen to me now?" was one the nurse had heard repeatedly over her years of nursing home practice as residents began to understand that they might not return home. She had begun to view the question as a marker of transition that demanded her concentrated attention to what mattered most for the resident.

Elizabeth didn't understand why her leg wouldn't move even though she worked so hard in therapy; she tried to hide the twitching, which she had never experienced before. The twitching and her attempts to move her leg took a lot of energy, and she often said

that she was tired. She never stopped saying that she wanted to "go home," but at some point the nurse suspected that the meaning of "going home" had changed for Elizabeth. The nurse asked her "Where is home?" and Elizabeth responded that she wasn't sure. Shortly thereafter, Elizabeth stopped asking to go to the bungalow, and she expressed wishes for a peaceful death.

It became clear that Elizabeth was not getting better as her heart failure became more debilitating and blood sugar swings continued despite precise insulin dosing and measured carbohydrate intake. At this time, the doctor suggested hospice. Elizabeth and her husband listened to the description of hospice services, and she signed the hospice papers. While under hospice care, she stopped troubling over her failed effort to move her left leg, continued to have blood sugar swings, and never stopped trying to hide the twitching.

Appearances mattered to Elizabeth, and she continued to care about how she looked. One time she told the nurse that she wore her pink shirt as often as she could because her husband liked it. She asked to have her roots done, and the nurse took her to the beauty shop one floor away. When she returned, her husband took her picture. She was wearing her pink shirt, and her husband later included the picture in a memorial collage that was created when she died. The long loving relationship between Elizabeth and her husband was most important to both of them in her last days. She giggled with him while recalling fun times they had over the years, and she asked for hugs, an uncharacteristic request that became increasingly familiar to her husband during this time.

Elizabeth and her roommate told each other stories, shared chocolates, and looked out for each other as well as they could. Her roommate called her "sweet pea." On the day Elizabeth died, the roommate asked Elizabeth's husband and the nurse if she could pray with them.

Elizabeth had been in the nursing home about 3 months before she died. The course of her story shifted from one of expectation for familiar normalcy in her bungalow with her husband to one of peaceful going home. The nurse in this situation of caring for Elizabeth was attentively present to the shifting story, following Elizabeth's lead to pursue meaning during the last months of her life.

Phase three of the story inquiry process requires that the nurse become familiar with the existing literature about the complicating health challenge—in this case, transitioning from independent to nursing home living. For the purposes of this chapter, only the beginnings of a literature review are reported. However, the practicing nurse interested in a particular health challenge will stay abreast of related literature and eventually develop a broad literature base informing ongoing interpretation of stories and physiological bodily responses. To begin this literature search, the phrases *nursing home transition* and *elder* were searched together.

Brandburg (2007) conducted an integrated literature review intended to synthesize the state of the science regarding transition to a nursing home for older adults. The 13 articles that met the inclusion criteria led to the creation of a "transition process framework" with the foundational concepts of initial reaction, transitional influences, adjustment, and acceptance. Brandburg (2007) reported that the initial reaction and adjustment phases of the process require approximately 6 months. During that time, people move from disorganization to reorganization and relationship building. They also move from a sense of homelessness to recognition of a new home where new relationships are developed and old ones are cultivated. She describes the "final" or acceptance phase as one in which "reflecting on the transition experience in light of personal values helped many older adults accept their new home because they could find meaning in their present situation" (p. 55).

The theme of home that was noted by Brandburg (2007) was strongly described by Heliker and Scholler-Jaquish (2006) in a study of 10 newly admitted nursing home residents

who were interviewed multiple times over their first 3 months of residency. Residents responded to the directive: "Tell me a story about what it is like for you to come here and live." Data from 32 interviews lasting from 15 to 60 minutes were analyzed using a hermeneutical phenomenological approach. Three themes emerged: becoming homeless, getting settled, learning the ropes, and creating a place. The first theme, becoming homeless, contributed to the researchers' conclusion that "one cannot separate home, memories, and friends from one's very identity. Each continuously shapes and is shaped by the other" (p. 41). Getting settled and learning the ropes was a theme characterized by residents' shift from unknown to known, invisible to visible. Creating a place was a theme related to creating meaning in this new life situation. In their conclusion, the authors note the important place of story: "The challenge for nursing home staff is to create situations, a clearing for sharing stories . . . that facilitate the cocreation of new meanings. . . . A staff that listens to what matters to residents can interpret a plan of care that is meaningful" (p. 41).

Listening was the major theme in a brief by Maynes (2004). She shared the story of a patient she met on a short hospitalization, during which his cancer diagnosis was confirmed and he was evaluated as having a "poor prognosis." The nurse listened to the quiet man and honored his wish to return "home" to the farm country where he was raised. On the day he was to be transferred, the nurse went to his bedside to say good-bye, thankful that he would be returning to the place he loved. When she approached the bed, she realized that he had died. "I sat next to him, put his hand in mine, and whispered 'good-bye'" (p. 32).

Elizabeth's short nursing home stay fits most clearly with the initial reaction phase described by Brandburg (2007) and the becoming homeless theme described by Heliker and Scholler-Jaquish (2006), both of whom call attention to the meaning of home. The idea of "home" emerges strongly from the literature and story sources. Both Elizabeth and the man in Maynes's (2004)

Continued

Practice Exemplar cont.

brief feel the pull of "home" as they approach death. Merging Elizabeth's story with the relevant literature prepared the stage for the next step of the story inquiry process: refining the name of the health challenge.

Phase four suggests that the nurse refine the name of the health challenge, if necessary. There may be some times when the original name is confirmed as adequately expressive of the challenge, and there are other times when the convergence of the reconstructed story with the existing literature demands that the health challenge name be refined. We believe that "naming" is most important for the continuing work, and we advocate that the health challenge name be neither too high nor too low in level of abstraction. Names that are too high may be difficult to apply to practice situations, and names that are too low may be meaningful for only a few people. Considering Elizabeth's story and the existing literature, the name of the complicating health challenge was changed to "struggling to go home." This health challenge name is consistent with the original name of transitioning from independent to nursing home living, but it captures more clearly what matters most about the transition. It is neither so high that it cannot be applied in practice nor so low that it applies to only a narrow subset of people. Because it is in the middle, it may also have applicability to other populations, such as people who have been evacuated from their homes due to natural disasters or families of premature newborns who demand extended hospital stays.

Phase five of the story inquiry process focuses on the developing story plot through identification of high points, low points, and turning points. Turning points are shifts in what is happening to create a revision in the storyteller's forward view. These are situations or events that move the story along. High and low points note times when things are going well or not so well. Table 24-1 records the turning points, high

Table 24 • 1 — Turning Points, High Points, and Low Points in Elizabeth's Story

Story Event	TP	HP	LP
Difficulty moving leg beginning in January			x
Change in leg pain, temperature, and color—leading to hospitalization	x		x
Decision not to amputate	x	x	
Clot was dissolved	x	x	
Return to nursing home for rehabilitation	x		
Diagnosed with flu	x		x
Couldn't move leg though she tried			x
Husband's four-times-daily visits		x	
Inability to perform usual activities with physical therapist in bungalow—aware she may not return	x		x
Blood sugar swings, confusion, and twitching			x
"What's going to happen to me now?"			x
Stopped asking about going to bungalow and began talking about peaceful death	x		
Signed hospice papers	x		
Getting roots done, giggling with husband, sharing chocolate with roommate		x	

TP = turning point; HP = high point; LP = low point.

Practice Exemplar cont.

points, and low points in Elizabeth's reconstructed story. Turning points may also be high points or low points, but this is not always the case. Sometimes turning points exist with no particular value assigned by the person living the story. In Elizabeth's story, turning points can be summarized as: (1) diagnosed health issues, (2) treatment milestones, and (3) the hospice decision. High points are (1) "favorable" (according to Elizabeth) treatment milestones and (2) relationship-centered moments of joy. Low points are (1) limitations in physical movement, (2) unfamiliar bodily experiences with and without diagnoses, and (3) uncertainty. As the practicing nurse collected more stories of this nature, comparison, contrast, and synthesis of turning points, high points, and low points would be possible, and the evidence from stories could contribute to the knowledge base guiding practice with people who are transitioning into a nursing home. One last phase of analysis considers the evidence from stories to identify how people get through the health challenge.

Phase six asks that the practicing nurse identify how an individual moved toward resolving the health challenge. This phase of practice inquiry may be most instructive for the nurse's continuing work with a particular population because it taps the inherent wisdom of people living the challenge to understand how they got by. The question facing the nurse analyzing Elizabeth's reconstructed story is: How does Elizabeth move toward resolving the complicating health challenge of struggling to go home? Elizabeth put all her

effort into her recovery so that her therapists called her their "energizer bunny." When her efforts failed and her bodily experience indicated that she was on a different path, she signed the hospice papers. Finally, Elizabeth enjoyed moments with her husband and her roommate and chose to do things that kept her appearance as she liked. Movement toward resolving recounted in the reconstructed story included the approaches of (1) devoting energy to recovery, (2) accepting hospice, (3) experiencing the joy of relationship, and (4) attending to self through personal appearance. The range of ways Elizabeth moved toward resolving reflects the dynamic and complex nature of story. What is characterized as movement toward resolving emerges as the story unfolds. At a higher level of abstraction, these approaches used by Elizabeth, may be conceptualized as (1) focusing energy to heal, (2) accepting the inevitable, (3) appreciating relationship, and (4) attending to self. At this higher level of abstraction, the four approaches extracted from the reconstructed story have implications for people who are struggling to go home, regardless of the context of their situation. The story describes how one person created ease and offers an invitation to consider how others in similar situations may create ease as they move toward resolving a health challenge of struggling to go home. Once again, there is guidance for nursing practice in the wisdom of people living health challenges. The nurse could use what is learned from this story analysis to guide current practice and frame further inquiry.

■ Summary

This chapter has introduced the reader to story as an essential element of evidence guiding nursing practice. The authors hope that practicing nurses can use the story inquiry process to access story evidence for the precious contribution it can make to nursing

knowledge. Each nurse at the bedside, in the clinic, or in the office is uniquely positioned to gather and analyze practice stories. The middle-range story theory is proposed as a framework for structuring story-gathering and analysis.

References

Banks-Wallace, J. (2002). Talk the talk: Storytelling and analysis rooted in African-American oral tradition. *Qualitative Health Research, 12*(3), 410–426.

Benner, P. (1984). *From novice to expert.* Menlo Park, CA: Addison-Wesley.

Boykin, A., & Schoenhofer, S. (1991). Story as a link between nursing practice, ontology and epistemology. *IMAGE: Journal of Nursing Scholarship, 23,* 245–248.

Boykin, A., & Schoenhofer, S. (2001). The role of nursing leadership in creating caring environments in health care delivery systems. *Nursing Administration Quarterly, 25*(3), 1–7.

Brandburg, G. (2007). Making the transition to nursing home life: A framework to help older adults adapt to the long-term care environment. *Journal of Gerontological Nursing, 33*(6), 50–56.

Charon, R. (2006). *Narrative medicine: Honoring the stories of illness.* New York: Oxford University Press.

Charon, R. (2012). At the membranes of care: Stories in narrative medicine. *Academic Medicine, 87*(3), 342–347.

Charon, R., & Montello, M. (2002). *Stories matter: The role of narrative in medical ethics.* New York: Routledge.

Chinn, P. L., & Kramer, M. K. (1999). *Theory and nursing integrated knowledge development.* St. Louis, MO: C. V. Mosby.

Crichton, J., & Koch, T. (2007). Living with dementia: Curating self-identity. *Dementia, 6*(3), 365–381.

Diamond, J. (2000). *Narrative means to sober ends: Treating addiction and its aftermath.* New York: Guilford Press.

Ford, K., & Turner, D. (2001). Stories seldom told: Pediatric nurses' experiences of caring for hospitalized children with special needs and their families. *Journal of Advanced Nursing, 33,* 288–295.

Hain, D. (2007). What matters most?: Promoting adherence by understanding health challenges faced by hemodialysis patients. *American Kidney Fund: Professional Advocate, 7*(1), 3.

Hain, E. (2008). Cognitive function and adherence of older adults undergoing hemodialysis. *Nephrology Nursing Journal, 35*(1), 23–29.

Hain, D., Wands, L. M., & Liehr, P. (2011). Approaches to resolve health challenges in a population of older adults undergoing hemodialysis. *Research in Gerontological Nursing, 4*(1), 53–62.

Heliker, D. (2007). Story sharing: Restoring the reciprocity of caring in long-term care. *Journal of Psychosocial Nursing and Mental Health Services, 45*(7), 20–23.

Heliker, D., & Scholler-Jaquish, A. (2006). Transition of new residents: Basing practice on resident's perspective. *Journal of Gerontological Nursing, 32*(9), 34–42.

Holm, A.-K., Lepp, M., & Ringsberg, K. C. (2005). Dementia: Involving patients in storytelling—a caring intervention. A pilot study. *Journal of Clinical Nursing, 14,* 256–263.

Keady, J., Williams, S., & Hughes-Roberts, J. (2007). Making mistakes: Using co-constructed inquiry to illuminate meaning and relationships in the early adjustment to Alzheimer's disease—a single case study approach. *Dementia, 6*(3), 343–364.

Kelley, M., & Lowe, J. (2012). The health challenge of stress experienced by Native American adolescents. *Archives in Psychiatric Nursing, 26*(1), 71–73.

Liehr, P., Meininger, J. C., Vogler, R., Chan, W., Frazier, L., Smalling, S., & Fuentes, F. (2006). Adding story-centered care to standard lifestyle intervention for people with Stage One hypertension. *Applied Nursing Research, 19,* 16–21.

Liehr, P., Nishimura, C., Ito, M., Wands, L.M. & Takahashi, R. (2011). A lifelong journey of moving beyond wartime trauma for survivors from Hiroshima and Pearl Harbor. *Advances in Nursing Science, 34*(3), 215–228.

Liehr, P., & Smith, M. J. (2000). Using story theory to guide nursing practice. *International Journal of Human Caring, 4,* 13–18.

Liehr, P., & Smith, M. J. (2008). Story theory. In M. J. Smith & P. Liehr (Eds.), *Middle range theory for nursing* (2nd ed.). (pp. 205–224). New York: Springer.

Maynes, R. (2004). Going home again. *Nursing 2004, 34*(4), 32.

Mehl-Madrona, L. (2007). *Narrative medicine: The use of history and story in the healing process.* Rochester, VT: Bear & Company.

Newman, M. A. (1999). The rhythm of relating in a paradigm of wholeness. *Image: Journal of Nursing Scholarship, 31,* 227–230.

Newman, M. A., Sime, A. M., & Corcoran-Perry, S. A. (1991). The focus of the discipline of nursing. *Advances in Nursing Science, 14*(1), 1–6.

Nightingale, F. (1969). *Notes on Nursing.* New York: Dover.

Parse, R. R. (1981). *Man-living-health: A theory of nursing.* New York: Wiley.

Peplau, H. (1991). *Interpersonal relations in nursing.* New York: Springer.

Polanyi, M. (1958). *The study of man.* Chicago: University of Chicago Press.

Sierpina, M., & Cole, T. R. (2004). *Care Management Journals, 5*(3), 175–182.

Ramsey, A. R. (2012). Living with migraine headache: A phenomenological study of women's experiences. *Holistic Nursing Practice, 26*(6), 297–307.

Smith, M. J., & Liehr, P. (1999). Attentively embracing story: A middle-range theory with practice and research implications. *Scholarly Inquiry for Nursing. Practice: An International Journal, 13,* 187–204.

Smith, M. J., & Liehr, P. (2003). The theory of attentively embracing story. In M. J. Smith & P. Liehr (Eds.),

Middle range theory for nursing (1st ed.) (pp. 167–188). New York: Springer.

Smith, M. J., & Liehr, P. (2005). Story theory: Advancing nursing practice scholarship. *Holistic Nursing Practice, 19*(6), 272–276.

Smith, M. J., & Liehr, P. (2014a). *Middle range theory for nursing* (3rd ed.). New York: Springer.

Smith, M. J., & Liehr, P. (2014b). Story theory. In M. J. Smith & P. Liehr (Eds.), *Middle range theory for nursing* (3rd ed.) (pp. 225–252). New York: Springer.

Wands, L. M. (2013). "No one gets through it OK": The health challenge of coming home from war. *Advances in Nursing Science, 36*(3), 186–199.

Watson, J. (1997). The theory of human caring: Retrospective and prospective. *Nursing Science Quarterly, 10,* 49–52.

Williams, L. (2007). Whatever it takes: Informal caregiving dynamics in blood and marrow transplantation. *Oncology Nursing Forum, 34*(2), 379–387.

Chapter 25

The Community Nursing Practice Model

MARILYN E. PARKER,
CHARLOTTE D. BARRY,
AND BETH M. KING

Introducing the Theorists
Overview of the Model
Application of the Model
Practice Exemplar
Summary
References

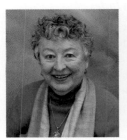

Marilyn E. Parker

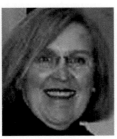

Charlotte D. Barry

Introducing the Theorists

Marilyn E. Parker is professor emerita at the Christine E. Lynn College of Nursing at Florida Atlantic University and recently retired professor from the University of Kansas School of Nursing. She earned degrees from Incarnate Word College (BSN), the Catholic University of America (MSN), and Kansas State University (PhD). Her overall career mission is to enhance nursing practice, scholarship, and education through nursing theory, using both innovative and traditional means to improve care and advance the discipline.

As principal investigator for a program of grants to create and use a new community nursing practice model, Dr. Parker has provided leadership to develop transdisciplinary school-based wellness centers devoted to health and social services for children and families from underserved multicultural communities, to teach university students from several disciplines, and to develop research and policy to promote community well-being.

Dr. Parker's active participation in nursing education and health care in several countries led to her 2001 Fulbright Scholar Award to Thailand, where she continues collaboration with Thai colleagues. Her commitment to caring for underserved populations and to health policy evaluation led to being named a National Public Health Leadership Institute Fellow and to being elected a distinguished practitioner in the National Academies of Practice in Nursing. Dr. Parker is a fellow in the American Academy of Nursing.

Charlotte D. Barry is a professor and master teacher at the Florida Atlantic University Christine E. Lynn College of Nursing. Dr. Barry graduated from Brooklyn College, New York, with an associate's degree in nursing; holds a bachelor's degree in health administration, a master's degree in nursing from Florida Atlantic University, and a PhD from the University of Miami, Florida. She is nationally certified in school nursing and in 2013 was recognized as one of the best 25 Nursing Professors in Florida. Dr. Barry is a fellow in the American Academy of Nursing.

The focus of Dr. Barry's scholarship has been caring for persons in schools and communities. As a coprincipal investigator with Dr. Parker, Dr. Barry cocreated the community nursing practice model from the transdisciplinary practice unfolded at several school-based wellness centers. Her current research includes the usefulness of the community nursing practice model to guide practice in global communities including the United States, Uganda, and Haiti. Building on the school-based wellness center in Uganda, a replica program is being developed in a rural community in Haiti.

Dr. Barry provides leadership in many community and professional organizations including Sigma Theta Tau, Iota XI Chapter, the International Association for Human Caring, the National Association of School Nursing, and the Florida Association of School Nurses. She also serves on the Board of the South Florida Haiti Project and the Broward County School Health Advisory Committee.

Overview of the Model

The *community nursing practice model* (CNPM) began with and continues to be a blend of the ideal and the practical. The ideal was the commitment to develop and use nursing concepts to guide nursing practice, education, and scholarship and a desire to develop a nursing practice as an essential component of a college of nursing. The practical was the effort to bring this CNPM to life within the context and structures of an existing community health care system. The model reflects the mission of the Christine E. Lynn College of Nursing at Florida Atlantic University and the concept of nursing held by its faculty: *Nursing is nurturing the wholeness of persons and environments in caring* (Florida Atlantic University College of Nursing Philosophy and Mission [FAU], 1994/2012).

The concepts and relationships of the model are the guiding forces for community practice. Through various participatory-action approaches, including ongoing shared reflection, intuitive insights, and discoveries, the CNPM has evolved and continues to develop. The education of university students and the conduct of student and faculty research have been integrated with nursing and social work practice. Throughout the early development and ongoing refinement of the model, there has been nurturing of collaborative community partnerships, evaluation and development of school and community health policy, and development of enriched community.

Foundations of the Model

Essential values that form the basis of the model are (1) persons are respected; (2) persons are caring, and caring is understood as the essence of nursing; and (3) persons are whole and always connected with one another in families and communities. These essential, or transcendent, values are always present in nursing situations, while other actualizing values guide practice in certain situations.

The principles of primary health care from the World Health Organization (WHO; 1978) are the actualizing values. These additional concepts of the model are (1) access, (2) essentiality, (3) community participation, (4) empowerment, and (5) intersectoral collaboration. Concepts of nursing practice that have emerged include transitional care and enhancing care. The CNPM illuminates these values and each of the concepts in four interrelated themes: nursing, person, community, and environment, along with a structure of interconnecting services, activities, and community partnerships (Parker & Barry, 1999). An inquiry group method has been designed and is the primary means of ongoing assessment and evaluation (Barry, Lange, & King, 2011; Campbell et al., 2001; Clark et al., 2003; Parker, Barry, & King, 2000; Ryan, Hawkins, Parker, & Hawkins, 2004; Sadler, Newlin, & Jenkins, 2011).

Nursing

The unique focus of nursing is nurturing the wholeness of persons and environments in caring (FAU, 1994/2012). Nursing practice, education, and scholarship require creative integration of multiple ways of knowing and understanding through knowledge synthesis within a context of value and meaning. Nursing knowledge is embedded in the nursing situation, the lived experience of caring between the nurse and the one receiving care. The nurse is authentically present for the other, to hear calls for caring and to create dynamic nursing responses. The school-based wellness centers in the community become places for persons and families to access nursing and social services where they are: in homes, work camps, schools, or under trees in a community gathering spot. Nursing is dynamic and portable; there is no predetermined nursing and often no predetermined access place (Dyess & Chase, 2012; Parker, 1997; Parker & Barry, 1999).

Nursing practice is further described within the context of transitional care and enhancing care. Transitional care is that in which clients and families are provided essential health care while being referred to a more permanent source of health care in the community. Transitional care, an ideal for nursing and social work practice, is sometimes not possible owing to immigration status, a complex and confounding health-care system, or other issues of the family.

Enhancing care describes nursing and social work that is intended to assist the client and family who need care in addition to that provided by a local health-care provider.

Person

Respect for person is present in all aspects of nursing, with clients, community members, and colleagues. Respect includes a stance of humility that the nurse does not know all that can be known about a person and a situation, acknowledging that the person is the expert in his or her own care and knowing his or her experience. Respect carries with it an openness to learn and grow. Values and beliefs of various cultures are reflected in expressions of caring. The person as whole and connected with others, not the disease or problem, is the focus of nursing.

Persons are empowered by understanding choices, how to choose, and how to live daily with choices made. The person defines what is necessary to well-being and what priorities exist in daily life of the family. Nursing and social work practice based on practical, sound, culturally acceptable, and cost-effective methods are necessary for well-being and wholeness of persons, families, and communities.

Early on, Swadener and Lubeck's (1995) work on deconstructing the discourse of risk was a major influence on practice. *At risk* connotes a deficiency that needs fixing; a doing to, rather than collaborating with. Thinking about children and families "at promise" instead of "at risk" inspires an approach to knowing the other as whole and filled with potential.

Respect and caring in nursing require full participation of persons, families, and communities in assessment, design, and evaluation of services. Based on this concept, an inquiry group method is used for ongoing appraisal of services. This method is defined as a "route of knowing" and "a route to other questions." Each person is a coparticipant, an expert knower in his or her experience; the facilitator is the expert knower of the process. The facilitator's role is to encourage expressions of knowing so that calls for nursing and guidance for nursing responses can be heard. In this way, the essential care for persons and families can be known, and care can be designed, offered, and evaluated (Barry, 1998; Barry, Lange, & King, 2011; Gordon, Barry, Dunn, & King, 2011; Parker et al., 2000).

Community

Community, as understood within the model, was formed from the classical definition offered by Smith and Maurer (1995) and from Peck's (1987) existential, relational view. According to Smith and Maurer, a community is defined by its members and is characterized by shared values. This expanded notion of community moves away from a locale as a defining characteristic and includes self-defined groups who share common interests and concerns and who interact with one another.

Community, offered by Peck (1987), is a safe place for members and ensures the security of being included and honored. His work focuses on building community through a web of relationships grounded in acceptance of individual and cultural differences among faculty and staff and acceptance of others in the widening circles, including colleagues within the practice and discipline, other health-care colleagues from varied disciplines, grant funders, and other collaborators. The notion of transdisciplinary care is an exemplar of this approach to community. Another defining characteristic of community, according to Peck, is willingness to risk and tolerate a certain lack of structure. The practice guided by the model reflects this in fostering a creative approach to program development, implementation, evaluation, and research.

Practice within the model, whether unfolding in a clinic or under a tree where persons have gathered, provides a welcoming and safe place for sharing stories of caring. The intention to know others as experts in their self-care while listening to their hopes and dreams for well-being creates a communion between the client and provider that guides the development of a nurturing relationship. Knowing the other in relationship to their communities, such as family, school, work, worship, or play, honors the complexity of the context of persons' lives and offers the opportunity to understand and participate with them.

Environment

The notion of environment within the CNPM provides the context for understanding the wholeness of interconnected lives. The environment, one of the oldest concepts in nursing described by Nightingale (1859/1992), is not only the immediate effects of air, odors, noise, and warmth on the reparative powers of the patient but also indicates the social settings that contribute to health and illness such as those identified as the social determinants of health (WHO, 2007, 2012). Another nursing visionary, Lillian Wald, witnessed the hardships of poverty and disenfranchisement on the residents of the lower Manhattan immigrant communities. She developed the Henry Street Settlement House to provide a broad range of care that included direct physical care up to and including finding jobs, housing, and influencing the creation of child labor laws (Zaiger, 2013).

Chooporian (1986) reinspired nurses to expand the notion of environment not only to include the immediate context of patients' lives but also to think of the relationship between health and social issues that "influence human beings and hence create conditions for heath and illness" (p. 53). Reflecting on earth caring, Schuster (1990) urged another look at the environment, inviting nurses to consider a broader view that included nonhuman species and the nonhuman world. Acknowledging the interrelatedness of all living things energizes caring from this broader perspective into a wider circle. Kleffel (1996) described this as "an ecocentric approach grounded in the cosmos. The whole environment, including inanimate elements such as rocks and minerals, along with animate animals and plants, is assigned an intrinsic value" (p. 4). This perspective directs thinking about the interconnectedness of all elements, both animate and inanimate. Teaching, practice, and scholarship require a caring context that respects, explores, nurtures, and celebrates the interconnectedness of all living things and inanimate objects throughout the global environment.

Structure of Services and Activities

The CNPM is envisioned as three concentric circles around a core. Envisioning the CNPM as a watercolor representation, one can appreciate the vibrancy of practice within the CNPM, the amorphous interconnectedness of the core and the circles, and the "certain lack of structure" draws attention to the beauty in creating responses to unique calls for nursing. The CNPM calls into the circles others to create programs and environments that nurture well-being (Fig. 25-1).

The Community Nursing Practice Model: Concentric Circles of Empathetic Concern

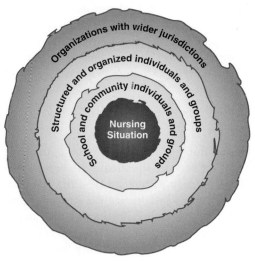

Fig 25 • 1 The community nursing practice model: Concentric circles of empathic concern. ©Florida Atlantic University.

Core Services

Core services, created from the results of inquiry group methodology (Barry, Gordon, & Lange, 2007; Barry et al., 2011; Parker et al., 2002), are provided to nurture the wholeness of persons and environments through caring. The unique experiences of staff and faculty with the hopes and dreams for well-being of those receiving care create the substance of the core: respecting self-care practice; honoring lay and indigenous care; inviting participation and listening to clients' stories of health and well-being; providing care that is essential for the other; supporting caring for self, family, and community; providing care that is culturally competent; and collaborating with others for care. These services, provided to children, students, school staff, and families from the community, occur in the following (and frequently overlapping) categories of care:

1. *Design and coordinate care:* examples include referrals, navigation to other health services, home visits, and concepts of transitional and enhancing care are illuminated here through the development of collaborative relationships

2. *Primary prevention and health education:* examples include assessment of child-development milestones, pre- and postnatal wellness, breast health, testicular health, and stress reduction

3. *Secondary prevention/health screening/early intervention:* examples include screenings for hearing and vision, height/weight/BMI, cholesterol, blood sugar, blood pressure, clinical breast examinations, lead levels, assessment, administration of immunizations, and early management of health issues

4. *Tertiary prevention/primary care:* assessment, diagnosis, treatment, and care management for chronic health issues, crisis intervention, and behavioral support

First Circle

The first circle of the CNPM depicts a widening circle of concern and support for the well-being of persons and communities. This circle includes persons and groups in each school and community who share concern for the well-being of persons served at the centers. This includes participants in inquiry groups, parents/guardians, school faculty, and noninstructional staff, after-school groups, parent/teacher organizations, and school advisory councils. The services provided within this circle might include the following:

1. *Consultation and collaboration:* building relationships and community, answering inquiries on matters of health and well-being, providing in-service and health education, serving on school committees, reviewing policies and procedures

2. *Appraisal and evaluation:* conducting community assessments, appraising care provided, evaluating outcomes, and promoting programs that enhance well-being for individuals and communities

Second Circle

The second circle draws attention to the wider context of concern and influence for well-being and includes structured and organized groups whose members also share concern for the education and well-being of the persons served at the centers but within a wider range or jurisdiction such as a district or county. Examples of these policy-making or advising groups include the school district and county public health department, voluntary organizations such as the Red Cross, and funders who offer support for school and community caring. The services provided in this circle include the following:

1. *Consultation and collaboration:* building relationships and community with members of these groups; contributing to policy appraisal, development, and evaluation; leading and serving on teams and committees responsible for overseeing the care of students and families; providing school nurse education
2. *Research and evaluation:* assessing school health services, describing research findings for best practices related to school and community health, and designing research projects focused on school/community health issues, and/or school/community nursing practice.

Third Circle

The third circle includes state, regional, national, and international organizations with whom we are related in various ways. Services within this circle are focused on:

1. *Consultation and collaboration:* building relationships and community with members and collaborating about scholarship, policy, outcomes, practice, research, educational needs of school nurses and advanced practice nurses; sustainability through ongoing and additional funding
2. *Appraisal and evaluation:* school nursing and advanced practice faculty organizations offer a milieu for discussion and appraisal of the services provided at the centers (Organizations in this circle may include national and international organizations such as universities, religious organizations, the Centers for Disease Control and Prevention,

Department of Health and Human Services, Ministry of Health, World Health Organization, national professional organizations and boards, licensing agencies, and various non-governmental organizations [NGOs], such as Partners in Health and Doctors Without Borders.)

Connection of Core to Concentric Circles

Connections of the core to the concentric circles of services illuminate the complexity of the practice within the CNPM. The core service of *consultation and collaboration* is a primary focus of practice, beginning with nursing and social work colleagues and extending to participating clients, families, policymakers, funders, and legislators. This value-laden service has been essential to the viability and sustainability of this CNPM. It promotes the stance of humility that guides the respectful question throughout the circles: How can we be helpful to you? The answer directs the creation of respectful, individualized care and program development. Essential health-care services are created within the core and extend into the first circle.

Connections to the second circle unfold from the collaborating relationships with colleagues in the health department, school district, and other groups taking the lead with school and community health. Committees of center administrators and staff meet regularly to discuss school and community health issues and to seek consensus on possible solutions. Health-care providers are consultants for medical questions and referrals, and school nurse education may also be provided for nurses to prepare them for community nursing practice.

Like the other circles, the third circle depicts the breadth of relationships developed at meetings and through publications and presentations at local, regional, national, and international conferences. Administration and faculty have been widely recognized for the contribution made to the health and well-being of children and families.

Application of the Model

The model has been used as the framework for research, education, and practice across disciplines and with diverse foci. Some examples include the study of nursing language in electronic records; a framework for curriculum development for a master's program in advanced community nursing at Naresuan University, Phitsanulok, Thailand; and the use of the model by faculty of nursing at Mbarara University of Science and Technology, Mbarara, Uganda, to develop study of advanced community nursing and to design and operate the first school-based community nursing wellness center in Uganda.

The CNPM guides a diverse, complex, and transdisciplinary practice of nursing and social work in school-based community wellness centers serving children and families from diverse multicultural communities. The collaborative approach of the CNPM fosters relationships and acceptance by local communities and providers as essential component to the health-care system. The CNPM was featured in a major community nursing text (Clark, 2003) and a school nursing practice text (Gordon & Barry, 2006).

The CNPM has been the guiding framework for a wide range of theses and dissertations and in software development. In the field of computer science engineering, the CNPM has been used to give voice to nursing through the development of a web-based classification system, which quantifies the qualitative language of nursing, specifically the concepts of caring, knowing, connection, and respect. The researchers analyzed nursing situations based on the CNPM to develop an electronic record that quantified the transcendent values of the CNPM (Chinchanikar, 2009; Dass, 2011; Parker, Pandya, Hsu, Noel, & Newlin, 2008; Tripathi, 2010). A first patent application has been published by the US Patent Office (U.S. Patent No. 2013/0311203A1; Parker, Pandya, Hsu, & Huang, 2013). The research includes use of caring theory and nursing language research based on the community caring practice model as a framework for patient human–robot interaction (Huang, Tanioka, Locsin, Parker, & Masory, 2011)

Sternberg (2009) identified the CNPM as the theoretical perspective grounding her research exploring the experience and meaning of transnational motherhood. Her findings illuminated the themes of sacrifice, suffering, and hoping for a better life for their children as the essence of their mothering from a distance. The author affirms the usefulness of the CNPM in guiding this research to understand the experience of these women living as whole caring individuals.

Similarly the findings of Conrad's (2010) dissertation research identified the usefulness of the CNPM as a framework to provide care to culturally diverse populations. The intention to respect each individual and to respect his or her health-care beliefs and practices can be the grounding for the creation of nursing responses that nurture the other's hopes and dreams for well-being. Pope's (2011) historical research was grounded in the core beliefs of the CNPM, and her findings identified the need for interconnectedness to facilitate community partnership and enhancement of relationships.

Application in Nursing Education

Barry, Blum, Eggenberger, Palmer-Hickman, and Mosley (2010) focused on the transcendent values of respect, caring, and wholeness of persons in the nursing situation through the use of simulation to enhance nursing education. Through simulation, the students were guided to come to know the human face of homelessness, to understand the whole context of the person's life, and, through compassion, to come to see their faces reflected back. The specific goals of the simulation were to understand the fullness of the lived experience of homelessness and to understand the full experience of caring for Mildred, the simulated woman who was homeless.

Ladd, Grimley, Hickman, and Touhy (2013) built on the simulation model grounded in the CNPM to develop a teaching–learning nursing situation related to end-of-life care.

Focusing on coming to know the individual and family, students studied ways of nurturing wholeness. Reflective analysis was incorporated to promote the student's self-awareness of their own values and beliefs and the relation of these to nursing care.

Barry, Blum, and Purnell (2007) used the CNPM to assist nursing's students understanding of the lived experience of victims of Hurricane Katrina. The students went door to door asking individuals how they could be helpful and listening to calls for nursing. Many times the call was to listen to an individual's story of survival and displacement; for others, it was facilitating getting a child enrolled in school. The students reached out into the community for resources and brought them back to the individuals. Through this immersion experience, the students were able to live and feel the connectedness to others and community and to experience the meaning of nurturing the wholeness of the other through caring.

Application in Practice

The transcendent values of respect and caring provide the underpinnings of the inquiry group method used by the CNPM to identify health concerns and community strengths and assets. Several studies have identified the usefulness of the inquiry group method as a valuable tool not only to gather perspectives from community residents and partners to understand and identify health needs and services but also to resolve problems (Clark, 2003; Kasle, Wilhelm, & Reed, 2002; Plonczynski et al., 2007; Sadler et al., 2011). This method has also been linked to increasing the likelihood of acceptance of change by communities (Campbell et al., 2001). The value of including community partners and stakeholders in decision making was supported by the research of Dyess and Chase (2012).

The actualizing values of access, essentiality, community participation, empowerment, and intersectoral collaboration guide nursing practice in the CNPM. An example of these values in action can be found in the study by Barry et al. (2011). They used the CNPM as the framework to develop a breast health promotion outreach for underserved women. The inquiry group method was used to establish the participant as the expert of her own care with dialogue and inclusiveness grounded in the values of respect, caring, and wholeness of persons. The value of community voice to enhance the care of the underserved is highlighted in the research of Sternberg and Lee (2013). Their research compared the frequency of depressive symptoms of premenopausal Latinas born in the United States to Latina immigrants and found that immigrant Latinas rated themselves slightly higher on the Centers for Epidemiologic Studies Depression Scale.

Tables 25-1 and 25-2 highlight the research and studies focusing on the transcendent and actualizing values of the CNPM.

Table 25 • 1   Illumination of the Transcendent and Actualizing Values of the Community Nursing Practice Model

Value Category	Description	References
Transcendent Values: Present in all nursing situations		
Respect	Refers to honoring the inherent dignity and uniqueness of each individual	Barry, Gordon, & Lange (2007); Barry, Lange, & King (2011); Chinchanikar (2009); Dass (2011); Tripathi (2010)
Caring	Understand that to be human is to be caring and also that caring is the essence of nursing	Barry, Gordon, & Lange (2007); Barry, Lange, & King (2011); Chinchanikar (2009); Dass (2011); Huang, Tanioka, Locsin,

Table 25 • 1	Illumination of the Transcendent and Actualizing Values of the Community Nursing Practice Model—cont'd	
Value Category	**Description**	**References**
		Parker, & Masory (2011); Parker, Pandya, Hsu, Noell, & Newlin (2008); Tripathi (2010)
Wholeness	Views persons as whole in the moment and always connected with others in families and communities	Barry, Gordon, & Lange (2007); Barry, Lange, & King (2011); Chinchanikar (2009); Dass (2011); Tripathi (2010)
Actualizing Values: Guides practice in specific nursing situations		
Access	Views as ongoing and constant availability of health care that is competent, culturally acceptable, respectful and cost-effective	Barry, Blum, Eggenberger, Palmer-Hickman, & Mosley (2010); Barry, Gordon, & Lange (2007); Sternberg (2009); Sternberg & Lee (2013); Larson, Sandelowski, & McQuiston, (2012)
Essentiality	Described from the client's view as what is necessary for well-being	Barry, Blum, Eggenberger, Palmer-Hickman, & Mosley (2010); Barry, Blum, & Purnell, M. (2007); Ladd, Grimley, Hickman, & Touhy (2013)
Community participation	Described as the active engagement with members of a community fostered by openness to listen to calls for nursing and to create nursing responses	Barry, Lange, & King (2011); Plonczynski et al., (2007)
Empowerment	Understood as the client's awareness of making individual choices that influence health and well-being	Barry, Gordon, & Lange (2007); Barry, Lange, & King (2011)
Intersectoral collaboration	Refers to the openness to seek and honor the expertise of providers and agencies to potentiate the outcomes of services essential to well-being	Barry, Gordon, & Lange (2007); Barry, Lange, & King (2011); Pope, B. (2011)

Table 25 · 2 Overview of publications

Application to Research

Authors	Application of Model	Study Design/Focus/ Hypothesis
Chinchanikar (2009, master's thesis/engineering)	Framework for study	Document indexing framework for automating classification of nursing knowledge and language
Tripathi, S. (2010, master's thesis/engineering)	Framework for study	Development of a knowledge based decision making and analyzing system for the nurses to capture and manage the nursing practice
Dass (2011, master's thesis/engineering)	Framework for study	Development of a nursing knowledge management system
Huang, Tanioka, Locsin, Parker, & Masory (2011).	Framework for study	Development of a patient human–robot interaction.
Sternberg (2009, doctoral dissertation/nursing)	Part of the framework for study	Qualitative research that explored the experiences of Latinas living transnational motherhood
Conrad (2010, doctoral dissertation)	Identified as faculty practice model	Evidence-based project that compared faculty practice models through comprehensive literature review of evidence based documents
Pope (2011, doctoral dissertation)	Drew grounding concepts from the model of interconnectedness to facilitate partnerships and enhancement of relationships	Social history research study that explored the eugenic policies of the Progressive Era and the Social Security Act of 1935, specifically the maternal and child health services as it relates to nursing

Application to Education

Authors	Application of Model	Study Design /Focus/ Hypothesis
Barry, Blum, Eggenberger, Palmer-Hickman, & Mosley (2010)	Used transcendent values of respect, caring, and wholeness of person in a nursing situation	Development of a simulation to guide students in understand the "face" of homeless individuals and families
Ladd, Grimley, Hickman, & Touhy, (2013).	Used model to further develop nursing simulation/situation	Simulation development related to nursing situations at the end of life
Barry, Blum, & Purnell (2007)	Used model to help students understand the lived experience of Hurricane Katrina	Immersion experience with victims of Hurricane Katrina

Application to Practice

Authors	Application of Model	Study Design/ Focus/Hypothesis
Barry, Lange, & King (2011)	Framework for study	Qualitative descriptive study which developed a community outreach program for breast health promotion for underserved women

Table 25 · 2	Overview of publications—cont'd	
Application to Research		
Authors	**Application of Model**	**Study Design/Focus/ Hypothesis**
Parker, Pandya, Hsu, Noell, & Newlin (2008)	Framework for collaborative project with computer science engineers.	Used the model concepts to illuminate nursing's voice in an electronic record
Plonczynski et al. (2007)	Identified use of inquiry group method and correlated to participatory action	Discussed use of inquiry group method to be used by groups to define and resolve problems
Sadler, Newlin, Johnson-Spruill, & (2011)	Used inquiry group method	Longitudinal study examining the faith community values, disease threats, and barriers to self-care
Gordon, Barry, Dunne, & King (2011)	Framework for study	Described the process of bringing community partners in a school health program together to clarify a vision of health literacy
Sternberg & Lee (2013)	Further research based on original dissertation	Secondary analysis of longitudinal study which compared frequency of depressive symptoms of premenopausal Latinas women born in the United States compared with Latina immigrants

PRACTICE EXEMPLAR

The following is an exemplar of the usefulness of using the inquiry group method as a "route to knowing." As part of a community assessment, the inquiry group methodology was used to determine the hopes and dreams for well-being of community members in rural Haiti. Community members were gathered together at a primary school, and introductions were made using a language facilitator. Then the assertions were discussed that the three facilitators were experts in the method and in nursing but that each participant was expert in his or her self-care and care of the family and community. The following question was asked: "How can we be helpful to you?" One man responded with a story of caring for his wife who was in a prolonged labor. He described how he carried her down from the mountain, her back against his back, and hired a motorbike to take her to the closest hospital 45 minutes away. His call for nursing was heard loud and clear. We need a hospital so that our families don't have to suffer so much.

Another teacher told a story of his concern for his baby, Grace, 8 months old. He said she had a temperature and cough and that he and his wife were worried about her. He asked if we would examine her when the meeting was over. We agreed and were brought to his home on the school campus. We were invited inside and met his wife and baby. At first glance, the baby looked very well nourished; she was alert, smiling in response to interactions, and laughing when we babbled to her. The mother told us she was nursing her and that Grace had been able to nurse as usual. With a stethoscope, we listened to her chest and took her temperature the old-fashioned way—with the back of our hands. Her chest was clear, by our estimation she did not have a fever, and her skin showed no sign of dehydration. We instructed the parents to watch for signs of deterioration and to seek medical help. They said they had neither local access to a doctor nor transportation to seek help elsewhere. And another call was heard—to develop a school-based wellness center for health promotion and primary care.

■ Summary

The fundamental beliefs and commitment to the discipline and unique practice of nursing provided for both creating and sustaining the CNPM. This CNPM provides the environment in which nursing and social work is practiced from the core beliefs of respect, caring, and wholeness. Nurses and social workers are encouraged to reach out through the concentric circles, strengthening and widening the web of relationships with colleagues, clients, and community members. Through use of this CNPM, the ideals of the discipline are brought into the reality of care for wholeness and well-being of persons and families in multicultural communities.

References

Barry, C. (1998). The celebrity chef cooking club. A peer involvement feeding program promoting cooperation and community building. *Florida Journal of School Health, 9*(1), 17–20.

Barry, C. D., Blum, C. A., Eggenberger, T. L., Palmer-Hickman, C., & Mosley, R. (2009). Understanding homelessness using a simulated nursing experience. *Journal of Holistic Nursing Practice, 23*(4), 230–237.

Barry, C., Blum, C. A., & Purnell, M. (2007). Caring for individuals displaced by Hurricanes Katrina and Wilma: The lived experience of student nurses. *International Journal for Human Caring, 11*(2), 67–73.

Barry, C. D., Gordon, S. C., & Lange, B. (2007). The usefulness of the community nursing model in school based community wellness centers: Narratives from the U.S. and Africa. *Research and Theory for Nursing Practice: An International Journal, 21*(3), 174–184.

Barry, C. D., Lange, B., & King, B. (2011). Women alive: Gather underserved women upstream for a comprehensive breast health program. *Southern Online Journal of Nursing Research, 11*(1). Retrieved from http://www.resourcenter.net/images/SNRS/Files/SOJNR_articles2/Vol11Num01Art07.html.

Campbell, M. K., Meier, A., Carr, C. Enga, Z., James, A., Reedy, J., & Zheng, B. (2001). Health behaviour changes after colon cancer: A comparison of findings from face to face and on-line focus groups. *Family & Community Health, 24*(3), 88–103.

Chinchanikar, S. V. (2009). Automated nursing knowledge classification using indexing (master's thesis). Available from ProQuest Dissertations and Theses database. (UMI No.1466377)

Chooporian, T. (1986). Reconceptualizing the environment. In P. Mocia (Ed.), *New approaches to theory development* (pp. 39–54). New York: National League for Nursing Press.

Clark, M. J. (2003). *Community health nursing: Caring for populations.* Upper Saddle River, NJ: Prentice-Hall.

Clark, M. J., Cary, S., Grover, D., Ceballos, R., Sifuentes, M., & Trieu, S. (2003). Involving communities in community assessment. *Public Health Nursing, 20*(6), 456–463.

Conrad, S. N. (2010). Best faculty practice plan model for a small college of nursing (doctoral dissertation). Available from ProQuest Dissertations and Theses database. (UMI No.3413204)

Dass, S. (2011). A web-based automated classification system for nursing language based on nursing theory (master's theory). Available from ProQuest Dissertations and Theses database. (UMI No. 1507507)

Dyess, S. M., & Chase, S. (2012). Sustaining health in faith community nursing practice: Emerging processes that support the development of middle range theory. *Holistic Nursing Practice 26*(4), 221–227.

Florida Atlantic University Christine E. Lynn College of Nursing. (1994/2012). Mission and philosophy. In Faculty handbook. Boca Raton, FL: Author.

Gordon, S., & Barry, C. (2009). Delegation guided by school nursing values: Comprehensive knowledge, trust and empowerment. *Journal of School Nursing, 25*(5), 352–360.

Gordon, S., Barry, C. Dunne, D., King, B. (2011). Clarifying a vision for health literacy: A holistic school-based community approach. *Holistic Nursing Practice, 25*(3), 120–126.

Huang, S., Tanioka, T., Locsin, R., Parker, M., & Masory, O. (2011, November). Functions for a caring robot in nursing. Proceedings of the 7th IEEE International Conference on Natural Language Processing and knowledge in engineering (KLP_KE 2011), Tokushima, Japan.

Kasle, S., Wilhelm, M. S., & Ree, K. L., (2002). Optimal health and wellbeing for women: Definitions and strategies derived from focus groups of women. *Women's Health Issues 12*(4), 178–190.

Kleffel, D. (1996). Environmental paradigms: Moving toward an ecocentric perspective. *Advances in Nursing Science, 18*(4), 1–10.

Ladd, C., Grimley, K., Hickman, C., & Touhy, T. (2013). Teaching end of life nursing using simulation. *Journal of Hospice & Palliative Nursing, 15*(1), 41–51.

Larson, K., Sandelowski, M., & McQuiston, C. (2012). "It's a touchy subject": Latino adolescent sexual risk behaviors in the school context. *Applied Nursing Research, 25,* 231–238.

Nightingale, F. (1859/1992). *Notes on nursing: Commemorative edition with commentaries by contemporary nursing leaders.* Philadelphia: J. B. Lippincott.

Parker, M. E. (1997). Emerging innovations: Caring in action. *International Journal for Human Caring, 1*(2), 9–10.

Parker, M. E., & Barry, C. D. (1999). Community practice guided by a nursing model. *Nursing Science Quarterly, 12*(2), 125–131.

Parker, M. E., Barry, C. D., & King, B. (2000). Use of inquiry method for assessment and evaluation in a school-based community nursing project. *Family and Community Health, 23*(2), 54–61.

Parker, M. E., Pandya, A., Hsu, S., & Huang, S. (2013). U.S. Patent No. 2013/0311203A1. Washington, DC: U.S. Patent and Trademark Office.

Parker, M. E., Pandya, A., Hsu, S., Noell, D., & Newlin, K. (2008). Assuring nursing's voice in the electronic health record. IEEE International Conference on Natural Language and Knowledge Development Engineering, Beijing, China. Proceedings (NLP-KE 107). Piscataway, NJ: Institute of Electrical and Electronics Engineers.

Peck, S. (1987). *The different drum: Community making and peace.* New York: Simon & Schuster.

Plonczynski, D., Ehrlich-Jones, L., Fischer Robertson, J., Rossetti, J., Munroe, D., Koren, M. E., et al. (2007). Ensuring a knowledgeable and committed gerontological nursing workforce. *Nursing Education Today, 27*(2), 113–121.

Pope, B. (2011). Maternal health policy: Nursing's legacy and the social security act 1935 (doctoral dissertation). Available from ProQuest Dissertations and Theses database. (UMI No. 3462566)

Ryan, E., Hawkins, W., Parker, M. E., & Hawkins, M. (2004). Perceptions of access to U. S. health care of Haitian immigrants in South Florida. *Florida Public Health Review, 1,* 36–43.

Sadler, L., Newlin, K., & Johnson-Spruill, I. (2011). Beyond the medical model: Interdisciplinary programs of community engaged health research. *Clinical and Translational Science, 4*(4), 285–297.

Schuster, E. (1990). Earth caring. *Advances in Nursing Science, 13*(1), 25–30.

Smith, C., & Mauer, F. (1995). *Community health nursing: Theory and practice.* Philadelphia: W.B. Saunders.

Sternberg, R. M. (2009). Latinas experiencing transnational motherhood (doctoral dissertation). Available from ProQuest Dissertations and Theses database. (UMI No. 3401817)

Sternberg, R. M., & Barry, C. (2011). Transnational mothers crossing the border and bringing their healthcare needs. *Journal of Nursing Scholarship, 43*(1), 64–71.

Sternberg, R. M., & Lee, K. (2013). Depressive symptoms of midlife Latinas: Effect of immigration and sociodemographic factors. *International Journal of Women's Health. 3*(5), 301–308.

Swadener, B., & Lubeck, S. (1995). *Children and families "at promise." Deconstructing the discourse on risk.* Albany: State University of New York Press.

Tripathi, S. (2010). Knowledge based evaluation of nursing care practice model (master's thesis). Available from ProQuest Dissertations and Theses database. (UMI No. 1485670)

World Health Organization, Alma-Ata. (1978). *Primary health care.* Geneva, Switzerland: Author.

World Health Organization. (2012). World conference on the social determinants of health: Meeting report. Geneva, Switzerland: World Health Organization Press.

World Health Organization. (2007). A conceptual framework for action on the social determinants of health. Geneva, Switzerland: World Health Organization.

Zaiger, D. (2013). Historical perspectives of school nursing. In J. Selekman (Ed.), *Comprehensive textbook of school nursing* (2nd ed., pp. 2–25). Philadelphia: F. A. Davis.

Rozzano Locsin's Technological Competency as Caring in Nursing

Knowing as Process and Technological Knowing as Practice

ROZZANO C. LOCSIN

Introducing the Theorist
Overview of the Theory
Application of the Theory
Practice Exemplar
Summary
References

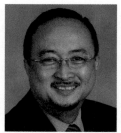

Rozzano C. Locsin

Introducing the Theorist

Rozzano C. Locsin is Professor Emeritus of Nursing at Florida Atlantic University's Christine E. Lynn College of Nursing, and inaugural International Nursing Professor at the Institute of Health Biosciences, University of Tokushima, in Tokushima, Japan. His program of research focuses on life transitions in the health–illness experience. He holds baccalaureate and master's degrees in nursing from Silliman University in the Philippines and a Doctor of Philosophy degree from the University of the Philippines. Dr. Locsin was a Fulbright Scholar in Uganda in 2000, a recipient of the 2004 to 2006 Fulbright Alumni Initiative Award to Uganda and the Fulbright Senior Specialist in Global and Public Health and International Development Award. He was inducted as a Fellow of the American Academy of Nursing in 2006, and received the prestigious Edith Moore Copeland Excellence in Creativity Award from Sigma Theta Tau International Honor Society of Nursing and two lifetime achievement awards from premier schools of nursing in the Philippines. In addition, Locsin received the first University Researcher of the Year Award in 2006 in the Scholarly/Creative Works category as Professor at Florida Atlantic University. Published in 2001, his edited book *Advancing Technology, Caring, and Nursing* introduced the germinal work of relating technology with caring in nursing. His middle-range nursing theory, *Technological Competency as Caring in Nursing: A Model for Practice,* was published by Sigma

Theta Tau International Press in 2005. In 2007, his coedited book *Technology and Nursing: Practice, Process and Issues* illustrated the importance of technology in nursing practice. A fourth book, *A Contemporary Process of Nursing: The (Unbearable) Weight of Knowing in Nursing,* was published in 2009. This book provides essential chapters defining and describing the concept of "knowing persons." Dr. Locsin's interest in global nursing and care initiatives enhances his appreciation of the dynamic nature of humans and of nursing as the practice of continuously knowing persons through emerging technologies within a caring framework.

Overview of the Theory

There is a great demand for a practice of nursing based on an authentic intention to know human beings fully as persons and as participants in their care rather than as objects of our care. Nurses want to use creative, imaginative, and innovative ways of affirming, appreciating, and celebrating humans as whole persons. In present-day health and human care, advancing technologies claim a stronghold. Often the best way to realize intended nursing care outcomes is the excellent and competent use of nursing technologies (Locsin, 1998). Frequently perceived as the practice of using machines in nursing (Locsin, 1995), technological competency as caring in nursing is the process of knowing persons as whole (Locsin, 2001), while frequently engaging technological advancements.

Contemporary definitions of technology include (1) a means to an end, (2) an instrument, (3) a tool, or (4) a human activity that increases or enhances efficiency (Heidegger, 1977). Conceptualizing caring and technology within nursing practice is challenging. However, viewing them in harmonious coexistence is crucial so that mutual caring occurs, fostering the understanding of technological competency as an expression of caring in nursing (Locsin, 2005).

The purpose of this chapter is to explain "knowing persons through technological competency as a process of nursing," a framework of nursing that guides its practice, grounded in the theoretical construct of *technological competency as caring in nursing* (Locsin, 2005). This model of practice illuminates the harmonious relationship between technological competency and caring in nursing. In this model, the emphasis of nursing is on the person, a human being whose hopes, dreams, and aspirations are focused on living life fully as a caring person (Boykin & Schoenhofer, 2001).

As a model of practice, *technological competency as caring in nursing* (Locsin, 2005) is as valuable today as it has been in the past and will continue to be in the future. Technological advances in health care demand expertise with technology. Often, such expertise is perceived as the antithesis of caring, particularly in situations in which the focus of attention is on the technology rather than on the person. Nonetheless, it is the premise of this chapter that being technologically competent is being caring.

Technological competency as caring in nursing is a middle-range theory illustrated in the practice of nursing and grounded in the harmonious coexistence between technology and caring in nursing. The assumptions of the theory are informed by Boykin and Schoenhofer's (2001) work and include the following:

- Persons are caring by virtue of their humanness.
- Persons are whole or complete in the moment.
- Knowing persons is a process of nursing that allows for continuous appreciation of persons moment to moment.
- Technology is used to know wholeness of persons moment to moment.
- Nursing is a discipline and a professional practice.

The ultimate purpose of technological competency in nursing is to acknowledge that the person is the focus of nursing and that various technologies can and should be used in the service of knowing the person.

This acknowledgment of persons brings together the relatively abstract concept of wholeness-of-person with the more concrete concept of technology. Such acknowledgment compels the redesigning of nursing processes—ways of expressing, celebrating, and appreciating the practice of nursing as continuously knowing persons as whole moment to moment.

In this practice of nursing, technology is used not to know the person as object to be controlled and manipulated but rather to know who the person is as an experiencing subject in her or his wholeness. Appropriately, knowing person as object alludes to an expectation of knowing empirical aspects and facts about the composite person, whereas knowing person as subject requires the understanding of an unpredictable, irreducible person who is more than and different from the sum of his or her empirical parts. In this way, technology is used to understand the uniqueness and individuality of persons as humans who continuously unfold and who, therefore, require continuous knowing (Locsin, 2005).

Persons as Whole and Complete in the Moment

One of the earlier definitions of the word *person* appeared in Hudson's 1988 publication claiming that the "emphasis on inclusive rather than sexist language has brought into prominence the use of the word 'person'" (p. 12). The origin of the word *person* is from the Greek word *prosopon*, which means the actor's mask of Greek tragedy; of Roman origin, *persona* indicated the role played by the individual in social or legal relationships. Hudson (1988) also declares that "an individual in isolation is contrary to an understanding of 'person'" (p. 15). A necessary appreciation of persons requires the view that humans are whole or complete in the moment. As such, there is no need to fix them or to make them complete again (Boykin & Schoenhofer, 2001). There is nothing missing that requires nurses' intervening to make persons "whole or complete" again, or for nurses to assist in this completion. Persons are complete in the moment. Their varying situations of care call for creativity, innovation, and imagination from nurses so that they may come to know the nursed as a "whole" person. The uniqueness of the person emerges in the response to being called forth in particular situations.

Inherent in humans as unpredictable, dynamic, and living beings is the regard for self-as-person. This appreciation is like the human concern for security, safety, self-esteem, and self-actualization popularized by Maslow (1943) in his quintessential theoretical model

on the hierarchy of needs. More important, however, is the understanding that being human is being a person, regardless of biophysical parts or technological enhancements.

Because the future may require relative appreciation of persons, if the ultimate criterion of being human today is being wholly natural, organic, and functional, then being human may not be so easy to determine or appreciate. The purely natural human being may be rare. The understanding that technology-supported life is artificial, and therefore is not natural, stimulates discussions among practitioners of nursing (Locsin & Campling, 2005), particularly when the subject of concern is technology-dependent care and technological competency as an expression of caring in nursing. Hudson (1988) suggests that "false comfort may be offered whenever it is implied that this life and this body are significantly less important than the 'spiritual body' and the 'next life'. . . the time has come to enhance an awareness of the post human or spiritual future" (p. 13). What structural requirements will the next-generation human possess? Today, some humans have anatomic and/or physiological components that are already electronic and/or mechanical, such as mechanical cardiac valves, self-injecting insulin pumps, cardiac pacemakers, or artificial limbs, all appearing as excellent facsimiles of the real. Yet the idea of a "whole person" and being natural continues to persist as a requirement of what a human being should be.

How Are Persons Known?

Often, questioning in order to know the person is limited to inquiry about his or her body parts. For example, "How are your knees?" instead of "How are you doing with your knees?" Of what purpose is the question? Is it to know the person or to know the condition of the specific component part? Perhaps inadvertently, unconsciously, or both, one inquires about the body part because of a culturally founded reason or because the customary focus on another's bodily features defines that person.

How are persons known as human beings? Historically, humans were depicted through drawings and paintings. Colorful artworks represented the human being in imaginative ways as conceptualized by painters and illustrators. Artists and their works became commodities, and Leonardo da Vinci may top this list as, perhaps, the most prized of illustrators and painters. Studying the human being as an object allowed Leonardo to illustrate the composite of the human being through dissected remains. Illustrations such as these may have influenced Michelangelo in his creation of masterful artworks such as *David* and *Moses*. The clarity, definition, and fidelity of these representations reveal the utmost appreciation of the human being. Yet the question remains: Does the human being become a person, or is he always a person? Is the composition of the human being the ultimate descriptor, characteristic, and quality of a whole and complete person? What happens when the human being has no limbs, or has limbs that are not functional? Is this human being a person?

Consider the case of a baby born without limbs but otherwise alive and well. When the baby became ill, he was rushed to a hospital. To the chagrin of the nurses and physicians, they were at first unable to care for the baby. Their main question was "How can we initiate IV when there are no extremities?" They may also have wondered, "On growing up, will this baby be concerned about what it is like to have no limbs, or will he wish he had limbs so he could 'go' places like others?" (Barnard & Locsin, 2007, p. 17).

Consider also the "Girl With Eight Limbs" (PBS) from a province in India, who was subjected to intense surgical intervention to remove the other "nonfunctional" limbs that were putting her life in a precarious situation. What does this girl think now? "Am I complete or incomplete? Am I normal or abnormal, just because I am like everyone else—with two upper limbs and two lower limbs?" (PBS).

In an episode of the television series *The Twilight Zone*, a woman perceived herself as so hideous that she thought she was unworthy to be seen; she had to hide her face behind a veil. She was shunned by her family. It was an unbearable life for her and for her family as well. In the end, the moral of the story focused on the adage "beauty is in the eye of the beholder" (Serling, 1960). The people who shunned the woman had faces like those of pigs, while she had more "human-like" features. In fact, she was a beautiful human woman whom everyone found to be ugly, embarrassing, pitiful, and a misfit and was advised to move to a distant colony with a small population of people like her. This particular story addresses the impact of prejudice in considering what a person ought to be. In essence, it marginalizes those who are not like others and in doing so prevents the understanding of nursing as the process of knowing persons as whole and complete in the moment.

In a recent Associated Press news article, "The Androgynous Pharaoh? Akhenaten Had Feminine Physique" (*USA Today*, May 2, 2008), writer Alex Dominguez presented Dr. Irwin Braverman's findings on the controversial "feminine" features of the pharaoh Akhenaten. Dominguez wrote, "Akhenaten wasn't the most manly pharaoh, even though he fathered at least a half-dozen children. In fact, his form was quite feminine, which has puzzled experts for years. And he was a bit of an egghead." The pharaoh had "an androgynous appearance. He had a female physique with wide hips and breasts, but he was male and he was fertile and he had six daughters," Braverman is quoted as saying. "But nevertheless, he looked like he had a female physique." Apparently, what constitutes "knowing" whether a human being is a man or a woman is the physical appearance. This makes Braverman's study of the Pharaoh Akhenaten most meaningful.

An example of person as object, known as a composite of physical elements, is the legendary Frankenstein monster, an entity assembled from various human parts. The monster was created and made human in the sense of being a composite of parts but also in the sense of his essence of being energy (electricity).

The Process of Knowing Persons

Persons possess the prerogative and the choice of whether to allow nurses to know them fully. Entering the world of the other is a critical requisite to knowing as a process of nursing. Establishing rapport, trust, confidence, commitment, and the compassion to know others fully as persons is integral to this crucial positioning.

Wholeness is the idealized condition or situation of the one who is nursed. This idealization is held within the nurse's understanding of persons as complete human beings "in the moment." Expressions of this completeness vary from moment to moment. These expressions are human illustrations of living and growing. Using technology alone and focusing on the received technological data rather than on continually "knowing" the other fully as person can lead to the nurse thinking of the person as an object who needs to be completed and made whole again. Paradoxically, because of the idea that humans are unpredictable, it is not entirely possible for the nurse to fully know another human being—except in the moment and only if the person allows the nurse to know him or her by entering into the other's world.

In this perspective, the condition in which the nurse and the other allow knowing each other exists as the nursing situation, the shared lived experience between the nurse and nursed (Boykin & Schoenhofer, 2001).

In this relationship, trust is established that the nurse will know the other fully as person; the trust that the nurse will not judge the person or categorize the person as just another human being or experience but rather as a unique person who has hopes and aspirations that are singularly his or her own.

It is the nurse's responsibility to know the person's hopes and aspirations. Technological competency as caring allows for this understanding. In doing so, the nurse also sanctions the other (the nursed) to know him or her as person. The expectation is that the nurse is to use multiple ways of knowing competently in using technologies to know the other fully as person.

The nurse's responsibility is immeasurable in creating conditions that demand technological competency and care. In creating a nursing situation of care, there is a requisite competency to know persons fully, to understand, and to appreciate the important nuances of the person's dreams and desires.

There are many ways of interpreting the concept of "person as whole." We will look at three interpretations that shape the popular understanding of the concept. One of these interpretations is the mind–body dualism ascribed to Descartes, which describes the connection between mind and body. In nursing, the mind–body–spirit connection is popularized by Jean Watson (1985) in her theory of transpersonal caring. Another version of the mind–body connection, the simultaneity paradigm (Parse, 1998), categorizes the human–environment mutual connection as the relationship that best serves the nursing perspective and grounds theoretical frameworks and models of practice, including many of those in caring science. These contemporary and popular elucidations regard humans as the focus of nursing and knowing persons in their wholeness as the practice of nursing.

Knowing persons as the process of nursing is a dynamic encounter between the nurse and nursed in which nursing situations unfold toward an encompassing practice of knowledge-based nursing. The meaning of the process is characterized by listening, knowing, being with, enabling, and maintaining belief as described by Swanson (1991). The following descriptions exemplify the process of knowing persons as nursing within the theory of technological competency as caring in nursing:

- *Knowing:* The process of knowing a person is guided by technological knowing in which persons are appreciated as participants in their care rather than as objects of care. The nurse enters the world of the other. In this process, technology is used to magnify the aspect of the person that requires revealing—a representation of the real person. The person's state may change moment to moment—the person is dynamic and alive, and his or her actions cannot be predicted. This provides the opportunity for nurses to continuously know the person as whole.
- *Designing*: Both the nurse and the one nursed (patient) plan a mutual care process from which the nurse can organize a rewarding nursing practice that is responsive to the patient's desire for care.
- *Participative engaging*: This encounter provides a simultaneous practice of conjoined

activities that are crucial to knowing persons. This stage of the process is characterized by alternating rhythms of implementation and evaluation. The evidence of continuous knowing, implementation, and participation is reflective of the cyclical but recursive process of knowing persons.

• *Furthering knowing*: The continuous, circular and recursive process of knowing persons demonstrates the ever-changing, and dynamic nature of fundamental ways of knowing in nursing. Knowledge about the person that is derived from knowing, designing, and participative engagement further informs the caring practice of the nurse, thereby acknowledging the recursive process of knowing persons.

Figure 26-1 describes the process of knowing persons.

Notice in the model of practice shown in the figure that knowing is the primary process. "Knowing nursing means knowing in the realms of personal, ethical, empirical, and aesthetic—all at once" (Boykin & Schoenhofer, 2001, p. 6). Knowledge about the person that is derived from knowing, designing, participative engaging and furthering knowing additionally informs the nurse in appreciating the patient. In knowing persons, one comes to understand that more knowing about the person and about his or her being allows the nurse to affirm, support, and celebrate his or her dreams and aspirations in the moment. Supporting this process of knowing is the understanding that persons are unpredictable, that they simultaneously conceal and reveal themselves as persons from one moment to the next (Parse, 1998).

The nurse can know the person fully only in the moment. This knowing occurs only when the person allows the nurse to enter his or her world. When this happens, the nurse and nursed become vulnerable as they move toward further continuous knowing.

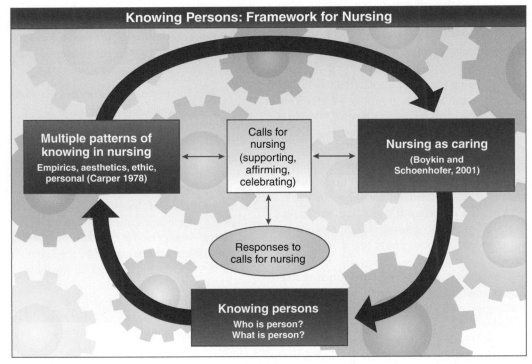

Loscin, R. (2005).Technological Compentency as Caring in Nursing: A Model for Practice. Sigma Theta Tau International Press, Indianapolis, IN

Fig 26 • 1 Nursing as knowing persons. *(From Locsin, R. (2005).* Technological Competency as Caring in Nursing: A Model for Practice. *Indianapolis, IN: Sigma Theta Tau International Press.)*

Vulnerability allows participation so that the nurse and nursed continue knowing each other moment to moment. Daniels (1998) explained that in such situations, the "nurse's work is to ameliorate vulnerability" (p. 191). Demonstrating vulnerability in caring situations enables others to recognize it, participate in mutual vulnerability, and share in the humanness of being vulnerable. Further, Daniels declared that "vulnerable individuals seek nursing care, and nurses seek those who are vulnerable" (p. 192). By entering the world of the one nursed, the nurse shares "power with" rather than having "power over" the patient through a created hierarchy (Daniels, 1998). The nurse does not know more about the person than the person knows about him- or herself. No one knows the lived experience of the patient better than the patient.

Nonetheless, there is the possibility that the nurse will be able to predict and prescribe for the one nursed. When this occurs, these situations forcibly lead the nurse to appreciate persons more as object than as person. Such a situation can occur only when the nurse is assumed to "have known" the one nursed. Although it can be assumed that with the process of "knowing persons as whole," opportunities to continuously know the other become limitless, there is also a much greater likelihood that having "already known" the one nursed, the nurse will predict and prescribe activities for the one nursed, ultimately causing objectification of the person (see Fig. 26-2).

To Know and Knowing

The verb *know* has common definitions. Of these definitions, some are appropriate descriptions that explain the intended use of the word in nursing, thereby facilitating its understanding for the purpose and process of competently using technologies in nursing. These definitions are as follows:

- To perceive directly with the senses or mind
- To be certain of, regard, or accept as true beyond doubt
- To be capable of, have the skills to
- To have thorough or practical understanding of, as through experience of

- To be subjected to or limited by
- To recognize the character or quality of
- To be able to distinguish, recognize
- To be acquainted or familiar with
- To see, hear, or experience

While the verb *know* sustains the notion that nursing is concerned with activity and that the one who acts is knowledgeable (in the sense of understanding the rationales behind the activities), the word *knowing* is a key concept that alludes to the focus of an action from a cognitive perspective requiring description. *Knowing* perfectly describes the ways of nursing—transpiring continuously as explicated from the framework of *knowing persons*. It is the use of the word *knowing* in which the process of nursing as *knowing persons* is lived. The framework for practice clearly shows the circuitous and continuous process of knowing persons as a practice of nursing.

We hope that nurses practice nursing from a theoretical perspective rather than from tradition or from blind obedience to instructions and directions. Nevertheless, processes of nursing that are derived from extant theories of nursing continue to dictate and prescribe how a nurse should nurse. Contrary to this popular conception, *knowing persons* as a model of practice using technologies of nursing achieves for the nurse an appreciation of expertise and the knowledge of persons in the moment. Technologies allow nurses to know about the person only as much as the person permits the nurse to know. It can be true that technologies detect the anatomical, physiological, chemical, and/or biological conditions of a person. This identifies the person as a living human being. However, with knowing persons, the nurse is allowed to understand and anticipate the ever-changing person from moment to moment.

The purpose of knowing the person is derived from the nurse's intention to nurse (Purnell & Locsin, 2000)—a continuing appreciation of the person as ever-changing and never static: one who is a dynamic human being. The information derived from knowing the person is only relevant for the moment, for the person's "state" can change moment to moment. Importantly, knowing the "who or what" of persons helps nurses realize that a person is more than simply the physiochemical and anatomical being. Knowing persons allows the nurse to know "who and what" is the person. "Who" is the subjective knowing of the person as whole and "what" is objective knowing of the person as parts.

Knowing When Using Technology

From such a view, it may seem that the process of knowing is possible only when using technologies in nursing. This perception, which is not necessarily true, is supported by the idea that nursing is technology when technology is appreciated as anything that creates efficiency, whether this is an instrument or a tool, such as machines, or the activity of nurses when nursing. Sandelowski (1993) has argued about the metaphorical depiction of nursing as technology, or with technology as nursing, and the semiotic relationship of these concepts. Locsin and Purnell (2007) have declared that accompanying the nurse's rapture with technologies in nursing is the consequent suffering or the price of advancing dependency on technologies that critically influence contemporary human lives. With increased use of technologies and ensuing technological dependency experienced by recipients of care, the imperative is to provide technological competency as caring in nursing (Locsin, 2005).

Regardless, the idea of knowing persons guiding nursing practice is novel in the sense that there is no ideal prescription; rather there is the wholesome appreciation of an informed practice that allows the use of multiple ways of knowing such as described by Phenix (1964) and expanded by Carper (1978). These ways of knowing involve the empirical, ethical, personal, and aesthetic. Aesthetic expressions document, communicate, and perpetuate the appreciation of nursing as transpiring moment to moment. Popular aesthetic expressions include storytelling; poetry; visual expressions as in drawings, illustrations, and paintings; and aural renditions such as music. Encountering aesthetic expressions again allows the nurse and the nursed to relive the occasion anew. Reflecting on these experiences using the fundamental patterns of knowing (Carper, 1978) enhances learning, motivates the furtherance of knowledgeable practice, and increases the valuing of nursing as a professional practice grounded in a legitimate theoretical perspective of nursing.

The use of technologies in nursing is consequent to the contemporary demands for nursing actions requiring technological knowing (Locsin, 2009). Technological knowing is demanded for the ultimate purpose of knowing the real person. Technological knowing is defined as the practice of using technologies of care to know the one nursed. Important along with technology use in nursing is the condition that the one nursed allows himself or herself to be known as a person.

Technological competency in nursing fosters the recognition of persons as participants in their care rather than as objects of care. The idea of *participation in their care* stems from active engagement, in which the nurse enters the world of the one nursed through available appropriate technologies, attempting to know the nursed more fully in the moment. In this practice, the assumption is understood that the one nursed allows the nurse to enter his or her world so that together they may mutually support, affirm, and celebrate each other's being. In this relationship of the knower and the one known, technology provides the efficiency and the valuing that marks their mutual and momentary reality (Locsin, 2009).

Technology currently encompasses the bulk of functional activities that nurses are expected to perform, particularly when the practice is in a clinical setting. Clinical nursing is firmly rooted in the clinical health model (Smith, 1983) in which the organismic and mechanistic views of humans as persons convincingly dictate the practice of nursing. Nevertheless, the process of knowing persons will prevail, for the model of technological competency as caring in nursing provides the nurse the fitting stimulation and motivation (and the prospective autonomy to judge critically) a mode of action that desires an appreciation of persons as whole.

The model articulates continuous knowing. Continuing to know persons deters objectification, a process that ultimately regards human beings as "stuff" to care about, rather than as knowledgeable participants in their care.

Participating in his or her care frees the person from having to be "assigned" care that he or she may not want or need. This relationship signifies responsiveness of the cared for by the person who is caring for (Hudson, 1988). Continuous knowing results when findings obtained through consequent knowing further increase the desire to know "who" and "what" the person is. Continuous knowing overpowers the motivation to prescribe and direct the person's life. Rather, it affirms, supports, and celebrates his or her hopes, dreams, and aspirations as a participating human being.

Technological Knowing

Technological knowing in nursing illustrates the shared practice of using technologies to know persons as whole and using technologies of care for the purpose of understanding persons more fully. The circuitous and recursive engagement that occurs in technological knowing includes:

• Appreciating the person's humanness
• Engaging in mutual knowing—between the nurse and nursed

• Participating in dynamic relating within caring nursing relationships
• Furthering knowing of persons

Through technological knowing, further knowing of persons is achieved. Because it is a circuitous and recursive process, consequently, the practice of technological knowing begins anew. The following model (Fig. 26-2) illustrates the way of technological knowing in nursing.

Calls and Responses for Nursing

Calls for nursing are illuminations of the persons' hopes, dreams, and aspirations. Calls for nursing are individual expressions by persons who seek ways toward affirmation, support, and celebration as person. The nurse appreciates the uniqueness of persons in his or her nursing. In doing so, the nurse sustains and enhances the wholeness of the human being, while facilitating the realization of the persons' completeness through "acting for or with" the person. This is a way of affirming, supporting, and celebrating the person's wholeness.

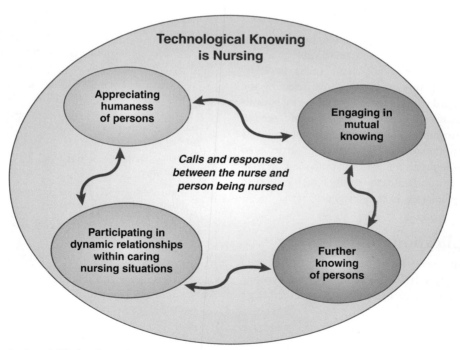

Fig 26 • 2 Technological knowing in nursing.

The nurse relies on the person for calls for nursing. These calls are specific mechanisms that the persons use, allowing the nurse to respond with authentic intentions to know them fully as persons in the moment. Calls for nursing may be expressed in various ways, often as hopes and dreams, such as the hope to be with friends while recuperating in the hospital, the desire to play the piano when the fingers are well enough to function effectively, or simply the ultimate desire to go home or to die peacefully. As uniquely as these calls for nursing are expressed, the nurse knows the person continuously moment to moment. Nursing responses to these calls may to monitor patterns of information, such as those derived from an electrocardiogram to know the physiological status of the person in the moment or to administer lifesaving medications, to institute transfer plans, or to refer patients for services to other health-care professionals.

The entirety of nursing is to direct, focus, attain, sustain, and maintain the person. In doing so, hearing calls for nursing is continuous and momentarily complete. Knowing persons allows the nurse to use technologies in articulating calls for nursing. The empirical, personal, ethical, and esthetic ways of knowing that are fundamental to understanding persons as whole increase the likelihood of knowing persons in the moment.

Unpredictable and dynamic, human beings are ever-changing moment to moment. This characteristic challenges the nurse to know persons continuously as a whole, rejecting the traditional concept of possibly knowing persons completely at once, to prescribe and predict their expressions of wholeness. In continuously knowing persons as whole through articulated technologies in nursing, the nurse can perhaps intervene to facilitate patients' recognition of their wholeness in the moment.

Applications of the Theory

Locsin's theory is relatively new. Applications of the theory of technological competency as caring in nursing have been documented, although

mostly anecdotal references exist as these are shared and its utility explained. Through these anecdotes received in various occasions, especially after presentations and conversations and through personal communications via e-mail, these positive declarations continue to provide and affirm that the theory is useful particularly in nursing practice demanding technological proficiency such as in critical care settings. Likewise, during class presentations and in scholarly/academic conferences, students and participants express their claims that the theory resonates well in their practice, affirming their understanding of nursing, and confirming their appreciation of knowing persons through technologies as practice. However, there has been an absence of comments from practitioners who have signified that the theory has guided their practice, or of any researcher who has claimed that he or she has used the theory as framework in any study. Nevertheless, the claims that the theory has affirmed one's practice exist (Fig. 26-3).

Future Research

- Experiences of 'caring for'
- Lived experiences of being 'cared for'
- Ethics and technological dependence
- Cloning and bionic parts and the experience of being with
- Design and development of instrument to measure technological competency as caring in nursing
- Testing of instrument to measure patient experience with technologies
- Genetics and the future of humans as posthumans
- Burnout phenomenon and the prospective use of robots in the practice of nursing
- Nursing administration calls to care for nurses in high-tech environments
- Universality of technological competency as caring in varying nursing settings

Fig 26 • 3 Future research.

Practice Exemplar: Knowing Persons in the Moment

The following is a nursing situation involving a nurse's act to direct her care to what was important for her patients.

One of my patients requested a new IV on her opposite arm, even though the one she had was safely infusing her IV fluids. I was extremely far behind, but I knew that her IV would not get changed until much later if at all, as shift change was occurring, and she did not have veins that were easily accessed. I requested the vein finder instrument from the supervisor and successfully inserted a new IV. My patient was so happy and told me that no one else had been able to "get a vein" on the first try. It seemed like a simple task, but it made such a difference to her. I can appreciate that through competent use of the vein finder instrument, I was able to allow my patient to use her dominant hand instead of limiting her range of motion because of the IV location. She was able to experience herself as more "whole" through the use of her dominant extremity. This was such a simple an act, and yet it mattered to her quality of life in the moment for both her and me.

This nurse explains, "As I reflect on Locsin's theory, I can appreciate that as nurses we strive to know our patients as whole." According to Locsin (2010), "Nurses want to use creative, imaginative, and innovative ways of affirming, appreciating, and celebrating humans as whole persons" (p. 461). This desire will often lead nurses to understand that these "intentions" can be realized through "expert, competent use of nursing technologies" (p. 461).

■ Summary

The purpose of this chapter is to describe and explain "knowing persons as whole," a framework of nursing guiding a practice grounded in the theoretical construct of *technological competency as caring in nursing* (Locsin, 2005). This framework of practice illuminates the harmonious relationship between technological competency and caring in nursing. In this model, the focus of nursing is the person. The chapter introduces technological knowing, a way of knowing in nursing engaging the competent use of technologies of care to come to know persons as whole. Through technological knowing, both the nurse and one nursed are appreciated as whole persons whose hopes, dreams, and aspirations matter most in living their lives fully as whole persons.

Critical to understanding the phenomenon of technological competency as caring in nursing are the conceptual descriptions of technology, caring, and nursing. Assumptions about human beings as persons, nursing as caring, and technological competency are presented as foundational to the process of knowing persons as whole in the moment—a process of nursing grounded in the perspective of technological competency as caring in nursing.

The process of knowing persons as whole is explicated as technological knowing—efficiency in using clinical nursing practices. The model of practice is illustrated through the understanding of technology and caring as coexisting in nursing.

The process of knowing persons is continuous. In this process of nursing, with calls and responses, the nurse and nursed come to know each other more fully as persons in the moment. Grounding the process is the appreciation of persons as whole and complete in the moment, of human beings as unpredictable, of technological competency as an expression of caring in nursing, and of nursing as critical to health care.

References

Barnard, A., & Locsin, R. (2007). *Technology and nursing: Concepts, practice, and issues*. London: Palgrave-Macmillan.

Boykin, A., & Schoenhofer, S. (2001). *Nursing as caring: A model for transforming practice*. Boston: Jones and Bartlett; New York: National League for Nursing Press.

Carper, B. (1978). Fundamental patterns of knowing in nursing. *Advances in Nursing Science, 1*(1), 13–24.

Daniels, L. (1998). Vulnerability as a key to authenticity. *Image: Journal of Nursing Scholarship, 30*(2), 191–192.

Heidegger, M. (1977). *The question concerning technology*. New York: Harper and Row.

Hudson, R. (1988). Whole or parts—a theological perspective on "person." *The Australian Journal of Advanced Nursing, 6*(1), 12–20.

Hudson, G. (1993). Empathy and technology in the coronary care unit. *Intensive Critical Care Nursing, 9*(1), 55–61.

Locsin, R. (1995). Machine technologies and caring in nursing. *Image: Journal of Nursing Scholarship, 27*(3), 201–203.

Locsin, R. (1998). Technologic competence as expression of caring in critical care settings. *Holistic Nursing Practice, 12*(4), 50–56.

Locsin, R. (2001). Practicing nursing: Technological competency as an expression of caring in nursing. In: *Advancing technology, caring, and nursing*. Westport, CT: Auburn House/Greenwood.

Locsin, R. (2005). *Technological competency as caring in nursing: A model for practice*. Indianapolis, IN: Sigma Theta Tau International.

Locsin, R. (2009). Painting a clear picture: The technological knowing of persons as contemporary process of nursing. In R. Locsin & M. Purnell (Eds.),

A contemporary process of nursing: The (un)bearable weight of knowing persons in nursing. New York: Springer.

Locsin, R., & Campling, A. (2005). Techno sapiens and posthumans: Nursing, caring and technology. In R. Locsin (Ed.), *Technological competency as caring in nursing: A model for practice*. Indianapolis, IN: Sigma Theta Tau International.

Locsin, R., & Purnell, M. J. (2007). Rapture and suffering with technology in nursing. *International Journal for Human Caring, 11*(1), 38–43.

Maslow, A. H. (1943). A theory of human motivation. *Psychological Review, 50,* 370–396.

Parse, R. R. (1998). *The human becoming school of thought*. Thousand Oaks, CA: Sage.

Phenix, P. H. (1964). *Realms of meaning*. New York: McGraw-Hill.

Purnell, M., & Locsin, R. (2000). *Intentionality: Unification in nursing*. Unpublished manuscript, Florida Atlantic University College of Nursing, Boca Raton, Florida.

Reader's Digest Association. (1987). *Reader's Digest illustrated encyclopedic dictionary* (p. 932). Pleasantville, NY: The Reader's Digest Association.

Sandelowski, M. (1993). Toward a theory of technology dependency. *Nursing Outlook, 41*(1), 36–42.

Serling, R. (1960). Season 2, Episode 6 of *The Twilight Zone*, "Eye of the Beholder." CBS.

Smith, J. (1983). *The idea of health: Implications for the nursing professional*. New York: Teachers College Press.

Swanson, M. (1991). Dimensions of caring interventions. *Nursing Research, 40,* 161–166.

Watson, J. (1985). *Nursing: Human science and human care*. East Norwalk, CT: Appleton-Century-Crofts.

Chapter 27

Marilyn Anne Ray's Theory of Bureaucratic Caring

MARILYN ANNE RAY
AND MARIAN C. TURKEL

Introducing the Theorist
Overview of the Theory
Application of the Theory
Practice Exemplar
Summary
References

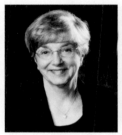

Marilyn Anne Ray

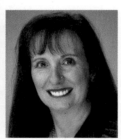

Marian C. Turkel

Introducing the Theorist

Marilyn Anne (Dee) Ray, RN, PhD, CTN, FAAN, is a Professor Emerita at Florida Atlantic University (FAU), Christine E. Lynn College of Nursing, in Boca Raton, Florida. She holds a bachelor of science and a master of science in nursing from the University of Colorado in Denver, Colorado; a master of arts in cultural anthropology from McMaster University in Hamilton, Canada; and a doctorate from the University of Utah in transcultural nursing. She retired as a colonel in 1999 after 30 years of service with the U.S. Air Force Reserve Nurse Corps. As a transcultural nursing scholar and certified advanced transcultural nurse (CTN-A), she has published widely on the subjects of caring in organizational cultures, caring theory and inquiry development, transcultural caring, and transcultural and communitarian ethics. She has held faculty positions at the University of California San Francisco, the University of San Francisco, McMaster University, the University of Colorado, and FAU and Scholar positions at FAU and Virginia Commonwealth University. Ray has enjoyed many diverse teaching and learning assignments around the world. She is featured in Who's Who in America, Who's Who in the World (2010–2015), is a Fellow of the American Society for Applied Anthropology, and is a Fellow of the American Academy of Nursing. She is a review board member of the *Journal of Transcultural Nursing* and *Qualitative Health Research* and a reviewer for the *International Journal of Human Caring*. Ray has conducted phenomenological, ethnographic, and grounded theory research on different topics related to nursing administration and practice, and in the U.S. military. Ray's initial research revolved around the culture of organizations that included technological, political, legal, and economic structures and issues related to caring in complex organizations resulting in the development of the *theory of bureaucratic caring* in 1981. Her research over the past 2 decades, conducted with Dr. Marian Turkel, has used both qualitative and quantitative research methods to study and design patient and professional questionnaires of the complex nurse–patient relational caring process and its impact on economic and patient outcomes in hospitals. Ray and Turkel (2012) advanced the theory of relational caring complexity. Ray (2010) also developed the model of transcultural caring dynamics in nursing and health care in her book by the same name. In her role as professor emerita, Ray is actively engaged in mentoring new faculty members and guiding doctoral students, both in the United States and abroad, whose studies focus on the research of administrative and clinical caring practice, including the clinical nurse leader role, patient safety, the ethical practice of nursing, and transcultural nursing.

Overview of the Theory

This chapter presents a discussion of contemporary nursing culture and shares theoretical views in nursing and those related to the author's theoretical vision and development of professional nursing. The theory of bureaucratic caring is discussed first as a grounded theory (both substantive and formal) and then as a holographic theory. Within this chapter, Dr. Marian Turkel, Director of Professional Nursing Practice and Magnet Holy Cross Hospital, Fort Lauderdale, Florida, integrates the relevance of the theory in administrative and clinical practice.

The Generation of Bureaucratic Caring Theory

The theory of bureaucratic caring was generated in a hospital organization from a qualitative research study using three research approaches more than 30 years ago (Ray, 1981). The theory has been published in the book by Ray (2010),

A Study of Caring Within an Institutional Culture: The Discovery of the Theory of Bureaucratic Caring. Data analysis involved the description of the hospital as a culture (*ethnography*), the meaning of caring in the life world (*phenomenology*), and the discovery of conceptual categories and subcategories and theories of the structure and process of caring in the complex organization (*grounded theory method*). Substantive theory called *differential caring* was generated from the diversity and dominant meanings of caring expressed by participants on different units in the hospital. Formal theory was discovered and developed from insight and interpretation of the initial qualitative data and data related to complex systems, such as tenets of bureaucracy. The culture of the hospital was a dynamic unity illustrating caring as not only humanistic (physical), ethical, spiritual/religious, social-cultural, and educational but also as part of the structural—political, economic, legal, and technological—characteristics of a complex organization. These codetermining processes related to the thesis of caring and the antithesis of bureaucracy were synthesized into the theory of bureaucratic caring (Fig. 27-1). The initial research revealed that economic and political patterns of meaning were more dominant followed by the technical and legal dimensions and finally the social and ethical/spiritual dimensions within the complex system of the hospital. Subsequently, the model was pictured with coequal dimensions. After additional research and continued reflection on what was occurring in science and in nursing science, Ray revisited the theory and discovered that the theory itself incorporated many concepts from the *new sciences of complexity* (the science of change, interconnectedness, wholeness [holography] and emergence). The theory, as shown in Figure 27-2, was subsequently revealed as holographic (Coffman, 2006, 2010, 2014; Ray, 2006; Ray & Turkel, 2010; Turkel, 2007; holography is explained further later in this chapter). The current holographic model depicts the primacy of caring as spiritual–ethical and the other dimensions as equal, indicating the holistic nature of the interface between the spiritual and ethical and the bureaucratic dimensions. In the

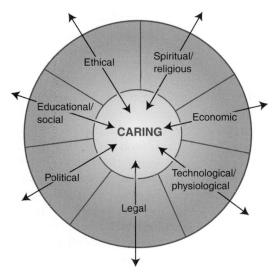

Fig 27 • 1 Grounded theory of bureaucratic caring (differential caring and bureaucratic caring theories).

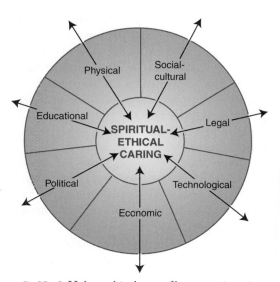

Fig 27 • 2 Holographic theory of bureaucratic caring.

holographic model, caring (the center of the model) is highlighted as spiritual and ethical in relation to the physical (humanistic), the social–cultural and educational, and the more structural dimensions of a complex organization: the political, economic, legal, and technological. Thus, spiritual–ethical caring honors the good of caring, commits to the moral position of caring and virtue, the ethics of compassion, integrity, courage, and humility, (University of San Francisco Curriculum, 2013). Moreover,

spiritual-ethical caring engages the theological, the virtues of faith, hope, and love; the process is creative and shows the integration of the networks of relationships in complex organizational or bureaucratic systems. This holographic model shows overall that spiritual–ethical caring is multidimensional, complex, holistic, and dynamic. Interactions and symbolic systems of meaning by nurses and others are formed and reproduced from the constructions or dominant values held and evolving within the human-environment organization. In some respect, the holographic model depicts that "*we* are the organization." The theory of bureaucratic caring as a holographic model will facilitate and increase our understanding of the practice of nursing in complex contemporary health-care environments.

Holographic Emergence in the Theory of Bureaucratic Caring

The holographic paradigm in complexity science(s) and emergent in the theory of bureaucratic caring recognizes the following:

• that the ontology or "what is" of the universe or creation is the interconnectedness of all things;
• that reality is composed of neither wholes nor parts but of wholes/parts or holons, the whole is in the part and the part in the whole;
• that the epistemology or knowledge that exists is *in* the relationship rather than in the objective world or the subjective experience of it;
• that uncertainty is inherent in the relationship because everything is in process and emerging; and
• that information and choice hold the key to grasping the holistic and complex nature of the meaning of holography or the whole (Cannato, 2006; Davidson, Ray, & Turkel, 2011; Harmon, 1998; Peat, 2003; Wilber, 1982).

Holography thus means that the implicate order (the whole) and explicate order (the part) are interconnected, that everything is a holon, including humans, in the sense that everything is a whole in one context and a part in another—each part being in the whole and the whole being in the part (Cannato, 2006; Peat, 2003). For example, "The molecule depends on the atom, the cell depends on the molecule, and all depend on the stability of the interconnected system in order to thrive" (Cannato, 2006, p. 98). All cycles of activities are linked coherently together; the more energy is stored within systems, the more sub-cycles there are. It is the relational and reciprocal aspect of relationship itself, information and choice, that makes it holistic rather than mechanistic, which subsequently opens all systems to diversity and emergence (integrated sets of possibilities; Davidson & Ray, 1991; Ray, 1998a, 1998b; Thoma, 2003). Holistic science is a human–environmental mutual process and a dynamic unity and a transformative or emergent process. Holistic science (and art) thus captures the idea that all systems, including health-care systems, are living systems, are both wholes and parts, and depend on networks of relationships, information, choice, and communication flow.

The human–environmental mutual process is not a new idea to nursing. It was a central theoretical perspective of Martha Rogers (1970; Smith, 2011) and central to beliefs in anthropology and transcultural nursing advanced by Leininger (1991), and it was a foundation for other theories, such as those of Parse, Newman, and Reed (Alligood, 2014). This notion is seen again at a different time and through a different lens. In the author's work, the focus is on the caring patterns of the nurse–patient relationship within the bureaucratic context of a hospital. The Bureaucratic Caring Theory, already considered paradoxical (bureaucratic caring), identified the linkage between caring as humanistic, social–cultural, educational, and spiritual–ethical and the organizational hospital system as political, economic, legal, and technological. Caring is a relational pattern; it is the flow of nurses' and others' own experiences in the structural context of the organization. This simultaneous process illuminates the idea that the whole and parts are one and the same; all cycles of activities are linked coherently together, but

each may be doing different things at different paces; all the parts are participating in the whole, and the whole is participating as a part in different contexts of meaning (Davidson et al., 2011; Rogers, 1970; Smith 2011; 2013a; 2013b). Information (caring and system data) unfolds and emerges at the same time in the same space without contradicting itself. The theory of bureaucratic caring as a holographic theory furthers the vision of nursing and organizations as complex, dynamic, relational, integral, informational, and emergent—open to sets of possibilities because of the synchronicity of interacting parts and the whole. Everything interconnects; we are all creative manifestations of the oneness of the environment (context), moving in relationship, and continually transforming (emerging—growing and developing; Thoma, 2003). Because of the knowledge of complexity science/s as holography (holistic science and art), we all need to become more aware of the meaning of participatory life and ways of relating to the reality of complex organizations or bureaucracies. Rather than continuing mechanistic approaches of prediction and control that may have worked to some extent to gain precise knowledge in the past, we must now give way to new understanding. Nurses and other professionals must be open to change, to the integral nature of the dynamic unity of the human and environment, and to phenomena that are coherent and emergent wholes (body, mind, spirit, and context) that make up our world of caring, health, healing, and well-being (Davidson et al., 2011; Rogers, 1970; Smith, 2011).

Contemporary Nursing Practice as Complex, Dynamic, Relational, Caring, and Emergent: Foundations of the Theory of Bureaucratic Caring

The practice of nursing is dynamic, always changing, and emerging with new possibilities as people relate to each other. Contemporary nursing practice, however, continues to occur in organizations that are generally bureaucratic or systematic in nature. Although there has been much discussion about the "end of bureaucracy" to cope better with 21st-century innovation and work life within complex systems (Leavitt, 2005; Perrow, 1986; Sorbello, 2008a, 2008b), bureaucracy remains a valuable *tool* to identify and understand the fundamentally different structural principles that undergird coordinated and relational organizational systems. Bureaucracies are organizational systems that can be viewed as cultures. Organizational cultures have a rich heritage and have been studied as both *formal and informal systems* since the 1930s in the United States (Bolman & Dial, 2008; Brenton & Driskill, 2005; Morgan, 1997; Porter-O'Grady & Malloch, 2003, 2007; Ray, 1981, 1984, 1989a, 2006, 2010a, 2010b, 2010c; Ray in Coffman, 2006, 2010, 2014 ; Ray & Turkel, 2010, 2012; Swinderman, 2005, 2011; Turkel & Ray, 2000, 2001; 2004; Wheatley, 2006). *Informal organizational culture* integrates codes of ethics and conduct encompassing commitment, identity, character, coherence, and a sense of community in social-cultural interaction and the social environment. The informal organizational culture is considered essential to the successful functioning or the administering of the *formal organization:* political power and authority, technology and technological computation, economic exchange and legal methods and judgments. Thus, the *formal organization* comprises political, economic, legal, and technical systems within organizational cultures (the typical phenomena of bureaucracies). Bureaucracies themselves create their own cultural orientations, patterns, goals, rituals, languages, and norms within the structural elements of the political, economic, legal, and technological dimensions (Britain & Cohen, 1980; Ray, 2013).

What distinguishes "organizations as cultures" from other paradigms, such as organizations as machines, brains, or other images (Morgan, 1997), is its foundation in anthropology or the study of how people *act* in communities or formalized structures and the *significance or meaning* of work life (Brenton & Driskill, 2005; Cuilla, 2000; Louis, 1985). Organizational cultures, therefore, are viewed as social constructions, symbolically formed

and reproduced through interaction (Sawyer, 2005).

The beliefs about work emerge in organizations through relationships and organizational mission and policy statements. A nation's prevailing tenets and expectations about the nature of work, leisure, and employment are pivotal to the work life of people; hence, there is interplay between the macrocosm of a national/global culture and the microcosm of specific organizations (Eisenberg & Goodall, 1993; Schein, 2004; Wheatley, 2006). In recent years, organizational cultures have emerged as globalizing corporate systems with multiple descriptions of meaning. However, economics, or the "bottom line," is the potent equalizer of most macro- and microcultures (Eisler, 2007; Henderson, 2006). There is an ever-greater concentration of economic and political power in a handful of corporations, which separate their interests (usually profit-driven) from the interests of humans, which are life-centered (Eisler, 2007; Henderson, 2006; Ray, 2010c; Ray, Turkel, & Cohn, 2011; Turkel & Ray, 2000, 2001).

Health care and its activities are tightly interwoven into the social and economic fabric of nations. Values that drive a nation are experienced in the health-care arena. For example, for the most part, "cost and profit" have transformed health care in the United States. As health-care organizations continually are affected by issues of cost and profit and prompt healthcare systems to undergo immense change, such as the health-care reforms of the Patient Protection and Affordable Care Act in the United States (January 5, 2010). Over recent years, confidence in major health-care institutions and their leaders have fallen so low as to put the legitimacy of executives who manage health-care systems at risk. Trust is a major issue (Ray, Turkel, & Marino, 2002; Ray & Turkel, 2012, 2014). Old rules of loyalty and commitment to employees, investment in the worker, fairness in pay, and the need to provide good benefits are in jeopardy. Health-care systems have fallen victim to the corporatization of human enterprise. Consequently, the conflict between health care as a business and caring as a human need has resulted in a crisis in professional nursing, patient safety issues, and the quality of care provided by health-care organizations (Anderson & McDaniel, 2008; Davidson et al., 2011; Eisler, 2007; Institute of Medicine, 2010).

The actual work of nurses, although undervalued in terms of both cost and worth (Ray, 1987a; Ray & Turkel, 2012; Turkel & Ray, 2000, 2001), is currently being evaluated in terms of issues of patient safety and clinical nurse leadership (Page, 2004). Since the Institute of Medicine (2010) report, a resurgence of interest is taking place in the meaningfulness of work and patient safety in many hospitals. Nursing education and the clinical nurse leader role are highlighted as bridges to quality (Sherman, Edwards, Giovengo, & Hilton, 2009). As such, the language of trust and morally worthy work (Cuilla, 2000; Ray et al., 2002; Ray & Turkel, 2012, 2014) is beginning to replace the language of downsizing and restructuring at the same time that mergers and acquisitions still hold sway in contemporary corporate environments. Cuilla (2000) stated that "[t]he most meaningful jobs are those in which people directly help others [provide care] or create products that make life better for people" (p. 225). Although the traditional work of nurses is defined as directly helping others through *knowledgeable* caring (Watson, 2008), contemporary nurses' work and its meaning is also defined by and within the organizational context—the structural dimensions of political, economic, legal, and technological systems (Ray, 1989a, 2006, 2013; Ray & Turkel, 2012; Turkel, 2007). Urging nurses, physicians, and administrators to find cohesion among these dimensions in organizations and the dynamics of unity of human beings (body, mind, and spirit integration) call for the reinvention of work (Fox, 1994). In health care, there is a movement underway for advancing interprofessional education and practice (Keller, Eggenberger, Belkowitz, Sarsekeyeva, & Zito, 2013). Incorporating business principles and creativity of caring, the "work of the soul" or inner work of spiritual–ethical relational caring leads to more emancipatory praxis

and relational self-organization (Ray, 1994a, 1998a; Ray et al., 2002; Ray & Turkel, 2014) means leading in a new way (Porter-O'Grady & Malloch, 2007; Ray, 2010a, 2010b, 2010c; Ray & Turkel, 2012, 2014; Turkel, 2014; Turkel & Ray, 2004, 2012). Spiritual–ethical caring is a witness to the power and depth of transformation in nursing and complex organizations: reseeing the good of nursing, searching for meaning in life and society, creating caring organizations, and finding new meaning in the complexities of work itself.

Organizational Cultures as Transformational Bureaucracies

The transformation of nursing toward a greater understanding of relational self-organization and creativity (work of the soul—spiritual–ethical caring) is not necessarily a new pursuit for the profession; what it reveals is a focus on and movement from invisibility to visibility. Identifying professional nurse caring work as having spiritual–ethical value and being an expression of one's soul or one's creative self at work and at the same time, understanding and identifying nurses' value as an economic resource replaces the notion of nursing as performing only machinelike tasks.

Bureaucracy, still considered by some as a machinelike metaphor, as we have identified, continues to play a significant role in the meanings and symbols of health-care organizations (Coffman, 2006; 2014; Perrow, 1986; Ray, 2010a, 2010b, 2013; Ray & Turkel, 2012, 2014). The social theorist Max Weber (1999) actually predicted that the future belonged to the bureaucracy and not to the working class. Weber, who saw bureaucracy as an efficient and superior form of organizational arrangement, predicted that the bureaucratization of enterprise would dominate the world (Bell, 1974; Weber, 1999). This, of course, is witnessed by the current globalization of commerce and technical information systems. In terms of global commerce, recent acquisitions and mergers of industrial firms and even health-care systems, especially in the United States, are larger and hold more power than some world governments. Yet, to maintain the integrity of large scale, for-profit corporations, often governments have to step in with increased regulation and infuse systems with monetary guarantees. Information technology systems often are in the hands of a few who direct and guide knowledge. The concept of bureaucratization is thus a worldwide phenomenon (Ray, 1989, 2010a, 2010b, 2010c). Although they are considered less effective than other forms of organization, Britain and Cohen (1980) stated that

"[l]ike it or not, humankind is being driven to a bureaucratized world whose forms and functions, whose authority and power must be understood if they are ever to be even partially controlled. . . . The study of bureaucracies is, in effect, the study of the most salient and powerful organizations of the contemporary world. (p. 27).

As bureaucracies grow, so too will the importance of family, kin, community, organizational life, culture, ethnicity, and what is now termed *panethnicity*, and an understanding of diversity within wholeness, ethics, healing, and caring (Britain & Cohen, 1989; Ray, 2010a, 2010b, 2010c).

The *characteristics of bureaucracies* are as follows:

- A division of labor based on roles, departments, leadership, and authority
- A hierarchy of offices [bureaus or units] with diverse social-cultural orientations
- A set of general policies and rules that govern performance
- A separation of the personal from the official
- A selection of personnel on the basis of technical/professional qualifications
- A movement toward interprofessionalism and collaboration
- Equal treatment of all employees or standards of fairness, ethical applications, and reimbursement
- Employment viewed as a career by participants
- Protection of dismissal by tenure or evaluation (from Eisenberg & Goodall, 1993; Leavitt, 2005; Perrow, 1986).

Bureaucracy thus incorporates within the human and ethical dimension the political (power and authority), legal (policies and rules), economic (cost systems), and technical (professional, informational, and computational) dimensions. At the same time, bureaucracies integrate the whole social and cultural system. Bureaucracy, although condemned by some as associated with red tape and inflexibility, continues to provide the most reasonable way in which to view systems and facilitate the preservation and understanding and transformation of organizations. In the past 2 decades, there has been a call for decentralization and the "flattening" of organizational structures—to become less bureaucratic and more participative or heterarchical (Porter-O'Grady & Malloch, 2005, 2007). Many firms have begun to hold to new principles that honor creativity and imagination, and a vision of spiritual and ethical caring and healing (Morgan, 1997; Turkel & Ray, 2004; Ray & Turkel, 2014). Even nursing has advanced in a more collaborative or decentralized manner by its focus on patient-centered nursing and a movement from more centralized control and administration to more decentralized self-governance (Allen, 2013; Nyberg, 1998; Wheatley, 2006). But creative views still need to be marked with understanding of structural systems of bureaucracy as globalization, information, and economics sweep the world.

Leadership models, which are fundamentally hierarchical because of the need for order, continue to head the short-lived participative movement toward decentralization. Even the new clinical nurse leader role sets a nursing leader apart from his or her peers in terms of knowledge and role responsibility. Power is still in the hands of a few. As local and global economic markets rule, there is a call for creating a "caring economics" and a need to be creative and ethical in terms of the worldwide technological and economic transformation taking place (Eisler, 2007; Ray, 1987a, 2010c; Ray & Turkel, 2012, 2014; Turkel, 2001, 2013a, 2013b). We have to look at the social, psychological, and spiritual factors that shape our societies and organizations. As a result, the concept of bureaucracy does not seem as bad as was once thought because it addresses human, and in many respects, humane action. It can be considered as a much less radical paradigm than the business paradigm that focuses only on competition and response to market forces, subsequently eradicating standards of fairness or social justice for humans in the workplace (Ray & Turkel, 2014).

Caring as the Unifying Focus of Nursing

Caring in nursing speaks of relationships, compassion, human dignity, ethics, justice, and competent and knowledgeable caring practice (Ray, 1981, 1989b, 2010a, 2010b, 2013; Roach, 2002; Smith, Turkel, & Wolf, 2013; Turkel, 1997; Watson, 2005, 2008). Caring science and art is holistic, humane, and dynamic; thus, it facilitates growth and development of human persons and helps to make things work in health-care agencies. As such, caring science and art is considered by many nurse scholars to be the essence of nursing (Boykin & Schoenhofer, 2001; 2013; Boykin, Schoenhofer, & Valentine, 2013; Leininger, 1981a, 1981b, 1991, 1997; Ray, 1989a, 1989b, 1994a, 1994b; Ray & Turkel, 2012; Smith et al., 2013; Watson, 1985, 1988, 1997, 2008). Although not uniformly accepted, Newman, Sime, and Corcoran-Perry (1991) and Newman (1992) characterized the social mandate of the discipline of nursing as caring in the human health experience. Newman, Smith, Pharris, and Jones (2008) further emphasized her initial idea that relationship is the focus and health is the rhythmic fluctuations of the life process, as well as caring, consciousness, mutual process, patterning, presence, and meaning. Caring and health thus are influential concepts. The expression "caring" in the human health experience emphasizes the social mandate to which nursing has responded throughout its history and encompasses the scope of the discipline (Roach, 2002; Watson, 2008). Caring, with multiple meanings, however, is manifested in different and complex ways in the nursing discipline and profession (Morse et al., 2013; Smith et al., 2013).

Evolution and Development of the Theory of Bureaucratic Caring

Facing the challenge of the economic and patient safety crises in health care and nursing, the disillusionment of registered nurses about the disregard for their caring services, and the concern of the nursing profession and the public about the effects of the shortage of nurses (Institute of Medicine, 2010), working for the good of the profession and preservation of the nurse–patient caring relationship is imperative. Running away from the chaos of hospitals or misunderstanding the meaning of work life cannot become the norm. Wherever nurses go, they will be "haunted" by bureaucracies, some functional, many problematic. What, then, is the deeper reality of nursing practice? The following is a presentation of theoretical views that relate to the theory of bureaucratic caring, culminating in a vision for understanding the deeper significance of nursing life as holistic, spiritual and ethical, relational, cultural, contextual, and the dynamics of complexity.

Complexity and Nursing Theory

To understand this significance, and holographic nature of the theory of bureaucratic caring, an overview of complexity science(s) is necessary. "Complexity theory is a scientific theory of dynamical systems collectively referred to as the sciences of complexity" (Ray, 1998a, p. 91). They illuminate the nature and creativity of science itself. Revolutionary approaches to new scientific theory development have transpired, such as quantum theory and actually "beyond the quantum," the science of wholeness, holographic and chaos theories, fractals or the idea of self-similarity, networks of relationships and complex information systems, and the concepts of choice and self-organization/relational self-organization (Bar-Yam, 2004; Battista, 1982; Briggs & Peat, 1989, 1999; Davidson & Ray, 1991; Davidson et al., 2011; Lindberg, Nash, & Lindberg, 2008; Peat, 2003; Ray, 1998a; Ray & Turkel, 2012; Wheatley, 2006; Wilber, 1982).

Complexity theory is replacing other theories, such as Newtonian physics and even Einstein's beliefs and those of other scientists as well, that the physical world is governed by laws and order. New scientific views illustrate that the fundamental force in the universe is dynamic (always changing), chaotic, nonlinear, nonpredictable, relational, moving toward self-organization, and open to possibilities. As such, phenomena that are antithetical actually coexist—determinism with uncertainty and reversibility with irreversibility (Nicolis & Prigogine, 1989; Peat, 2003). "Opposing things can happen at the same time, in the same space, without contradicting each other" (Thoma, 2003, p. 17). Thus, both linear and nonlinear and simple (e.g., gravity) and complex (economic and cultural) systems exist together (for example, the paradoxical nature of the theory of bureaucratic caring). One of the tools or metaphors in the studies of complexity is chaos theory. Chaos deals with life at the edge, or the notion that the concept of order exists within disorder at the system communication or choice point phases where old patterns disintegrate or new patterns emerge (Davidson & Ray, 1991; Davidson et al., 2011; Lindberg et al., 2008; Newman et al., 2008; Ray, 1994a, 1998b, 2011; Ray et al., 1995). This new science, which signifies interrelationship of mind and matter, interconnectedness and choice, carries with it a moral responsibility and the quest toward wisdom, which includes awareness, information systems, networks of relationships, patterns of energy, creativity, information about the environment and emergence (Davidson & Ray, 1991; Davidson et al., 2011; Fox, 1994). The conception of the interconnectedness and relational reality of all things, the interdependence of all human–environmental phenomena, and the discovery of order in a chaotic world demonstrate the pioneering story of 20th-century science and how the insightful idea of belongingness and relationality (a powerful nursing concept) is shaping the science of the 21st century (Peat, 2003).

Within nursing, certain nursing theorists have embraced the notion of nursing as complexity in which consciousness, human–environmental mutual relationship, caring, and choice-making are central concepts (Davidson & Ray, 1991; Davidson et al., 2011; Lindberg et al., 2008; Newman, 1986, 1992; Newman et al., 2008; Ray, 1994a, 1998a; Rogers, 1970). Given the nature of nursing as unitary, holistic, relational, and caring, and of health as expanding consciousness (Newman et al., 2008; Pharris, 2006), there is a coherent link between the importance of theory as wakefulness (awareness) and professional practice. Ray and Turkel hold the position that nurses do need to be exposed to ideas and need diverse nursing theories to stimulate thinking. The only way that nursing can critique itself is by understanding the intellectual views of scholars in the complex world of nursing science, research, education, and practice. Theories, as the integration of knowledge, research, and experience, highlight the way in which scholars and practitioners of nursing interpret their world and the context where nursing is lived. Theories in this sense are also philosophies or ideologies that serve a practical purpose. Thus, the idea that theories are the pure viewing of truth (wakefulness or awareness; van Manen, 1982) and that they can be judged in light of their practical consequences (Bohman, 2005) underscores the importance of nursing theory as both a scholarly enterprise and a wise practice that identifies and participates in the complexities of inquiry about relationships, knowledgeable caring, health, healing, complex organizations, and the universe.

Description of Bureaucratic Caring Theory

In the original qualitative study of caring in the organizational context conducted by Ray (1981, 1984, 1989a, 2010b), the research revealed that nurses and other professionals struggled with the paradox of serving the bureaucracy and serving humans, especially patients, through caring. Caring, however, had multiple meanings and was expressed differently in terms of the way a particular unit was organized. The system phenomena of political, economic, legal, and technological became integrated into the meaning system of caring just as the humanistic, social, educational, ethical, and spiritual. The discovery of bureaucratic caring resulted in both substantive theory (grounded in the context of meaning) and formal theory (integrated from the substantive theory and general understanding of dimensions of complex bureaucracies; Ray, 1981, 1984, 1989a, 2010b).

The bureaucracy represented a living system. Caring was expressed not only in the more interpersonal relational patterns of humanness and compassion but also in the official structures of the bureaucracy, especially the political and economic structures, and both expressions were infused into the meaning system of professionals. Even patients saw the "system" as affecting how they understood caring in their own healthcare experiences (Ray, 1981, 1989a, 2010b; Ray & Turkel, 2001–2004, 2012, 2014; Ray et al., 2011). The substantive theory (grounded) emerged as *differential caring theory* and showed that caring in the complex organization of the hospital was complex and differentiated itself in terms of meaning by its specific context— dominant caring dimensions related to areas of practice or units wherein professionals worked and patients resided. Differential caring theory showed that professionals and patients on different units espoused different and dominant caring meanings based on their professional roles and personal and organizational goals and values. For example, participants in the oncology unit espoused caring as intimate and spiritual; in contrast, participants in the intensive care unit espoused caring as more technological; and in administration, participants espoused caring as maintaining economic viability. The formal theory of bureaucratic caring symbolized a dynamic structure of caring, which was synthesized from a dialectic using the tenets of the philosophy of Hegel (*thesis, antithesis,* and *synthesis*); the dialectic between the thesis of caring as humanistic, social, educational, ethical, and religious/spiritual (dimensions of humanism, morality, and spirituality), and the antithesis of caring as economic, political, legal, and technological (dimensions of bureaucracy; Coffman, 2014; Ray, 1981, 1989a, 2006; 2010a, 2010b; Ray et al., 2011; Ray & Turkel, 2010, 2012, 2014; Turkel, 2007).

The Theory of Bureaucratic Caring as Holographic Theory

How can the theory of bureaucratic caring be viewed as a holographic theory? As previously discussed, the theory arose initially from interpretations and choices that were made about the meaning and structure of caring in organizational life. The process parallels ideas from complexity sciences and specifically holography: consciousness or awareness; intentionality of the mutual human–environmental caring relationships; quality of the caring transactions; and the effective ability to analyze, negotiate, make choices, and reconcile paradoxes between caring and the system demands. The humanistic nurse–patient care needs and professional responsibilities in terms of the structural considerations of the system (political, economic, legal, and technological dimensions) were always emerging from sets of caring possibilities. Awareness of belongingness/interconnectedness, the mutual human–environmental relationship, the implicate (the whole) and explicate (the part) order (*the whole is reflected in the part, and part reveals the whole*), respect for the good of all things, and communication, choice and emergence—all of these are central to holistic science. Similarly, as revealed through this research, these concepts were central to the interpretation of caring as a whole in the complex organization. The dialectic of caring (the thesis, the *implicate order,* or the whole of caring as humanistic and spiritual-ethical) in relation to the various organizational structures (the antithesis of the system, *explicit order,* or part, the organization as political-economic-technical-legal) is reconciled and transformed by a synthesis of the polar opposites into the theory of bureaucratic caring. The synthesis of the theory of bureaucratic caring shows that everything is interconnected, even humanistic spiritual–ethical caring and the organizational system. The whole is in the part, and the part is in the whole; therefore, nursing in the system is a holon, and the theory is holographic.

Transforming the Organization

The theory of bureaucratic caring reveals that knowledge of holistic caring interconnectedness is possible to motivate nurses to continue to embrace the human dimension within the current political, economic, legal, and technologic bureaucratic environment of health care. Can higher ground thus be reclaimed for the 21st century? Higher ground requires that we make excellent and ethical choices at the "edge of chaos" where possibilities exist in relationships and systems/organizations to either transform or disintegrate (Peat, 2003). Understanding of spiritual–ethical caring in the holographic theory of bureaucratic caring helps us to connect at our deepest level. Nurses and others in complex systems can reclaim higher ground by doing the "work of the soul" (understanding and engaging creatively, spiritually, and lovingly, and taking ethical responsibility for self and other and the organizational system). Our choice(s) depends on a commitment and ethical social action to cocreate caring-healing relationships and communities (Ray & Turkel, 2014; Turkel & Ray, 2004). The model (see Fig. 27-2) presents a vision of nursing as spiritual–ethical caring, but it is also based on the reality of practice. Through continuous research and observation, the model emphasizes a direction toward the unity of experience. *Spirituality* involves creativity and choice and refers to genuineness, vitality, and depth. It is revealed in attachment, love, and community and comprehended within each of us as intimacy and an unfolding of virtue and the sacred art of divine love (Cannato, 2006; Harmon, 1998; Ray, 1997a, 1997b; 2010a; Secretan, 1997). *Ethics* deals with our moral accountability to self and caring for self, and responsibility to one another and to the organizations within which we work. Secretan states: "Most of us have an innate understanding of soul, even though each of us might define it in a very different and personal way"(p. 27).

As such, Fox (1994) calls for the theology of work—a redefinition of work as spiritual and ethical. Because of the crisis in our work life mainly due to economic and political constraints, and in general our relationship to work, we are challenged to reinvent it. For nursing, this is important because work puts us in touch with others, not only in terms of personal gain, but also at the level of service to humanity or the community of patients/clients and other professionals. Work must be spiritual and ethical, with recognition of the creative spirit at work in us. Nurses must be the "custodians of the human spirit" (Secretan, 1997, p. 27).

The ethical imperatives of caring that join with the spiritual relate to questions or issues about our moral obligations to others. The ethics of caring involve never treating people simply as a means to an end or as ends in themselves but rather as beings that have the capacity to make choices about the meaning of life, health, healing, and caring. Ethical content—principles of doing good, doing no harm, allowing choice, being fair, and promise-keeping—functions as the compass directing our decisions to sustain humanity in the context of the bureaucracy—the political, economic, legal, and technological issues and situations within organizations. Roach (2002) pointed out that ethical caring is operative at the level of discernment of principles, in the *commitment* needed to carry them out, and in the *decisions or choices* to uphold human dignity through love and compassion. Furthermore, Roach (2002) remarked that health is a community responsibility, an idea that is rooted in ancient Hebrew ethics. The expression of human caring as an ethical act is inspired by spiritual traditions that emphasize charity. For nursing, spiritual–ethical caring does not question whether or not to care in complex systems but intimates how sincere deliberations and ultimately the facilitation of ethical choices for the good of others can or should be accomplished. By integrating knowledgeable caring creatively, by staying intentional and conscious of dynamic movements within the circle of life, love, and relationships, and by leading in a new way in complex systems/bureaucracies, nurses are engaging in new and exciting work (Davidson et al., 2011; Eisler, 2007; O'Grady & Malloch, 2007; Ray, 1997b; Ray et al., 2002; Ray & Turkel, 2012, 2014; Turkel & Ray, 2004). The theory of bureaucratic caring as a holistic science and art bears witness to the power and depth of transformation: reseeing the good of nursing as spiritual and ethical, believing in human potential, continually searching for meaning in life, creating caring organizations, cocreating new possibilities, and finding new meaning in the complexities of work life itself. The scientist Sheldrake remarked:

> The recognition that we need to change the way we live [work] is gaining ground. It is like waking up from a dream. It brings with it a spirit of repentance, seeing in a new way, a change of heart. This conversion is intensified by the sense that the end of the age of oppression is at hand. (1991, p. 207)

Application of the Theory

The theory of bureaucratic caring illuminated in this chapter is a response to the end of the age of oppression. The theory is holistic with a practical purpose, thus responding to the call for a *translational science,* translating caring theory into practice or facilitating theory-guided practice (Ray & Turkel, 2012; Smith et al., 2013). Ray (1989a, p. 31) warned that the "transformation of American and other health-care systems to corporate enterprises emphasizing competitive management and economic gain seriously challenges nursing's humanistic philosophies and theories, and nursing's administrative and clinical policies." As nurses know, for more than 30 years, there has been an intense focus on operating costs and the bottom line in the American health-care environment, and caring is often not valued within the organizational culture. However, caring scientists, nurse researchers, nurse leaders, and nurses in practice have sought out principles of caring science (Watson, 2008), transcultural caring dynamics (Ray, 2010), and relational caring complexity (Ray & Turkel, 2012). The application of the theory of bureaucratic caring as a framework to guide practice and ethical decision making (Ray, 2010a, 2010b; Ray & Turkel, 2012; Ray et al., 2012; Smith et al., 2013; Turkel, 2007, 2013b) will transform a complex organization to a community of caring where caring for self, thoughtfulness for others through compassion, integrity, courage, and humility can thrive (Smith et al., 2013; University of San Francisco, 2013). Nurses must be encouraged to continue the struggle not only to be caring but

to respond with confidence to the economic issues and engage the political, legal, and technological questions and trials facing them. With hospital system goals of decreasing length of stay and increasing staffing ratios, nurses need to be committed to establishing trust and initiate a caring relationship during their first encounter with a patient. As this relationship is being established, nurses need to focus on "being, knowing, and doing all at once" (Turkel, 1997, 2013) within what Watson (2008; 2013) calls the "caring moment." From a patient perspective, "being there" means completing a task while simultaneously engaging caringly with them. This approach to practice means not only viewing the patient as a person in all of his or her complexity but viewing the patient and the needs of professional nursing competently within the complex organizational environment.

As a holographic and translational science, we can see that the economic, political, technological, legal, and spiritual–ethical, humanistic dimensions of bureaucratic caring, and in general, the theory of bureaucratic caring can be used to guide practice. Staff nurses can hold close their core value that caring is the essence of nursing and can still retain a focus on meeting the issues of the bottom line (economics). Empirical studies have firmly established a link between caring and positive patient outcomes (Watson, 2009). And positive patient outcomes are needed for organizational survival in this competitive and political era of health care. Given this, professional nursing practice must embrace and illuminate the caring philosophy in relation to complex organizational phenomena. As expressed, explicitly linking caring to patient and organizational outcomes is integral. For the first time since the inception of value-based purchasing, one third of hospital reimbursement will be linked to patient satisfaction data and two-thirds to patient quality/safety data. This is the time for the economic value of caring to be actualized with the organization (Ray & Turkel, 2009).

Moving away from just focusing on patient care to the economic justification of nursing and health-care systems has prompted professionals to desire a fuller understanding of just how to preserve humanistic caring within the educational, business, or corporate (economic and political) culture (Miller, 1989; Nyberg, 1998, 2013; Turkel, 2007, 2013a; Boykin, Schoenhofer, &Valentine, 2013; see also Watson Caring Science Institute, www .wcsi.org). In terms of application, the theory thus, has been used as a foundation for additional research and observational studies of the nurse–patient caring relationship and system issues, such as in public health administration, curriculum development, correctional facility health care, technology and information technology, economics of caring, the clinical nurse leader role, the charge nurse role, ethics and the moral community, legal caring, pediatric pain, and medication errors in complex organizations, perioperative do not resuscitate orders, the transtheoretical development of relational caring complexity theory, and nursing administration—the role of the nurse in shared governance (Al-Ayed, 2008; Allen, 2013, Coffman, 2006; Cross, 2014; Eggenberger, 2011a, 2011b; Gibson, 2008; Gomez, 2008; Manworren, 2008; McCray-Stewart, 2008; O'Brien, 2008; Ray, 1987b, 1993, 1997a, 1998a, 1998b; Ray et al., 2002; Sorbello, 2008a; Stedman, 2013; Swinderman, 2011; Ray & Turkel, 2010, 2012; Turkel, 1997, 2007; Turkel & Ray, 2000, 2001, 2009).

Over the past three decades, Ray and Turkel have conducted research and used dimensions of the theory of bureaucratic caring to examine the paradox between the concept of human caring and political, economic, legal and technological dimensions in complex organizations, and more specifically studies of the economics of caring. Their research showed that staff nurses value the caring relationship between nurse and patient. However, nurses are practicing in an environment where the economics and costs of health care permeate discussions and clinical decisions. The focus on costs is not a transient response to shrinking reimbursement; instead, it has become the catalyst for change within health-care organizations. Between 2002 and 2004, Relational Caring Questionnaires were distributed to registered nurses, patients, and administrators in five hospitals (Ray & Turkel, 2005, 2009, 2012). Overall

mean scores on the questionnaires were then compared to economic and patient outcome data. It is of interest to note that the hospital with the highest mean score of 3.30 for the professional questionnaire had the lowest number (3.36) of full-time employees per adjusted occupied bed and the lowest number of patient falls. The hospital with the highest patient mean score of 4.50 had the lowest cost ($1,265) per adjusted patient day. These findings validate what registered nurses verbalized in the qualitative research, "Living the caring values in everyday practice makes a difference in nursing practice and patient outcomes" (Ray & Turkel, 2009). Through their focused research on economic caring, they advanced the theory of relational caring complexity (Ray & Turkel, 2012), which is beginning to be used to improve the practice of nursing. It is a challenge for nurses to combine the science and art of caring within the complex health-care environment. However, these research efforts illustrate how this can be done to help reshape organizations and the health-care system in the United States and other countries, such as Canada, Australia, Japan, China, Columbia, Chile, and some countries in Scandinavia, the Middle East, and Africa.

Application of Theory of Bureaucratic Caring to Excellence in Contemporary Professional Nursing Practice

In addition to the earlier discussion of application of the theory to practice, the American Nurses Credentialing Center (ANCC) Magnet Recognition Program® recognizes excellence in professional nursing practice. Organizations provide written narratives and sources of evidence related to the development, dissemination, and enculturation of best practices, quality care, technical skill, and patient preference. This emphasis on *professional* nursing practice within the Magnet Recognition Program has resulted in organizations integrating evidence-based practice, nursing research, and professional models of care delivery informed by nursing theory into the practice setting.

In the past, organizations provided sources of evidence and written narratives illustrating the dissemination, enculturation, and sustainability of the Fourteen Forces of Magnetism across the organization (ANCC, 2005). A new model was developed in 2008 (ANCC, 2008) and a revision to this model was released in 2014. The new model has five components that contain the Forces of Magnetism. The five components include transformational leadership; structural empowerment; exemplary professional nursing practice; new knowledge, innovation, and improvements; and empirical quality results. The theory of bureaucratic caring can be integrated into each of these components.

Transformational leadership reflects nursing leadership that is transformational and visionary. The chief nurse executive (CNE) uses the theory of bureaucratic caring as the theoretical framework when creating the nursing strategic plan and achieving the goal of balancing caring and economics in clinical and administrative decision making. The economic dimension of the theory of bureaucratic caring and tenets from relational caring complexity serve as research-based references for the CNE in advocating how the limited resources within the organization will be allocated. Nursing leaders may not be able to change reimbursement from the government, but they can influence organizational decision making for the improvement of the quality of care and caring. Transformational leaders use ideas from direct care registered nurses to improve the work environment, which can include formal integration of self-care practices (Ray & Turkel, 2012; Turkel & Ray, 2004).

Structural (professional and organizational) empowerment represents professional engagement, commitment to professional development, teaching and role development, commitment to community involvement, and recognition of nursing. The CNE can advocate for involvement in the conferences sponsored by the International Association for Human Caring (humancaring.org), where nurses at all levels have an opportunity to disseminate caring scholarship and hear examples of how caring theory has been used to change practice and inform education and research. Upon return from conferences, direct-care registered nurses can make presentations to boards of trustees on how caring

science and theory make a difference in practice in terms of organizational, registered nurse, and patient outcomes. Ongoing education including interactive dialogue and reflective practice related to the theory and self-care practices can be part of internal professional development for nurses at all levels in the organization. As part of community involvement, registered nurses are integral to community caring. Being in the community requires integration of the social, political, and cultural dimensions of the theory. Having a formal practice theory supports the professional image of nursing within the organization and makes visible the outcomes and contributions of nursing practice to the organization (Turkel, 2007).

Exemplary professional practice includes having a *professional practice model* and care delivery system in place in complex organizations for registered nurses. Sources of evidence relate to how the theory of bureaucratic caring could be selected and used to guide practice. Nursing situations reflecting professional and interprofessional clinical decision making, and examining staffing patterns balancing caring and economics serve as examples of evidence to support a professional model of care. For consultation and resources, reference can be made to external consultation with nursing scholars as theorists, dissertation supervisors, or consultants, and how attendance at professional conferences or other contacts, for example, through Webinars or using Skype or Adobe Connect make a difference in nursing research, practice, and patient outcomes.

Under autonomy as a principle of the *Code of Ethics With Interpretive Statements* (American Nurses Association, 2001) for nurses, the component of spiritual–ethical caring illustrates how nurses promoting self-organization serve as advocates for patients and families. The educational dimension of the theory advances the care delivery system as the professional nurse develops innovative, individualized, evidence-based patient education initiatives. Organizations truly focused on innovation or transformational leadership can expand the theory to be interdisciplinary or interprofessional and serve as the interdisciplinary plan of care for the patient, the family, and the health-care system as a whole.

The component of new knowledge, innovation, and improvements includes quality improvement. Unit-based patient care projects, evidence-based best practice, and qualitative and quantitative findings related to the theory serve as exemplars included under this component.

The fifth component of the Magnet Recognition Program®, empirical outcomes recognizes the contribution of nursing in terms of patient, nursing, and organizational outcomes. Results from theory-guided research and evidence-based projects related to the dimensions of the theory of bureaucratic caring validating the difference in patient and organizational outcomes serve as evidence for this component.

Relevance of the Theory of Bureaucratic Caring to Nursing Education

The theory is relevant to nursing education because of its focus on caring in nursing practice and the conceptualization of the health-care system (Coffman, 2006, 2010, 2014). When developing the curriculum for a baccalaureate program, the faculty at Nevada State College combined Ray's theory of bureaucratic caring with theoretical constructs from Watson (1985) and Johns (2000) as a conceptual framework. According to this framework, the holographic theory of caring recognizes the interconnectedness of all things and that everything is a whole in one context and a part of the whole in another context. Spiritual–ethical caring, the focus for communication, infuses all nursing phenomena including physical, social–cultural, legal, technological, economic, political, and educational forces (Nevada State College, 2003, p. 2).

Turkel (2001) used the theory to guide curriculum development in the master's of science program in nursing administration at Florida Atlantic University. Dimensions from the theory, including ethical, spiritual, economic, technological, legal, political, and social, served as a framework for the exploration of current health-care issues. The economic dimension of the theory was a central component in several courses. Students analyzed the current economic and reimbursement structure of health care from the perspective of a caring lens.

Another example illuminates the creativity of faculty. For example, a professor from the University of San Francisco (2013) is implementing ways to use virtue ethics (a component of the School of Nursing curriculum) and complexity science and highlight the theoretical model for teaching and learning spiritual–ethical caring and complex systems.

The application of the theory of bureaucratic caring and the practice exemplar illustrate that the foundation for professional nursing is the blending of the humanistic and empirical/organizational aspects of care—understanding caring science and art in complex organizations. In today's environment, the nurse needs to integrate caring, knowledge, and skills "all at once" (being, knowing, and doing). Given political and economic constraints, the art of caring cannot occur in isolation from meeting the physical needs of patients and incorporating the dimensions of the economic, political, technological, spiritual-ethical caring dimensions. When caring is defined solely as science or as art—empirical or esthetic nursing, respectively—neither is adequate to reflect the reality of current practice. Nurses must be able to understand and articulate the politics and the economics of as well as caring in nursing practice and health care. Classes that examine the environment of practice generally, and the politics and the economics of health care in relation to caring, must be integrated into nursing education and staff development curricula. Nurses need to search continually for different approaches to professional practice that will incorporate caring in an increasingly political, technical, and cost-driven environment. Doing more with less no longer works; nurses must "move outside of the box" to create innovative practice models informed by nursing theory. Nurses need to, in essence, move nursing from being viewed as a "bed rate" in hospitals to nursing as a human caring science and practice AND valued as a central economic resource within an organization and the health-care system.

Administrative nursing research needs to continue to focus on the relationship among nursing, caring, patient outcomes, and complex organizational economic outcomes. Ongoing research is required to firmly establish the nurse–patient relationship as an economic resource in the new paradigm of evidence-based practice of health-care delivery (Ray & Turkel, 2008, 2012, 2014; Turkel, 2013a). Findings from additional qualitative and quantitative research studies will continue to support the theory of bureaucratic caring as a middle-range theory, a holographic practice theory, and a general/universal theory.

Nurses need ongoing education related to the politics, and economics and costs associated with health care as well as knowledge of complex technological organizational environments. Lack of knowledge in these areas allows others outside of nursing to continue to make the political and economic decisions concerning the practice of nursing. Having an in-depth knowledge of the politics and economics of health care allows nurses to use innovation and creativity to both challenge and transform the system. A new theory-guided model created for nursing practice that supports human caring in relation to the organization's economic, technical, and political values is an exemplar of such innovation The multiple dimensions of the theory of bureaucratic caring serve as a philosophical/theoretical framework to inform both contemporary and future

research and theory-guided nursing practice. Having this in-depth knowledge allows nurses to continually question and transform complex health-care organizations.

Ray and Turkel (2012) continue to advance their collaborative ideas related to theory development, caring science, and the paradox between caring and economics within complex systems. A metatheory (Ritzer, 1991) emerged from the integration of the following: the theory of bureaucratic caring (Ray, 1981, 2006), *Struggling to Find a Balance: The Paradox Between Caring and Economics* (Turkel 1997, 2001), and relational complexity (Ray & Turkel, 2012; Turkel & Ray, 2000). The metatheory is relational caring complexity, and it reveals the complexity of today's nursing practice situation while providing a foundation for emerging professional practice models focused on caring and healing, and innovative transdisciplinary research looking at caring and economics. Continually giving voice to the value of caring in nursing within and a part of complex organizations allows for spiritual–ethical caring to occur.[1]

---

[1]For additional practice exemplars please go to bonus chapter content available at FA Davis http://davisplus.fadavis.com

---

Practice Exemplar

The following exemplar from the practice setting was previously published by Turkel (2007).* The situation reflects the lived experiences of how the theory of bureaucratic caring serves as a framework for nursing practice and guides decision making.

Megan Smith, RN, MSN, was recently hired as the chief nurse executive (CNE) for a 500-bed inner-city hospital. The payer mix for this patient population was once private insurance, but now it is approximately 75% Medicare and Medicaid. When Megan met with the nursing staff, they stated, "We are not valued or treated with respect. The administrators only see us as numbers. We are implementing a new computerized documentation system, getting new monitors, being told that patient safety is important and getting ready for a survey from

the Joint Commission. With all the rules and regulations, it is stressful to find time to actually care for our patients. Plus we need more help."

Megan was committed to being an advocate for nursing while realizing the professional accountability of considering the economic, political, and technological perspectives of her decision making. Megan promised the nurses that she would review the budget and follow-up with their concerns. She explained to the nurses that providing safe, high-quality patient care in a caring and compassionate manner was the top priority for the organization.

Later that week, Megan met with the chief executive officer (CEO) to share the concerns of the nursing staff. Her first priority was to increase the number of registered nurses and to

Practice Exemplar cont.

hire two additional clinical nurse specialists. The CEO was reluctant to spend the additional financial resources. Megan explained that increasing the number of registered nurses would decrease the number of falls and pressure ulcers and increase compliance related to patient safety. Additional registered nurses would increase satisfaction for both nurses and patients, as the nurses would have more time to focus on developing caring relationships with patients and their families. In addition, the registered nurses would have time to focus on providing patient teaching and discharge planning. Megan presented the CEO with quantitative data to demonstrate the costs associated with falls, pressure ulcers, and patients returning to the emergency department (ED) within 48 hours postdischarge because of inadequate education or discharge planning. The request for additional registered nurses and clinical nurse specialists was approved. Six months later, the number of falls, pressure ulcers, medication errors, and return visits to the ED had decreased. Scores on the patient satisfaction survey related to nurses informing patients, showing concern, and checking patient identification bands increased.

The additional clinical nurse specialists served as mentors to increase the technical skills of the inexperienced graduate nurses and to demonstrate how the use of technology in terms of cardiac monitoring would enhance the caring interactions between the registered nurse and patient. Customized programing of the new clinical documentation system afforded nurses the opportunity to document interventions related to specific dimensions of the theory of bureaucratic caring.

Permission to use this practice exemplar was granted by Zane Robinson Wolf, RN, PhD, FAAN, editor of International Journal for Human Caring, *January 15, 2014.*

Summary

The values of nursing are deepening, and as a discipline and profession, nursing is expanding its consciousness (Newman et al., 2008; Ray & Turkel, 2014). Nursing is being shaped by the historical revolution occurring in science, social sciences, and theology as well as the revolution of its own commitment to caring science, health care for all, and understanding of holism and complex systems (Baer, 2013; Davidson & Ray, 1991; Davidson et al., 2011; Lindberg et al., 2008; Newman et al., 2008; Ray, 1998a, 2006, 2010a, 2010b; Reed, 1997; Watson, 2005). Freeman (in Appell & Triloki, 1988) pointed out that human values are a function of the capacity to make choices and called for a paradigm giving recognition to awareness and choice. As noted in this chaper, a revision toward this end is taking place in nursing based upon the science/s of complexity and a new holographic scientific worldview, as well as specific theories of nursing, especially this holographic theory of bureaucratic caring.

Nursing has the capacity to make creative and moral choices for a preferred future. Constructs of consciousness and choice are central and demonstrate that phenomena of the universe, including society and what happens in nursing, organizations and societies arise from the choices that are or are not made (Davidson et al., 2011; Harmon, 1998; Newman et al., 2008). The theory of bureaucratic caring has reinforced, caring as the primordial construct and consciousness of nursing within complex bureaucratic systems. In nursing, the critical task is to comprehend the meaning of the networks and complexity of relationships, between what is given in culture (the norms) and what is chosen (the moral and spiritual). In nursing, the unitary-transformative paradigm and the state of the science (Newman, et al., 2008), and various theories of Rogers, Newman, Leininger, Watson, Parse, and Ray's holographic theory of bureaucratic caring are challenging nurses to become more aware and understand their future in terms of the complexity of human–environment relationship. The unitary-transformative paradigm of nursing and its holographic tenets are consistent with new science/s of complexity. However, the other reality of nursing is that there continues to be threats by the business/economic model over its long-term human interests for facilitating health, healing and well-being of patients, nurses and other professionals, and organizations (Davidson & Ray, 1991; Davidson et al., 2011; Lindberg et al., 2008; Ray, 1994a, 1998; Ray & Turkel, 2012; Reed, 1997; Smith, 2004; Vicenzi, White, & Begun, 1997). However, the creative, intuitive, ethical, and spiritual mind is unlimited. Through "authentic conscience" (Harmon, 1998), we must find hope in our creative powers.

This presentation of the theory of bureaucratic caring is a creative enterprise. The theory reflects spiritual and ethical caring, bureaucratic system principles, and incorporation of tenets of the new sciences of complexity highlighting holography. Holographic theory illuminates holistic science and art, the interconnectedness of all things, human–environment integral relationships, scientific chaos theory, holographic patterning (the whole is in the part, and the part in the whole), informational networks, relational self-organization, transformation, change, choice, and emergence (Bar-Yam, 2004; Davidson & Ray, 1991; Davidson et al., 2011; Lindberg et al., 2008; Ray, 1991, 1994, 1998a, 2010a, 2010b; Turkel & Ray, 2000, 2001; Thoma, 2003). In the theory of bureaucratic caring, everything is infused with spiritual–ethical caring (the center of the model) by its integrative and relational connection to the structures of complex organizations. Spiritual–ethical caring is both a part and a whole, and every part secures its purpose and meaning from each of the other parts that can also be considered wholes. In

other words, the theoretical model shows how spiritual–ethical caring is involved with qualitatively different yet similar processes or systems, be they political, economic, technological, or legal. The systems, when integrated and presented as open and interactive, are a whole and must operate as such by conscious choice, especially by the ethical choice making of nursing, which always has, or should have, the interest of humanity at heart.

Envisioning the theory of bureaucratic caring as holographic from its initial substantive and formal grounded theories shows that through research, creativity, and imagination, nursing can build the profession it wants. Nurses are calling for opportunities for expression of their own spiritual and ethical existence, a reinvention of work. Nurses are also calling for understanding of the nurse–patient caring relationship *in* complex organizations. The new scientific, spiritual–ethical, and experiential approach to nursing theory as holographic will have positive effects—and that reality has been illustrated in this presentation. The union of complexity science, ethics, and spirituality will engender a new sense of hope for transformation in the work world. This transformation toward relational caring organizations and communities of caring *can* occur in the economic and politically driven atmosphere of today. The deep values that underlie caring and choice to do good for the many will be felt both inside and outside organizations. We must awaken our consciences and act on this awareness and no longer surrender to injustices and oppressiveness of systems that focus primarily on the good of a few (Ray & Turkel, 2014). "Healing a sick society [work world] is a part of the ministry of making whole" (Fox, 1994, p. 305). The holographic theory of bureaucratic caring—idealistic yet practical, visionary yet real—can give direction and impetus to lead the way.

References

Al-Ayed, B. (2008). *Applying bureaucratic caring theory in medication errors phenomena.* Unpublished manuscript, University of Jordan, Amman, Jordan.

Allen, S. (2013, September). *An ethnonursing study of the cultural meanings and practices of clinical nurse council leaders in shared governance.* Unpublished doctoral dissertation, University of Cincinnati, Cincinnati, Ohio.

Alligood, M. (Ed.). (2014). *Nursing theorists and their work* (8th ed.). St. Louis: Mosby-Elsevier.

American Nurses Association. (2001). *Code of Ethics for Nurses With Interpretive Statements.* (2001). Silver Spring, MD: Author.

American Nurses Credentialing Center. (2005). *Magnet recognition program: Application manual.* Silver Spring, MD: American Nurses Credentialing Center.

American Nurses Credentialing Center. (2008). *Magnet recognition program: Application manual.* Silver Spring, MD: American Nurses Credentialing Center.

Anderson, R., & McDaniel, R. (2008). Taking complexity science seriously: New research, new methods. In C. Lindberg, S. Nash, & C. Lindberg (Eds.), *On the edge: Nursing in the age of complexity.* Bordentown, NJ: Plexus Press.

Appell, G., & Triloki, N. (Eds.). (1988). *Choice and morality in anthropological perspective.* Albany: State University of New York Press.

Baer, E. (2012). Key ideas in nursing's first century. *American Journal of Nursing, 112*(5), 48–55.

Bar-Yam, Y. (2004). *Making things work: Solving complex problems in a complex world.* Boston: Knowledge Press.

Battista, J. (1982). The holographic model, holistic paradigm, information theory, and consciousness. In K. Wilber (Ed.), *The holographic paradigm and other paradoxes* (pp. 143–150). Boulder, CO: Shambhala.

Bell, D. (1974). *The coming of post-industrial society.* New York: Basic Books.

Bohman, J. (2005). Toward a critical theory of globalization: Democratic practice and multiperspectival inquiry. In M. Pensky (Ed.), *Globalizing critical theory.* Lanham: Rowman & Littlefield.

Bolman, L., & Dial, T. (2008). *Reframing organizations: Artistry, choice, and leadership* (4th ed.). San Francisco: Jossey-Bass.

Boykin, A., & Schoenhofer, S. (2001). *Nursing as caring: A model for transforming practice* (2nd ed.). Sudbury, MA: Jones and Bartlett.

Boykin, A., & Schoenhofer, S. (2013). Caring in nursing: Analysis of extant theory. In M. Smith, M. Turkel, & Z. Wolf (Eds.), *Caring in nursing classics: An essential resource.* New York: Springer

Boykin, A., Schoenhofer, S., & Valentine, K. (2013). *Practical strategies for transforming healthcare systems: Creating a culture of caring.* New York: Springer Publishing.

Brenton, A., & Driskill, G. (Eds.). (2005). *Organizational culture in action.* Thousand Oaks, CA: Sage.

Briggs, J., & Peat, F. (1989). *Turbulent mirror.* New York: Harper & Row.

Briggs, J., & Peat, F. (1999). *Seven lessons of chaos.* New York: HarperCollins.

Britain, G., & Cohen, R. (1980). *Hierarchy and society: Anthropological perspectives on bureaucracy.* Philadelphia: ISHI.

Cannato, J. (2006). *Radical amazement.* Notre Dame, IN: Sorin Books.

Chinn, P., & Kramer, M. (2011). (8th ed.). *Integrated theory and knowledge development in nursing.* St. Louis: Mosby-Elsevier.

Coffman, S. (2006). Ray's theory of bureaucratic caring. In A. M. Tomey & M. Alligood (Eds.), *Nursing theorists and their work* (6th ed.). St. Louis: Mosby.

Coffman, S. (2010). Ray's theory of bureaucratic caring. In A. M. Tomey & M. Alligood (Eds.), *Nursing theorists and their work* (7th ed.). St. Louis: Mosby-Elsevier.

Coffman, S. (2014). Ray's theory of bureaucratic caring. In M. Alligood (Ed.), *Nursing theorists and their work* (8th ed.). St. Louis: Mosby-Elsevier.

Corbin, J. & Strauss, A. (2007). *Basics of qualitative research: Techniques and procedures for developing grounded theory* (3rd ed.). Thousand Oaks, CA: Sage.

Cross, L. (2014). CNRA and do not resuscitate (dnr) orders in the operating room and the application of the theory of bureaucratic caring. Master's of science research project.

Cuilla, J. (2000). *The working life: The promise and betrayal of modern work.* New York: Times Books/Random House.

Davidson, A., & Ray, M. (1991). Studying the human-environment phenomenon using the science of complexity. *Advances in Nursing Science, 14*(2), 73–87.

Davidson, A., Ray, M., & Turkel, M. (Eds.). (2011). *Nursing, caring, and complexity science: For human-environment well-being.* New York: Springer (AJN 2011 Book of the Year Award).

Dolan, J. (1985). *Nursing in society: A historical perspective.* Philadelphia: W. B. Saunders.

Eggenberger, T. (2011a). *Holding the frontline: The experience of being a charge nurse in an acute care setting.* Unpublished doctoral dissertation, Florida Atlantic University, The Christine E. Lynn College of Nursing, Boca Raton, FL.

Eggenberger, T. (2011b). Response to Chapter 4, Ray, M., M., Turkel & J. Cohn, Relational caring complexity: The study of caring and complexity in health care hospital organizations. In A. Davidson, M. Ray, & M. Turkel (Eds.), *Nursing, caring, and complexity science: For human-environment well-being.* (pp. 118–124). New York: Springer.

Eisenberg, E., & Goodall, H. (1993). *Organizational communication.* New York: St. Martin's Press.

Eisler, R. (2007). *The real wealth of nations.* San Francisco: Berrett-Koehler.

Fox, M. (1994). *The reinvention of work.* San Francisco: Harper.

Gibson, S. (2008). Legal caring: Preventing re-traumatization of abused children through the caring nursing interview using Roach's Six Cs. *International Journal for Human Caring,*

Harmon, W. (1998). *Global mind change* (2nd ed.). San Francisco: Berrett-Koehler.

Henderson, H. (2006). *Ethical markets: Growing the green economy.* White River Junction, VT: Chelsea Green.

Institute of Medicine. (2010, October 5). *The future of nursing: Leading change, advancing health.* Retrieved February 18, 2013, from www.iom.edu/Reports/2010/the-future-of-nursing-leading-change-advancing-health.aspx

Johns, C. (2000). *Becoming a reflective practitioner.* Oxford: Blackwell Science.

Keller, K., Eggenberger, T., Belkowitz, J, Sarsekeyeva, M., & Zito, A. (2013). Implementing successful interprofessional communication opportunities in academia: A qualitative analysis. *International Journal of Medical Education, 4*, 253–259.

Leavitt, H. (2005). *Top down: Why hierarchies are here to stay and how to manage them more effectively.* Boston, MA: Harvard Business School Press.

Leininger, M. (1981a). The phenomenon of caring: Importance, research questions and theoretical considerations. In M. Leininger (Ed.), *Caring: An essential human need* (pp. 3–15). Thorofare, NJ: Slack.

Leininger, M. (Ed.). (1981b). *Caring: An essential human need.* Thorofare, NJ: Slack.

Leininger, M. (1991). *Culture care diversity and universality: A theory of nursing.* New York: National League for Nursing Press.

Leininger, M. (1997). Transcultural nursing research to transform nursing education and practice: 40 years. *Image: Journal of Nursing Scholarship, 29,* 341–354.

Lindberg, C., Nash, S., & Lindberg, C. (Eds.). (2008). *On the edge: Nursing in the age of complexity.* Bordentown, NJ: PlexusPress.

Louis, M. (1985). An investigator's guide to workplace culture. In P. Frost, L. Moore, M. Louis, C. Lundberg, & J. Martin (Eds.), *Organizational culture.* Beverly Hills: Sage.

Manworren, R. (2008). *A pilot study to test the feasibility of using human factors engineering methods to measure factors that compete or influence nurses' abilities to relieve acute pediatric pain* (Application of the bureaucratic caring theory). The University of Texas at Arlington, School of Nursing, Arlington, Texas.

McCray-Stewart, D. (2008). *Application of bureaucratic caring theory.* Administrator, State of Georgia Correctional Facility (Prison System).

Miller, K. (1989). The human care perspective on nursing administration. *Journal of Nursing Administration, 25*(11), 29–32.

Morgan, G. (1997). *Images of organization* (2nd ed.). Thousand Oaks, CA: Sage.

Morse, J., Solberg, S., Neander, W., Bottorff, J., & Johnson, J. (2013). Concepts of caring and caring as a concept. In M. Smith, M. Turkel, & Z. Wolf (Eds.), *Caring in nursing classics: An essential resource.* New York: Springer.

Nevada State College. (2003, August 19). *Nursing curriculum organizing framework.* Henderson, NV: Author.

Newman, M. (1986). *Health as expanding consciousness.* St. Louis: Mosby.

Newman, M. (1992). Prevailing paradigms in nursing. *Nursing Outlook, 40,* 10–14.

Newman, M., Sime, A., & Corcoran-Perry, S. (1991). The focus of the discipline of nursing. *Advances in Nursing Science, 14*(1), 1–6.

Newman, M., Smith, M., Pharris, M., & Jones, D. (2008). The focus of the discipline revisited. *Advances in Nursing Science, 31*(1), E16–27.

Nicolis, G., & Prigogine, I. (1989). *Explaining complexity.* New York: W. H. Freeman.

Nyberg, J. (1998). *A caring approach in nursing administration.* Niwot, CO: University Press of Colorado.

O'Brien, K. (2008). *Application of bureaucratic caring theory in public health nursing.* Director of Public Health Nursing, State of Colorado, Denver, CO.

Page, A. (Ed.). (2004). *Keeping patients safe: Transforming the work environment of nurses.* Institute of Medicine Report. Washington, DC: The National Academic Press.

Peat, F. (2003). *From certainty to uncertainty: The story of science and ideas in the twentieth century.* Washington, DC: Joseph Henry Press.

Pensky, M. (Ed.). (2005). *Globalizing critical theory.* Lanham, MD: Rowman & Littlefield.

Perrow, C. (1986). *Complex organizations: A critical essay* (3rd ed.). New York: McGraw-Hill.

Pharris, M. (2006). Margaret A. Newman's theory of health as expanding consciousness and its applications. In M. Parker (Ed.), *Nursing theories & nursing practice* (2nd ed., pp. 217–234). Philadelphia: F. A. Davis.

Porter-O'Grady, T., & Malloch, K. (2005). *Introduction to evidence-based practice in nursing and health care.* Sudbury, MA: Jones and Bartlett.

Porter-O'Grady, T., & Malloch, K. (2007). *Quantum leadership* (2nd ed.). Sudbury, MA: Jones and Bartlett.

Ray, M. (1981). *A study of caring within the institutional culture.* Unpublished doctoral dissertation, University of Utah, Salt Lake City.

Ray, M. (1984). The development of a nursing classification system of caring. In M. Leininger (Ed.), *Care, the essence of nursing and health* (pp. 95–112). Thorofare, NJ: Slack.

Ray, M. (1987a). Health care economics and human caring: Why the moral conflict must be resolved. *Family and Community Health, 10*(1), 35–43.

Ray, M. (1987b). Technological caring: A new model in critical care. *Dimensions of Critical Care Nursing, 2*(3), 166–173.

Ray, M. (1989a). The theory of bureaucratic caring for nursing practice in the organizational culture. *Nursing Administration Quarterly, 13*(2), 31–42.

Ray, M. (1989b). Transcultural caring: Political and economic caring visions. *Journal of Transcultural Nursing, 1*(1), 17–21.

Ray, M. (1993). A study of care processes using Total Quality Management as a framework in a USAF regional hospital emergency service and related services. *Military Medicine, 158*(6), 396–403.

Ray, M. (1994a). Complex caring dynamics: A unifying model of nursing inquiry. *Theoretic and Applied Chaos in Nursing, 1*(1), 23–32.

Ray, M. (1994b). Communal moral experience as the starting point for research in health care ethics. *Nursing Outlook, 41*, 104–109.

Ray, M. (1997a). The ethical theory of existential authenticity. *Canadian Journal of Nursing Research, 22*(1), 111–126.

Ray, M. (1997b). Illuminating the meaning of caring: Unfolding the sacred art of divine love. In M. Roach (Ed.), *Caring from the heart: The convergence of caring and spirituality* (pp. 163–178). New York: Paulist Press.

Ray, M. (1998a). Complexity and nursing science. *Nursing Science Quarterly, 11*, 91–93.

Ray, M. (1998b). The interface of caring and technology: A new reflexive ethics in intermediate care. *Holistic Nursing Practice, 12*(4), 71–79.

Ray, M. (2006). Marilyn Anne Ray's theory of bureaucratic caring. In M. Parker (Ed.), *Nursing theories, nursing practice* (2nd ed.). Philadelphia: F. A. Davis.

Ray, M. (2010a). *Transcultural caring dynamics in nursing and health care.* Philadelphia: F. A. Davis.

Ray, M. (2010b). *A study of caring within an institutional culture: The discovery of the theory of bureaucratic caring.* Saarbrücken, Germany: Lambert Academic.

Ray, M. (2010c). Creating caring organizations and cultures through communitarian ethics. *Journal of the World Universities Forum, 3*(5), 41–52.

Ray, M. (2013). The theory of bureaucratic caring. In M. Smith, M. Turkel, & Z. Wolf (Eds.). (2013). *Caring in nursing classics: An essential resource* (pp. 309–320). New York: Springer. (Resource book online).

Ray, M., DiDominic, V., Dittman, P., Hurst, P., Seaver, J., Sorbello, B., & Ross, M. (1995). The edge of chaos: Caring and the bottom line. *Nursing Management, 26*(9), 48–50.

Ray, M., & Turkel, M. (2000–2004). *Economic and patient outcomes of the nurse-patient relationship.* Grant funded by the Department of Defense, Tri-Service Nursing Research Program, Bethesda, MD.

Ray, M., & Turkel, M. (2009). Relational caring questionnaires. In J. Watson (Ed.), *Assessing and measuring caring in nursing and health science* (2nd ed.). New York: Springer.

Ray, M., & Turkel, M. (2010). *Marilyn Anne Ray's theory of bureaucratic caring.* In M. Parker & M. Smith (Eds.) *Nursing theories & nursing practice* (3rd ed., pp. 472–494). Philadelphia: F. A. Davis.

Ray, M., & Turkel, M. (2012). A transtheoretical evolution of caring science within complex systerms. *International Journal for Human Caring. 16*(2), 28–49.

Ray, M., & Turkel, M. (2014). The theory of emancipatory nursing praxis: The theory of relational caring complexity. *Advances in Nursing Science, 37*, 132–146.

Ray, M., Turkel, M., & Cohn, J. (2011). Relational caring complexity: The study of caring and complexity in health care hospital organizations. In A. Davidson, M. Ray, & M. Turkel (Eds.), *Nursing, caring, and complexity science: For human-environment well-being.* New York: Springer.

Ray, M., Turkel, M., & Marino, F. (2002). The transformative process for nursing in workforce redevelopment. *Nursing Administration Quarterly, 26*(2), 1–14.

Reed, P. (1997). Nursing: The ontology of the discipline. *Nursing Science Quarterly, 10*, 76–79.

Ritzer, G. (1992). *Metatheorizing.* Newbury Park, CA: Sage.

Roach, M. S. (2002). *The human act of caring* (rev. ed.). Ottawa, Canada: Canadian Hospital Association Press.

Rogers, M. (1970). *An introduction to the theoretical basis of nursing.* Philadelphia: F. A. Davis.

Sawyer, R. (2005). *Social emergence: Societies as complex systems.* New York: Cambridge University Press.

Schein, E. (2004). *Organizational culture and leadership* (3rd ed.). San Francisco: Jossey-Bass.

Secretan, L. (1997). *Reclaiming higher ground.* New York: McGraw-Hill.

Shaffer, F. (1985). *Costing out nursing: Pricing our product.* New York: National League for Nursing Press.

Sherman, R., Edwards, B., Grovengo, K., & Hilton, N. (2009). The role of the clinical nurse leader in promoting a health work environment at the unit level. *Critical Care Nursing Quarterly, 32*(4), 264–271.

Sheldrake, R. (1991). *The rebirth of nature.* New York: Bantam.

Smith, M. (2004). Review of research related to Watson's theory of caring. *Nursing Science Quarterly, 17*(1), 13–25.

Smith, M. (2011). Philosophical and theoretical perspectives related to complexity science in nursing. In A. Davidson, M. Ray, & M. Turkel (Eds.), *Nursing, caring, and complexity science: For human-environment well-being.* New York: Springer.

Smith, M., Turkel, M., & Wolf, M. (Eds.). (2013). *Caring in nursing classics: An essential resource.* New York: Springer. (Resource book online)

Smith, M. (2013a). Caring and the science of unitary human beings. In M. Smith, M. Turkel, & Z. Wolf (Eds.), *Caring in nursing classics: An essential resource* (pp. 43–57). New York: Springer. (Resource book online)

Smith, M. (2013b). Theoretical perspectives on caring. In M. Smith, M. Turkel, & Z. Wolf (Eds.), *Caring in nursing classics: An essential resource* (pp. 117–126). New York: Springer. (Resource book online)

Smith, M., Turkel, M., & Wolf, Z. (2013). *Caring in nursing classics: An essential resource.* New York: Springer.

Sorbello, B. (2008a). *Clinical nurse leader (SM) stories: A phenomenological study about the meaning of leadership at the bedside*. Doctoral dissertation proposal, Florida Atlantic University, the Christine E. Lynn College of Nursing, Boca Raton, Florida.

Sorbello, B. (2008b). Finance: It's not a dirty word. *American Nurse Today, 3*(8), 32–35.

Stanley, J. (2006). In command of care: Clinical nurse leadership explored. *Journal of Research in Nursing, 11*(91), 20–39.

Stedman, M. (2013). *The experience of caring and non-caring patient encounters of graduate registered nurses: A phenomenological study*. (Doctoral Dissertation) ProQuest. UMI: 3572912.

Swanson, K. (1991). Empirical development of a middle-range theory of caring. *Nursing Research, 40*, 161–166.

Swinderman, T. (2011). Technological change in health care electronic documentation as facilitated through the science of complexity. In A. Davidson, M. Ray, & M. Turkel (Eds.), *Nursing, caring, and complexity science: For human–environment well-being* (pp. 309–319). New York: Springer.

Swinderman, T. (2005). The magnetic appeal of nurse informaticians: Caring attractor for emergency. PhD dissertation, Florida Atlantic University.

Thoma, H. (2003). Holistic science: All at the same time. *Resurgence, 1*(216), 15–17.

Turkel, M. (1997). *Struggling to find a balance: A grounded theory study of the nurse-patient relationship in the changing health care environment*. Unpublished doctoral dissertation, University of Miami, Florida (Microfilm #9805958).

Turkel, M. (2001). Struggling to find a balance: The paradox between caring and economics. *Nursing Administration Quarterly, 26*(1), 67–82.

Turkel, M., & Ray, M. (2000). Relational complexity: A theory of the nurse-patient relationship within an economic context. *Nursing Science Quarterly, 13*(4), 307–313.

Turkel, M. (2007). Dr. Marilyn Ray's theory of bureaucratic caring. *International Journal for Human Caring, 11*(4), 57–74.

Turkel, M. (2013a). Caring leadership and administration. In M. Smith, M. Turkel, & Z. Wolf (Eds.), *Caring in nursing classics: An essential resource* (pp. 465–472). New York: Springer. (Resource book online)

Turkel, M. (2013b). Caring based practice models. In M. Smith, M. Turkel, & Z. Wolf (Eds.), *Caring in nursing classics: An essential resource* (pp. 395–430). New York: Springer. (Resource book online)

Turkel, M. (2014). Response to Chapter 10: Valuing, prizing and growing: Outcomes reframed. In A. Boykin, S. Schoenhofer, & K. Valentine (Eds.),

Practical strategies for transforming healthcare systems: Creating a culture of caring. New York: Springer.

Turkel, M., & Ray, M. (2000). Relational complexity: A theory of the nurse-patient relationship within an economic context. *Nursing Science Quarterly, 13*(4), 307–313.

Turkel, M., & Ray, M. (2001). Relational complexity: From grounded theory to instrument development and theoretical testing. *Nursing Science Quarterly, 14*(4), 281–287.

Turkel, M., & Ray, M. (2004). Creating a caring practice environment through self-renewal. *Nursing Administration Quarterly, 28*(4), 249–254.

Turkel, M., & Ray, M. (2009). Caring for "Not so picture perfect patients": Ethical caring in the moral community of nursing. In R. Locsin & M. Purnell (Eds.), *A contemporary nursing process: The (un) bearable weight of knowing persons* (pp. 225–249). New York: Springer.

Van Manen, M. (1982). Edifying theory: Serving the good. *Theory Into Practice, 31*, 45–49.

Vicenzi, A., White, K., & Begun, J. (1997). Chaos in nursing: Make it work for you. *American Journal of Nursing, 97*, 26–32.

Watson, J. (1985). *Human science, human care: A theory of nursing*. East Norwalk, CT: Appleton & Lange.

Watson, J. (1997). The theory of human caring: Retrospective and prospective. *Nursing Science Quarterly, 10*(1), 175–181.

Watson, J. (1988). New dimensions of human caring theory. *Nursing Science Quarterly, 1*, 175-181.

Watson, J. (2005). *Caring science as sacred science*. Philadelphia: F. A. Davis.

Watson, J. (2009). Caring science and human caring theory: Transforming personal/professional practices in nursing and healthcare. In D. Graber (ed.). *Journal of Health and Human Services Administration. Symposium Issue*. 31(4), 466–482.

Watson, J. (2008). *The philosophy and science of caring* (2nd rev. ed.). Boulder, CO: University Press of Colorado.

Watson, J. (2013). New dimensions of human caring theory. In M. Smith, M. Turkel, & Z. Wolf (Eds.), *Caring in nursing classics: An essential resource* (pp. 181–191). New York: Springer.

Weber, M. (1999). The ideal bureaucracy. In M. Matteson & J. Ivancevich (Eds.), *Management and organizational behavior classics* (7th ed.). Chicago: Irwin McGraw-Hill.

Wheatley, M. (1999). *Leadership and the new science* (2nd ed.). San Francisco: Berrett-Koehler.

Wiggins, M. (2006). Clinical nurse leader. Evolution of a revolution. The partnership care delivery model. *Journal of Nursing Administration, 36*(7/8), 341–345.

Wilber, K. (Ed.). (1982). *The holographic paradigm and other paradoxes*. Boulder, CO: Shambhala.

Chapter 28

Troutman-Jordan's Theory of Successful Aging

MEREDITH TROUTMAN-JORDAN

Introducing the Theorist
Overview of the Theory
Applications of the Theory in Research
Practice Exemplar
Summary
References

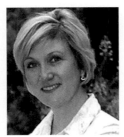

Meredith Troutman-Jordan

Introducing the Theorist

Dr. Troutman-Jordan began her nursing career after graduating from Presbyterian Hospital School of Nursing in Charlotte, North Carolina. She earned her BSN from Queens College, and her master's degree is in Psychiatric Mental Health Nursing from the University of North Carolina at Charlotte. Her doctoral degree is in nursing science from the University of South Carolina at Columbia. She is certified as psychiatric mental health clinical nurse specialist from the American Nurses Credentialing Center.

Dr. Troutman-Jordan received her inspiration for development of a middle-range theory of successful aging from her clinical practice with older adults in home care. The theory (Flood, 2002, 2006a) originated early during Dr. Troutman-Jordan's doctoral studies, and her subsequent research has been based on testing and refining this theory and developing and testing an instrument to measure successful aging. Her current research involves investigating the effect of health promotion interventions on successful aging and other health indicators.

Overview of the Theory

Although there is an array of theories detailing what successful aging is or how it can be accomplished, there remains rather limited theoretical work that provides practical guidelines for promoting successful aging. Therefore, the impetus for developing the theory of successful aging was enhanced understanding of successful aging, captured from the older adult's perspective, and identification of foci for interventions to foster successful aging.

One goal of *Healthy People 2020* is to improve the health, function, and quality of life of older adults (HealthyPeople.gov, 2012). Objectives include increasing the proportion of older adults with one or more chronic health conditions who report confidence in managing their conditions and reducing the number of older adults who have moderate to severe functional limitations. Optimal health and well-being of older adults across multiple domains—physical health; mobility; social, spiritual, and emotional well-being—is consistent with successful aging. Although there are commonly used definitions of old age, there is no general agreement on the age at which a person becomes old; the United Nations agreed cutoff is 60+ years to refer to the older population (World Health Organization, 2013). So the Healthy People 2020 goal aims to improve health and quality of life of individuals aged 60 and older. Similarly, the theory of successful aging was intended for this age group.

Development of the theory of successful aging began with a concept analysis of successful aging that clarified the phenomenon. The concept analysis was sparked by the question, "What was it that could make such a dramatic difference for two older adults with similar health, environmental, and social situations?" Although in similar circumstances, one might give up, for example, refusing help from others or trying to do for oneself, avoiding health-care measures, withdrawing from relationships, or becoming embittered. Another could maintain an optimistic, intrepid attitude and find meaning, purpose, and satisfaction in life, for example, accepting physical changes, actively managing chronic health conditions, and staying socially engaged. Many of us have encountered similar older adults. So the question became, "What describes the state of being of the more favorably aging individual, and how can nurses help older adults move toward this state of being?

Walker and Avant's (1995) framework was used for this concept analysis, resulting in a conceptual definition for successful aging: an individual's perception of a favorable outcome in adapting to the cumulative physiological and functional alterations associated with the passage of time, while experiencing spiritual connectedness, and a sense of meaning and purpose in life. Older adults encountered in clinical practice and research have validated this idea, emphasizing the importance of both coping mechanisms that mediate chronic illness and the older adult's perspective of his own aging. Over the course of several years, the theory of successful aging was developed.

Existing knowledge obtained deductively from the Roy adaptation model (Roy & Andrews, 1999) was synthesized with ideas from Tornstam's (1996) sociological theory of gerotranscendence and other literature on the concepts of successful aging. Adaptation is a process in which individuals use conscious awareness and choice to assimilate to their environment (Roy, 2013). The theory was established based on the following assumptions derived from and based on the literature:

- Aging is a progressive process requiring from simple to increasingly complex adaptation.
- Aging may be successful or unsuccessful, depending on where a person is along the continuum of progression from simple to more complex adaptation and the extensive use of coping processes.
- Successful aging is influenced by the aging person's choices.
- The self is not ageless (Tornstam, 1996).
- Aging people experience changes, which uniquely characterize their beliefs and perspectives as different from those of younger adults (Flood, 2006a).

Roy Adaptation Model

The Roy adaptation model was used in the development of the theory because of the theoretical fit of the successful aging assumptions within the Roy model. The Roy adaptation model is based on Helson's (1964) adaptation theory and von Bertalanffy's (1968) general systems theory. Roy (1997) referenced Erikson's (Erikson, Erikson, & Kivnick, 1986) developmental theory and stated that specific medical problems may arise with age and consideration should be given to the age of the patient. Scientific and philosophical assumptions underlying the Roy adaptation model inform the theory of successful aging and are explicated in the chapter on the Roy adaptation model in this text (Chapter 10).

There are three adaptation levels (the condition of life processes, according to Roy, 2013) that represent the condition of the life processes: integrated, compensatory, and compromised. One who is aging successfully has integrated adaptation levels; he or she has effectively functioning coping mechanisms and experiences physical, mental, and spiritual well-being. A compensatory adaptation level in someone who is aging successfully might be seeking social support from friends and family after an episode of acute illness. An older adult with compromised adaptation could be someone who experiences a cerebrovascular accident and refuses physical therapy or social support from family, becomes hopeless, depressed, stops eating, and ends up at increased risk for a thrombus related to immobility. Within the context of the theory of successful aging, this person could still age successfully if he adapts to health and other circumstances according to his optimum potential. This person can be best supported through a multidisciplinary approach including nursing, medicine, social work, physical therapy, pastoral care, and nutrition counseling to promote successful aging.

The Theory of Successful Aging

The theory of successful aging describes the process by which individuals use various coping mechanisms to progress toward desirable adaptation to the collective physiological and functional changes occurring over their lifetime, while maintaining a sense of spirituality, connectedness, and meaning and purpose in life. The theory of successful aging is comprised of various degrees of *coping processes*, the complex dynamics within the person according to Roy & Andrews (1999). Every older adult has *some* capacity for coping, and this is unique to the individual. Consider various older adults you have encountered in clinical practice; each individual had potential for some growth through enhanced adaptation. For some people, this might have been rather limited; perhaps they tended to "see the glass as half full,"

but you have probably encountered others who managed to persevere through considerable health, financial, or psychosocial challenges.

Three coping processes make up the foundation of the theory: functional performance mechanisms, intrapsychic factors, and spirituality. These coping processes, shown in Figure 28-1, describe the ways one responds to the changing environment (Flood, 2006a). Constructs within each of these coping processes are measurable output (cognitive, behavioral, or affective) responses, which provide feedback to the person and are thus interconnected by arrows. Solid arrows denote those exchanges that occur initially, and broken arrows indicate exchanges that occur subsequently (Flood, 2006a).

Functional Performance Mechanisms

Functional performance mechanisms describe the use of conscious awareness and choice as an adaptive response to cumulative physiological and physical losses with subsequent functional deficits occurring because of aging. Simply put, this foundational coping process captures the typical age-related declines that occur, such as decreasing vascular flexibility, increasing stiffness, and rise in blood pressure, and what people do to manage them, if anything. Everyone will experience change as a part of aging. Think of an older adult you know or that you recently worked with. What is one age-related physiological or functional change he or she experienced? How did he or she respond to this change?

Indicators of the functional performance mechanism coping process are health promotion activities, physical health, and physical mobility. Therefore, by assessing an older adult's participation in health promotion activities (e.g., annual health examinations, good nutrition), physical health state (history of illnesses, current chronic and acute disease processes), and physical mobility (e.g., gait stability and speed, use of assistive devices), the nurse determines the adaptive state of his or her functional performance mechanisms. Each of these output responses is a manifestation of the human adaptive response of functional performance

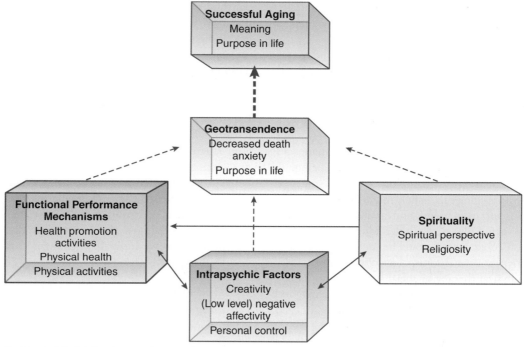

Fig 28 • 1   Model for theory of successful aging.

mechanisms. A broad array of functional performance mechanisms is possible, and the mix and extent of functional performance mechanism indicators is perhaps limitless. Therefore, each older adult is unique, and increasingly complex across the life span, as changes occur over time. As individuals, older adults could be viewed as unique histories to be explored, understood, and valued by the nurse.

Intrapsychic Factors

Intrapsychic factors describe the innate and enduring character features that may enhance or impair an individual's ability to adapt to change and to problem-solving (Flood, 2006a). Intrapsychic factors refer to an older adult's use of these inherent character traits to respond to environmental stimuli. Output responses indicative of intrapsychic factors include creativity, low levels of negativity, and personal control.

To assess an older adult's intrapsychic factors, the nurse could engage him or her in a discussion about creative activities he or she enjoys or explore problem-solving skills that have been

useful. For example, the nurse might note, "You did a pretty impressive job supporting three children after losing your husband. How did you manage?"

Creativity

There are numerous creativity assessments, and the best way for measuring or assessing creativity is debated. Some well-known methods of measuring creativity include the Torrance (1974) Tests of Creative Thinking, Guilford's (1967) Alternative Uses Tasks, and Wallach and Kogan's (1965) Creativity Test. Although the Torrance tests require a fee and special training to administer, the others do not. These tests as well as others can be accessed free online (www.indiana.edu/~bobweb/Handout/d3 .ttct.htm). Administering one of these assessments might stimulate conversation with the older adult, which could lead to discussion on problem-solving skills and/or exploration of enjoyable, creative leisure activities. Furthermore, these tests might even be fun for the older adult.

Positive and Negative Affect

Isen, Daubman, and Nowicki (1987) proposed that positive affect should be viewed as influencing the way in which material is processed, suggesting that good feelings increase the tendency to combine material in new ways and see the relatedness between divergent stimuli. Similarly, the theory of successful aging proposes that low levels of negative affectivity enhance or increase creativity.

The nurse might recognize the need to evaluate personal control or negative affectivity. The extent of these features presented over time could facilitate or detract from successful aging. *Negative affect* is defined as a general dimension of subjective distress and unpleasurable engagement that includes a variety of unpleasant mood states, such as anger, contempt, disgust, guilt, fear, and nervousness (Watson & Clark, 1984). Low negative affect is characterized by a state of calmness and serenity. Watson and Clark (1984) described negative affectivity as a mood-dispositional dimension that reflects pervasive individual differences in negative emotionality and self-concept. Negative affect is not simply the opposite or lack of positive affect; in fact, the two are quite distinct and nearly independent of each other (Naragon & Watson, 2009). Therefore, one could experience positive affect and still have quite frequent or extensive negative affect. Consider someone who is emotionally responsive to events, who could have positive or negative affect quite profoundly and frequently. Is this person more often (and more deeply) in a state of scorn, irritation, or disgust? Or is this person more frequently and intensely calm, relaxed, and contented?

A nurse might gauge degree of negative affectivity by administering the Positive and Negative Affect Schedule (PANAS; Watson, Clark, & Tellegen, 1988), a 20-item self-report measure of positive and negative affect that includes two subscales. The negative affect subscale includes descriptors such as distressed, guilty, and afraid. Individuals self-rate the extent to which they feel these emotions at the time they complete the PANAS, or they may respond based on the degree of their feelings over the past week (Watson et al., 1988). The PANAS is in the public domain and can be obtained from the article in which the authors published its initial use (Participation and Quality of Life Project, 2012).

Assessing degree of negative affectivity in the older adult could be an initial step toward increasing self-awareness of feelings and how often and intensely they are experienced. A tool such as the PANAS might be used to initiate a conversation about this self-awareness, with subsequent counseling or referral to a therapist if indicated.

Personal Control

Personal control reflects individuals' beliefs regarding the extent to which they are able to control or influence outcomes (MacArthur Research Network on SES and Health, 2008). Personal control expectancies relate to judgments about whether actions can produce a given outcome (e.g., a widow's expectations about how she will manage her household after losing her spouse, or a man's expectations of his ability to reduce body mass index to a normal range). Greater levels of personal control are proposed to contribute to successful aging. Although personal control can vary depending on the specific domain of interest (e.g., health versus marital longevity or occupational success), it can also be considered from a more global perspective.

Pearlin and Schooler's (1978) Mastery Scale has become perhaps the most widely used measure of personal control in health research. This tool could be quite useful in clinical practice as well, and it was used in the MacArthur Successful Aging Study (MacArthur Research Network on SES and Health, 2008). The Mastery Scale consists of seven items that are answered on a 4-point Likert scale.

Nurses may encounter patients who demonstrate little personal control, verbalizing helplessness with limited or no ability to effect change in his or her life. For example, a person with a perception of limited personal control might state, "Well, I am 67; it's too late to change" or "I am too old to exercise with my arthritis"

Although low levels of personal control do not enhance the likelihood of successful aging, their presence is not entirely detrimental. The breadth and extent of personal control (or lack thereof) must be considered. If the older adult has little sense of control over her ability to hike Mount Everest, this may be realistic, depending on her physical health, mobility, and past or present health promotion activities such as exercise involvement. But, more important, *this task may not be relevant* if the older adult does not need or aspire to climb Mount Everest. Therefore, the individual and his or her aspirations must be considered.

Think of an older adult with little sense of control over learning about a new medication. Perhaps this person does feel empowered to mentor her grandchildren or complete some household project. Focusing on areas of greater personal control could help increase the older adult's confidence in the ability to self-manage other areas of health and well-being.

Older adults vary widely in their adaptation to functional performance mechanisms as well as in their intrapsychic factors. One 77-year-old man may be post–cerebrovascular accident (CVA; physical health) but actively engage in physical therapy and walking around his farm for exercise (mobility, health promotion). This man might view his CVA as a challenge (low levels of negative affect) rather than a frustration and threat to his masculinity. He might be determined to overcome (high levels of personal control) and use gardening as a (creative) means of range of motion exercise. A similar 77-year-old man could also be post CVA and resist physical therapy because it is "too painful and difficult," believing there is little he can do at his age to help the situation. This man might avoid visitors, stop physical therapy, and refuse to ambulate, remaining in a wheelchair. Thus, two individuals in similar situations could respond quite differently, depending on their intrapsychic factors, resulting in very different aging trajectories.

Spirituality

Another foundational coping mechanism is spirituality, which is proposed to interact with intrapsychic factors and functional performance mechanisms in a way that is facilitative of successful aging. *Spirituality* encompasses the personal views and behaviors that express a sense of relatedness to something greater than oneself; the feelings, thoughts, experiences, and behaviors arising from the search for the sacred (Flood, 2006a). Spirituality is essential to successful aging; the sense of connection and beliefs about a higher power the older adult has help shape his values, beliefs, and behaviors while living, especially in terms of what he believes happens after death. Acceptance of the reality of death and one's own mortality are part of being able to age successfully.

Output responses representative of spirituality are spiritual perspective, prayer, and religiosity. Spiritual perspective refers to beliefs in the existence of something beyond what is concrete and immediate without devaluing the self (Reed & Larson, 2006). A spiritual perspective is considered to be an important resource for helping people transcend difficulties faced in aging (Reed & Rousseau, 2007) and may or may not include religious expression (Reed & Larson, 2006).

Indicators of spiritual perspective are connectedness (with others, nature, the universe, or God), belief in something greater than the self, in an intangible domain, or a positively life-affirming faith, and a constant, dynamic creative energy (Haase, Britt, Coward, Leidy, & Penn, 1992). Although these attributes can be considered aspects of inherent spirituality, it is the *realization and development* of these features that are represented by the term spiritual perspective (Haase et al., 1992). Moreover, spiritual perspective is believed to enable and motivate one to find meaning and purpose in life (Banks, 1980; Hiatt, 1986; Highfield & Caison, 1983; Hungleman, 1985; Jourard, 1974; Moberg, 1971), key indicators of successful aging (Troutman, 2011).

The nurse could assess spiritual perspective by administering the Spiritual Perspective Scale (Reed, 1986), a 10-item, self-administered or structured-interview formatted scale which measures one's perspectives on the extent to which spirituality permeates his life and he engages in spiritually related interactions. Other means of assessing spirituality include inquiring about the older adult's engagement in prayer or meditation; church (or other religious function) attendance; and discussing and/or encouraging religious rituals (what these mean to the older adult, ways these practices might be healthful, etc.).

Integrated use of foundational coping processes is unique for each individual and is the initial adaptive process of successful aging. People who are more creative and who have lower levels of negative affectivity and greater degrees of personal control will have more effective adaptation of functional performance mechanisms; they will be more likely to engage in health promotion activities and maintenance of physical mobility. Physical health can be affected by intrapsychic factors, the relationship between immune function and emotions, for example. Physical health also affects intrapsychic factors (such as how one responds psychologically to illness or accident).

The elements of successful aging interact and reciprocate, creating a strong, flexible web of support. More creativity, less negative affectivity, and greater personal control enhance spirituality through greater spiritual perspective and more religiosity. If one is more creative, then he is more receptive to new ideas and innovative problem-solving methods. Lower negative affectivity also makes one more accepting of circumstances and people, able to consider a broader range of possible outcomes to a situation, and it increases the possibility of pleasant, positive interactions with others. Greater personal control means that someone is more likely to be proactive in health promotion activities, problem-solving, and disease management. A stronger or deeper sense of spirituality contributes to one's valuation of self and sense of responsibility to appreciate and be responsible for blessings in life such as health, relationships, and resources.

Gerotranscendence

Gerotranscendence is a shift in metaperspective, from a materialistic and rationalistic perspective to a more mature and existential one that accompanies the process of aging (Tornstam, 2005). Experiencing gerotranscendence means one develops a new outlook on and understanding of life, with broad existential changes; changes in one's view of the present self and the self in retrospect; and developmental changes (related to existential changes and changes in the self; Tornstam, 2011). Gerotranscendence is associated with positive aging (Tornstam, 2005) and has been theorized as a precursor to successful aging (Tornstam, 1994).

Gerotranscendence occurs when there is a major shift in the person's worldview, where a person examines their place within the world and in relation to others (Tornstam, 1997). This means there is a radical change of one's outlook on life from a concern with mundane issues to a concern with universal values (Tornstam, 1989). The older adult examines values held, and these may change from what they were when that person was younger. Three levels of age-related change occur with gerotranscendence.

Cosmic dimension

The level of the cosmic dimension of life relates to the feeling of being part of and at one with the universe. There is a redefinition of one's sense of his or her place in the physical world as well as the more global universe. Furthermore, an increased understanding of the spirit of the universe results in a redefinition of the perception of time and, therefore, lessens one's concerns regarding the future (Tornstam, 1989). Thus, one has decreased concern or fear of death because of a sense of continuity with the universe; a newfound recognition of meaning and sense of purpose in the greater scheme of things occurs.

Self Dimension

A second level of gerotranscendent change deals with one's self-perception. Gerotranscendence is believed to cause a new understanding of fundamental questions regarding one's existence and a change in the way one perceives one's self and the world. The dimension of perception of self concerns how one perceives self and the surrounding world. Tornstam (1999) observed that many older adults look at their bodies with aversion, perceiving them as an indication of overall decline, and concluding that both their mind and their sense of self-worth have likewise declined. The gerotranscendent person, in contrast, recognizes the separateness of spiritual growth and development apart from physical deterioration. Tornstam suggests this ability to separate physical and spiritual concerns provides a new feeling of freedom, which might result in finding the courage to be oneself and to no longer fear both social norms and expected roles. The gerotranscendent person feels freedom to self-discover new and perhaps unexpected aspects of himself. The individual may also show an increase in time spent alone in meditation or contemplation.

Social Dimension

The third level of change experienced in gerotranscendence deals with an increase in a sense of interrelatedness with others. The gerotranscendent person will begin to have greater need to view self as a social being and will reevaluate the meaning behind relationships with family, friends, and other relationships. There is a stronger sense of needing to feel part of the human race. Tornstam suggests this need results in an increased feeling of kinship or connection with past and future generations, along with a decreased interest in superficial or casual social interactions. So the gerotranscendent older adult may become more open and responsive to other people while at the same time becoming more selective with whom they engage and interact.

Tornstam (1989, 1997) asserts gerotranscendence is closely associated with wisdom because gerotranscendence and wisdom both involve a transcendence beyond right and wrong, accompanied by an increased broadmindedness and tolerance, usually followed by an increase in life satisfaction. In the theory of successful aging, indicators of gerotranscendence are decreased death anxiety, engagement in meaningful activities, changes in relationships with others, self-acceptance, and wisdom.

Gerotranscendence could be assessed using the Gerotranscendence Scale (GS) (Tornstam, 1994). The GS consists of 10 items designed to capture what Tornstam (2005) calls "retrospective change" (p. 93), or how older adults see they have changed since age 50. The GS is brief and easily administered; it may also provide an opportunity to initiate discussions about gerotranscendence with older adults. Another means of assessing gerotranscendence is by evaluating the older adult's affective and emotional response to specific interventions. For example, does the older adult seem to enjoy solitude? Does he or she talk about death without fear, and as a transition, rather than an endpoint? If the nurse finds that an older adult patient does these things, then she could initiate further conversation with the patient about his perspectives and feelings or even describe the topic of gerotranscendence as Wadensten (2005) did finding that older adults recognized features of gerotranscendence in themselves.

A reasonable and well-balanced integration of the outputs of each foundational coping process for each individual, rather than an ideal amount or combinations of features from within the foundational coping processes, must be present in order for the aging person to experience gerotranscendence. The successful ager does not necessarily have ideal physical health; he or she likely has one or more age-related chronic conditions but manages them as well as possible, participating in health promotion activities (such as physical activity and good nutrition) and maintaining physical mobility to the best of his or her ability. This person finds innovative ways to deal with struggles and may be involved in more traditional creative activities such as painting or woodwork. On most days, the successful ager maintains low negative affectivity, seeing the glass as "half full rather than half empty." The successfully aging individual feels empowered to influence his own health and aging (personal control), though he recognizes that God or some Higher Power has a role in life also. The balance of intrapsychic factors enhances the older adult's spirituality. These foundational coping mechanisms increase the possibility of experiencing gerotranscendence, in which the older adult has a major shift in metaperspective and reevaluates where he is in the larger scheme of the world and what lies beyond. There may be pervasive change, as the older adult self-examines values, aspirations, and fundamental existential beliefs. When these foundational coping processes and gerotranscendent changes, greater life satisfaction and a sense of purpose and meaning in life ensue. This person is aging successfully.

Nurses could assess successful aging with the Successful Aging Inventory (SAI), a 20-item questionnaire with a 5.9 grade reading level. Each statement is brief, positively worded, and numbered 0 to 4 with higher values indicating more frequent/stronger responses. For example, one statement includes "I have been able to cope with the changes that have occurred to my body as I have aged." Respondents indicate the point to which they agree or disagree with the statement or the extent to which they believe the statement applies to them. Higher scores are indicative of more successful aging.

Applications of the Theory in Research

A growing number of studies have used or expanded on the theory of successful aging. One of these (Flood & Scharer, 2006) investigated the relationship between functional performance, creativity, and successful aging.

Although the creativity intervention (storytelling, writing poetry, reminiscing) did not increase creativity levels or successful aging, racial differences were observed, with Black participants scoring higher on creativity and successful aging compared with White participants. A subsequent study (Flood, 2006b) examined the relationships between creativity, depression, and successful aging. Level of depressive symptoms had a moderating effect on the relationship of creativity to successful aging; that is, the presence of depressive symptoms weakened the relationship between creativity and successful aging. Significant differences in creativity, depressive symptoms, and successful aging were found by racial group and education level, with Black participants having higher creativity levels and more depressive symptoms, compared with White ones.

McCarthy (2009) used the theory of successful aging as a guiding framework to investigate adaptation, transcendence, and successful aging. She found that adaptation and gerotranscendence were significant predictors of successful aging, which was measured with the SAI. And, together, adaptation and transcendence accounted for almost half of the variance in successful aging. Thus, McCarthy's study provided support for the theory of successful aging and demonstrated sound psychometric properties for the SAI. Other research has also used the theory (Barnes, 2012; Cozort, 2008; White, 2013), providing validation.

Practice Exemplar

Mr. P., a 69-year-old male, suddenly and unexpectedly lost his wife after she had a pulmonary embolus. He had known her since she was 15. Mr. P. had a third-grade education, limited literacy, and a very modest income. He was devastated by this loss. Although he had recently become the primary homemaker because of Mrs. P.'s surgery and declining health, he had rather advanced macular degeneration, postherpetic neuralgia, and arthritis. Despite these limitations, he had been his wife's primary caregiver, maintained the home, and still preached occasionally at the church where he had been a pastor. After her death, although it was a struggle, he managed to walk in the parking lot of a church near his home every day with the aid of a cane. Remaining in the home was very important to him; his ability to be as independent

Continued

Practice Exemplar cont.

as possible permitted him a greater sense of personal control. Therefore, he let his daughters help by delivering meals and doing his laundry regularly, although he "really didn't like" to give up these tasks or rely on others. But he recognized that he had to make this concession to remain in his home. He had figured out innovative ways to live alone without his wife; for example, he placed toiletries in bottles of certain shapes and sizes because he could no longer see well enough to read labels to determine contents. He devised an organization system for storing food items in the kitchen so that he could locate things by memory. He carried "a big stick" when he went walking in case he encountered any strange dogs. Mr. P. noticed that if he tried to focus on "what I do have and not what I don't" that it seemed easier to cope day to day.

Although the loss of his wife was almost unbearable, Mr. P. grew to accept the notion that "it was her time, and the Lord took her," and he found comfort and strength in prayer and listening to prerecorded sermons several times a week. Mr. P. found himself thinking of his wife often, as he now lived alone. Sometimes he talked to her because he sensed she could hear him. He began to enjoy having his home to himself, after having raised six children there, and the freedom of "not having to set an example for anyone." Sometimes he would put on his nightclothes early and eat cereal for dinner. Despite his chronic health conditions and the loss of his wife, Mr. P. grew to enjoy his solitude

and the freedom to "just be myself," although he derived great satisfaction from spending time with his grandchildren.

Superficially, Mr. P. might seem like an average, or perhaps disadvantaged, older adult. Despite his health limitations and significant loss, he continues to engage in health promotion and strives to maintain his mobility. He demonstrates creativity in the efforts and modifications to do these things. He also makes decisions that optimize his sense of personal control and makes a conscious effort to have low levels of negative affect through positive self-talk. His spirituality has deepened since the death of his wife; he now sees death as a transition to some other state of being rather than an end. Similarly, he finds a new appreciation of his life and his views of the world, with a newfound sense of who he is, his purpose, and the meaning in his life.

Mr. P. appears to be aging successfully. The nurse could encourage continued walking (health promotion and maintenance of physical mobility) and regular contact with his primary care provider. Likewise, his strategies to problem-solve related to home maintenance and activities of daily living could be commended to encourage their continuation. The nurse could encourage continued time spent in prayer and assist Mr. P. to negotiate transportation to church services. Mr. P. might also benefit from introduction to the idea of gerotranscendence and time spent reminiscing or quietly reflecting.

■ Summary

The theory of successful aging offers a framework for understanding a multidimensional, complex phenomenon and for planning nursing interventions geared toward promoting successful aging in various groups, making successful aging a possibility for a broader range of older adults. The theory provides an empirically supported (Cozort, 2008; Flood, 2006b; Flood & Scharer, 2006; McCarthy, 2009; Troutman, Bentley, & Nies, 2011; Troutman, Nies, & Mavellia, 2011) organizing framework for assessment, planning, interventions, and evaluation of older adults that is individualized to the needs and situations of unique individuals and sensitive to the importance that the older adult places on various aspects of aging.

References

Banks, R. (1980). Health and the spiritual dimensions: Relationships and implications for professional preparation programs. *Journal of School Health, 50,* 195.

Barnes, J. (2012). *Successful aging: A correlational study identifying the relationship between successful aging and purpose in life.* Unpublished Honors Thesis, Lenoir Rhyne University, Hickory, North Carolina.

Cozort, R. (2008). *Revising the Gerotranscendence Scale for use with older adults in the Southern United States and establishing psychometric properties of the Revised Gerotranscendence Scale.* Doctoral dissertation, University of North Carolina, Greensboro.

Erikson, E., Erikson, J., & Kivnick, H. (1986). *Vital involvement in old age.* New York, NY: Norton.

Flood, M. (2002). Successful Aging; A concept analysis. *Journal of Theory Construction and Testing, 6*(2), 105–108.

Flood, M. (2006a). A mid-range theory of successful aging. *Journal of Theory Construction and Testing, 9*(2), 35–39.

Flood, M. (2006b). Exploring the relationships between creativity, depression, and successful aging. *Activities, Adaptation, and Aging, 31*(1), 55–71.

Flood, M., & Scharer, K. (2006). Creativity enhancement; Possibilities for successful aging. *Issues in Mental Health Nursing, 27,* 1–21.

Guilford, J. P. (1967). *The nature of human intelligence.* New York: McGraw-Hill.

Haase, J., Britt, T., Coward, D., Leidy, N., & Penn, P. (1992). Simultaneous concept analysis of spiritual perspective, hope, acceptance, and self-transcendence. *Image: Journal of Nursing Scholarship 24*(2), 141–147.

HealthyPeople.gov. (2012). Older adults. Retrieved September 9, 2012, from www.healthypeople.gov /2020/topicsobjectives2020/overview.aspx?topicId=31

Helson, H. (1964). *Adaptation-level theory: An experimental and systematic approach to behavior.* New York, NY: Harper & Row.

Hiatt, J. (1986). Spirituality, medicine, and healing. *Southern Medical Journal, 79,* 736–743.

Highfield, M., & Caison, C. (1983). Spiritual needs of patients: Are the recognized? *Cancer Nursing, 6,* 187–192.

Hungleman, J., Kenkel-Rossi, W., Klassen, L., & Stollenwerk, R. (1985). Spiritual well-being in older adults: Harmonious interconnectedness. *Journal of Religion & Health, 24,* 147–153.

Isen, A., Daubman, K., & Nowicki, G. (1987). Positive affect facilitates creative problem-solving. *Journal of Personality and Social Psychology, 52*(6), 1122–1131.

Jourard, S. (1974). *Health personality.* New York: Macmillan.

MacArthur Research Network on SES and Health. (2008). *Research: Psychosocial notebook; Personal control.* Retrieved October 7, 2012, from http://www.macses.ucsf.edu/research/psychosocial/control.php

McCarthy, V. (2009). *Exploring a new theory of successful aging among low-income older adults in an independent and assisted living community.* Doctoral dissertation, University of Louisville, Kentucky.

Moberg, D. (1971). *Spiritual well-being: Background and issues.* Washington, DC: White House Conference on Aging.

Naragon, K., & Watson, D. (2009). Positive affectivity. In S. Lopez (Ed.), *The encyclopedia of positive psychology* (pp. 707–711). Hoboken, NJ: Wiley-Blackwell.

The Participation and Quality of Life Project. (2012). *Positive and Negative Affect Schedule (PANAS).* Retrieved October 4, 2012, from www.parqol.com/page.cfm?id=87

Pearlin, L., & Schooler, C. (1978). The structure of coping. *Journal of Health & Social Behavior, 18,* 2–21.

Reed, P. G. (1986). Religiousness in terminally ill and healthy adults. *Research in Nursing & Health, 9*(1), 35–41.

Reed, P. G., & Larson, C. (2006). Spirituality. In J. Fitzpatrick & M. Wallace (Eds.), *Encyclopedia of nursing research* (pp. 565–567). New York, NY: Springer.

Reed, P. G., & Rousseau, E. (2007). Spiritual inquiry and well-being in life-limiting illness. *Journal of Religion, Spirituality, & Aging, 19*(4), 81–98.

Roy, C. (1997). Future of the Roy Model: Challenge to redefine adaptation. *Nursing Science Quarterly, 10,* 42–48.

Roy, C. (2013). Key definitions: The Roy adaptation model. Retrieved October 22, 2013, from www.bc.edu /content/bc/schools/son/faculty/featured/theorist/Roy _Adaptation_Model/Key_Definitions.html

Roy, C., & Andrews, H. (1999). *The Roy adaptation model* (2nd ed.). Stamford, CT: Appleton & Lange.

Tornstam, L. (1994). Gerotranscendence: A theoretical and empirical exploration. In L. Thomas, & S. A. Eisenhandler (Eds.), *Aging and the religious dimension* (pp. 203–225). Westport, CT: Greenwood.

Tornstam, L. (1996). Caring for the elderly. Introducing the theory of gerotranscendence as a supplementary frame of reference for care of the elderly. *Scandanavian Journal of Caring Sciences, 10,* 144–150.

Tornstam, L. (1997). Gerotranscendence-a theory about mating into old age. *Journal of Aging and Identity, 2,* 17–36.

Tornstam, L. (1989). Gero-transcendence: A meta-theoretical reformulation of the disengagement theory. *Aging: Clinical and Experimental Research, 1,* 55–63.

Tornstam, L. (2005). *Gerotranscendence: A developmental theory of positive aging.* New York: Springer.

Tornstam, L. (2011). Maturing into gerotranscendence. *Journal of Transpersonal Psychology, 43*(2), 166–180.

Torrance, E. P. (1974). *Torrance Tests of Creative Thinking.* Bensenville, IL: Scholastic Testing Service.

Troutman, M. (2011). Mid-range theory of successful aging. In J. Lange (Ed), *The nurse's role in promoting optimal health of older adults: Thriving in the wisdom years* (pp. 4–16). Philadelphia, PA: F.A. Davis.

Troutman, M., Bentley, M., & Nies, M. A. (2011). Measuring successful aging in Southern Black older adults. *Educational Gerontology, 37*(1), 38–50.

Troutman, M., Nies, M. A., & Mavellia, H. (2011). Perceptions of successful aging in Southern Black older adults. *Journal of Psychosocial Nursing and Mental Health Services, 49*(1), 28–34.

von Bertalanffy, L. (1968). *Organismic psychology and systems theory.* Worchester, MA: Clark University Press.

Wadensten, B. (2005). Introducing older people to the theory of gerotranscendence. *Journal of Advanced Nursing, 52,* 381–388.

Walker, L., & Avant, K. (1995). *Strategies for theory construction in nursing* (3rd ed., pp. 37–54). Norwalk: Appleton & Lange.

Wallach, M. A., & Kogan, N. (1965). *Modes of thinking in your children: A study of the creativity-intelligence distinction.* New York: Holt, Rinehart & Winston.

Watson, D., & Clark, L. A. (1984). Negative affectivity: The disposition to experience aversive emotional states. *Psychological Bulletin, 96,* 465–490.

Watson, D., Clark, L. A., & Tellegen, A. (1988). Development and validation of brief measures of positive and negative affect: The PANAS scales. *Journal of Personality and Social Psychology,* 54(6), 1063–1070.

White, A. J. (2013, November). *The relationship between post-menopausal women's successful aging, global self-esteem, and sexual quality of life.* Paper presented at the Sigma Theta Tau International 42nd Biennial Convention, Indianapolis, IN.

World Health Organization. (2013). Definition of an older or elderly person. Retrieved October 22, 2013, from www.who.int/healthinfo/survey/ageingdefnolder/en

Chapter 29

Barrett's Theory of Power as Knowing Participation in Change

ELIZABETH ANN MANHART BARRETT

Introducing the Theorist
Overview of the Theory
Applications of the Theory
Practice Exemplar
Summary
References

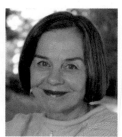

Elizabeth Ann Manhart Barrett

Introducing the Theorist

Elizabeth Ann Manhart Barrett, RN, LMHC, PhD, FAAN, is Professor Emerita, Hunter College, City University of New York; a research consultant; a Health Patterning Therapist; in private practice in New York City; and co-president of Power-Imagery Partners. From the University of Evansville in Indiana, she holds a BSN, summa cum laude, an MA, and an MSN; she earned a PhD in nursing science from New York University. Dr. Barrett has more than 40 years of experience as a practitioner, educator, researcher, and administrator at universities and medical centers in New York and Indiana. She is one of the founders and first president of the Society of Rogerian Scholars.

Dr. Barrett's scholarly endeavors have evolved from her commitment to carry forward Martha E. Rogers's Science of Unitary Human Beings. The primary focus of her research has been the Barrett *theory of power as knowing participation in change*® and the Power as Knowing Participation in Change Tool (PKPCT). Colleagues have conducted more than 100 studies using the theory and/or measurement instrument. The PKPCT has been translated into Japanese, Korean, Swedish, Danish, Portuguese, French, and German. Dr. Barrett has authored nearly 100 publications including articles and book chapters and has coedited three books. Two years after she crafted the first Rogerian practice methodology, she edited *Visions of Rogers' Science-Based*

Nursing, which received the *American Journal of Nursing* Book of the Year Award. This was one of the first books to provide chapters on research, education, and practice focused entirely on one nursing conceptual framework/nursing theory. Dr. Barrett has presented her work on power in Australia, Scotland, Canada, the Netherlands, Germany, South Korea, and the Philippines as well as throughout the United States. Her article in *Nursing Science Quarterly* that won the best paper award for 2012 was the lead article in an issue devoted to her work. She currently is writing a book on the power theory for the general public. Dr. Barrett's websites can be viewed at www.drelizabethbarrett.com and www.powerimagery.com.

Overview of the Theory

Certain things happen that sometimes change the entire direction of our lives. So it was that I transplanted myself from Indiana to begin doctoral studies with Martha E. Rogers at New York University more than 35 years ago. Studying with Martha changed my professional and personal thinking, values, and actions as she became my teacher, my dissertation advisor, and later my colleague and friend. And so the power theory journey began and continues to this day. The passion and excitement I experienced in those early days is still with me and moves onward, primarily through the work of other nurses.

Rogers wove the conceptual framework of the science of unitary human beings (SUHB) as threads in the irreducible, unpredictable tapestry of the universe and many, like myself, continue to weave this changing fabric of our participatory world. In this chapter, I describe the flow from Rogers's science to the power theory to the research and practice applications. Figure 29-1 provides an overview of this process. Although it appears to be linear, in truth, it is a nonlinear, evolving, mutual process. Figure 29-1 also serves as an outline that tracks the unfolding of the theory and practice developments described in this chapter. It will be helpful to refer to it frequently.

Theoretical Underpinnings

Butcher and Malinski discuss the theoretical matrix of the postulates and principles of the SUHB in depth elsewhere in this book, and so only a cursory overview will be presented here. Keep in mind that development of the power theory required theoretical consistency with the postulates and principles of Rogerian science. This is one of the most difficult and yet critically important aspects involved in creating both theoretical and practice applications of the SUHB.

The postulates of the SUHB are energy fields, openness, pattern, and pandimensionality. We don't have **energy fields;** we are energy fields. There are two fields: the human and the environment. The environment encompasses all that the individual or group is not. These basic units of the living and nonliving are irreducible; they are unitary (Rogers, 1992). Parse (1998) defined unitary as ever changing, indivisible, and unpredictable.

We live in a universe of **openness,** so fields are open—all the way, all the time. There are no boundaries. Pattern is the distinctive defining characteristic of energy fields. **Pattern** is what makes you you and me me. Pattern cannot be directly observed; we observe manifestations of pattern. **Pandimensionality** is a way of perceiving reality; it is a nonlinear domain without temporal or spatial attributes (Rogers, 1992)

The three principles of the SUHB are about change. **Resonancy** is how change takes place: from long, slow waves to short, fast waves. **Helicy** is the nature of change, and **integrality** is the mutual process of humans and their environments (Phillips, 1994). These four postulates and three principles are the blueprint. All work developed from this theoretical perspective needs to be consistent with them.

Concepts of Barrett's Theory of Power as Knowing Participation in Change®

Rogers did not write about power in the SUHB, but she did emphasize that human beings can *knowingly* participate in change. Even though continuous participation in change is a given, participation in that change

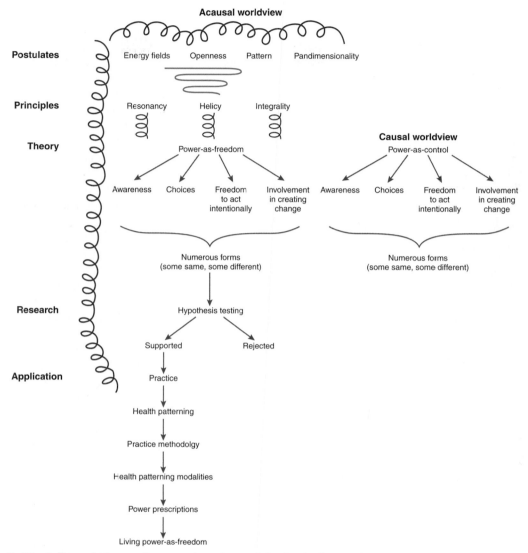

Fig 29 • 1 Barrett's theory of power as knowing participation in change. *(Copyright © Elizabeth Ann Manhart Barrett, RN, LMHC; PhD; FAAN.)*

may not take place in a *knowing* manner. I searched for a definition of power that would be consistent with the postulates and principles of the SUHB and connect with the literature where, for centuries, the primary propositions maintained that power was about change and about causality, although there was some meager support for an acausal view of power. Finally, the light bulb turned on. Power is the capacity to participate *knowingly* in change. Initially, I connected this definition with the literature in terms of change, but not in terms of causality because my purpose was to derive an acausal theory of power consistent with Rogers's conceptual model. This acausal theory was differentiated from other causal power theories that can be summarized by May's (1972) definition that power is the ability to cause or prevent change. Only much later did it become clear that the definition of power as the capacity to participate *knowingly* in change also described causal ideas of power.

Through readings in various relevant areas and synthesizing my own ideas, the conceptual manifestations of the inseparable dimensions of power were identified as **awareness, choices, freedom to act intentionally,** and **involvement in creating change.** These concepts were validated as consistent with the SUHB through a judges' study with New York University faculty, who were considered knowledgeable in Rogerian thought.

Power is the capacity to participate knowingly in change by being aware, making choices, feeling free to act intentionally, and involvement in creating change. In a nutshell, power is being aware of what one is choosing to do, feeling free to do it, and doing it intentionally (Barrett, 1986, 1989, 1990a, 2010). The theory describes power in groups as well as in individuals. The inseparable association of a person's or a group's power strengths or weaknesses is known as their Power Profile.

Power-as-Freedom and Power-as-Control

While my initial interest was in developing an acausal view of power, I was often puzzled regarding why the four dimensions of awareness, choices, freedom to act intentionally, and involvement in creating change seemed to also describe power from a causal perspective. After many years and for the second time, the power light bulb turned on. One day while walking down the street, I realized that the power theory did indeed describe two *types* of power. The difference is simply that one reflects an acausal worldview and the other reflects a causal worldview. We live in two worlds, and power as a phenomenon that exists in the universe lives in both of them. So I named these two **types** of *power—power-as-freedom* and *power-as-control.* For example, in the extreme situation of murder, if the murderer is aware of what she is choosing to do and feels free to act on that intention and is, actually, involved in creating that change, this is power as surely as the acausal type of power that does not interfere with another person's freedom. Freedom is incompatible with causality because causality allows for control, prediction,

and reduction. Some of the **forms** in which power manifests can be for purposes of control, such as money that can be used to control people, places, or things. On the other hand, money can be used for purposes of freedom through such things as philanthropy, education, meeting basic needs, but never interfering with the freedom of others. Knowledge can also be used for purposes of control or freedom.

I would further suggest that we can view the many variations of power theories, such as social power, political power, positional power, personal power, empowerment, and others as *forms* in which power manifests. They can be further understood in terms of the definition of power with its four dimensions of awareness, choices, freedom to act intentionally, and involvement in creating change, along with the 12 characteristics used to measure power as *knowing* participation in change. It is important to note that these new insights changed nothing I had previously written concerning power, but they expanded the theory to describe how power operates in the two worlds we live in—the causal and acausal worlds. Of course, although practice applications continue to focus on power-as-freedom, clients more easily understand how to live power-as-freedom when it is contrasted with power-as-control, the usual way people understand power and witness it in our everyday world. Power-as-control is often described in terms of force, dominance, or manipulation in subtle or not-so-subtle varieties of control. Figure 29-2 contrasts these two worldviews.

The Power as Knowing Participation in Change Tool (PKPCT, Version II)

Following a second judges' study, a paper-and-pencil research instrument using semantic differential technique was developed to measure power as *knowing* participation in change. The PKPCT, Version II consists of the four power dimensions, each measured by 12 bipolar adjective pairs randomly reversed and randomly ordered for each dimension. A thirteenth adjective pair is not included in the score because it is a retest reliability item that is used only for research purposes. A complete accounting of the

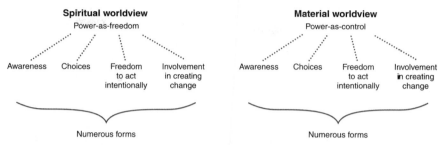

Barrett's Theory of Power as Knowing Participation in Change: Spiritual and Material Worldviews

Fig 29 • 2 Barrett's theory of power as knowing participation in change: spiritual and material worldviews. *(Copyright © Elizabeth Ann Manhart Barrett, RN-BC, LMHC; PhD; FAAN.)*

tool development, along with a copy of the PKPCT, Version II and the Scoring Guide is presented elsewhere (Barrett, 1990b, 2003), so only a brief summary is discussed here to aid understanding of how it is used in practice. Although the adjective pairs appear to be linear, in truth they are not to be conceptualized in that manner when one attempts to move from the less powerful adjective to the more powerful adjective. "In a world where time and space exist, the words *from* and *to* would be a linear process. However, in a pandimensional universe, change takes place throughout the human and environmental fields that are without spatial or temporal attributes" (Phillips, 2010, p. 57).

After a pilot study of 267 men and women, revised versions of the PKPCT, Version I and Version II, were further tested in a national study using a volunteer sample of 625 men and women with participants from every state. The response rate was 61%, and the sample comprised men and women with a minimum of a high school education who were diverse in terms of age (21–60 years), marital status, city size, geographic residence, and occupation. This sample was used to test the dissertation hypothesis that human field motion and power were correlated. I reasoned that the greater the effortless, rhythmic flow of human field motion in one's life, the greater one's capacity to participate knowingly in creating change. The hypothesis was supported with two statistically significant moderately strong canonical correlations of .61 and .16. Reliability, measured

as the variances of factor scores, ranged from .63 to .99; and validity coefficients, computed as factor loadings, ranged from .56 to .70 (Barrett, 1986, 1990b, 2003). The findings from these studies provided support for using the theory and measurement tool in nursing practice. Most other researchers who have used the PKPCT, Version II computed reliability using Chronbach's alpha with the majority reporting higher coefficients than what I had found (Caroselli & Barrett, 1998; Kim, 2009).

Although I use Version II in my practice and most researchers select this version as well, Version I also has acceptable reliability and validity (Barrett, 1986). The difference is that in Version I the power dimensions are measured in relation to self, family, and work.

Applications of the Theory
Research

I have completed eight additional studies, both quantitative and qualitative, most with colleagues, both funded and unfunded. In 1998, Caroselli and I published a review of the power as knowing participation in change research literature (Caroselli & Barrett, 1998); and Kim (2009) published an update of the power as knowing participation in change research in 2009. Currently, more than 90 studies have been conducted using the theory and/or measurement instrument. The tool has been translated into Japanese, Korean, Swedish, Danish, Portuguese, French, and German. These translations allow for testing a basic premise of the power theory that the capacity to participate knowingly in change is a quality of all people, regardless of race, ethnicity, nationality, or country of residence.

Practice Methodology

Shortly before finishing my doctoral studies, I completed a postgraduate program in holistically oriented psychotherapy to enhance the knowledge gained through a MSN in psychiatric/mental health nursing and experience teaching students and working in mental health settings. So I began a private nursing practice called Health Patterning as an alternative to traditional psychotherapy.

Soon I developed the first practice methodology for Rogerian nursing practice (Barrett, 1988). In the revised version, it consisted of two processes: pattern manifestation knowing and voluntary mutual patterning (Barrett, 1998). Butcher (2006) modified the methodology to include Cowling's (1990, 1997) methodology from his theory of unitary pattern appreciation. Incorporating Butcher's revision, the two phases are termed *pattern manifestation knowing and appreciation* and *voluntary mutual patterning*. There is no sequential order; both processes are continuously shifting and/or going on simultaneously.

Phase I: Pattern Manifestation Knowing and Appreciation

My first question when someone sits down in my office is "What do you want?" I'm interested in knowing what changes people want in their lives since that will be the focus of the health patterning sessions. Relevant historical information will unfold as our dialogue proceeds; I do not take a typical initial health history.

Phase II: Voluntary Mutual Patterning

Another initial question is "Where do you see yourself in your life right now?" If a person is having difficulty zeroing in, I might ask, "If you only had one sentence rather than 45 minutes, what would you say?" As you can see, the three principles of change are operating as we mutually explore the nature of change in their lives

(helicy) as well as the mutual process through which the change occurs (integrality) and how that change evolves (resonancy) as we focus our intention on creating change without attachment to outcomes or results. Intentions, aims, or directions are consistent with the acausal postulates and principles of the SUHB, whereas setting goals involves end points and, like outcomes, end points are not appropriate. Clients learn quickly that there is no causal "If I do this, then that will happen." They are often relieved to learn that the way this works is that "If I do this, then I will see what happens." The phenomenology of the moment is present-oriented with little focus on the past, which is gone, or the future, which hasn't been created yet, nevertheless recognizing that we are actually using our power to participate in creating that future at every moment. There is no focus on pathology or diagnosis. The idea of power as *knowing* participation in change helps people change limiting beliefs, disturbing emotions, and other difficulties in living. Most people easily understand ideas of wholeness, unitary human beingness, and the mutual process with the entirety of their environment, including other people, places, and things. We are not in charge of how things turn out as that involves everyone and everything else participating, knowingly or unknowingly, in the mutual process. Our power concerns what we think, feel, say, and do.

Health Patterning

Quite simply, health patterning is exploring with people ways to make the changes they want to make. More formally, health patterning is a power enhancement therapy that guides people to use their power-as-freedom to participate *knowingly* in creating the changes they want to make in their lives by becoming increasingly aware, making more powerful choices, feeling free to act on their intentions, and involving themselves in creating change. It is not talk therapy. It is pattern manifestation *knowing* and appreciation and voluntary mutual patterning coming alive in a moment-by-moment unfolding process. How is that different from talk therapy? The focus is not on simply "talking about"; rather, the focus is on the person's intentions and involvement in participating *knowingly* in change. There are no labels, no agendas, and no expectations.

My clients, for the most part, are people who want some sort of change in their lives that they haven't been able to accomplish, even when the change means accepting what cannot be changed in ways they desire. Often there is a crisis revolving around one or more of four major areas of life: oneself, health, relationships or career. My intention is to teach people how to find the authority and clarity in themselves by becoming aware of their intentions, by making choices from the options that are open to them, and learning to give themselves the freedom to carry through on their choices as they go about creating change in their lives.

After initiating a dialogue of meaning and asking clients to identify what they want to accomplish in our work together by telling me specifically three things, I ask clients to complete the PKPCT. I tell them nothing about the tool except how important it is to follow the instructions. It is important that they respond to the items honestly and frankly in order to get an accurate, meaningful reading. I point out that the tool is a reflecting mirror; it reflects back to people who they tell it they are. Afterward, I inquire about their notion about what the tool is assessing; they are usually shocked to learn it is power. This provides an opportunity to teach them the power theory by briefly describing the definition, the two types, the four dimensions, and a few examples of the numerous forms in which both types of power manifest. In the following session, I will have scored the power tool and can discuss the person's Power Profile strengths and weaknesses as well as ways our work together may enhance their Power Profile and facilitate accomplishment of what they are seeking through health patterning. For those who do not wish to complete the tool, there are many other optional modalities.

This process is quite different from using the PKPCT in quantitative research in which the interest is in group scores and what is learned is about the group, and group scores

can be compared with scores of other groups, and all the other possibilities available through quantitative methods. In Health Patterning, the PKPCT scores provide the Power Profile for one individual. This is a qualitative, phenomenological process. I do not tell or show the person his or her scores. The scores are used only to help the nurse or clinician assess the relative strengths and weaknesses not only of the four dimensions but also of the 12 opposite adjective pairs used to measure the dimensions. These 12 characteristics are pattern manifestations of power and often represent a person's belief systems concerning power. Dwelling with this data is quite a complex process. In the power-imagery process (described later in the chapter), sophisticated algorithms fine-tune the mechanics of the method. The point here is that using the tool with an individual is a mutual process of the client and the nurse; a computer cannot duplicate this human encounter. Power enhancement occurs when the weaker areas are reversed toward their stronger opposites using various health patterning modalities and Power Prescriptions.® This is not the work of a day, yet the power tool can be a valuable entrée to defining the person's Power Profile of greater and lesser areas of strength and providing direction for working with different modalities, such as creating a shift to the opposite, for example, from chaotic to orderly or from constrained to free.

Health Patterning Modalities

When clients, like all of us, are attempting to create an intended change, it is helpful for them to understand the acausal nature of the universe and appreciate the patterning manifesting in their experiences, perceptions, and expressions (Cowling, 1997). Interestingly, clients grasp simple examples of acausality quickly as they, like most of us, have learned that wanting something to happen, certainly does not mean that it will. It is often a relief to realize none of us is the sole generator of what occurs in our lives, and yet we can use our power to *knowingly* participate in the relative present. That's where health patterning modalities come in, yet these avenues for creating change in a *knowing* way are not magic bullets. Nor does one size fit all.

Even though the battle between free will and determinism is believed to go back as far as the pre-Socratics and continues to rage on, the SUHB and Barrett's power theory accept the acausality of free will as a given. Power-as-freedom is just that—freedom to powerfully create change without interfering with the freedom of someone else. Nor is power-as-freedom about forcing yourself to do something you don't want to do; rather, it is about making aware choices, feeling free to carry out those choices, and then doing so in a way that is true to your values, such as those that pertain to health and well-being. This approach requires practice methods and modalities to be consistent with this worldview. It does not, however, require clients to view the world in this way.

Health patterning modalities are *general* approaches used to help people use their power in new ways. The general focus includes *lifestyle changes, struggles with illness, difficulties in living, and enhancement of power-as-freedom through involvement in the healing encounter.* These modalities are selected within the context of what is happening in a person's life and in relation to the nurse's knowledge and skill in using them as well as the client's personal preferences. They take place in a life affirming, caring environment, described by Rogers as unconditional love.

Examples of health patterning modalities include imagery, Therapeutic Touch (TT), meditation, dream reading, love-power resonance, centering, prayer, power-imagery process, Power Profile process, and techniques of will. Imagery exercises can often be created from the content of what comes up during the session. However, here is an exercise that can be used to focus on any intention that the client wants to manifest. The title is health patterning, and it incorporates light, sound, color, and motion. These are modalities Rogers believed would be frequently used in the future. The intention for this health patterning imagery is a change the person wants to make in her life.

Health Patterning Imagery Exercise

Sit up straight. Get comfortable. Close your eyes. Find yourself breathing in an even and regular way with long, slow out-breaths through your mouth and briefer in-breaths through your nose. Breathe out with a long, slow breath through your mouth, releasing pain and suffering, and through your nose breathe in love and light. After breathing out with another slow, releasing breath letting go of any distress you may be experiencing, breathe in the blue of the sky and the gold of the sun in beautiful blue-golden light. Breathe out slowly one more time and then breathe any way you like.

Now, see and know that your hands are made of sky and earth. With these hands, you are able to weave your own life. Know that you are able to weave your own life with the threads and colors you choose. See and recognize the working out of the health patterning that your own weaving is creating. In doing so, know that by freely making choices with awareness, you are finding your own way to powerfully participate knowingly in bringing about change. Now think of your intention to create a specific change.

> *Breathe out one time. See yourself choosing with awareness.*
>
> *Breathe out one time. See yourself acting freely.*
>
> *Breathe out one time. See how you are involving yourself in participating in creating the change you want to see in your life.*

Breathe out and open your eyes.

It is important after completion of any imagery exercise to ask the client how she is feeling. If the person is uncomfortable in any way, it is necessary to continue voluntary mutual patterning to explore her experience, perception, and expression until comfort returns.

Health patterning modalities can be used in most situations that nurses encounter. People often come to me seeking relief from emotional pattern manifestations related to physical illness. Other people come with conditions that include pattern manifestations such as anxiety, depression, grief, anger, fear, guilt, troubling human field image, meaninglessness, creative blocks, substance use dependency, disease prevention, eating disorders, many types of pain, pre–post surgical procedures, prosperity or employment career concerns, spiritual distress, end-of-life issues, or a combination of these or other difficulties in living. The focus is on people as unitary wholes with their unique perceptions, experiences, and expressions. The practice arena is ripe with opportunities for nurses to research how the power theory can be used to advance practice by investigating ways health patterning modalities can promote healing.

Power Prescriptions

Power Prescriptions are the *specific* ways the health patterning modalities are used with a particular individual or group, as opposed to the *general* category of health patterning modalities. Again, they are designed to enhance power-as-freedom and are individualized depending on each person's wants and needs. As power-as-freedom grows, the person is less vulnerable to power-as-control tactics from others or from themselves with others and with themselves. This is one way people heal. With enhanced power-as-freedom, they find the strength to change limiting beliefs and behaviors.

Power Prescriptions are not like medical prescriptions. It is not as if you follow the prescribed regimen expecting a particular result. Rather than "if this, then that," the aim of Power Prescriptions is to guide people toward developing awareness, making more powerful choices, feeling free to act on their intentions, and becoming involved in creating specific changes in their lives.

Sometimes clients create their own Power Prescriptions. A client whom we will call Julia came to see me when she finished chemotherapy for non-Hodgkin's lymphoma. Sometimes she creates her own exercises that often come as images to her during Therapeutic Touch treatments. Along with other clients, she shares her remarkable story on my website (www.DrElizabethBarrett.com) as a way to contribute to the well-being of others. There you will find an example of an imagery exercise she created called "The Hapuna Chair." To access "The Hapuna Chair," click on "What I Do" on the menu bar. Then click "Real Stories. Real People. Real Power—Julia's Story" on the drop-down menu.

The Power-Imagery Process

The power-imagery process, or PIP as Gerald N. Epstein and I named it when we began developing it several years ago, basically works like this. A person completes the PKPCT. The findings, called the Power Profile, identify the stronger and weaker areas of power. Then, the client begins working through imagery exercises and techniques of will created to enhance the weaker areas in both the four power dimensions and the 12 power characteristics. This is a three-step, 21-day process designed to enhance people's power through imagery. In the first week, imagery exercises are focused on the four dimensions. In the second week, the focus is on the 12 characteristics. We call this process the Power Plan, which is a way to create a shift from lesser to greater power pattern manifestations, for example, from chaotic or orderly or from constrained to free. In the third week, the process involves the PowerGram exercises that put together the power dimension exercises from the first week with the exercises for the characteristics that were the focus during the second week. We have used this process with groups in the corporate and nonprofit worlds, with individuals in our private practices, and with group workshops. An online version is available at www.powerimagery.com. One nursing professor required her students to complete the online PIP as part of their professional development course.

504 SECTION VI • *Middle-Range Theories*

Practice Exemplar: True Stories of the Power-as-Freedom Journey of Two Friends

Although all nursing experiences are meaningful, some remain with us forever. So it was with Allison and Kay. Allison and Kay struggled with their own illnesses and yet maintained a healing partnership with each other even though their illnesses took quite different directions; it was a mutual process partnership that manifested love-power resonance. Although it was many years ago that these two young women crossed the threshold of my office door to begin health patterning, the memory lingers on. Love-power resonance was the glue that united the three of us.

Love-power resonance is a health patterning modality I developed to further understand the nurse–client healing process—a way to capture the meaning of the love that goes on between the nurse and client. It is well known that love heals—both the giver and the receiver—while hate destroys, and the absence of love hinders healing and can be deadly. Love is the most potent form of power-as-freedom, and hate may be the most intense emotion motivating extreme forms of power-as-control, such as abuse, oppression, and murder. Love and freedom are intimately connected, as are hate and control.

I believe that love is the fire that lights the power-as-freedom furnace. In love-power resonance, the frequency vibrations of both love and power accelerate one another, and healing manifests through resonating waves of change. The illusion of separation disappears, and the will is used for intentional healing events that enliven health. Love-power resonance teaches people to become "in power" in the same sense as being "in love," where two people become part of something greater than themselves and healing manifests through resonating waves of change. Helicy describes the nature of this change, resonancy describes how this change takes place, and integrality is the process whereby the change occurs (Phillips, 1994).

In love-power resonance, love is like power without effort—it just flows. It taps into

consciousness and spirituality, where consciousness is defined as the *Spirit* in all that is, was, and will be, and spirituality is defined as *experiencing* the Spirit in all that is, was, and will be. Phillips (2010) uses the term *energyspirit* to describe consciousness. I hypothesized that love-power resonance created an opportunity for change by accelerating the momentum of commitment to go forward with one's intentions, while acknowledging that the outcome is unknown and unpredictable.

First came Allison shortly after she had finished surgery, chemotherapy, and radiation for treatment of synovial sarcoma of the hip. Allison's picture and story are published on my website at www.drelizabethbarrett.com.

Pattern manifestation *knowing* and appreciation revealed that Allison was experiencing bilateral foot drop and that she was walking with an awkward gait that she perceived, experienced, and expressed as painful. It was apparent that this was affecting her human field image. After the chemotherapy, her latent genetic predisposition to Charcot-Marie-Tooth Disease (CMT) had emerged. Voluntary mutual patterning included discussion of this degenerative nerve demyelination disorder and how it had produced a progressive muscle atrophy of her legs, hands, and feet. A year later the sarcoma reoccurred, and she again underwent surgery and radiation. We worked together for another year, and since then she has come for a health patterning session occasionally for what she calls her "power boost."

Allison learned the power-as-freedom way using imagery exercises, techniques of will, prayer, and dream reading as her health patterning modalities, individualized as Power Prescriptions, to transcend the initial devastation she experienced with the cancer and CMT. She used a daily imagery exercise in which she imagined a magic wand tapping her legs, ankles, and feet and bringing the nerves to life. She remains cancer free, yet she still struggles with the pattern manifestations of CMT. She and her husband have two children,

Practice Exemplar: True Stories of the Power-as-Freedom Journey of Two Friends cont.

even though she was told if she had a child she would spend the rest of her life in a wheelchair.

By the end of our formal time together, Allison had decided to channel her fighting spirit and advocacy for others toward starting a foundation, the Hereditary Neuropathy Foundation (HNF), to search for a "cure" for CMT. HNF is now a thriving client advocacy and research-oriented nonprofit organization that provides educational information to persons living with CMT, professionals, and the general public. Allison had this to say: "Health patterning helped me view my illnesses as opportunities for learning how to deal with life circumstances, not as tragedies, but as experiences that helped me become a more powerful person" (www.drelizabethbarrett.com). You can find the HNF website at http://hnf-cure.org.

Allison met Kay as they entered the elevator of the building where they both lived. By the time they arrived at their floors, they had revealed to each other that they both had cancer; the seeds for love-power resonance between them had been planted. Soon Allison referred Kay to me.

Kay began her almost-continuous, 10-year battle with cancer when she was 21. First, cancer claimed her left breast, then the right breast, then it went to the spine and other bones and then the lungs and finally the brain.

Kay came to me for health patterning focused on Therapeutic Touch and imagery to relieve pain at the time the cancer had spread to her spine. Later, she became paraplegic and was told by her physicians that she would have to spend the rest of her life in a wheelchair. She refused to accept this ultimatum. When she was no longer able to come to my office, I began going to her home to give her TT treatments, and she also began to work with a physical therapist. During one of the TT treatments, she suddenly cried out, "I can feel sensations in my spine." As the tears rolled down her cheeks, she looked up at me and said, "This is what I prayed for." Soon she could walk with a

walker and for short distances with a cane, and that was the last she ever saw of a wheelchair. She shocked the physicians the first time she walked into their offices on her husband's arm, using just a cane.

During those sessions at Kay's apartment, Allison would often join us. Pattern manifestation *knowing* and appreciation and voluntary mutual patterning kept the sessions focused on a dialogue of meaning. Here's a brief sample of how the health patterning conversations would take place.

Kay: Why do we have to be sick when we want so much to be healthy?
Elizabeth: Are illness and health incompatible?
Allison: What is health, anyway?
Kay: I'm confused.
Elizabeth: I see health as a process of actualizing possibilities for well-being by participating knowingly in change.
Allison: Can health be different for different people?
Elizabeth: Yes. Health is a value that people define for themselves, so different people see it differently.
Kay: I've known people who are sick or at least have some disease, and I think they are healthy in what I've been seeing as the bigger picture.
Allison: Me, too.
Elizabeth: Illness can simply be a way a person's health is manifesting at a certain time, sometimes serving as a wake-up call or a trigger for transformation.
Kay: These new ideas are hopeful, and they are giving me courage.
Allison: It's hard not to ask, "why me?" Why do Kay and I have to struggle with these devastating diseases?
Elizabeth: Illness and disease can have many sources and many meanings, and sometimes those sources remain a mystery.
(Allison hands Kay a tissue to wipe her eyes.)

My efforts were not to get Kay to face her so-called death or work through stages of death and dying. My purpose was to help her live the way she chose, and live she did. She lived her dying in a power-as-freedom way that was uniquely her own.

Continued

On a few occasions, she asked me to tell her what I thought it would be like "at the end." I told her for me there is no end, as we never die; our energy simply transforms. We talked about the fact that some persons who have had a near-death experience describe a deep sense of peace and well-being and they sometimes describe passing through a tunnel of great darkness into a bright light on the other side, where a world of indescribable beauty awaits. She asked questions such as, "How can I stay alive while dying?" and "What about people without illness who are dying or may be almost already dead?"

Many times Kay talked about feeling a sense of closeness with her spirituality that for her connected healing with a sense of holiness. This was a new way she was experiencing her power-as-freedom, as a kind of prayerful reverence. She often asked me to pray with her. During this time, she also returned to her religious roots and developed a personal relationship with her God.

Kay needed frequent TT treatments, and it wasn't possible for me to go to her home that often. So I decided to offer her an opportunity to try a love-power resonance experiment.

I explained that imagery and TT are powerful nonlinear Power Prescriptions that do not depend on physical proximity and that healing possibilities are enhanced when we leave the visible realm of ordinary time and space and enter the invisible realm of pandimensionality, which is a domain where there are no temporal or spatial attributes. I invited Kay to meet with me over the phone for 5 minutes daily. We agreed that during this 5 minutes we would unite our intentions for her healing to manifest in whatever way that might happen. We were both clear that there could be no attachment to outcomes; yet the pattern manifestations that emerged included decreased pain, improved memory, less disturbed sleep, unlabored breathing, and an uplifted spirit. Over time, she came to understand that healing is far more than curing a disease; it is about healing the whole person, and it is not defined by the presence or absence of disease.

Some days, our 5-minute love-power resonance experiment consisted of a brief imagery exercise lasting less than a minute before doing healing at a distance with my hands hovering over a Polaroid photograph of her. The imagery often incorporated the powerful, pandimensional healing modalities of light, sound, color, and motion. Some days, I asked her to define a specific intention for her healing for that session. In keeping with our previous discussions, her intentions did not focus on outcomes.

For the first year, we did what we called "our thing" almost daily and after that three or four times a week. Kay found this love-power resonance experiment a meaningful way to maintain her optimistic courage and relieve pain and other symptoms despite the progression of the disease. She was an inspiration to me, and we shared what Parse calls "meaning moments" many times as she continued her healing journey. Although she didn't deny her illness, she was healthy in spite of it. Cancer may have ravaged her body, but not her soul—not her energy field.

Rumi (1988) described the transformation I witnessed as the months went by when he said: Journeys bring power and love back into you. If you can't go somewhere, move in the passageways of yourself. They are like shafts of light, always changing and you change when you explore them.

I asked Kay to remind herself that she was living her power-as-freedom by repeating daily the following power mantra: "I am free to choose with awareness how I participate in changes I intend to create." The days turned into weeks, months, and eventually over 2 years. She often would tell me during our 5-minute exchange that she was going into the hospital for another gamma knife treatment or radiation or chemotherapy, procedures she considered helpful and "no big deal," and amazingly she quickly bounced back to her optimistic self. Early on, Allison made a commitment to contact Kay several times a week and was a source of strength to Kay in ways that I could not be since they had both experienced cancer.

Practice Exemplar: True Stories of the Power-as-Freedom Journey of Two Friends cont.

Finally, Kay's husband called to tell me she had been admitted to the hospital. When I arrived, she was propped up in bed in a sitting position, but hunched over with her forehead near her chest. She was semiconscious and hadn't spoken for the 2 days she had been there, although her husband and parents thought she recognized them. Her family left the room so that we could have private time together. I asked her if she wanted to do "our thing," and she nodded her head. When I told her we were finished, I was amazed that she looked over at me with a slight smile. I held her hand. Soon her husband came into the room, and he and I were talking softly. All of a sudden, Kay rose up and called out her husband's name, saying, "I love you. I love you so very much." He was overcome with joy and ran out of the room to tell her parents and brother who returned immediately. Kay called out first to her father, "Daddy, Daddy, I love you" and then to her mother and brother. These were moments of love-power resonance. She passed on 3 days later having completed a 10-year healing journey. In the words of my imagery teacher of blessed memory Colette Aboulker-Muscat, "The bridge between us will always exist—now and forever" (Laura Goldstein, personal communication, January 10,

2004). For me, what I witnessed that day at the hospital was evidence that imagery, Therapeutic Touch, and prayer used during the love-power resonance experiment had made a difference in her healing.

The love-power resonance experiment was not a scientific experiment testing the principle of resonancy; it was simply a process of discovery that I sometimes experienced like a laser moving in unison between us, focused on our intention for her healing.

Love is a higher frequency vibration rippling through the universe; it has greater power to impact the universe than the lower frequency vibrations of negative phenomena. Everything we do makes a difference in terms of our mutual process with all that is. The more love we manifest, the stronger the power to bring peace and well-being to the world.

In closing, I am grateful that for more than 40 years, I have been privileged to be a professional nurse and to have experienced my profession by participating in the roles of practitioner, teacher, administrator, and researcher. Although all these roles were meaningful, practice has always been my first love, and Allison and Kay are two of the many clients that remain in my heart.

■ Summary

In this chapter a description of the flow from Rogers' science of unitary human beings to Barrett's power theory to research and practice applications is presented. Major assumptions include (1) power is a phenomenon that exists in the universe; (2) human beings are born with power; (3) no one can give power to another, and no one can take power away; and (4) human beings have free will and can *knowingly* participate in creating change.

The definition of power as the capacity to participate *knowingly* in change was derived from Rogers' conceptual model and describes both power-as-freedom and power-as-control.

The PKPCT measurement instrument and the research basis for practice are reviewed. Health patterning is a power enhancement therapy that guides people to use their power-as-freedom to participate *knowingly* in creating the changes they want to make in their lives by becoming increasingly aware, making more powerful choices, feeling free to act on their intentions, and involving themselves in creating change. Health Patterning modalities are individualized by using Power Prescriptions. A practice exemplar illustrates the way the theory is used to teach people how to live power-as-freedom.

References

Barrett, E. A. M. (1986). Investigation of the principle of helicy: The relationship of human field motion and power. In V. M. Malinski (Ed.), *Exploration on Martha Rogers' science of unitary human beings* (pp. 173–188). Norwalk, CT: Appleton-Century-Crofts.

Barrett, E. A. M. (1988). Using Rogers' science of unitary human beings in nursing practice. *Nursing Science Quarterly, 1,* 50–51.

Barrett, E. A. M. (1989). A nursing theory of power for nursing practice: Derivation from Rogers' paradigm. In J. Riehl (Ed.), *Conceptual models for nursing practice* (3rd ed., pp. 207-217). Norwalk, CT: Appleton & Lange.

Barrett, E. A. M. (1990a). Health patterning with clients in a private practice environment. In E. A. M. Barrett (Ed.), *Visions of Rogers' science-based nursing* (pp. 31-44). New York: National League for Nursing.

Barrett, E. A. M. (1990b). An instrument to measure power as knowing participation in change. In O. Strickland & C. Waltz (Eds.), *The measurement of nursing outcomes: Measuring client self-care and coping skills* (Vol. 4, pp. 159–180). New York: Springer.

Barrett, E. A. M. (1998). A Rogerian practice methodology for health patterning. *Nursing Science Quarterly, 11,* 94–96.

Barrett, E. A. M. (2003). A measure of power as knowing participation in change. In O. Strickland & C. Dilorio (Eds.), *Measurement of nursing outcomes: Self care and coping* (2nd ed., Vol. 3, pp. 21–39). New York: Springer.

Barrett, E. A. M. (2010). Power as knowing participation in change: What's new and what's next. *Nursing Science Quarterly, 23,* 47–54.

Butcher, H. K. (2006). Unitary pattern-based praxis: A nexus of Rogerian cosmology, philosophy, and science.

Visions: The Journal of Rogerian Nursing Science, 13, 41–58.

Caroselli, C., & Barrett, E. A. M. (1998). A review of the power as knowing participation in change literature. *Nursing Science Quarterly, 11,* 9–16.

Cowling, W. R. (1990). A template for unitary pattern-based nursing practice. In E. A. M. Barrett (Ed.), *Visions of Rogers' science based nursing* (pp. 45–65). New York: National League for Nursing.

Cowling, W. R. (1997). Pattern appreciation: The unitary science practice of reaching essence. In M. Madrid (Ed.), *Patterns of Rogerian knowing* (pp. 129–142). New York: National League for Nursing.

Kim, T. S. (2009). The theory of power as knowing participation in change. A literature review update. *Visions: The Journal of Rogerian Nursing Science, 16,* 40-47.

May, R. (1972). *Power and innocence: A search for the sources of violence.* New York: Dell.

Parse, R. R. (1998). *The human becoming school of thought: A perspective for nurses and other health professionals.* Thousand Oaks, CA: Sage.

Phillips, J. R. (1994). The open-ended nature of the science of unitary human beings. In M. Madrid & E. A. M. Barrett (Eds.). *Rogers' scientific art of nursing practice* (pp. 11–25). New York: National League for Nursing.

Phillips, J. R. (2010). The universality of Rogers' science of unitary human beings. *Nursing Science Quarterly, 23,* 55–59.

Rogers, M. E. (1992). Nursing science and the space age. *Nursing Science Quarterly, 5,* 27–34.

Rumi, (1988). *The branching moments* (J. Moyne & C. Barks, trans.). Providence, RI: Copper Beach Press.

Chapter 30

Marlaine Smith's Theory of Unitary Caring

MARLAINE C. SMITH

Introducing the Theorist
Overview of the Theory
Applications of the Theory
Practice Exemplar
Summary
References

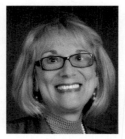

Marlaine C. Smith

Introducing the Theorist

Marlaine C. Smith is currently the Dean and Helen K. Persson Eminent Scholar at the Christine E. Lynn College of Nursing at Florida Atlantic University. Dr. Smith has been a nurse since 1972 and has practiced in acute care and public health settings in large metropolitan areas and a rural small town. She graduated from Duquesne University with a BSN, the University of Pittsburgh with two master's degrees in public health and nursing with a specialty in oncology and nursing education, and New York University with a PhD in nursing. Dr. Smith held faculty and academic administrative positions at Duquesne University, Penn State University, LaRoche College, and University of Colorado before her current position.

Dr. Smith is known for her work in two areas: metatheory, or the study of nursing theories and theoretical issues, and research related to healing through touch therapies. She has studied, written about, and conducted research related to Rogers's science of unitary human beings, Parse's man-living-health (now humanbecoming), Watson's theory of transpersonal caring, and Newman's health as expanding consciousness, and has written many commentaries on issues related to nursing theory development. She conducted five studies examining how the touch therapies of massage, therapeutic touch, hand massage, and simple touch can affect pain, symptom distress, quality of life, sleep, and other important outcomes for persons in acute and long-term care settings. The last completed study was funded by the National Institutes of Health, National Center for Complementary and Alternative Medicine.

Dr. Smith has been interested in transtheoretical work—that is, looking across nursing theories for points of convergence. The unitary theory of caring developed while studying the literature on caring in nursing, and then analyzing this literature through the theoretical lens of the science of unitary human beings. Dr. Smith was the recipient of the National League for Nursing's Martha E. Rogers Award for the Advancement of Nursing Science, is a Distinguished Alumna of New York University's Division of Nursing Alumni Association, and is a fellow in the American Academy of Nursing.

Overview of the Theory

A significant body of literature in nursing explicates caring as a phenomenon that is central to nursing's focus as a discipline and profession (Boykin & Schoenhofer, 1993, 2001; Leininger, 1977; Roach, 1987; M. C. Smith, Turkel & Wolf, 2013; Stevenson & Tripp-Reimer, 1990; Watson, 1979, 1985). At the same time, there has been a corresponding body of literature critiquing the assertion that caring is an identifying concept for the discipline and that the existing literature related to caring is ambiguous and provides no direction for meaningful inquiry (Morse, Solberg, Neander, Bottorf, & Johnson, 1990; Rogers in Smith, 1988; Paley, 2001; M. J. Smith, 1990). An analysis of the caring literature revealed that caring was a multidimensional concept that assumed multiple meanings depending on the framework within which it was situated or the lens from which it was viewed (M. C. Smith, 1999). Paley (1996) argued that a concept acquires its meaning within the context of the theory within which it resides. Concepts are theoretical niches, and to understand a concept fully, the theory in which the concept lives and derives its meaning must be clearly explicated. This chapter is the explication of a middle range theory of caring within the perspective of the unitary–transformative paradigm. For this reason, the theory is called *unitary caring*. This chapter contains a description of the theory development process, the assumptions

underpinning the theory, the concepts and propositions of the theory, the empirical referents of the theory, applications of the theory, and a practice exemplar that illustrates the major concepts.

Process of Theory Development

This process of developing a middle-range theory was guided by the question: "What is the substantive domain of caring knowledge from a unitary perspective?" Through a unitary lens the question was framed as: What is the quality of being in mutual process that is called "caring" within other theoretical contexts? This question was answered through a process of concept clarification that evolved from Paley's assertion that concepts were niches within theories. This concept clarification involved the following processes: (1) identifying the existing meanings of the concept in context, (2) identifying theoretical niches, (3) synthesis of the concept through identifying constitutive meanings, and (4) instantiation of the concept (M. C. Smith, 1999). Identification of the existing meanings of the concept occurred through reviewing the literature on caring that described it as a way of being. Exemplar sources (Boykin & Schoenhofer, 1993; Eriksson, 1997; Gadow, 1980, 1985, 1989; Gaut, 1983; Gendron, 1988; Leininger, 1990; Mayeroff, 1971; Montgomery, 1990; Rawnsley, 1990; Ray, 1981, 1997; Roach, 1987; Sherwood, 1997; Swanson, 1991; Watson, 1979, 1985) were reviewed in this process. From these sources semantic expressions, or phrases that captured the essential meaning of caring as a way of being, were listed. Next, the literature written by unitary scholars (Barrett, 1990; Cowling, 1990, 1993a, 1997; Krieger, 1979; Madrid, 1997; Madrid & Barrett, 1992; Newman, 1994; Quinn, 1992; Rogers, 1994) was examined for existing concepts that corresponded to the semantic expressions of caring. These were identified as theoretical niches in the unitary literature. Constitutive meanings, phrases that captured the meaning of a cluster of semantic expressions, were named using language consistent with a unitary perspective. Five constitutive meanings were developed (M. C. Smith,

1999). Since the initial publication, the work was expanded with assumptions and empirical referents (Cowling, Smith, & Watson, 2008) to form a middle-range theory. The theory is connected philosophically to the unitary–transformative paradigm, has five concepts that describe the phenomenon of caring from a unitary perspective, and can guide practice behaviors and research questions at the empirical level (M. J. Smith & Liehr, 2008).

Assumptions

Assumptions of the unitary theory of caring come from Rogers's science of unitary human beings (1970, 1994), Newman's theory of health as expanding consciousness (1994, 2008), and Watson's Theory of Transpersonal Caring (1985, 2005; Watson & Smith, 2002). To fully understand the meaning of the theory, readers will benefit from studying these sources.

1. Human beings are unitary or irreducible, in mutual process with an environment that is coextensive with the Universe, participating knowingly in patterning, and ever-evolving through expanding consciousness (Barrett, 1989; Newman, 1994; Rogers, 1992).
2. Caring is a quality of participating knowingly in human–environmental field patterning (M. C. Smith, 1999).
3. Caring is the process through which human wholeness is affirmed and that potentiates the emergence of innovative patterning and possibilities (Cowling et al., 2008, E44).
4. Caring is a manifestation and reflection of expanding consciousness potentiating greater meaning, insight, and transformative ways of relating to self and others (Cowling et al., Smith, & Watson, 2008).
5. Caring consciousness is resonating with the pandimensional universe (Rogers, 1994; Watson, 2005; Watson & Smith, 2002).

Concepts

After establishing the theoretical linkages to the unitary-transformative paradigm, the five concepts of this theory are explicated. The five concepts were developed from an analysis of literature on caring and similar concepts described by unitary scholars. The theoretical concepts have their underpinnings in each of the assumptions.

Manifesting Intentions

Manifesting intentions is the first concept in the unitary theory of caring; it was originally defined as creating, holding, and expressing thoughts, feelings, images, beliefs, desires, will, purpose and actions that affirm possibilities for human health and healing (Smith, 1999). From this point of view, the nurse is a healing environment, creating sacred space through her thoughts, feelings, intentions, and actions (Quinn, 1992). Understanding intentionality in this way comes with an assumption that underlying the world of form that is accessed by sensory perception, there is the primary reality that is pandimensional (Rogers, 1994) and beyond access through the five senses alone. David Bohm's (1980) concept of the holographic universe with implicate–explicate orders of reality is consistent with this point of view. The implicate order is the primary, unseen pattern, whereas the explicate order is the manifestation of this underlying pattern that is accessible through the senses. Caring is engaging with both orders of reality, holding intentions through affirmations and images, and expressing these intentions through actions. Thoughts, feelings, perceptions, and images are as potent as our words and actions. Intentions are meaningful energetic blueprints for transformation (M. C. Smith, 1999). What we hold in our hearts matters (Cowling et al., 2008, p. E46). Manifesting intentions encompasses actions that create healing environments, preserve dignity, humanity, and reverence for personhood, focus attention to and concern for the other, and facilitate authentic presence.

Appreciating Pattern

Appreciating pattern is the second concept in this theory. It is apprehending and understanding the mysteries of human wholeness and diversity with awe. This concept was referenced by both Dolores Krieger (1979) and Richard Cowling (1990, 1993a, 1993b, 1997), and defined by Cowling (1997) as "seeing underneath all that is fragmented to the real existence of wholeness and acknowledging that with awe" (p. 136). Cowling (1997) describes the process of approaching knowing the other with gratitude and enjoyment. This contrasts with a clinical problem-solving approach. While appreciating pattern is an existing concept in unitary theory, it corresponds to many important meanings within caring theories including valuing and celebrating the wholeness and uniqueness of persons, acknowledging pattern without attempting to change it, recognizing the person as perfect in the moment, being sensitive to the unfolding pattern of the whole, and coming to know the other. Pattern is reflected in meaning, so finding out what is meaningful to the other becomes primary in knowing pattern (Newman, 2008). Appreciating pattern is coming to know the uniqueness of the other. It is grasping the wholeness of the other (individual, family, and community) not through analysis, but through sensing, coexploring experiences, and listening to the other's story. This happens through letting go of preconceptions and the need to categorize, classify, diagnose, or judge. When we resist labeling and diagnosing we can glimpse the dynamic being that is sharing this moment with us. Appreciating pattern is being-with in wonder at this work of art before us, this life that reflects the diversity of creation.

Attuning to Dynamic Flow

Attuning to dynamic flow is the third concept in this unitary theory of caring. Attuning to dynamic flow is sensing of where to place focus and attention in mutual process. It was originally described as "dancing to the rhythms within continuous mutual process" (M. C. Smith, 1999, p. 23). Caring is flowing with the cocreated rhythms of relating in the moment. It happens by being truly present in the moment and is a back and forth movement of relationship building through a "vibrational sensing of where to place focus and attention" (M. C. Smith, 1999, p. 23). This includes expressions

of caring and unitary relating from the literature such as attuning to the subtle cues in the moment (Montgomery, 1990), shifting perspectives and patterns of response (Mayeroff, 1971), relating in a complex synchronized integration (Gendron, 1988), and experiencing energetic resonance (Quinn, 1992). It is hearing the call that may be spoken or unspoken. Newman (2008) describes the process of resonance as a way of knowing that presents itself through intuitive insights and feelings. Intellectualization can actually break this resonant field that is created through true presence. Caring is not taking the lead and telling the person what he or she needs to do. It is understanding where the other wants to go and moving with him or her in the struggle to get there. It is going to the relationship without an agenda, a plan, a bag of tricks, but trusting in the transformative power of healing presence.

Experiencing the Infinite

The next concept in the theory is experiencing the infinite. This concept is defined as "pandimensional awareness of coextensiveness with the universe occurring in the context of human relating" (M. C. Smith, 1999, p. 24). This is described by many caring theorists as spiritual union (Watson, 1985), Divine Love (Ray, 1997), or an actual caring occasion (Watson, 1985). Experiencing the Infinite is the recognition that the nurse–person relationship is sacred, we meet the Holy in it, and when we are with others in this way, there are no limits to the possibilities. Miracles happen! There are miracles of healing that happen with our patients every day that can be potentiated through love and caring. This can be recognizing who one really is, appreciating the Oneness of Being with all there is, and finding hope in the darkest of hours. All of this is mediated by our outlook, how we view our world, and what we entertain as possibilities. William Blake (1790–1793) said, "The tree which moves some to tears of joy is in the eyes of others only a green thing that stands in the way." Experiencing the infinite occurs in moments of grace, experiencing the presence of God in relationship with others. In those moments, there is an experience of connectedness to all-that-is extending beyond space–time boundaries that defies description in ordinary language.

Inviting Creative Emergence

The final concept in this theory of unitary caring is inviting creative emergence. It is attending the birth of innovative, emergent patterning through affirming the potential for change, nurturing the awareness of possibilities, imagining new directions, and clarifying hopes and dreams. This concept was taken from Quinn's (1992) description of healing and Newman's (1994, 2008) descriptions of transforming presence. Descriptions of caring in the literature that correspond to this concept are a "transformative experience wherein the constant birthing of love in caring actions is the growth of spiritual life within" (Roach, 1987), allowing a person to grow in his/her own time and way (Mayeroff, 1971), and calling to a deeper life, the spiritual life, of each person (Ray, 1997). Caring is inspiring the other to birth oneself anew in the moment. It might be through an activity, realization, decision, a new role, a new life pattern. The nurse creates a safe space for this new life to emerge through supporting, coaching, and providing confidence when it is lacking. This concept relates caring to healing. Caring is the vehicle through which healing occurs. Caring takes trust and patience. People change and grow in their own ways and in their own time. They know their way and we journey with them. This invitation for creative emergence is gentle and encouraging. Quinn (1992) calls it being a midwife to healing.

Propositions

The following are propositional statements that further clarify concepts of the theory. Manifesting intention is:

• Preparing self to participate knowingly in cocreating an environment for healing.
• Focusing images, thoughts and intentions for health and healing.

• Expressing intentions in actions that support health and healing.

Appreciating pattern is:

• Seeing wholeness in perceived fragmentation.
• Valuing uniqueness and diversity of patterning with wonder.
• Acknowledging what is without attempting to change or fix.
• Exploring what is meaningful in the moment.
• Coming to know by listening to the other's story.

Attuning to dynamic flow is:

• Being truly present in the flow of relating.
• Attending to the subtleties of meaning.
• Synchronizing rhythms of self with other.
• Trusting intuition in the mutual process.

Experiencing the infinite is:

• Acknowledging the sacred in human relating.
• Believing in limitless possibilities.
• Igniting hope in despair.
• Connecting to a pandimensional universe.

Inviting creative emergence is:

• Honoring the unique timing, pace and direction of change.
• Calling attention to possibilities and potentialities hidden from view.
• Inspiring new life to emerge in the moment.
• Trusting in the wisdom of knowing one's own way.

Empirical Indicators

An empirical indicator is a "concrete and specific real world proxy for a middle range theory concept" (Fawcett, 2000, p. 20). It is taking a conceptual abstraction and moving it to a place where it lives...where it can be seen, heard, felt, experienced, or measured. There are empirical indicators for both practice and research. Those for practice are useful in translating the theoretical concept to guides for nursing practice. Those for research can be used to generate research questions, develop measures of the concept, or develop paths of inquiry where the concept might be explicated through experiences. Each of the concepts is discussed at the empirical level.

Manifesting Intentions

As far as the concept of *manifesting intentions,* nurses enter a caring relationship with intention, through preparing to become the energetic environment that potentiates healing. Nurses prepare by centering or connecting to the True Self, going to that place within where it is possible to hear the still small voice. Nurses prepare by focusing on the present moment, leaving behind the thoughts racing in their heads that interfere with being truly present. Nurses prepare for caring by holding intentions that change the vibratory pattern of the energy field. Marcus Aurelius (171–175) said, "The soul becomes dyed by the color of its thoughts." The soul of our practice is dyed by our pattern of thinking. If we cultivate the habit of focusing, centering, and setting intentions before any encounter; we can create the space for caring and healing. This way of being-with can be developed through self reflection, expressing intentions through touch and energy work, centering exercises, spiritual practices such as meditation and prayer, mantra repetition, and experiences in nature (Cowling et al., 2008). The development of an inner life is critical for the full expression of caring in nursing. If caring is a way of being, nurses must develop these competencies as much as any other to evolve as caring beings. Rituals can structure the process of setting intentions that are manifest in the nursing situation. Watson (2008) gives an example of creating a handwashing ritual in which nurses use this daily practice as a way of centering and leaving behind any thoughts that might interrupt presence. Morning huddles are used in some settings as a ritual to come together as a team and set the intentions for the day. Nurses can develop rituals related to giving report that signify the duty to care (Cowling et al., 2008).

The concept of manifesting intentions can be studied. Activities such as centering, setting an intention, affirmations, meditations, prayers, values-based decision making, and use of mantras could be tested using any variety of outcomes associated with nurses or their clients. One could explore how nurse centering before care influences outcomes related to patient safety or how the handwashing ritual described above might improve patient satisfaction. One could study if there were healing outcomes associated with Reiki, Therapeutic Touch, or prayer because intentionality is integral to these practices.

Appreciating Pattern

In a unitary theory of caring, nurses would approach coming to know their patients in an entirely different way. The nursing process, or the problem-solving process, would not be consistent with caring from this point of view. It would involve knowing the other through using the sensory and extrasensory abilities to grasp wholeness. Nursing assessments would include exploring the unique life patterns of the person, exploring what is most important in the moment, and hearing the person's story. Perhaps the first questions that we ask our patients should be "What is important to you right now?" and "What matters most in this moment?" (Boykin & Schoenhofer, 2006). Cowling (1997) and Newman (1994, 2008) have both developed clear praxis methods that focus on pattern appreciation and pattern recognition. Nurses need to develop their abilities to appreciate pattern. Skills of pattern seeing, listening, grasping the essence, and art and music appreciation correspond to this ability of appreciating pattern (Cowling et al., 2008). In interdisciplinary team conferences, nursing is the voice that represents the wholeness of the person; no other discipline does this. Instead of describing a community by its census and health statistics, we can come to know it by asking its members to describe the essence of the community. Nurses can use bulletin boards in patient rooms as places that persons and families can display their uniqueness and what is most important to them.

Research related to pattern appreciation already exists (Cowling, 2005; Repede, 2009) Cowling's unitary pattern appreciation is a praxis method (combines research and practice) in which he and the participant/client explore patterning together; this is then captured and shared through aesthetic expressions. Through using Newman's praxis method, nurses engage persons in an exploration of the meaningful events and relationships in their lives toward recognizing pattern and making choices about those patterns.

Attuning to Dynamic Flow

Attuning to dynamic flow is lived in practice through sensing the readiness to begin to talk about sensitive issues or the willingness to take on a major life change. An example is staying engaged with a person and family members as they struggle together with the decision to transition to hospice care. Another example is knowing when a person needs the nurse to be tough, urging him to get out of bed and walk after surgery or to be soft, facilitating some quiet space for a person to be alone for awhile. Nurses need to cultivate their abilities related to this through sensing, hearing and moving with rhythms, presencing, and focusing. Learning to listen for shifts and pauses and learning to listen to and trust intuitive insights is important. There are hospital myths about the nurse who walks by a patient's room and knows that the patient is going to code. This may be an example of being sensitive to changes and shifts within a situation, attuning to the information that is embedded in the field of consciousness.

There are research possibilities related to this concept. It would be interesting to study how nurses attune to the dynamic flow of relationship with an unconscious person or a neonate. What are the cues that they pick up and act on? What are the ways that they sense beyond the senses to understand what is happening or what is being communicated to them? The study of intuition in practice is an example of an empirical indicator of this concept.

Experiencing the Infinite

One example of experiencing the infinite is seeing the sacred in mundane activities. It is recognizing the extraordinary in the ordinariness of our activities. This might be made concrete by practice rituals that can help us to recognize and celebrate the work of nursing. One such ritual that has been used is the "blessing of the hands." Another way to experience the infinite in practice is to validate its existence through nursing practice stories. We don't take the time to really appreciate the incredible moments experienced in caring with others. The sensitivity to experience the infinite in our practice may be developed through spiritual practice or a practice that fosters deep reflection. This could be meditation, prayer, centering, being in nature, or walking a labyrinth (Cowling et al., 2008, p. E48).

The research questions that are related to this concept might be studying nurses' and patients' stories of the extraordinary moments experienced in nursing practice.

Inviting Creative Emergence

There are many examples in nursing practice that can illustrate how caring can invite creative emergence. This can happen when we help women become mothers through teaching them the necessary skills to care for their babies and help them to grow, or when we connect people to resources in the community that allow them to live with greater ease in the midst of a family crisis. It is helping others live their lives differently and discover new ways of becoming.

The empirical indicators for research might be developing an instrument to measure satisfaction or pride associated with life changes. Studies could be structured to explore differences in outcomes when lifestyle change is approached with a nondirective model suggested by this concept, rather than a structured directive approach to lifestyle change.

Applications of the Theory

The middle-range theory of unitary caring has been advanced as a model for palliative care practice. Reed (2010), a palliative care clinical nurse specialist, has described how unitary caring is used as a guide for his practice. Reed's (2011) dissertation explored experiences in providing and receiving massage and simple touch at end of life. The study was a secondary analysis of qualitative interviews from persons with advanced cancer who had received massage or simple touch as part of their participation in a research study. Three themes were identified from the data that describe their experiences of receiving touch: (1) pattern recognition and wholeness,

(2) caring relationships, and (3) transformation and transcendence. These themes were related to unitary caring, the theoretical framework for the study.

Unitary caring is used as a guiding theory for studying nursing at St. Thomas University in Houston, Texas. This program has a unique curriculum model built on the tenets of unitary caring.

Practice Exemplar

Sue is a family nurse practitioner working in a community-based family practice with a physician colleague. She practices from a nursing model, using theories in the unitary-transformative paradigm as a guide for her practice. Beth is a 55-year-old attorney who has been seeing Sue for her primary care for some time. She is waiting in the examining room.

Sue has had a busy morning with time pressures and some difficult patient encounters. She is "backed up" with two patients waiting for her. She approaches the examining room and pulls out the chart. She smiles as she sees Beth's name. In front of the door, she pauses, closes her eyes, takes several deep breaths and centers herself, repeating her mantra. She sets an intention to be fully and authentically present with Beth in this encounter and to enter a relationship with her that facilitates their mutual well-being.

Sue opens the door and finds Beth sitting on the chair fully clothed. Sue approaches her warmly, holding out her hand and touching her on the shoulder. She pulls up her chair and puts the chart aside. "OK, Beth, what's going on? How are you?"

Beth talks rapidly, wringing her hands and tugging on her sleeve. "I was on vacation last week in North Carolina with my friends. We were having a relaxing time, and as I was getting out of the car I felt myself go into atrial fibrillation. My heart rate went way up like it does to about 270, and I felt just awful, like I couldn't breathe, lightheaded . . . I thought I was going to die."

"Oh, how scary . . . that's awful."

"I know. I ended up in the emergency room of this tiny hospital where they treated me with IV antiarrhythmic drugs, and finally my heart rate went down, and I converted to sinus rhythm in about 3 hours. But this is the third time that this has happened to me, and the second time when I've been away from home. I just need to get to the bottom of this. I'm frustrated and scared."

"Of course you are," Sue continues. "OK tell me how things are going with you generally and anything unusual that you were doing on vacation that might have precipitated this episode."

"Well, you know I had that episode of diverticulitis before I left for vacation, and you prescribed the Cipro for me. Well, I was not feeling great on vacation, the pain was better, but I had constipation, but took the Miralax and the fiber that I always take. We went on a boat trip the day before and I took some Dramamine, too. Also, my friends and I were drinking wine every night. That's all I can think of."

"What about home and work?"

Beth looks down at her hands. "Well, Bob still can't find a job, and things have been crazy at work. I just can't seem to get ahead of it. I have a major brief due in a couple of weeks . . . It was hard to leave for vacation. I love being with my friends, but I was torn about taking the time."

Sue pauses then says, "Tell me more about this feeling of being torn between what you love and what you have to do."

Practice Exemplar cont.

"I guess I'm in that space a lot lately, Sue." Beth begins crying. "I don't think I'm doing what I love to do . . . I feel like I'm not in control of my life."

Sue hands Beth some tissues and sits quietly with her, gently touching her arm as Beth sobs. In the moment Beth sobs for the loss of joy in her life now, and at the memory of her mother telling her she had to go into a practical career like law, not fiction writing. In the moment Sue imagines holding and rocking Beth in the space between them. In her mind's eye she whispers comforting words. In silence, they both experience an intimacy that is beyond language.

When Beth stops crying she looks up and asks, "What do I do now?"

"Let's take care of the A-fib issue first, Beth. Are you still on the same dose of the beta-blocker that your cardiologist prescribed?"

"Yes, Toprol 25 mg."

"OK. I want you to get in to see the cardiologist as soon as possible and discuss this with him. You have some options with ablation or other antiarrhythmics. You might want to talk with an electrophysiologist as well. I'll make a referral. Also, I just checked the side effects of Cipro, and atrial fibrillation is a rare side effect. So taking the Cipro could have triggered this event given your history. And of course Dramamine and alcohol could have contributed. And at the time this happened you were just getting over diverticulitis and weren't feeling great. But, we also need to focus on this distress that you are experiencing related to your work. I'd like you to do some journaling for a period of 2 weeks. Write down the things that you love, your passions, what makes your heart sing? Don't overthink it, Beth. If you have images or messages that come to you, jot them down. Make an appointment in 2 weeks, and we'll talk about what you discovered. OK?"

"Yes, OK." Beth nods tentatively.

"Before you leave I'm going to listen to your heart and check your blood pressure again. Hop up on the table." Sue auscultates Beth's heart sounds and measures her blood pressure. "Everything is fine. Your heart rate is regular at 60, and your blood pressure is OK, but a bit higher than we'd like it to be: 130/82. I know you experience some "white-coat hypertension." We'll check it again next week. You check it too at the machine in the grocery store and keep track. Bring that back in 2 weeks too."

Sue puts two hands on Beth's shoulders. "I'm in this with you. You'll figure this out. Change can be hard, but it's how we grow. Anything else that we need to talk about today?"

"No, I feel better . . . thanks, Sue."

"Thank you! I'll see you in 2 weeks."

(The encounter took 15 minutes.)

The five concepts of the unitary theory of caring were evident. First, *manifesting intention* was visible in the preparation before Sue entered the room. She was aware that she, as nurse, is an environment for healing (Quinn, 1992). Sue set an intention and entered the nursing situation being fully present to Beth. She shared her intentions with Beth when she said, "I'm in this with you," and in her use of touch and eye contact to communicate her desire to be present and in partnership with Beth. *Appreciating pattern* was evident as Sue asks Beth about what was going on with her, how she was, and if there was anything different about the time that led up to the episode of atrial fibrillation. Sue values the uniqueness of Beth's experience and Beth's own insights about events that led up to the episode, affirming that Beth's knowledge of her own pattern had validity. Intuitively, Sue asked the questions, "What about home and work?" and "Tell me more about this feeling of being torn between what you love to do and what you have to do." This second question emerged from Sue's tuning into meaning and resonating with the whole, illustrating the concept of *attuning to dynamic flow*. This led to the revelation of Beth's life pattern that could have remained undisclosed had Sue not attended to the intuitive flash. As Sue silently sat with Beth as she sobbed, they both experienced an intimacy beyond words, and a pandimensional awareness of past–present–future in the moment. This is an example of the concept of *experiencing the*

Continued

Practice Exemplar cont.

infinite. Finally, when Beth expresses that she is not doing what she loves, Sue is *inviting creative emergence* by asking her to attend to any cues she may receive about what she would love to do and to record this in a journal. She asks her to return for a follow-up visit in 2 weeks.

Often, the argument is advanced that "there is no time to care in this way," but this encounter took 15 minutes, no longer than a conventional, medically focused primary care visit. It isn't the time we have; it is what we do with that time that counts.

■ Summary

The unitary theory of caring provides a constellation of concepts that describe caring from a unitary perspective. The theory is constituted with five concepts: manifesting intentions, appreciating pattern, attuning to dynamic flow, experiencing the Infinite, and inviting creative emergence. Assumptions of the theory were explicated, each concept was described, and examples of empirical indicators for practice and research were offered. The unitary theory of caring is new; it can grow through those who invest in it through testing it in practice and research.

References

Aurelius, M. (171–175). *Meditations.*

Barrett, E. A. M. (1989). A nursing theory of power for nursing practice; Derivation from Rogers' paradigm. In J. Riehl (Ed.), *Conceptual models for nursing practice* (3rd ed., pp. 207–217). Norwalk, CT: Appleton & Lange.

Barrett, E. A. M. (1990). *Visions of Rogers' science-based nursing.* New York: National League for Nursing Press.

Blake, W. (1790–1793). *The Marriage of Heaven and Hell.*

Bohm, D. (1980). *Wholeness and the implicate order.* London: Routledge & Kegan Paul.

Boykin, A., & Schoenhofer, S. (1993). *Nursing as caring: A model for transforming practice.* New York: National League for Nursing Press.

Boykin, A., & Schoenhofer, S. (2001). *Nursing as caring: A model for transforming practice* (2nd ed.). Sudbury, MA: Jones and Bartlett.

Boykin, A., & Schoenhofer, S. (2006). Anne Boykin and Savina Schoenhofer's nursing as caring theory. In M. Parker (Ed.), *Nursing theories and nursing practice* (pp. 334–348). Philadelphia: F. A. Davis.

Cowling, W. R. (1990). A template for unitary pattern-based practice. In E. A. M. Barrett (Ed.), *Visions of Rogers' science-based nursing* (pp. 45–65). New York: National League for Nursing Press.

Cowling, W. R. (1993a). Unitary knowing in nursing practice. *Nursing Science Quarterly, 6,* 201–207.

Cowling, W. R. (1993b). Unitary practice: revisionary assumptions. In M. Parker (Ed.), *Patterns of nursing theories in practice.* New York: National League for Nursing Press.

Cowling, W. R. (1997). Pattern appreciation: The unitary science/practice of reaching for essence. In M. Madrid (Ed.), *Patterns of Rogerian knowing.* New York: National League for Nursing Press.

Cowling, W. R. (2000). Healing as appreciating wholeness. *Advances in Nursing Science, 22*(3), 16–32.

Cowling, W. R. (2005). Despairing women and healing outcomes: A unitary appreciative nursing perspective. *Advances in Nursing Science 28*(2), 94–106.

Cowling, W. R., Smith, M. C., & Watson, J. (2008). The power of wholeness, consciousness and caring: A dialogue on nursing science, art and healing. *Advances in Nursing Science, 31*(1), E41–E51.

Eriksson, K. (1997). Understanding the world of the patient, the suffering human being: The new clinical paradigm from nursing to caring. *Advanced Practice Nursing Quarterly, 3*(1), 8–13.

Fawcett, J. (2000). *Analysis and evaluation of contemporary nursing knowledge: Nursing models and theories.* Philadelphia: F. A. Davis.

Gadow, S. (1980). Existential advocacy: Philosophical foundations of nursing. In S. Spicker & S. Gadow (Eds.), *Nursing images and ideals.* New York: Springer.

Gadow, S. A. (1985). Nurse and patient: The caring relationship. In A. Bishop & J. Scudder (Eds.), *Caring, curing, coping: Nurse, physician, patient relationships.* Tuscaloosa, AL: University of Alabama Press.

Gadow, S. A. (1989). Clinical subjectivity: Advocacy with silent patients. *Nursing Clinics of North America, 24,* 535–541.

Gaut, D. A. (1983). Development of a theoretically adequate description of caring. *Western Journal of Nursing Research, 5*, 313–324.

Gendron, D. (1988). *The expressive form of caring* (Perspectives in Caring Monograph 2). Toronto: University of Toronto Faculty of Nursing.

Krieger, D. (1979). *The therapeutic touch: How to use your hands to help or heal*. Englewood Cliffs, NJ: Prentice-Hall.

Leininger, M. (1977). *Caring: The essence and central focus of nursing* (Nursing Research Report). Silver Spring, MD: American Nurses' Foundation.

Leininger, M. M. (1990). Historic and epistemologic dimensions of care and caring with future directions. In J. S. Stevenson & T. Tripp-Reimer (Eds.), *Knowledge about care and caring: State of the art and future developments*. Kansas City, MO: American Academy of Nursing.

Madrid, M. (1997). *Patterns of Rogerian knowing*. New York: National League for Nursing Press.

Madrid, M., & Barrett, E. A. M. (Eds.). (1992). *Rogers' scientific art of nursing practice*. New York: National League for Nursing Press.

Mayeroff, M. (1971). *On caring*. New York: Harper & Row.

Montgomery, C. (1990). *Healing through communication: The practice of caring*. Newbury Park, CA: Sage.

Morse, J. M., Solberg, S. M., Neander, W. L., Bottorff, J. L., & Johnson, J. L. (1990). Concepts of caring and caring as a concept. *Advances in Nursing Science, 13*, 1–14.

Newman, M. A. (1994). *Health as expanding consciousness*. New York: National League for Nursing Press.

Newman, M. A. (2008). *Transforming presence: The difference that nursing makes*. Philadelphia: F. A. Davis.

Paley, J. (1996). How not to clarify concepts in nursing. *Journal of Advanced Nursing, 24*, 572–578.

Paley, J. (2001). An archaeology of caring knowledge. *Journal of Advanced Nursing, 36*(2), 188–198.

Quinn, J. F. (1992). Holding sacred space: the nurse as healing environment. *Holistic Nursing Practice, 6*, 26–36.

Rawnsley, M. (1990). Of human bonding: The context of nursing as caring. *Advances in Nursing Science, 13*(2), 41–48.

Ray, M. A. (1981). A philosophical analysis of caring within nursing. In M. M. Leininger (Ed.), *Caring: An essential human need*. Thorofare, NJ: Slack.

Ray, M. A. (1997). Illuminating the meaning of caring: Unfolding the sacred art of divine love. In M. S. Roach (Ed.), *Caring from the heart: The convergence of caring and spirituality*. New York: Paulist Press.

Reed, S. (2010). A unitary caring conceptual model for advanced practice nursing in palliative care. *Holistic Nursing Practice, 24*(1), 23–34.

Reed, S. (2011). *Experiences in providing and receiving massage and simple touch at end of life*. Unpublished doctoral dissertation, University of Colorado Health Science Center School of Nursing, Denver.

Repede, E. (2009). Participatory dreaming: A conceptual exploration from a unitary appreciative inquiry perspective. *Nursing Science Quarterly 22*(4), 360–368.

Roach, S. (1987). *The human act of caring*. Ottawa: The Canadian Hospital Association.

Rogers, M. E. (1970). *An introduction to the theoretical basis of nursing*. Philadelphia: F. A. Davis.

Rogers, M. E. In M. J. Smith (1988). Perspectives on nursing science. *Nursing Science Quarterly, 1*, 80–85.

Rogers, M. E. (1992b). Nursing science and the space age. *Nursing Science Quarterly, 5*, 27–34.

Rogers, M. E. (1994). The science of unitary human beings: Current perspectives. *Nursing Science Quarterly, 7*, 33–35.

Sherwood, G. D. (1997). Metasynthesis of qualitative analysis of caring: Defining a therapeutic model of nursing. *Advanced Practice Nursing Quarterly, 3*(1), 32–42.

Smith, M. C., Turkel, M. C., & Wolf, Z. R. (2013). *Caring in nursing classics: An essential resource*. New York: Springer.

Smith, M. C. (1999). Caring and the science of unitary human beings. *Advances in Nursing Science, 21*(4), 14–28.

Smith, M. J. (1990). Caring: Ubiquitous or unique. *Nursing Science Quarterly, 3*, 54.

Smith, M. J., & Liehr, P. R. (2008). *Middle range theory for nursing* (2nd ed.). New York: Springer.

Swanson, K. M. (1991). Empirical development of a middle range theory of caring. *Nursing Research, 40*, 161–165.

Stevenson, J., & Tripp-Reimer, T. (Eds.). (1990, February). *Knowledge about care and caring: Proceedings of a Wingspread Conference.*. Kansas City, MO: American Academy of Nursing.

Watson, J. (1979). *Nursing: The philosophy and science of caring*. Boston: Little, Brown.

Watson, J. (1985). *Nursing: Human science and human care: A theory of nursing*. East Norwalk, CT: Appleton-Century-Crofts.

Watson, J. (2005). *Caring science as sacred science*. Philadelphia: F. A. Davis.

Watson, J. (2008). *Nursing: The philosophy and science of caring*. Boulder: University Press of Colorado.

Watson, J., & Smith, M. C. (2002). Caring science and the science of unitary human beings: a transtheoretical discourse for nursing knowledge development. *Journal of Advanced Nursing, 37*(5), 452–461.

Chapter *31*

Kristen Swanson's Theory of Caring

KRISTEN M. SWANSON

The Journey of Theory Development
Evolution of a Middle-Range
Theory of Caring
As It Progresses: Caring and Healing
The Journey Continues: The Couple's
Miscarriage Project
The Connection Between Caring
and Healing
Summary
References

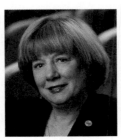

Kristen M. Swanson

In this latest revision, I have kept just about all of the content that was included in previous versions of this chapter and have added some updated materials. Most notably, I have added a bit of information about results of a recent randomized trial and some thoughts about the connections between the five caring categories and healing. For ease of reading, I have placed the new material in the section titled "As It Progresses: Caring and Healing."

The Journey of Theory Development

I have updated answers to questions posed by students and practitioners who have wanted to know more about the origins and progress of my research and theorizing on caring. I have situated myself as a nurse and as a woman so that the context of my scholarship, particularly as it pertains to caring, may be understood. I consider myself to be a second-generation nursing scholar. I was taught by first-generation nurse scientists (that is, nurses who received their doctoral education in fields other than nursing). My struggles for identity as a woman, nurse, and academician were, like many women of my era (the baby boomers), a somewhat organic and reflective process of self-discovery during a rapidly changing social scene (witness the women's and civil rights movements). Third-generation nursing scholars (those taught by nurses whose doctoral preparation is in nursing) may find my "yearning" somewhat odd. To those who might offer critique about the egocentricity of my pondering, I offer the defense of having been brought up during an era in which nurses dealt with such struggles as, "Are we a profession? Have we a unique body of knowledge? Are

521

we entitled to a space in the full (i.e., PhD-granting) academy?" I fully appreciate that questions of uniqueness and entitlement have not completely disappeared. Rather, they have faded as a backdrop to the weightier concerns of making a significant contribution to the health of all, keeping patients safe, educating and retaining a supply of nurses prepared to provide comprehensive patient-centered care to an aging population with increasingly complex and chronic health conditions, working collaboratively with consumers and other scientists and practitioners, practicing in a highly technological environment, embracing pluralism, and acknowledging the socially constructed power differentials associated with gender, race, poverty, and class.

Turning Point

In September 1982, I had no intention of studying caring; my goal was to study what it was like for women to miscarry. It was my dissertation chair, Dr. Jean Watson, who guided me toward the need to examine caring in the context of miscarriage. I am forever grateful for her foresight and wisdom.

I believe that the key to my program of research is that I have studied human responses to a specific health problem (miscarriage) in a framework (caring) that assumed from the start that a clinical therapeutic had to be defined. So, hand in glove, the research has constantly gone back and forth among "What's wrong and what can be done about it?" "What's right and how can it be strengthened?" "What's real to women (and most recently their mates) who miscarry and how might care be customized to that reality?" and "How can we measure the impact of caring-based interventions on couples' healing after miscarriage?" The back-and-forth nature of this line of inquiry has resulted in insights about the nature of miscarrying and caring that might otherwise have remained elusive.

Predoctoral Experiences

My preparation for studying caring-based therapeutics from a psychosocial perspective began in a cardiac critical care unit. After receiving my BSN at the University of Rhode

Island, I was wisely coached by Dean Barbara Tate to pursue a job at the brand-new University of Massachusetts Medical Center in Worcester. I was drawn to that institution because of the nursing administration's clear articulation of how nursing could and should be. It was exciting to be there from day one. We were all part of shaping the institutional vision for practice. It was phenomenal witnessing our collective capacity as nurses, physicians, respiratory therapists, and housekeepers to collaboratively make a profound difference in the lives of those we served. However, what I learned most from that experience came from the patients and their families. I realized that there was a powerful force that people could call on to get themselves through incredibly difficult times. Watching patients move into a space of total dependency and come out the other side restored was like witnessing a miracle unfold. Sitting with spouses in the waiting room while they entrusted the hearts (and lives) of their partners to the surgical team was awe-inspiring. It was encouraging to observe the inner reserves family members could call upon in order to hand over that which they could not control. I felt so privileged, humbled, and grateful to be invited into the spaces that patients and families created in order to endure their transitions through illness, recovery, and, in some instances, death.

After a year and a half at the University of Massachusetts, I was still a fairly new nurse and unclear what all of these emotional insights had to do with nursing. I saw them as something related to my spiritual beliefs and me, rather than about my profession. At that point, what mattered most to me as a nurse was my emerging technological savvy, understanding complex pathophysiological processes, and conveying that same information to others. Hence, I applied to graduate school. Approximately 2 years after completing my baccalaureate degree, I enrolled in the Adult Health and Illness Nursing program at the University of Pennsylvania.

While at Penn, I served as the student representative to the graduate curriculum committee and, as such, was invited to attend a 2-day retreat to revise the master's program. I distinctly remember listening in amazement to Dr. Jacqueline Fawcett as she spoke about health, environments, persons, and nursing; she claimed that these four concepts were the "stuff" that truly comprised nursing. I was hearing someone put voice to the inner stirrings I had kept to myself back in Massachusetts. It really impressed me that there were nurses who studied in such arenas. Shortly after the retreat, I received my MSN and was hired at Penn on a temporary basis to teach undergraduate medical-surgical nursing. I immediately enrolled as a postmaster's student in Dr. Fawcett's new course on the conceptual basis of nursing. It proved to be one of the best decisions I ever made, primarily because it helped me to figure out an answer to the constant question, "Why doesn't a smart girl like you enter medicine?" I finally knew that it was because nursing, a discipline that I was now starting to understand from an experiential, personal, and academic point of view, was more suited to my beliefs about serving people who were moving through the transitions of illness and wellness. It is safe to say that I was beginning to understand that my "gifts" lay not in the diagnosis and treatment of illness, but in the ability to understand and provide care to people as they lived through transitions of health, illness, and healing.

Doctoral Studies

Such insights made me want more; hence, I applied for doctoral studies and was accepted into the graduate program at the University of Colorado. My area of study, psychosocial nursing, emphasized such concepts as loss, stress, coping, caring, transactions, and person-environment fit. Having been supported by a National Institute of Mental Health traineeship, one requirement of our program was a hands-on experience with the process of undergoing a health promotion activity. Our faculty offered us the opportunity to carry out the requirement by enrolling ourselves in some type of support or behavior-change program of our own choosing. Four weeks into the same semester in which I was required to complete

that exercise, my first son was born. I decided to enroll in a cesarean birth support group as a way to deal with the class assignment and the unexpected circumstances surrounding his birth. It so happened that an obstetrician had been invited to speak to the group about miscarriage at the first meeting I ever attended. I found his lecture informative with regard to the incidence, diagnosis, prognosis, and medical management of spontaneous abortion. However, when the physician sat down and the women began to talk about their personal experiences with miscarriage and other forms of pregnancy loss, I was suddenly overwhelmed with the realization that there had been a one-in-five chance that I could have miscarried my son. Up until that point, it had never occurred to me that anything could have gone wrong with something so central to my life. I was 29 years old and believed, quite naively, that anything was possible if you were only willing to work hard at it.

Two profound insights came to me from that meeting. First, I was acutely aware of the American Nurses' Association (ANA) Social Policy Statement, that "[n]ursing is the diagnosis and treatment of human responses to actual and potential health problems" (ANA, 1980, p. 9). It was clear to me that whereas the physician had talked about the health problem of spontaneously aborting; the women were living the human response to miscarrying. Second, being in my last semester of course work, I was desperately in need of a dissertation topic. From that point on, it became clear to me that I wanted to understand what it was like to miscarry. The problem, of course, was that I was a critical care nurse and knew little about anything related to childbearing. An additional concern was that during the early 1980s, there was a strong emphasis on epistemology, ontology, and the methodologies to support multiple ways of understanding nursing as a human science; however, our methods courses were traditionally quantitative. Luckily, two mentors came my way. Dr. Jody Glittenberg, a nurse anthropologist, agreed to guide me through a predissertation pilot study of five women's experiences with miscarriage in order that I might learn about interpretive methods. Dr. Colleen Conway-Welch, a midwife, agreed to supervise my trek up the psychology-of-pregnancy learning curve.

Evolution of a Middle-Range Theory of Caring

Twenty women who had miscarried within 16 weeks of being interviewed agreed to participate in my phenomenological study of miscarriage and caring. These results have been published in greater depth elsewhere (Swanson, 1991; Swanson-Kauffman, 1985, 1986b).

Through that investigation, I proposed that caring consisted of five basic processes:

- **Knowing**
- **Being with**
- **Doing for**
- **Enabling**
- **Maintaining belief**

At that time, the definitions were fairly awkward and definitely tied to the context of miscarriage. In addition to naming those five categories, I also learned some important things about studying caring:

1. If you directly ask people to describe what caring means to them, you force them to speak so abstractly that it is hard to find any substance.
2. If you ask people to list behaviors or words that indicate that others care, you end up with a laundry list of "niceties."
3. If you ask people for detailed descriptions of what it was like for them to go through an event (i.e., miscarrying) and probe for their feelings and what the responses of others meant to them, it is much easier to unearth instances of people's caring and noncaring responses.
4. Although my intentions were to gather data, many of my informants thanked me for what I did for them.

As it turned out, a side effect of gathering detailed accounts of the informants' experiences was that women felt heard, understood, and attended-to in a nonjudgmental fashion.

In later years, this insight would become the grist for a series of caring-based intervention studies.

I have often been asked if my research was an application of Jean Watson's theory of human caring (Watson, 1979/1985, 1985/1988). Neither Dr. Watson nor I have ever seen my research program as an application of her work per se, but we do agree that the compatibility of our scholarship lends credence to both of our claims about the nature of caring. I have come to view her work as having provided a research tradition that other scientists and I have followed. Watson's research tradition asserts the following:

1. Caring is a central concept and way of relating.
2. Multiple methodologies are essential to understanding caring as a concept and way of relating.
3. It is important to study caring so that it may be better understood, consciously claimed, and intentionally acted upon to promote, maintain, and restore health and healing.

Refining the Theory Through Research

Postdoctoral Studies

Approximately 9 months after I completed the dissertation, my second son was born. He had a difficult start in life and spent a few days in the newborn intensive care unit (NICU). Through this event, I became aware that in my experience of childbearing loss (having a not-well child at birth), I, too, wished to receive the kinds of caring responses that my miscarriage informants had described. Hence, my next study, an individually awarded National Research Service Award postdoctoral fellowship (1985-1987), was inspired. With the mentorship of Dr. Kathryn Barnard, at the University of Washington, I spent over a year "hanging out" in the NICU at the University of Washington Medical Center (the staff gave me permission to acknowledge them and their practice site when discussing these findings).

The question I answered through the NICU phenomenological investigation was "What is it like to be a provider of care to vulnerable infants?" In addition to my observational data, I did in-depth interviews with some of the mothers, fathers, physicians, nurses, and other health-care professionals who were responsible for the care of five infants. The results of this investigation are published elsewhere (Swanson, 1990). With respect to understanding caring, there were three main findings:

1. Although the names of the caring categories were retained, they were grammatically edited and somewhat refined so as to be more generic.
2. It was evident that care in a complex context called upon providers to simultaneously balance *caring* (for self and other), *attaching* (to people and roles), *managing responsibilities* (self-, other-, and society-assigned), and *avoiding bad outcomes* (for self, other, and society).
3. What complicated everything was that each NICU provider (parent or professional) knew only a portion of the whole story surrounding the care of any one infant. Hence, there existed a strong potential for conflict stemming from misunderstanding others and second-guessing one another's motives. In many ways, this study foreshadowed much of the current emphasis in health care regarding communication, transparency, protecting the patient experience, and sustaining safety through avoidance of actions that result in bad outcomes.

While I was presenting the findings of the NICU study to a group of neonatologists, I received an interesting comment. One young physician told me that it was the caring and attaching parts of his vocation that brought him into medicine, yet he was primarily evaluated on and made accountable for the aspects of his job that dealt with managing responsibilities and avoiding bad outcomes. Such a schism in his role-performance expectations and evaluations had forced him to hold the caring and attaching parts of doing his job unexpressed. Unfortunately, it was his experience that those more person-centered aspects of his role could not be "stuffed" for too long

and that they often came hauntingly into his consciousness at 3 a.m. His remarks left me to wonder if the true origin of burnout is the failure of professions and care delivery systems to adequately value, monitor, and reward practitioners whose comprehensive care embraces *caring, attaching, managing responsibilities,* and *avoiding bad outcomes.*

Caring for Socially At-Risk Mothers

While I was still a postdoctoral scholar, Dr. Barnard invited me to present my research on caring to a group of five master's-prepared public health nurses. They became quite excited and claimed that the early draft of the caring model captured what it had been like for them to care for a group of socially at-risk new mothers. About 4 years before our meeting, these five advanced practice nurses had participated in Dr. Barnard's Clinical Nursing Models Project (Barnard et al., 1988). They had provided care to 68 socially at-risk expectant mothers for approximately 18 months (from shortly after conception until their babies were 12 months old). The purpose of the intervention had been to help the mothers take care of themselves and control of their lives so that they could ultimately take care of their babies. As I listened to these nurses endorsing the relevance of the caring model to their practice, I began to wonder what the mothers would have to say about the nurses. Would the mothers (1) remember the nurses and (2) describe the nurses as caring?

I was able to locate 8 of the original 68 mothers. They agreed to participate in a study of what it had been like to receive an intensive long-term advanced practice nursing intervention. The result of this phenomenological inquiry was that the caring categories were further refined and a definition of caring was finally derived.

Hence, as a result of the miscarriage, NICU, and high-risk mothers studies, I began to call the caring model a middle-range theory of caring. I **define caring as a "nurturing way of relating to a valued 'other' toward whom one feels a personal sense of commitment and responsibility"** (Swanson, 1991, p. 162). *Knowing,* striving to understand an event as it has meaning in the life of the other, involves avoiding assumptions, focusing on the one cared for, seeking cues, assessing thoroughly, and engaging the self of both the one caring and the one cared for. *Being with* means being emotionally present to the other. It includes being there, conveying availability, and sharing feelings while not burdening the one cared for. *Doing for* means doing for the other what he or she would do for himself or herself if it were at all possible. The therapeutic acts of doing for include anticipating needs, comforting, performing competently and skillfully, and protecting the other while preserving his or her dignity. *Enabling* means facilitating the other's passage through life transitions and unfamiliar events. It involves focusing on the event, informing, explaining, supporting, allowing and validating feelings, generating alternatives, thinking things through, and giving feedback. The last caring category is *maintaining belief,* which means sustaining faith in the other's capacity to get through an event or transition and face a future with meaning. This means believing in the other and holding him or her in esteem, maintaining a hope-filled attitude, offering realistic optimism, helping find meaning, and going the distance or standing by the one cared for, no matter how his or her situation may unfold (Swanson, 1991, 1993, 1999b, 1999c).

Developing and Testing Theory-Guided Practice Applications

As my postdoctoral studies were coming to an end, Dr. Barnard challenged me and claimed, "I think you've described caring long enough. It's time you did something with it!" We discussed how data-gathering interviews were often perceived by study participants as caring. Together we realized that, at the very least, open-ended interviews involved aspects of *knowing, being with,* and *maintaining belief.* We suspected that if *doing-for* and *enabling* interventions specifically focused on common human responses to health conditions were added, it would be possible to transform the

techniques of phenomenological data gathering into a caring intervention. That conversation ultimately led to my design of a caring-based counseling intervention for women who miscarried.

Soon, I was writing a proposal for a Solomon four-group randomized experimental design (Swanson, 1999b, 1999c). It was funded by the National Institute of Nursing Research and the University of Washington Center for Women's Health Research. The primary purpose of the study was to examine the effects of three 1-hour-long, caring-based counseling sessions on the integration of loss (miscarriage impact) and women's emotional well-being (moods and self-esteem) in the first year after miscarrying. Additional aims of the study were (1) to examine the effects of early versus delayed measurement and the passage of time on women's healing in the first year after loss and (2) to develop strategies to monitor caring as the intervention/process variable.

An assumption of the caring theory was that the recipient's well-being should be enhanced by receipt of caring from a provider informed about common human responses to a designated health problem (Swanson, 1993). Specifically, it was proposed that if women were guided through in-depth discussion of their experience and felt understood, informed, provided for, validated, and believed in, they would be better prepared to integrate miscarrying into their lives. The content for the three counseling sessions was derived from the miscarriage model, a phenomenologically derived model that summarized the common human responses to miscarriage (Swanson, 1999c; Swanson-Kauffman, 1983, 1985, 1986a, 1986b, 1988).

Women were randomly assigned to two levels of treatment (caring-based counseling and controls) and two levels of measurement (*early* = completion of outcome measures immediately, 6 weeks, 4 months, and 1 year postloss; or *delayed* = completion of outcome measures at 4 months and 1 year only). Counseling took place at 1, 5, and 11 weeks postloss. Analysis of variance was used to analyze treatment effects. Outcome measures included self-esteem (Rosenberg, 1965), overall emotional disturbance, anger, depression, anxiety, and confusion (McNair, Lorr, & Droppleman, 1981) and overall miscarriage impact, personal significance, devastating event, lost baby, and feeling of isolation (investigator-developed Impact of Miscarriage Scale).

A more detailed report of these findings is published elsewhere (Swanson, 1999b). There were 242 women enrolled, 185 of whom completed. Participants were within 5 weeks of loss at enrollment: 89% were partnered, 77% were employed, and 94% were Caucasian. Over 1 year, outcomes were as follows: (1) caring was effective in reducing overall emotional disturbance, anger, and depression and (2) with the passage of time, women attributed less personal significance to miscarrying and realized increased self-esteem and decreased anxiety, depression, anger, and confusion.

In summary, the Miscarriage Caring Project provided evidence that, although time had a healing effect on women after miscarrying, caring did make a difference in the amount of anger, depression, and overall disturbed moods that women experienced after miscarriage. This study was unique in that it employed a clinical research model to determine whether or not caring made a difference. I believe that its greatest strength lies in the fact that the intervention was based both on an empirically derived understanding of what it is like to miscarry and on a conscientious attempt to enact caring in counseling women through their loss. The greatest limitation of that study is that I derived the caring theory (developed from the intervention) and conducted most of the counseling sessions. Hence, it is unknown whether similar results would be derived under different circumstances. My work is further limited by the lack of diversity in my research participants. Over the years, I have predominantly worked with middle-class, married, educated, Caucasian women. I, as well as others, must make a concerted effort to examine what it is like for diverse groups of men and women to experience both miscarriage and caring.

Monitoring caring as an intervention variable was the second specific aim of the Miscarriage Caring Project. Three strategies were used to document that, as claimed, caring had occurred. First, approximately 10% of the intervention sessions were transcribed. Analysis was done by research associate Katherine Klaich, RN, PhD. As one of the counselors in the study, she found she could not approach analysis of the transcripts naively—that is, with no preconceived notions, as would be expected in the conduct of phenomenologic analysis. Hence, she employed both deductive and inductive content analytic techniques to render the transcribed counseling sessions meaningful. She began with the broad question, "Is there evidence of caring as defined by Swanson [1991] on the part of the nurse counselors?" The unit of analysis was each emic phrase that was used by the nurse counselor. Phrases were coded for which (if any) of the five caring processes were represented by the emic utterances. Each counselor statement was then further coded for which subcategory of the five processes was represented by the phrase. Twenty-nine subcategories of the five major processes were defined. With few exceptions (social chitchat), every therapeutic utterance of the nurse counselor could be accounted for by one of the subcategories.

The second way in which caring was monitored was through the completion of paper-and-pencil measures. Before each session, the counselor completed a Profile of Mood States (McNair et al., 1981) to document her presession moods (thus enabling examination of the association between counselor presession mood and self or client postsession ratings of caring). After each session, women were asked to complete Caring Professional Scale (Swanson, 2002). Having been left alone to complete the measure, women were asked to place the evaluations in a sealed envelope. In the meantime, in another room, the counselor wrote out her counseling notes and completed the Counselor Rating Scale, a brief five-item rating of how well the session went.

The Caring Professional Scale originally consisted of 18 items on a 5-point Likert-type scale. It was developed through the Miscarriage

Caring Project and was completed by participants in order to rate the nurse counselors who conducted the intervention and to evaluate the nurses, physicians, or midwives who took care of the women at the time of their miscarriage. The items included the following: "Was the health-care provider that just took care of you understanding, informative, aware of your feelings, centered on you?" The response set ranged from 1 (*yes, definitely*) to 5 (*not at all*). The items were derived from the caring theory. Three negatively worded items (abrupt, emotionally distant, and insulting) were dropped due to minimal variability across all of the data sets. For the counselors at 1, 5, and 11 weeks postloss, Cronbach alphas were .80, .95, and .90 (sample sizes for the counselor reliability estimates were 80, 87, and 76). The lower reliability estimates were because the counselors' caring professional scores were consistently high and lacked variability (mean item scores ranged from 4.52 to 5.0).

Noteworthy findings include the following:

1. Each counselor had a full range of presession feelings, and those feelings/moods were, as might be expected, highly intercorrelated.
2. For the most part, counselor presession mood was not associated with postsession evaluations.
3. The caring professional scores were extremely high for both counselors, indicating that, overall, the clients were pleased with what they received and, as claimed, caring was "delivered" and "received."
4. One of the counselors was a psychiatric nurse by background. She knew little about miscarriage before participating in this study and had recently experienced a death in her family. The only time her presession moods (in this case, depression and confusion) were significantly associated ($p \leq .05$) with any of the postsession ratings (both client caring professional score and counselor self-rating) was in Session I. During Session I, women discussed in-depth what the actual events of miscarrying felt like. It is possible that the counselor was so touched by and caught up in the sadness of the stories that her own vulnerabilities were a bit less veiled.
5. Session II, in which the two topics addressed were relationship oriented (who the woman could share her loss with and what it felt like to go out in public as a woman who had miscarried), was the only session in which the other counselor's vulnerabilities came through. This counselor had just gone through a divorce. Her postsession self-evaluation was significantly associated with her presession moods: depression ($p \leq .05$) and low vigor, confusion, fatigue, and tension (all at $p \leq .01$). Also, most notably, there was an association between this counselor's presession tension and clients' postsession Caring Professional scores ($p \leq .05$).

Clarifying Caring Through Literary Meta-analysis

I also conducted an in-depth review of the literature. This literary meta-analysis is published elsewhere (Swanson, 1999a). Approximately 130 data-based publications on caring were reviewed for that state-of-the-science paper. Through it I developed a framework for discourse about caring knowledge in nursing. Proposed were five domains (or levels) of knowledge about caring in nursing. I believe that these domains are hierarchical and that studies conducted at any one domain (e.g., Level III) assume the presence of all previous domains (e.g., Levels I and II). The first domain includes descriptions of the capacities or characteristics of caring persons. Level II deals with the concerns and/or commitments that lead to caring actions. These are the values nurses hold that lead them to practice in a caring manner. Level III describes the conditions (nurse, patient, and organizational factors) that enhance or diminish the likelihood of caring occurring. Level IV summarizes caring actions. This summary consisted of two parts. In the first part, a meta-analysis of 18 quantitative studies of caring actions was performed. It was demonstrated that the top five caring behaviors valued by patients were that the nurse (1) helps the patient to feel confident that adequate care was provided, (2) knows how to give shots and manage equipment, (3) gets to know the patient as a person, (4) treats the patient with respect, and (5) puts the patient first, no matter what. By contrast, the top five caring behaviors valued by nurses were (1) listens to the patient, (2) allows expression of feelings, (3) touches when comforting is needed, (4) perceives the patient's needs, and (5) realizes the patient knows him- or herself best. The second part of the caring actions summary was a review of 67 interpretive studies of how caring is expressed (the total number of participants was 2314). These qualitative studies were fully able to be classified under Swanson's caring processes. The last domain was labeled "consequences." These are the intentional and unintentional outcomes of caring and noncaring for patient and provider. In summary, this literary meta-analysis clarified what "caring" means, as the term is used in nursing, and validated the generalizability or transferability of Swanson's caring theory beyond the perinatal contexts from which it was originally derived.

From Theory and Research Back to Practice

In 2004, I was honored to be named a Robert Wood Johnson Foundation (RWJF) Executive Nurse Fellow. When I wrote the application, I set the goal to "leave the comfort of academia" and to make myself learn more about the world of nursing practice. I realized that if my work on caring was going to have relevance to nursing I needed to understand better what it was like to practice as a nurse in today's health-care environment. I was delighted that Susan Grant (at that time Vice President for Patient Care at the University of Washington Medical Center) agreed to mentor me. My personal mantra was that I wanted to "help create the conditions that enable nurses to work in accordance with their core values of caring, healing, and keeping their patients safe." The journey I took as an executive nurse fellow was extremely rewarding and, at the same time, daunting. The world of health care is undergoing rapid change. The vocabulary, pace, politics, technologies,

locations, and challenges of health care are changing at warp speed. I learned that in the healthiest practice settings caring must take place at the organizational level and at the point of care. Institutional caring practices take the form of continuous quality improvements that strive to achieve the Institute of Medicine's (2001) call for health care that is delivered in a safe, efficient, effective, timely, equitable, and patient-centered manner. Providers experience the rewards of knowing their work matters when they practice in organizations that are driven to constantly enhance safe, effective, and compassionate care for patients, families, and employees. As a result of lessons learned through the RWJF fellowship, I now routinely consult with health-care facilities where the mission is to create and sustain a culture of caring.

As It Progresses: Caring and Healing

The Journey Continues: The Couple's Miscarriage Project

In 2009, we completed a National Institutes of Health/National Institute of Nursing Research–funded randomized controlled trial of the effectiveness of three caring-based interventions against a control condition in enhancing the resolution of grief and depression for men and women during the first year after miscarriage. This study included four treatment arms: nurse caring (three nurse counseling sessions), self-caring (three home-delivered videotapes and journals), combined caring (one nurse counseling plus three videotapes and journals), and no intervention (control). All intervention materials were developed based on the Miscarriage Model and the Swanson Caring Theory. We enrolled and randomized 341 couples. Intervention findings are reported in depth elsewhere (Swanson, Chen, Graham, Wojnar, & Petras, 2009) and briefly summarized here. We learned that whereas resolution of women's grief was enhanced through any of our three caring-based interventions, resolution of men's grief was only helped by the combined and nurse-caring interventions. Women's depression resolved faster when they received the nurse caring intervention. Men's depression was not affected by receipt of three counseling sessions (there was no significant difference from the control group) and appeared to be slowed by receipt of the combined caring or self-caring interventions (their resolution of depression took longer than the control group). Additional research needs to be done to identify who is most likely to experience depression during the first year after miscarriage so that the right intervention may be offered.

The Connection Between Caring and Healing

It is hard to believe that the caring model was first proposed almost 30 years ago. There are now scientists, practitioners, and educators around the world who are applying the caring theory in their work. Reflecting back on the work we did to understand how couples evaluated our caring interventions, considering the lessons learned through consulting with nurses and other providers seeking to change the culture of care, and integrating the writings and findings of others who have explored the caring processes and their impact, I now propose that there are some logical links between the caring processes and healing outcomes. Using the language of provider to mean the one who is practicing caring and recipient to mean the one who is receiving caring, I offer the following model (Fig. 31-1) and thoughts about the connections between the caring processes and experiences of healing.

When providers strive to understand the recipient's experience (e.g., *knowing*), the recipient has the feeling of not only being *understood* but, possibly, also understanding their own experiences more fully. When the provider is able to *be with* the recipient through times of sorrow, frustration, suffering, and joy, the recipient feels *valued* by the provider and perceives that they and their experiences matter to the provider. When the provider seeks to *do for* the recipient what he or she would do independently if they had the knowledge, time, energy, capacity, or skills to do so, the recipient feels *safe and comforted*. When the provider enables the other's capacity to manage a situation by providing information, validation, and support, the recipient feels *capable* to get through the challenge before them. Lastly, and at the very core of caring, when the provider *maintains belief* in the other's capacity to come through an event or transition and face a future with meaning, the recipient feels *hopeful* (as opposed to hopeless). This hope does not mean that sickness, sorrow, fear, or loss will not unfold as it must; rather, it is hope that the recipient will be able to get through the situation and find meaning and purpose in whatever comes next. In summary, when a provider takes the time to *know, be with, do for, enable, and maintain belief* in the other, the recipient feels a sense of wholeness - that is they feel *understood, valued, safe and comforted, capable, and hopeful* for the future. I believe caring and healing is possible whenever a provider acts with the recipient's best interests

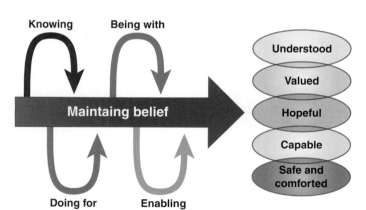

Fig 31 • 1 Swanson theory of caring and healing. *(Copyright © Kristen N. Swanson, 2013.)*

in mind. Caring can be enacted at the bedside, in the community, in the boardroom, or in the legislature. The measure of caring's worth is determined by whether it leads to the recipient feeling seen and intact (or enhanced) versus diminished and dismissed.

References

American Nurses' Association (ANA). (1980). *Nursing: A social policy statement.* Kansas City, MO: American Nurses' Association.

Barnard, K. E., Magyary, D., Sumner, G., Booth, C. L., Mitchell, S. K., & Spieker, S. (1988). Prevention of parenting alterations for women with low social support. *Psychiatry, 51,* 248-253.

Institute of Medicine of the National Academies. (2001). *Crossing the quality chasm: A new health system for the 21st century* (report brief). Retrieved January 29, 2008, from www.iom.edu/CMS/8089/5432/27184.aspx

McNair, D. M., Lorr, M., & Droppleman, L. F. (1981). *Profile of mood states: Manual.* San Diego, CA: Educational and Industrial Testing Service.

Rosenberg, M. (1965). *Society and the adolescent self-image.* Princeton, NJ: Princeton University Press.

Swanson, K. M. (1990). Providing care in the NICU: Sometimes an act of love. *Advances in Nursing Science, 13*(1), 60-73.

Swanson, K. M. (1991). Empirical development of a middle-range theory of caring. *Nursing Research, 40,* 161-166.

Swanson, K. M. (1993). Nursing as informed caring for the well-being of others. *Image, 25,* 352-357.

Swanson, K. M. (1999a). What's known about caring in nursing science: A literary meta-analysis. In: A. S. Hinshaw, S. Feetham, & J. Shaver (Eds)., *Handbook of clinical nursing research.* Thousand Oaks, CA: Sage.

Swanson, K. M. (1999b). The effects of caring, measurement, and time on miscarriage impact and women's well-being in the first year subsequent to loss. *Nursing Research, 48,* 6, 288-298.

Swanson, K. M. (1999c). Research-based practice with women who miscarry. *Image: Journal of Nursing Scholarship, 31,* 4, 339-345.

Swanson, K. M. (2002). Caring Profession Scale. In: J. Watson (Ed.), *Assessing and measuring caring in nursing and health science.* New York: Springer.

Swanson, K. M., Chen, H. T., Graham, J. C., Wojnar, D. M., & Petras, A. (2009). Resolution of depression and grief during the first year after miscarriage: A randomized controlled clinical trial of couples-focused interventions. *Journal Women's Health and Gender-based Medicine, 18*(8), 1245-1257. Retrieved from www.liebertonline.com/doi/abs/10.1089/jwh.2008.1202

Swanson-Kauffman, K. M. (1986a). A combined qualitative methodology for nursing research. *Advances in Nursing Science, 8*(3), 58-69.

Swanson-Kauffman, K. M. (1986b). Caring in the instance of unexpected early pregnancy loss. *Topics in Clinical Nursing, 8*(2), 37-46.

Swanson-Kauffman, K. M. (1985). Miscarriage: A new understanding of the mother's experience. *Proceedings of the 50th anniversary celebration of the University of Pennsylvania School of Nursing,* 63-78.

Swanson-Kauffman, K. M. (1988). The caring needs of women who miscarry. In M. M. Leininger (Ed.), *Care: Discovery and uses in clinical and community nursing.* Detroit, MI: Wayne State University Press.

Swanson-Kauffman, K. M. (1983). *The unborn one: The human experience of miscarriage.* Doctoral dissertation, University of Colorado Health Sciences Center, 1983. *Dissertation Abstracts International, 43,* AAT8404456.

Watson, M. J. (1985/1988). *Nursing: Human science and human care.* New York: National League for Nursing Press.

Watson, M. J. (1979/1985). *Nursing: The philosophy and science of caring.* Boulder, CO: Colorado Associated Press.

Index

Note: Page numbers followed by *f* refer to figures; page numbers followed by *t* refer to tables; page numbers followed by *b* refer to boxes.

A

Adaptation
  Johnson Behavioral System Model, 91–92
  Roy model of. *See* Roy Adaptation Model
Adaptive potential, in Modeling and Role-Modeling theory, 191–192, 192*f*
Administration
  Johnson Behavioral System Model application to, 99–100
  Neuman Systems Model application to, 176
Aesthetic knowing, 29, 214–215
Affiliation, 190–191
Aging
  in Theory of Accelerating Evolution, 240–241
  in Theory of Goal Attainment, 142
American Holistic Nurses Association, 210
Anger, in morbid grief, 194
Anti-coagulants, 45
Arousal, stress-related, 192, 192*f*
Assessing and Measuring Caring in Nursing and Health Sciences (Watson), 322
Attending Caring Team, 334–337
Attending Nurse Caring Model, 332–334
Awareness
  in nursing theory selection, 28
  in Quality Caring Model, 398
  in Theory of Health as Expanding Consciousness, 283

B

Barrett, Elizabeth Ann Manhart, 497–498. *See also* Theory of Power as Knowing Participation in Change
Barry, Charlotte D., 435–436. *See also* Community Nursing Practice Model
Basic Principles of Nursing Care (Henderson), 62
Bearing witness, 223
Behavioral System Model. *See* Johnson Behavioral System Model
Beliefs, 6, 24. *See also* Values
Bentov, Itzhak, 281, 282, 284
Boykin, Anne, 341–342. *See also* Nursing as Caring Theory
Bureaucracy, 466–468. *See also* Theory of Bureaucratic Caring

C

Care, Cure, and Core Model, 59–61, 59*f*
  practice application of, 63
Care/caring, 5
  Boykin and Schoenhofer's theory of. *See* Nursing as Caring Theory
  bureaucratic. *See* Theory of Bureaucratic Caring
  culture. *See* Theory of Culture Care Diversity and Universality
  Duffy's model of. *See* Quality Caring Model
  in Hall's model of nursing, 59*f*, 60
  in Human-to-Human Relationship Model, 76–77
  Leininger's theory of. *See* Theory of Culture Care Diversity and Universality
  Locsin's theory of. *See* Technological Competency as Caring
  in Nightingale's work, 49
  Smith's theory of. *See* Theory of Unitary Caring
  Swanson's theory of. *See* Theory of Caring
  Watson's theory of. *See* Theory of Human Caring
Caring Professional Scale, 527–528
Caring Science as Sacred Science (Watson), 322
Caritas nursing, 322, 323–324
Change, 12–13
  transition triggers, 364*f*, 365–366, 372–373
Choice points, in Theory of Health as Expanding Consciousness, 288–290, 289*f*, 290*f*
Christian feminist, 47
Client, 5
Client-nurse encounter, 5. *See also* Dynamic Nurse-Patient Relationship Theory; Nurse-patient/client relationship; Nurse-Patient Relationship Theory
Clinical Nursing: A Helping Art (Wiedenbach), 61–62
Collaborative care, 312–313
Collected Works of Florence Nightingale, 37, 49
Comfort Theory, 382–390
  application of, 385–389
  best policy in, 385, 388–389
  best practices in, 385, 388
  care plans in, 385
  coaching in, 385
  Comfort Contract in, 392
  comfort definition in, 384
  comfort interventions in, 384
  concepts of, 383–384, 384*f*
  contexts in, 382
  ease in, 382
  electronic data base in, 388–389
  health care needs in, 384–385
  health-seeking behaviors in, 384–385
  institutional advocacy in, 386–387
  institutional awards in, 387
  institutional integrity in, 385
  intention in, 386
  intervening variables in, 384
  nursing practice in, 386, 388
  practice exemplar of, 389–390
  relief in, 382

taxonomic structure of, 382–383, 383*f*
technical interventions in, 385
transcendence in, 382
value-added outcomes in, 386
wow moments in, 386
Comfort Theory and Practice (Kolcaba), 381
Communication
    integral, 224
    nonverbal, 198
    nursing discipline, 6
Community
    Community Nursing Practice Model, 437–438,
        439
    Humanbecoming Paradigm, 271–273
    Self-Care Deficit Theory, 117
    Theory of Health as Expanding Consciousness,
        294–295
Community Nursing Practice Model, 436–446
    application of, 441–442, 442*t*–445*t*
    community in, 437–438, 439
    core services in, 439, 440
    development of, 436
    in education, 441–442
    environment in, 438
    evaluation and, 440
    first circle services in, 439, 440
    foundations of, 436
    nursing in, 437
    person in, 437, 439
    policy development and, 439–440
    practice exemplar of, 445
    second circle services in, 439–440
    services in, 438–440, 439*f*
    third circle services in, 440
Compassion, 223
Complexity theory, 468–469
Concept development, 135–136
Conceptual models, 13
    analysis of, 31
    evaluation of, 31
Conceptual structures, of nursing discipline, 5–6
Conscious dying, 222
Consciousness. *See* Theory of Health as Expanding
        Consciousness
Contagionism, 45
Couple's Miscarriage Project, 529–530
*Creating a Caring Science Curriculum: Emancipatory
        Pedagogies* (Hills and Watson), 322
Crimean War, 40–44, 41*f*, 43*f*
Critical points, 368
Cultural feminism, 47
Culture. *See also* Theory of Culture Care Diversity and
        Universality
    nursing theory and, 15–16
    organization, 466–468
    in Theory of Goal Attainment, 141
    in Theory of Health as Expanding Consciousness,
        291
Curiosity, 20

D
Death
    grieving response to, 192–194, 194*t*
    in Theory of Integral Nursing, 222
Debriefing, 369
Developmental processes
    in Modeling and Role-Modeling theory, 194–195,
        195*t*
    in Theory of Integral Nursing, 211, 217–218, 220*f*
Disease, origin of, 45
Dissipative structures, theory of, 288, 289*f*
Diversity of Human Field Pattern Scale, 251
Domain, 4–5
Dossey, Barbara, 207–208. *See also* Theory of Integral
        Nursing
Dream Experience Scale, 251
Drives, 189–190, 190*t*
Duffy, Joanne, 393–394. *See also* Quality Caring Model
Dying
    conscious, 222
    in Theory of Integral Nursing, 222
*Dynamic Nurse-Patient Relationship: Function, Process and
        Principles, The* (Orlando), 82
Dynamic Nurse-Patient Relationship Theory, 82
    practice applications of, 82–84

E
Education, 6
    Community Nursing Practice Model, 441–442
    of Florence Nightingale, 38–39
    Humanbecoming Paradigm and, 273
    Johnson Behavioral System Model and, 99
    Neuman Systems Model and, 175–176
    on nurse-patient relationship, 69
    Nursing as Caring Theory and, 350
    theory-guided nursing practice and, 33
    Theory of Bureaucratic Caring and, 477
    Theory of Culture Care Diversity and Universality
        and, 313
    Theory of Goal Attainment and, 140
    Theory of Human Caring and, 335
    Theory of Integral Nursing and, 225
    Transitions Theory and, 371
Emancipation, of women, 47
Emancipatory knowing, 29–30
Empathy, in Human-to-Human Relationship Model,
        78
Energyspirit, 244
Environment, 5
    Community Nursing Practice Model, 438
    Johnson Behavioral System Model, 93, 95–96
    Modeling and Role-Modeling Theory, 189–191
    Neuman Systems Model, 171–172, 171*f*
    Nightingale model, 45–46
    Quality Caring Model, 439
    Roy Adaptation Model, 158
    Theory of Integral Nursing, 213–214, 213*f*, 220*f*, 224
Epigenesis, in Modeling and Role-Modeling theory,
        195

Equanimity, 223
Equilibrium, 192, 192*f*
Erickson, Helen, 185–186. *See also* Modeling and
    Role-Modeling Theory
Ethical knowing, 29
Ethnonursing, 304. *See also* Theory of Culture Care
    Diversity and Universality
Evidence-based practice, 144

F

Family Health Theory, 139
Feminism
    cultural, 47
    in Nightingale's caring, 46–48
    in Transitions Theory, 363
Fermentation, 45
*Florence Nightingale Today: Healing, Leadership, Global
    Action* (ANA), 37
Four-quadrants perspective, 215–220, 215*f*, 216*f*, 220*f*
    collective exterior ("Its"), 216*f*, 217, 219, 220*f*, 224
    collective interior ("We"), 216*f*, 217, 219, 220*f*,
        222–224
    individual exterior ("It"), 216*f*, 217, 219, 220*f*, 224
    individual interior ("I"), 216, 216*f*, 219, 220*f*, 222
Functional performance mechanisms, 485–486, 486*f*

G

General System Theory, 134
Generating Middle Range Theory: Evidence for Practice
    (Roy), 154
Geotranscendance change, 486*f*, 489–491
Goal attainment. *See* Theory of Goal Attainment
Goal Attainment Scale, 137
Grand theories, 13
    analysis of, 31
    evaluation of, 31
    interactive-integrative. *See* Johnson Behavioral System
        Model; Modeling and Role-Modeling Theory;
        Neuman Systems Model; Roy Adaptation
        Model; Self-Care Deficit Theory; Theory of Goal
        Attainment; Theory of Integral Nursing
    unitary-transformative. *See* Paradigm Science of
        Unitary Human Beings; Theory of Health as
        Expanding
Grieving response, 192–194, 193*f*, 194*t*
Growth needs, 192

H

Hall, Lydia, 56–57. *See also* Care, Cure, and Core Model
Healing
    Quality Caring Model, 399
    Science of Unitary Human Beings, 243
    Theory of Caring, 530–531, 530*f*
    Theory of Human Caring, 328
    Theory of Integral Nursing, 212, 212*f*, 213*f*, 221
Health, 5
    Johnson Behavioral System Model, 96–97
    Modeling and Role-Modeling theory, 191

Neuman Systems Model, 172
Roy Adaptation Model, 158–159
Theory of Goal Attainment, 143
Theory of Integral Nursing, 213, 213*f*, 220*f*, 224
Health Goal Attainment instrument, 139
Health patterning, 500–501
    modalities, 501–503
Henderson, Virginia, 56
    basic nursing care components of, 58–59, 63–64
    nursing definition of, 58–59, 62–63
Hierarchy, 92
Holistic person, in Modeling and Role-Modeling
    theory, 190–191, 197
Home, family, 46–48
Homeorrhesis, 91
Homo pandimensionalis, 244
Honesty, 20
Hope, 77
Humanbecoming Paradigm, 264–274
    art of, 269–273
    change in, 268
    community settings of, 271–273
    eighty/twenty (80/20) model of, 272
    language in, 268
    in nursing education, 285
    nursing in, 264–265
    nursing practice in, 270, 271–273
    parish nursing in, 272–273
    philosophical assumptions of, 266–267
    postulates of, 267–268
    principles of, 267–268
    reality construction in, 268
    relating in, 268
    research in, 268–269
    resources on, 273
    true presence in, 269–270
Human Becoming School of Thought, The (Parse), 266
Human Field Image Metaphor Scale, 252
Human Field Motion Test, 251
Human-to-Human Relationship Model, 76–79
    practice applications of, 79
Humanuniverse, 266
Hygiene, Nightingale on, 47
Hypnotherapeutic techniques, 198

I

Imagination, 4
Impoverishment, stress-related, 192, 192*f*
Individuation, 190–191
Instincts, 189–190, 190*t*
Integral Nursing. *See* Theory of Integral Nursing
Intention
    Comfort Theory, 386
    Nursing as Caring Theory, 343
    Technological Competency as Caring, 455–456
    Theory of Integral Nursing, 211, 224
    Theory of Unitary Caring, 511, 515
Intentional dialogue, in Story Theory, 424
Intentionality, in Science of Unitary Human Beings, 244

Interactive-integrative paradigm, 12
Interdisciplinary practice, 20
International Caritas Consortium, 330
International Research on Caritas as Healing (Nelson and
    Watson), 322
Interpersonal Relations in Nursing (Peplau), 67
Interpretation, in Human-to-Human Relationship
    Model, 78
Intervention in Psychiatric Nursing (Travelbee), 78
Interventions
    Comfort Theory, 385–386
    Johnson Behavioral System Model, 97–98
    Modeling and Role-Modeling theory, 186, 187*t*
    Neuman Systems Model, 173–174
    Theory of Health as Expanding Consciousness,
        292
    Transitions Theory, 364*f*, 367–369, 377
Intrapsychic factors, 486
Intuition, 190, 224

J

Johnson, Dorothy, 89–90. *See also* Johnson Behavioral
    System Model
Johnson Behavioral System Model, 90–98
    achievement subsystem in, 93*t*
    action in, 95
    in administration, 99–100
    affiliative subsystem in, 93*t*
    aggressive/protective subsystem in, 93*t*
    applications of, 98–102
    behavioral set in, 95
    choice in, 95
    concepts of, 92–98
    conceptual set in, 95
    core principles of, 90–92
    dependency subsystem in, 93*t*
    diagnostic classifications in, 97
    dialectical contradiction principle of, 92
    in education, 99
    eliminative subsystem in, 93*t*
    environment in, 95–96
    functional requirements in, 95
    goal in, 95
    health in, 96–97
    hierarchic interaction principle of, 92
    imbalance and instability in, 96
    ingestive subsystem in, 94*t*
    nursing interventions in, 97–98
    nursing process in, 97–98
    person in, 92, 94
    practice exemplar of, 100–102
    reorganization principle of, 91–92
    research on, 98–99, 99*b*
    restorative system in, 94*t*
    set point in, 91
    sexual system in, 94*t*
    stabilization principle of, 91
    subsystems in, 94–95, 108*t*–109*t*
    wholeness and order principle of, 90–91
Justice-making, 38

K

King, Imogene M., 133–134. *See also* Theory of Goal
    Attainment
Knowing, 29
    aesthetic, 29, 214–215, 214*f*
    emancipatory, 29
    empirical, 214, 214*f*
    ethical, 29, 214*f*, 215
    paranormal, 241–242
    personal, 29, 214, 214*f*
    sociopolitical, 214*f*, 215
    Technological Competency as Caring, 450–457,
        454*f*
    Theory of Integral Nursing, 214–215, 214*f*, 220,
        220*f*
Knowledge, structure of, 11–14
Kolcaba, Katherine, 381–382. *See also* Comfort Theory
Kuhn, Thomas , 12

L

Language, 6
    grammatical persons of, 215–216
Legitimate nursing, 108, 114
Leininger, Madeleine, 303–304. *See also* Theory of
    Culture Care Diversity and Universality
Liehr, Patricia, 423. *See also* Story Theory
Life orientation, need satisfaction and, 194
Listening, deep, 223
Literature, 6. *See also* Research
    meta-analysis of, 528–529
Living a Caring-based Program (Boykin), 341
Locsin, Rozzano C., 449–450. *See also* Technological
    Competency as Caring
Loeb Center for Nursing and Rehabilitation, 63

M

Man-Living-Health: A Theory of Nursing (Parse), 266
Marriage, 46
Meaning, 222–224
    grasping of, 248
    in Nursing as Caring Theory, 344–346
    philosophical, 222
    psychological, 222
    in Quality Caring Model, 401
    spiritual, 222
    in Theory of Health as Expanding Consciousness,
        286–288
Medical model, 25
Meeting the Realities in Clinical Teaching (Wiedenbach),
    57
Meleis, Afaf I., 50, 361–362. *See also* Transitions
    Theory
Metaparadigm, 5
    in Theory of Integral Nursing, 213–214, 213*f*
Middle-range theories, 13, 31–32, 138. *See also* Comfort
    Theory; Community Nursing Practice Model;
    Quality Caring Model; Story Theory;
    Technological Competency as Caring; Theory of
    Bureaucratic Caring; Theory of Caring; Theory of

Power as Knowing Participation in Change;
Theory of Self-Transcendence; Theory of
Successful Aging; Theory of Unitary Caring;
Transitions Theory
  analysis of, 31
  development of, 138
  evaluation of, 31–32
Mindfulness, 222
Miscarriage Caring Project, 526–528
Modeling and Role-Modeling Theory, 186–204
  adaptive potential in, 191–192, 192*f*
  data collection in, 187, 188*t*
  data interpretation in, 197–198
  data processing in, 197–198
  developmental processes in, 194–195, 195*t*
  drives in, 189–190, 190*t*
  environment in, 189–191
  epigenesis in, 195
  health in, 191
  human needs in, 192–194, 193*f*
  hypnotherapeutic techniques in, 198
  instincts in, 189–190, 190*t*
  intervention aims and goals in, 186, 187*t*
  modeling process in, 187, 188*t*
  nursing in, 191
  person in, 189–191, 190*t*, 197
  philosophical assumptions in, 188–191
  practice applications of, 198–201, 199*t*–201*t*
  practice exemplars of, 202–204
  proactive nursing care in, 198
  role-modeling process in, 187–188
  sequential development in, 195
  social justice in, 191
  theoretical constructs in, 191–196, 192*f*, 193*f*
  theoretical linkages in, 195–196
  theoretical propositions in, 187–188, 188*t*
  trusting-functional relationship in, 190, 196–197,
    196*t*
Morbid grief, 194

N

Narrative. *See* Story Theory
Narrative means to sober ends (Diamond), 423
*Narrative Medicine: The Use of History and Story in the
    Healing Process* (Mehl-Madrona), 423
Nature of Nursing, The (Henderson), 62
Needs
  Comfort Theory, 384–385
  growth, 192
  life orientation and, 194
  Modeling and Role-Modeling theory, 192–194, 193*f*
  Quality Caring Model, 399–400
Neuman, Betty, 165–166. *See also* Neuman Systems
    Model
Neuman Systems Model, 166–181, 168*f*
  in administration, 176
  archive for, 179
  client-client system in, 168*f*, 169–171, 169*f*
  client variables in, 169*f*, 170–171

  concepts of, 167
  created environment in, 172
  in education, 175–176
  environment in, 171–172, 171*f*
  flexible line of defense in, 168*f*, 169, 169*f*, 171*f*
  health in, 172
  lines of resistance in, 168*f*, 169–170, 169*f*, 171*f*
  normal line of defense in, 168*f*, 169, 169*f*, 171*f*
  nursing process in, 172–174, 173*f*
  practice applications of, 174–175, 178–179
  practice exemplar of, 179–181
  prevention intervention in, 173–174
  spirituality in, 170–171
  website for, 179
Newman, Margaret, 279–281. *See also* Theory of Health
    as Expanding Consciousness
NICU study, 524–525
Nightingale, Florence, 37–53, 38*f*, 44*f*
  assumptions of, 50
  biographies of, 37
  Crimean War nursing of, 40–44, 41*f*, 43*f*
  early life of, 38–39
  education of, 38–39, 44–45
  feminist context of, 46–48
  medical milieu of, 44–46
  nurse definition for, 51
  nursing definition for, 4, 51, 52*f*
  nursing ideas of, 48–52
  nursing's goal for, 50–51
  patient for, 51
  spirituality of, 39–40, 43
  Theory of Integral Nursing and, 209
  travel by, 39
  21st century legacy of, 52–53
Non-nursing functions, 62
Notes on Nursing: What It Is and What It Is Not
    (Nightingale), 4, 38, 46, 49
Not knowing, 214*f*, 215
Nurse-patient/client relationship. *See also* Nurse-Patient
    Relationship Theory
  Nursing as Caring Theory, 344
  Orlando's theory of, 82–84
  Quality Caring Model, 397–399, 397*f*
  Theory of Goal Attainment, 140
  Theory of Health as Expanding Consciousness,
    290–292
  Theory of Human Caring, 326–327
  Travelbee's theory of, 76–79
Nurse-Patient Relationship Theory, 67–74
  communication skills in, 70
  components of, 69
  listening skills in, 69–70
  orientation phase of, 70–71
  phases of, 70–71
  practice exemplar on, 73–74
  research on, 71–72
  resolution phase of, 71
  self-awareness in, 69
  supervisory education for, 69
  working phase of, 71

Nurse Performance Goal Attainment, 139
Nurse presence
   Humanbecoming Paradigm, 269–270
   Nursing as Caring Theory, 344
   Theory of Health as Expanding Consciousness, 285–286
   Theory of Integral Nursing, 222
Nursing, 5. *See also* Nursing discipline; Nursing theory *and specific nursing theories*
   caring in, 5
   in Community Nursing Practice Model, 437
   genderization of, 47–48
   Hall's conceptualization of, 59–61, 59*f*
   Henderson's definition of, 58–59, 62–63
   in Humanbecoming Paradigm, 264–265
   legitimate, 108, 114
   in Modeling and Role-Modeling theory, 191
   Nightingale's definition of, 4, 51
   Peplau's definition of, 69
   relationship in, 5
   in Self-Care Deficit Theory, 115–116
   task-based, 3–4
   Wiedenbach's conceptualization of, 57–58
Nursing: Concepts of Practice (Orem), 107
Nursing: Human Science and Human Care (Watson), 321
Nursing: The Philosophy and Science of Caring, Revised New Edition (Watson), 322
Nursing agency, 108, 116–117
Nursing and Anthropology (Leininger), 304
Nursing as Caring: A Model for Transforming Practice (Boykin and Schoenhofer), 341, 343
Nursing as Caring Theory, 342–355
   in administration, 349–350
   applications of, 347–351
   assumptions of, 343–347
   call for nursing in, 344, 346
   caring in, 343
   in education, 350
   historical perspective on, 342–343
   intention in, 343
   lived meaning in, 344–346
   nurse-client relationship in, 344
   nursing focus in, 343
   nursing practice in, 347–349
   nursing response in, 344
   nursing situation in, 343–344
   person in, 344, 346
   practice exemplar of, 351–355
   research in, 351
Nursing discipline, 4–6. *See also* Nursing theory *and specific nursing theories*
   communication networks of, 6
   conceptual models in, 13
   conceptual structures of, 6
   domain of, 4–5
   education of, 6
   grand theories in, 13. *See also* Grand Theories
   imagination in, 4
   language of, 6
   literature of, 6

   middle-range theories in, 13, 31–32, 138
   paradigms of, 11–13
   practice-level theories in, 13–14
   relationship in, 5
   structure of knowledge in, 11–14
   symbols of, 6
   syntactical structures of, 6
   tradition of, 6
   values and beliefs of, 6
Nursing education. *See* Education
Nursing Knowledge Development and Clinical Practice (Roy), 154
Nursing practice. *See also* Practice applications; Practice exemplar
   Humanbecoming School of Thought, 270, 271–273
   Johnson Behavioral System Model, 99–100
   Nursing as Caring Theory, 347–349
   Science of Unitary Human Beings, 244–249
   scope of, 20
   theory-guided, 7–9, 14, 23–25, 32–33
      administrative support for, 32
      education for, 33
      feedback for, 33
      practice evaluation for, 33
      practice implementation for, 32
      theory selection for, 32
   Theory of Bureaucratic Caring, 464–468, 473–475
   Theory of Integral Nursing, 221–224
   Theory of Power as Knowing Participation in Change, 500–503
   Transitions Theory, 370–371
Nursing process
   Johnson Behavioral System Model, 97–98
   Neuman Systems Model, 172–174, 173*f*
   Roy Adaptation Model, 160
   Self-Care Deficit Theory, 114–116, 116*f*
   Technological Competency as Caring, 453–454
   Theory of Goal Attainment, 139–140
Nursing science, evolution of, 9–11
Nursing theory, 3–16. *See also specific theories and models*
   communication of, 6
   complexity and, 472–474
   conceptual structure and, 6
   contextual development of, 21
   culture and, 15–16
   definitions of, 6–7
   domain of, 4–5
   education and, 6
   evaluation of, 19–22, 25–27, 30–32
      criteria for, 30
      frameworks for, 31–32
      guidelines for, 31
      questions for, 21–22, 25–27, 31–32
   functional components of, 31
   future development of, 14–16
   grand. *See* Grand Theories
   imagination and, 4
   implementation of, 32–33
   language and symbols of, 6
   middle-range. *See* Middle-Range theories

nursing conceptualization in, 21
practice and, 7–9, 14, 23–24. *See also* Nursing practice;
    Practice applications; Practice exemplar
practice-level, 13–14
purpose of, 7–9
questions for, 21–22
research and, 8. *See also* Research
selection of, 23–33
    evaluation and, 30–32
    implementation and, 32–33
    practice and, 24–25
    questions about, 25–27
    reflective exercise for, 28–30
significance of, 22, 24–25
sources for, 21–22
structural components of, 31
study guide for, 19–22
syntactical structure and, 6
tradition and, 6
values and beliefs and, 6

O

Object attachment, 192–194, 193*f*
Observation, in Human-to-Human Relationship
    Model, 78
Occupations, for women, 47, 48
Ordered to Care: The Dilemma of American Nursing
    (Reverby), 46
Orem, Dorothea E., 105–106. *See also* Self-Care Deficit
    Theory
Organization-disorganization paradigm, 12
Orlando, Ida Jean, 82. *See also* Dynamic Nurse-Patient
    Relationship Theory

P

Paradigm, 11–13
Paranormal phenomena, 241–242
Parker, Marilyn E., 437. *See also* Community Nursing
    Practice Model
Parse, Rosemarie Rizzo, 263–264. *See also*
    Humanbecoming Paradigm
Particulate-deterministic paradigm, 12
Peplau, Hildegard, 67–69. *See also* Nurse-Patient
    Relationship Theory
Person, 5
    Community Nursing Practice Model, 437, 439
    Humanbecoming Paradigm, 270–271
    Johnson Behavioral System Model, 92, 94
    Modeling and Role-Modeling theory, 189–191, 190*t*,
        197
    Nursing as Caring Theory, 344, 346
    Self-Care Deficit Theory, 108
    Technological Competency as Caring, 450–451,
        454*f*
    Theory of Integral Nursing, 213, 213*f*, 220*f*,
        222–224
Personal control, 487–488
Personal knowing, 29
Postmodern Nursing and Beyond (Watson), 321–322

Power as Knowing Participation in Change Tool, 251,
    495, 498–499. *See also* Theory of Power as
    Knowing Participation in Change
Power-imaginary process, 503
Power Prescriptions, 503
Practice, 5. *See also* Nursing practice; Practice
    applications; Practice exemplar
Practice applications. *See also* Practice exemplar;
    Research
    Care, Cure, and Core Model, 63
    Comfort Theory, 385–389
    Community Nursing Practice Model, 441–442
    Dynamic Nurse-Patient Relationship Theory, 82–84
    Henderson's conceptualization of nursing, 62–63
    Human-to-Human Relationship Model, 79
    Modeling and Role-Modeling Theory, 198–201,
        199*t*–201*t*
    Neuman Systems Model, 174–175, 178–179
    Nurse-Patient Relationship Model, 71–73
    Prescriptive Theory, 61–62, 61*f*
    Roy Adaptation Model, 160
    Science of Unitary Human Beings, 242–255
    Self-Care Deficit Theory, 118–125, 119*t*–122*t*
    Technological Competency as Caring, 458
    Theory of Bureaucratic Caring, 472–475
    Theory of Caring, 526–528
    Theory of Culture Care Diversity and Universality,
        313–315
    Theory of Goal Attainment, 138–144
    Theory of Health as Expanding Consciousness,
        292–295
    Theory of Human Caring, 329–332
    Theory of Integral Nursing, 225
    Theory of Power as Knowing Participation in Change,
        499–503
    Theory of Self-transcendence, 414–415
    Theory of Successful Aging, 491
    Theory of Unitary Caring, 515–516
    Transitions Theory, 369–371
    Wiedenbach's conception of nursing, 61–62, 61*f*
Practice exemplar
    Care, Cure, and Core Model, 64–65
    Comfort Theory, 389–390
    Community Nursing Practice Model, 445
    Dynamic Nurse-Patient Relationship Theory, 84–85
    Henderson's conceptualization of nursing, 63–64
    Human-to-Human Relationship Model Theory,
        80–81
    Johnson Behavioral System Model, 100–102
    Modeling and Role-Modeling theory, 202–204
    Neuman Systems Model, 179–181
    Nurse-Patient Relationship Theory, 73–74
    Nursing as Caring Theory, 351–355
    Quality Caring Model, 403–407
    Roy Adaptation Model, 160–163
    Science of Unitary Human Beings, 270–271
    Self-Care Deficit Theory, 126–129
    Story Theory, 427–431, 430*t*
    Technological Competency as Caring, 459
    Theory of Bureaucratic Caring, 475–477

Theory of Culture Care Diversity and Universality, 315–316
Theory of Goal Attainment, 145–147
Theory of Health as Expanding Consciousness, 295–297
Theory of Human Caring, 332–337
Theory of Integral Nursing, 226–230
Theory of Power as Knowing Participation in Change, 504–507
Theory of Self-transcendence, 416–417
Theory of Successful Aging, 491–492
Theory of Unitary Caring, 516–518
Transitions Theory, 371–378
Unitary Pattern-Based Praxis method, 255–258
Wiedenbach's conceptualization of nursing, 63
Prescriptive theory, 57–58, 61–62
practice applications of, 61–62, 61*f*
Prevention in Neuman Systems Model, 173–174, 173*f*
Prigogine, Ilya, 288, 289*f*

Q

Qualitative Research Methods in Nursing (Leininger), 304
Quality Caring Model, 394–407
affiliation needs in, 399–400
applications of, 400–403
assumptions of, 396–397
attentive reassurance in, 399
caring factors in, 399–400
caring relationships in, 397–399, 397*f*
collaborative relationships in, 398, 400
concepts of, 396
development of, 394–3957, 395*f*
encouraging manner in, 399
feeling cared for emotion in, 397, 400
healing environment in, 399
human needs in, 400
institutional use of, 407
meaning in, 399
mutual problem-solving in, 399
nurse's role in, 397
practice exemplar of, 403–407
propositions of, 396
relationship-centered professional encounters in, 396
self-caring in, 396
Quarantine, 45
Queen Victoria, 48

R

Rapport, in Human-to-Human Relationship Model, 78
Ray, Marilyn Anne, 461–462. *See also* Theory of Bureaucratic Caring
Reaction paradigm, 12
Reciprocal interaction paradigm, 12
Reed, Pamela, 411–412. *See also* Theory of Self-transcendence
Relationship, 5. *See also* Nurse-Patient Relationship Theory
Hall's model of nursing, 60–61
Modeling and Role-Modeling Theory, 189–191, 196–197, 196*t*

Quality Caring Model, 397–399, 397*f*
Theory of Human Caring, 326–327
Theory of Integral Nursing, 220–221
Religion, 223. *See also* Spirituality
Research. *See also* Practice applications
Humanbecoming Paradigm, 268–269
Johnson Behavioral System Model, 98–99, 99*b*
Neuman Systems Model, 176–178, 178–179
nurse-patient relationship, 71–72
Nursing as Caring Theory, 351
Science of Unitary Human Beings, 242–255, 249–255
Syrian Muslim ethnonursing, 314–315
Technological Competency as Caring, 458*f*
theory-based, 8
Theory of Culture Care Diversity and Universality, 310–313, 311*f*, 314
Theory of Goal Attainment, 141–143
Theory of Health as Expanding Consciousness, 291–295
Theory of Integral Nursing, 225
Theory of Power as Knowing Participation in Change, 499–500
Theory of Self-transcendence, 414–415
traditions of, 14
Transitions Theory, 369–370
Rhythmical Correlates of Change, 242
Rogers, Martha E., 237–238, 281–282, 283. *See also* Science of Unitary Human Beings
Role modeling. *See* Modeling and Role-Modeling Theory
Roy, Sister Callista, 153–154. *See also* Roy Adaptation Model
Roy Adaptation Model, 154–163
assumptions of, 155, 156*t*
cognator-regulator processes in, 156
concepts of, 155–159
environment in, 158
health in, 158–159
historical development of, 154–155
interdependence mode in, 157, 158
modes in, 157–158
nursing process in, 160
people in, 155–158
physiologic-physical mode in, 157
practice applications of, 160
practice exemplar of, 160–163
role function mode in, 157, 158
self-concept-group identity mode in, 157–158
stabilizer-innovator processes in, 156
Theory of Successful Aging and, 484–485
Roy Adaptation Model, The (Roy), 154
Roy Adaptation Model-based Research: Twenty-five Years of Contributions to Nursing Science, 154

S

Schoenhofer, Savina, 342. *See also* Nursing as Caring Theory
Science, evolution of nursing as a, 9–11
Science of Unitary Human Beings, 238–258
applications of, 242–255
Barrett's practice method and, 245

Butcher's practice method and, 245–249
Cowling's practice constituents and, 245
energy fields in, 238–239
healing in, 243
helicy in, 240
homeodynamics in, 239–240
integrality in, 240
intentionality in, 244
nursing practice and, 243*b*
openness in, 239
pandimensionality in, 239
pattern in, 239
postulates of, 238–239
practice exemplar of, 270–271
practice methods and, 244–249
research applications of, 249–255
resonancy in, 240
spirituality in, 244
theories from, 240–242
Theory of Accelerating Evolution from, 240–241
Theory of Emergence of Paranormal Phenomena
        from, 241–242
Theory of Rhythmical Correlates of Change from, 242
therapeutic touch in, 243, 244
Unitary Pattern-Based Praxis method and, 245–249
website for, 243*b*
worldview of, 238
Self-care, 190
    integral, 222
    for nurse, 221
Self-Care Deficit Theory, 107–130
    agent in, 109
    basic conditioning factors in, 109–110, 109*f*
    caregiver in, 109
    community groups in, 117
    concepts of, 109
    deliberate action in, 111
    dependent-care theory in, 107–108
    developmental self-care requisites in, 113
    estimative capabilities in, 111–112
    family in, 117
    foundational capabilities and dispositions in, 111
    health deviation self-care requisites in, 113
    multiperson situations and units in, 117
    nursing agency in, 108, 116–117
    nursing system definition in, 114–116, 116*f*
    nursing systems theory in, 108–109
    power components in, 111
    practice applications of, 118–125, 119*t*–122*t*
    practice exemplar of, 126–129
    productive operation capabilities in, 111–112
    self-care agency in, 111, 111*f*
    self-care deficit theory in, 107
    self-care definition in, 110–111
    self-care requisites in, 112–113
    self-management in, 125
    structure of, 109*f*
    therapeutic self-care demand in, 112
    transitional capabilities in, 111–112
    universal self-care requisites in, 112–113

Self-care knowledge, 190
Self-care resources, 190
*Self-Care Theory in Nursing: Selected Papers of Dorothea
        Orem*, 106
Simultaneity paradigm, 12
Simultaneous action paradigm, 12
Skills, 25
Smith, Marlaine C., 511–512. *See also* Theory of Unitary
        Caring
Smith, Mary Jane, 421. *See also* Story Theory
Social justice, in Modeling and Role-Modeling theory,
        191
Spinsterhood, 46, 48
Spirituality
    Florence Nightingale, 39–40, 43
    Modeling and Role-Modeling theory, 191
    Neuman Systems Model, 170–171
    Reed's studies of, 413. *See also* Theory of Self-
        transcendence
    Science of Unitary Human Beings, 244
    Theory of Integral Nursing, 223
    Theory of Successful Aging, 486*f,* 488–489
Standardized nursing languages, 139–140
Story. *See also* Story Theory
    in Modeling and Role-Modeling theory, 196*t,* 197
Story path, 425–426, 425*f*
Story Theory, 421–431
    assumptions of, 423
    concepts of, 423, 423*f*
    ease in, 426
    emergence of, 422–423
    foundations of, 423–424, 423*f*
    intentional dialogue in, 424
    practice exemplar of, 427–431, 430*t*
    self-in-relation in, 424–426, 425*f*
    story path in, 425–426, 425*f*
Stress response, in Modeling and Role-Modeling
        theory, 191–192, 192*f*
Study guide, 19–22
Suffering, 77
    in Theory of Integral Nursing, 222–224
Suggestions for Thought (Nightingale), 43
Sunrise enabler, in Theory of Culture Care Diversity and
        Universality, 310–312, 311*f*
Swain, Mary Ann, 186. *See also* Modeling and Role-
        Modeling Theory
Swanson, Kristen M., 521–522. *See also* Theory of
        Caring
Sympathy, in Human-to-Human Relationship Model,
        78
Syntactical structures, of nursing discipline, 5–6
Syrian Muslims, ethnonursing study of, 314–315

T
Technological Competency as Caring, 450–459
    applications of, 458
    calls for nursing in, 457–458
    change in, 458
    continuous knowing in, 455–456
    definition of, 450

future research in, 458*f*
intention in, 455–456
knowing persons in, 450–457, 454*f*
nursing process in, 453–454
nursing response in, 457–458
practice exemplar of, 459
purpose of, 450
situation of care in, 452–457
technological knowing in, 457, 457*f*
trust in, 452, 453
wholeness ideal in, 453
Temporal Experience Scale, 252
Textbook of the Principles and Practice of Nursing
        (Henderson), 58, 62
Theoretical Nursing: Development and Progress (Meleis),
        362
Theory. *See* Nursing theory *and specific nursing theories*
Theory for Nursing: Systems, Concepts, Process, A (King),
        133
Theory of Accelerating Evolution, 240–241
Theory of Bureaucratic Caring, 462–477
    application of, 472–475
    caring in, 468
    description of, 469–470
    development of, 468–472
    generation of, 462–463, 463*f*
    holographic emergence in, 463–464, 463*f*
    as holographic theory, 470–472
    leadership models in, 467–468
    in nursing education, 475
    nursing practice in, 464–468, 473–475
    organizational cultures in, 466–468
    organizational transformation in, 470–472
    practice exemplar of, 475–477
Theory of Caring, 521–531, 530*f*
    at-risk mothers study and, 525–526
    caring knowledge in, 528–529
    Caring Professional Scale in, 527–528
    Couple's Miscarriage Project study and, 529–530
    evolution of, 524
    healing, connection to, 530–531, 530*f*
    literature meta-analysis in, 528–529
    Miscarriage Caring Project study and, 526–528
    NICU study and, 524–525
    practice applications of, 526–528
    refinements of, 524–526
Theory of Culture Care Diversity and Universality,
        304–317
    care modalities in, 307–308
    collaborative care in, 312–313
    cultural care diversities in, 306–307
    cultural commonalities in, 306–307
    culture care accommodation/negotiation in, 307–308,
        310
    culture care preservation/maintenance in, 307–308, 310
    culture care restructuring/repatterning in, 308
    development of, 304–305
    domain of inquiry in, 311–312
    generic care in, 307, 309, 312

goal of, 309
health in, 310
in nurse education, 313
orientational definitions in, 309–310
practice applications of, 313–315
practice exemplar of, 315–316
professional care in, 307, 309
purpose of, 308
rationale for, 306
research in, 310–313, 311*f*, 314
sunrise enabler in, 310–312, 311*f*
Syrian Muslim ethnonursing research in, 314–315
theoretical assumptions of, 308–310
theoretical tenets of, 306–308
worldview in, 307, 310
Theory of Dependent Care, 107–108
Theory of Dissipative Structures, 288, 289*f*
Theory of Emergence of Paranormal Phenomena,
        241–242
Theory of Goal Attainment, 133–147
    conceptual framework of, 135–136, 135*f*
    documentation system in, 137
    Goal Attainment Scale in, 137
    multicultural applications of, 141
    nursing process in, 139–140
    philosophical foundation of, 134
    practice applications of, 138–144
        client perspective and, 143
        in client systems, 140, 142–143
        with clients across life span, 142
        evidence-based, 144
        in multicultural settings, 141
        in multidisciplinary settings, 140–141
        recommendations for, 144
        in work settings, 143–144
    practice exemplar of, 145–147
    research applications of, 141–143
    standardized nursing languages in, 139–140
    transaction process model in, 136–137, 136*f*
Theory of Group Power within Organizations, 139
Theory of Health as Expanding Consciousness
    applications of, 284–291
    assumptions underlying, 282
    community-level application of, 294–295
    consciousness stages in, 290*f*
    cross-culture relevance of, 291
    development of, 282–284
    disruption-related choice points in, 288–290, 289*f*,
        290*f*
    expanding consciousness in, 284–285
    focusing process in, 291–292
    insights in, 288–290, 289*f*
    levels of awareness in, 283
    meaning in, 286–288
    nurse-client interaction in, 290–292
    nurse-family interaction in, 291–292
    nursing practice and, 292–295
    pattern in, 286–288, 292
    philosophical influences on, 281–282

practice exemplar of, 295–297
presence in, 285–286
research as praxis, 291–295
resonance in, 285–286
Toward a Theory of Health presentation and, 282
unitary-transformative paradigm in, 283–284
Theory of Human Caring, 322–337
   Attending Nurse Caring Model and, 332–334
   carative factors in, 323–324
   caring (healing) consciousness in, 328
   Caring Moment in, 326
   caring occasion in, 328
   Caring Science orientation in, 323
   clinical *caritas* processes in, 324–325
   conceptual elements of, 323
   in customer service, 335–336
   development of, 322–323
   in education, 335
   in hospitals, 331
   implications of, 328–329
   International Caritas Consortium and, 330
   practice applications of, 329–332
   practice exemplar of, 332–337
   reading of, 325–326
   transpersonal caring relationship in, 326–327
   Watson Caring Science Institute and, 329–330
Theory of Integral Nursing, 208–230
   application of, 225
   AQAL (all quadrants, all levels) in, 217–220, 220*f*
   communication in, 224
   content components of, 212–220
   context in, 220–221
   development in, 211, 217–218, 220*f*
   development of, 210
   in education, 225
   environment in, 213–214, 213*f*, 220*f*, 224
   four-quadrants perspective in, 215–220, 215*f*, 216*f*,
      220*f*, 222–224
   in global health, 226
   healing in, 212, 212*f*, 213*f*, 221
   health in, 213, 213*f*, 220*f*, 224
   integral dialogues in, 208–209
   integral process in, 208
   integral worldview in, 208
   intentions of, 211, 224
   meaning in, 222–224
   metaparadigm in, 213–214, 213*f*
   nurse in, 213, 213*f*, 220–221, 220*f*, 222
   nursing practice and, 221–224
   patterns of knowing in, 214–215, 214*f*, 220, 220*f*
   person in, 213, 213*f*, 220*f*, 222–224
   philosophical assumptions of, 211–212
   philosophical foundation of, 208, 209
   in policy guidance, 225–226
   practice exemplar in, 226–230
   questions in, 208
   relationship-based care in, 220–221
   relationship-centered case in, 220
   research on, 225

structure of, 220, 220*f*
transpersonal dimension in, 223
Theory of Integral Nursing (Dossey), 225
Theory of Nursing Systems, 108–109. *See also* Self-Care
   Deficit Theory
Theory of Power as Knowing Participation in Change,
   495–507, 497*f*
   applications of, 499–503
   concepts of, 496–499
   control, power as, 498
   freedom, power as, 498, 504–507
   practice exemplar of, 504–507
   practice methodology for, 500–503
   research on, 499–500
   underlying basis of, 496
Theory of Rhythmical Correlates of Change, 242
Theory of Self-Care, 107. *See also* Self-Care Deficit
   Theory
Theory of Self-transcendence, 412–418
   applications of, 414–415
   concepts of, 413–414, 414*f*
   personal factors in, 416–417
   practice exemplar of, 416–417
   research in, 414–415
   self-transcendence in, 413, 414*f* 417
   vulnerability in, 413, 414*f*
   well-being in, 413–414, 414*f*
Theory of Successful Aging, 483–492, 486*f*
   applications of, 491
   creativity in, 486
   development of, 483–485
   functional performance mechanisms in, 485–486, 486*f*
   geotranscendance and, 486*f*, 489–491
   intrapsychic factors in, 486, 486*f*
   model for, 486*f*
   negative affect and, 487
   personal control and, 487–488
   positive affect and, 487
   practice exemplar of, 491–492
   Roy Adaptation Model and, 484–485
   spirituality in, 486*f*, 488–489
Theory of Unitary Caring, 510–518
   applications of, 515–516
   appreciating pattern in, 511–512, 514–515
   assumptions of, 511
   caring concept in, 510
   concepts of, 511–513
   creative emergence in, 515
   development of, 510–511
   dynamic flow attunement in, 512, 515
   empirical indicators in, 513–515
   Infinity in, 512–513, 515
   manifesting intentions in, 511, 514
   practice exemplar of, 516–518
   propositions of, 513
Therapeutic touch, 244
Tomlin, Evelyn, 186
Totality paradigm, 12
Touch, therapeutic, 244

Towards a Theory for Nursing: General Concepts of Human Behavior (King), 133
Tradition, 6
Transaction process model, 136–137, 136*f*
Transcultural nursing, 306. *See also* Theory of Culture Care Diversity and Universality
Transcultural Nursing: Concepts, Theories, and Practices (Leininger), 304
Transitional objects, 193
Transitions Theory, 362–378
    applications of, 369–371
    assumptions of, 363
    change triggers, 364*f*, 365–366, 372–373
    concepts of, 363–367, 365*t*
    in education, 371
    feminist postcolonialism and, 363
    intervention within, 364*f*, 367–369, 377
    lived experience and, 362–363
    in nursing practice, 370–371
    origins of, 362–363
    practice exemplar of, 371–378
    properties of transition, 364*f*, 365, 373–376
    propositions of, 363–367
    research involving, 369–370
    responses, patterns of, 364*f*, 366–367, 368*t*, 376–377
    role theory in, 362
    situation-specific theories, development of, 371
    triggers of transition, 363–366, 364*f*
Transparency, in Theory of Integral Nursing, 222
Transpersonal Caring Theory. *See* Theory of Human Caring
Travelbee, Joyce, 76. *See also* Human-to-Human Relationship Model
Troutman-Jordan, Meredith, 485. *See also* Theory of Successful Aging
True presence, in Humanbecoming Paradigm, 269–270

Trusting-functional relationship, 190–191
    mind-set establishment for, 196, 196*t*
    nurturing space creation for, 196–197, 196*t*
    story facilitation for, 196*t*, 197
Turkel, Marian C., 464

U

Unitary field pattern portrait research method, 253–255, 254*f*
Unitary Pattern-Based Praxis method, 245–249
    pattern manifestation knowing and appreciation in, 245–248
    practice exemplar of, 255–258
    voluntary mutual patterning in, 248–249
Unitary-transformative paradigm, 12

V

Values, 6, 24
    Johnson Behavioral System Model, 97
Veritivity, 155
Visions of Rogers' Science-Based Nursing (Barrett), 495–496

W

Watson, Jean, 321–322. *See also* Theory of Human Caring
Ways of knowing, 29
Wholeness
    Johnson Behavioral System Model, 90–91
    Theory of Health as Expanding Consciousness, 285–286
Wiedenbach, Ernestine, 55–56
    nursing conceptualizations of, 57–58
    prescriptive theory of, 57–58, 61–62, 63
Wilber, Ken, 211
Women Founders of the Social Sciences, The (McDonald), 49